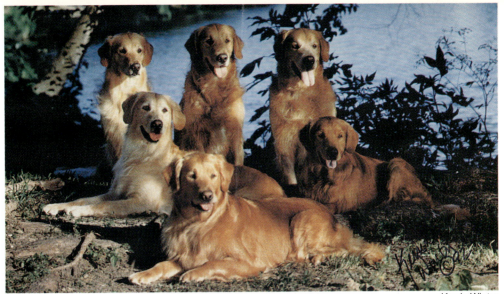
Kerrin Winter

Medical & Genetic Aspects of Purebred Dogs

Edited by Ross D. Clark, DVM
and
Joan R. Stainer

FORUM PUBLICATIONS, INC.
Fairway, Kansas
St. Simons Island, Georgia

Medical & Genetic Aspects of Purebred Dogs

EDITORS

Ross D. Clark, DVM
Woodland Animal Medical Center
Tulsa, Oklahoma

Joan R. Stainer
Lonesome Lane
Tulsa, Oklahoma

CONSULTING EDITOR
Art J. Quinn, DVM, Dipl. ACVO
Professor of Opthalmology
Oklahoma State University
Stillwater, Oklahoma

TECHNICAL EDITOR
Betsey A. Leedy, AKC Judge
Woodland Animal Medical Center
Tulsa, Oklahoma

ASSISTANT EDITOR
Susan Gaffney, DVM
Woodland Animal Medical Center
Tulsa, Oklahoma

PRODUCTION ART DIRECTOR
Candice S. Millard
Veterinary Forum
Fairway, Kansas

PROOFREADER
Lael Dalton
Assistant Editor
Veterinary Forum
Fairway, Kansas

Contents

Part I: Breed Specifics

ACKNOWLEDGMENTS

This edition represents 21 years of effort. Some of the original text from our first edition, written by breeders and their veterinarians is included. A list of these contributors can be found on page 662.

This second edition has been enhanced by the continued advice, photographs and counsel of Dr. Ralph Buckner.

We appreciate the efforts of Deborah Goddard, Paula Dempsey, Teresa Nash, Susan Dillin, Sherri Samel and Sarah Shuman in acquiring photographs.

We want to thank professional handlers Roy Lee and Shirley Murray, Carl Sanders and Walter Green, Mike Kemp, Bob and Delores Burkholder, Judy and Richard Cooper, Kenny and Ellie Rensick, Ron Buxton and Tom Spahn, Bruce Schultz, Linda Clark, Patricia Jenner and Art Montoya for taking the time to photograph dogs in their care.

— Ross Clark
Joan Stainer

FORWARD

The first edition of this book evolved from discussion between the two of us regarding the mutual lack of respect between breeders and veterinarians. Breeders gain much medical knowledge about their breed through extensive weekend discussions at dog shows and with fellow fanciers on the phone during the week. An unusual medical syndrome occurring on the East Coast on Thursday could easily be common discussion on the West Coast the following weekend. We hoped to combine the best information available to both groups into one definitive book so in the end the dog would benefit from the fact that breeders and veterinarians both have information previously available only in scattered breed publications and veterinary research journals.

With the advent of blood testing for genetic disorders, veterinarians will be better able to diagnose problems, but with 39 chromosome pairs in the canine, as compared to 23 pairs in the human, progress will be more difficult.

The combined knowledge and observations of breeders and veterinarians will still be critical for optimum care.

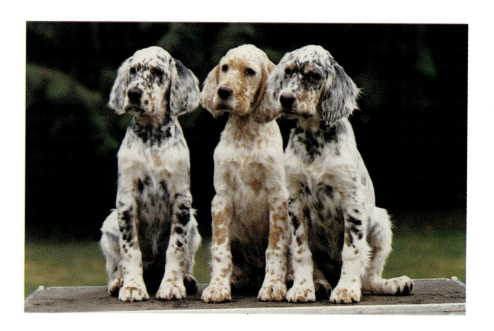

PREFACE

The process used to develop this book was to do a computer search of worldwide research journals and breed publications and to tap the knowledge of experienced breeders.

The fact that a breed shows many disorders may be more an indication of the extensive research done on that breed than on its comparative soundness.

Many genetic disorders are common to several breeds. We don't intend to convey severity or incidence by the length of text within a particular breed chapter.

PART I

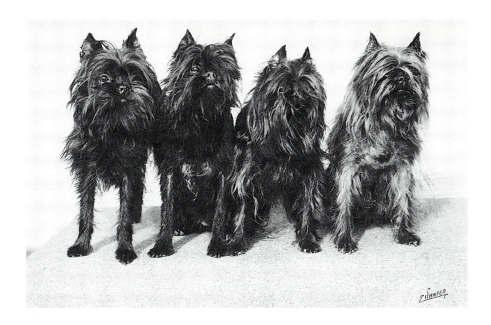

AFFENPINSCHER

ORIGIN AND HISTORY

The Affenpinscher, also known as the Monkey Pinscher or Monkey Terrier, appeared in Europe as early as the 17th century AD.[2] This sturdy little terrier provided the genetic foundation for some of the more common small breeds such as the Brussels Griffon.[1] The exact date and circumstances of its arrival in North America are not known; however, the breed was well established by the early 1900s. Affenpinschers were admitted to the AKC Stud Book and to show classification in 1936. Today 100 to 140 specimens are registered with the AKC each year.

DESCRIPTION

Originally bred as a varmint hunter, the Affenpinscher is an inquisitive, alert, and intelligent breed. Normally possessing a quiet disposition, it carries itself with a comical seriousness; when attacked, it can become extremely excited and will battle fearlessly with an aggressor.[1]

THE SHOW RING

The ideal Affenpinscher should be no more than 10 1/4 inches high at the shoulder and should weigh no more than 7 to 8 pounds.[2] The smaller animals are preferred.

Black, gray, silver or black and tan with symmetrical markings, or red, varying from a brownish red to an orangey tan, are seen as coat colors. Color is not a major consideration.[2]

The character of the coat is an important factor; it should be entirely stiff and wiry in texture. On the body, the coat should be short and dense; on the legs and around the eyes, nose and chin, it should be long, loose and shaggy.[2]

An Affenpinscher should reflect the sturdiness of its breed. Any tendency to frailty is discouraged. Its head should be round and not too heavy, with a well-domed forehead. Eyes should be round, of good size, black and very brilliant.[1] Ears are cropped to a point, rather small, but set high and erect. Muzzle must be short and rather pointed, with a black nose and prominent chin. The neck should be short and straight. The back should also be straight, with its length about equal to height at the shoulder.[2]

Front legs should be as straight as possible, and the hind legs should not have much bend at the hock. Feet should be small, round, compact, and turned neither in nor out.[2] The tail is docked short and carried high.

The total overall appearance of the Affenpinscher is more important than any individual characteristic.[2] There are no disqualifications in this breed.

BREEDING AND WHELPING

Affenpinscher litters average between two and four puppies, with a maximum of seven. Whelps range from 2 to 8 ounces each, the average weighing 3 to 5 ounces.

Tails should be docked at 3 to 5 days, close to the body, leaving about 1/3 inch. Male puppies should have descended testicles by 4 months, but some can pull up a testicle until 7 months.

First estrus is expected between 8 and 14 months.

DENTITION

Affenpinschers are seen with **ogliodontia** and must be checked for retention of puppy teeth. An undershot bite is the rule rather than an exception. The Standard calls for a level or slightly undershot bite with the teeth not showing.

RECOGNIZED PROBLEMS

Cushing's disease (hyperadrenal corticalism) has been reported in this breed.[3]

Breeders have reported incidences of **anasarca (walrus puppies)**, **patent ductus arteriosus**,[4] **Legg-Perthes** and whelps with **elongated soft palate** and **cleft palate**. **Patellar luxation** is seen in Affenpinschers.

Broken bones can be a problem in 4- to 10-month-old puppies because they have no fear and run and jump without thought.

Keratoconjunctivitis sicca (dry eye) has been reported in this breed.[5]

BEHAVIOR

The compatible nature and deep devotion of the Affenpinscher make it an admirable companion. It is exuberant, extremely curious, a barker and an outstanding watch dog.

OLD AGE

Corneal ulcers do occur in the breed with some individuals being prone to recurrence. **Urinary calculi** occur occasionally in older dogs. **Mitral valve insufficiency** may be seen in some individuals after 8 years of age.

References

1. Jones, A.F. and Hamilton F., Eds. *The World Encyclopedia of Dogs*. (Galahad Books: New York, 1971) 185, 495, 516.
2. American Kennel Club, *The Complete Dog Book*. 18th ed. (Howell Book House: New York, 1992) 422-423.
3. Affenpinscher column, *American Kennel Club Gazette*; August 1990.
4. Kirk, R.W., Ed.*Current Veterinary Therapy VI*. (W.B. Saunders: Philadelphia, 1977) 400-403.
5. Affenpinscher column, *American Kennel Club Gazette*; June 1990.

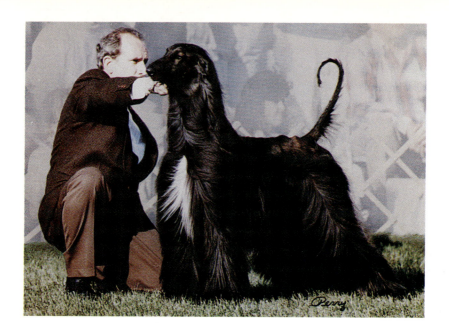

AFGHAN HOUND

ORIGIN AND HISTORY

The aloof, aristocratic Afghan Hound originated as a working dog in the mountains and deserts of Afghanistan, where it is still the hunting dog of the nomadic natives.

DESCRIPTION

The breed is characterized by its regal bearing, distinctive coat pattern and springy gait. These dogs are gentle but cautious with strangers. Sharpness or severe shyness (not to be confused with aloofness) is a fault. Because they are extremely sensitive to strange noises and unusual behavior, Afghans are excellent guard dogs.

If left alone, Afghans become extremely withdrawn and therefore are poor kennel dogs. They need human companionship daily or if this is impossible, the companionship of at least one other Afghan. The aloof behavior is typical of all sight hounds, which are bred to "sight and catch prey quickly." Because their vision is perfect for long-distance viewing, Afghans are most comfortable when they can evaluate situations from a distance. If they feel threatened they can move rapidly to safety.

In the Western Hemisphere, the Afghan is a popular breed in the show ring because of its aristocratic poise and dramatic appearance. Typically, an Afghan has long silky hair on top of its head, long ears framing an exotic face with a long muzzle and a flowing coat draping its body. The back is covered with short hair, forming a saddle. The pasterns are often bare, but the large

16

feet are well covered with hair. Because the long, heavy coat provides protection, dewclaw removal is a matter of preference.

An Afghan's hip bones give way to either a sickle-shaped tail or one with a ring on the end. The tail is covered with short hair or fringes, like a monkey's tail. The ring tail, often called the monkey tail, is most typical, but a sickle-shaped tail is not a fault. The characteristic ring tail develops as early as two months after birth.

THE SHOW RING

Afghan dogs should be 27 inches tall, plus or minus 1 inch and should weigh about 60 pounds. Bitches should be 25 inches and should weigh about 50 pounds. All colors are permissible. There are no breed disqualifications. Faults include coarseness; snipiness; overshot or undershot; round or light eyes; lack of topknot; a short, ewe or goose neck; roach back; sway back; lack of prominent hipbones; toeing in or out; weak or broken down pasterns; lack of saddle in adult dogs; sharpness or shyness.

DENTITION

The Standard asks for a level bite although a tight scissors closure is not to be penalized.[1] An overbite occurs as early as 2 months of age in approximately 20% of all puppies but usually disappears before the pup is 9 months old as the underjaw develops. A small percentage of overbites become permanent, frequently in dogs with unusually long muzzles.

Undershot bites seen in 4 to 5-month-old Afghans often conform spontaneously to the required bite. Undershot bites that develop at 9 to 14 months are seldom self-correcting. Jaw conformation is not easy to predict, and a level bite in a 4 to 7 month old Afghan still may become overshot or undershot. Level bites in 2- and 3-year-old dogs may change to a scissors, an overshot, or an undershot bite, especially in dogs with longer muzzles; however, malocclusions are not frequent. The Afghan breed Standard does not specify dentition requirements. Many of the dogs lack two to eight premolars.

BREEDING AND WHELPING

Maturation of the Afghan's personality, especially the male's, may not be complete until 4 years old. For this reason, a male should not be used for breeding before 18 months of age. Some breeders do not breed a dog until it is certified by the Orthopedic Foundation for Animals at 2 years. Males usually breed actively and require little assistance. They can remain potent until they are 10 to 12 years old. Bitches should not be bred until they are 2 years old. A healthy bitch with extended cycles can bear pups until she is 8 to 10 years old.

Onset of first estrus varies from 7 months to 2 1/2 years with intervals between cycles

17

ranging from 6 to 18 months. Afghans usually ovulate regularly, although a small number show a wide variation. For the safety of the puppies, a bitch should achieve the highest possible level of immunity before carrying a litter. A bitch should be immunized within two months before breeding, even if vaccinated only three to six months earlier. Freedom from external and internal parasites before whelping is essential. Vaccination and deworming on the same day are not recommended, because Afghans are often highly sensitive to this drug combination and can react unfavorably.

Signs of pregnancy appear late. The best time to determine whether a bitch is pregnant is 28 to 32 days after each service. Weight problems should always be avoided in Afghans, especially during pregnancy. Some pregnant bitches become ravenous and may gain too much weight. During the first three weeks after breeding, some pregnant Afghan bitches lose their appetites. In extreme cases loss of appetite may last up to four weeks, during which the animals may eat only one to three tablespoons of food daily. Sometimes food is refused for six to eight days. In such cases, vitamins and calcium phosphate in tablet form should be administered.

Afghan bitches whelp well and become naturally good mothers when allowed to whelp in seclusion. Privacy is important even at home. The whelping site should be removed from the bustle of everyday activities. Since this breed has retained a primitive sensitivity to strangers and strange places, the bitch should whelp in familiar surroundings.

Afghans seldom have serious problems whelping. Because some over-assisted Afghan bitches gladly relinquish all duties of motherhood, only essential help should be given. With a first litter, the bitch may not know how to lie while whelping, how to open the sac, how to cut the umbilical cord or how to clean the puppies. These functions are usually learned after the delivery of one or two puppies. Assistance, if needed, should be given by only one person, who should also change bedding and feed and exercise the mother until the puppies are weaned.

Post-whelping problems are seldom encountered. **Eclampsia** is rare. Although **mastitis** is not common, it should be carefully watched for. Problems with milk are infrequent.

Afghan bitches are naturally excellent mothers if the maternal instinct has not been impaired by human interference. They are extremely vocal, especially during delivery; their screaming often represents fear of the unknown rather than pain, although Afghans do scream in pain and much louder than any other breed.

GROWTH

At birth, most Afghan puppies weigh between 10 and 18 ounces. Given proper care, smaller ones (7 to 10 ounces) quickly catch up with their larger siblings. Many breeders supplement natural feedings of newborn puppies with tube feeding, particularly if the puppies are small or the litter is large. This provides additional food for weak puppies and satisfies larger puppies so that they do not usurp all the mother's milk.

There is no cause for concern if a puppy stays at the same weight or loses weight during the first two to four days. After that, however, a puppy should gradually gain until it reaches its ideal weight. Mature dogs may weigh from 55 to 70 pounds; mature bitches usually weigh between 40 and 55 pounds. Because the Afghan is one of the larger breeds, its growth is very slow and it may not reach full maturity until it is 4 years old.

Socialization of puppies should be achieved slowly but steadily. By the time it is weaned (4 1/2 to 6 weeks), the Afghan pup should appreciate human company. Seven to 14 months is a critical time in the development of the dog's personality. A change of home during this time can be damaging unless the dog is handled properly. If air travel to the new home is necessary, the puppy should be lightly sedated and handled with care and understanding when it reaches its new home. Respect for the Afghan's innate aloofness is particularly desirable at this time.

Umbilical hernias occur infrequently in Afghan puppies and many are self-repairing.

Young puppies and adolescents may appear gawky because of loose ligaments and tendons. To develop muscle tone and strengthen ligaments, a slowly accelerated program of exercise is recommended. A dog younger than a year old should never be exercised by strenuous road work. Also, because puppies are especially susceptible to injury, their play should be carefully supervised.

Because this breed matures slowly, patience is a prime virtue in owners of Afghans. As its bones develop, the puppy that looked beautifully balanced at 3 to 4 months of age becomes high in the rear and close in front. Growth of the front legs from the elbow to the pastern and of the upper arm exceeds the development of the rib cage. Consequently the elbows have little support. The chest appears narrow and pinched and the elbows may actually touch beneath it. The feet toe out. Later, as the chest deepens, the conformation of the chest becomes proper. However, some Afghans never develop the deep chest and remain close in front.

The same spurt of growth often occurs in the hind legs. The puppy appears high in the rear until growth of the hind legs equals that of the front legs. Infrequently a coat change occurs before the typical short hair of the Afghan puppy lengthens into the characteristic long, flowing adult coat. Special care in grooming is necessary to prevent serious matting as the puppy coat is lost.

A heavily coated puppy may not develop a saddle until 18 to 24 months — sometimes later. On a puppy with a light coat the saddle is apparent by the time the puppy is from 6 to 9 months old. Usually, this indicates that the mature coat will also be light. The mature coat should be silky with no cottony undercoat. Puppies, especially heavily coated ones, often have a fuzzy growth along the side of the muzzle, known as monkey whiskers. As the coat develops, the monkey whiskers are shed, revealing the characteristic long muzzle.

When mature dogs are exposed to anesthesia or heavy doses of medication that causes shedding, or when a bitch delivers puppies and later loses its coat, the entire coat growth cycle is repeated. The monkey whiskers and the dense coat on the back drop just as in puppies.

Newborn pups often have dark brown-to-black guard hairs that disguise the true color of the coat. This is especially true of apricot, cream or brindle coloring. If a dog is to have a mask, the mask will be noticeable at birth; however, a shaded mask may be difficult to see until the puppy is older. The domino pattern is a reversal of the usual markings. The domino puppy is born with a blue or black coat, a widow's peak and a white or light face (a reverse mask). The Afghan coat shows its true color by the time the puppy is 3 to 4 weeks old. Black or tan may occur in combination with red or silver (the light areas look white), or in tricolor patterning.

Spotting sometimes occurs on the feet of young puppies — in severe cases, on other parts of the body — but should disappear within 12 weeks. Except for a white spot on the chest, spots that remain beyond that time are mismarks and disqualify the dog from the show ring. Two to three months may be required for areas of incomplete pigmentation to fill. White and domino-patterned dogs may have winter nose, one that changes colors seasonally.

When a novice owner seeks a veterinarian's opinion on a litter of Afghans, the veterinarian should choose his comments carefully lest they be misconstrued as an evaluation of the puppies' conformation. Unless he is an expert on conformation, the veterinarian is wise to comment only on the health of the litter.

RECOGNIZED PROBLEMS
Afghan puppies have a peculiar sensitivity to older forms of hepatitis vaccine, as manifested by the **blue-eyed reaction.** This problem has been controlled by using the new vaccines developed to avoid blue eyes. Until pups have had their last inoculation, they should be isolated from the public. Afghans are sometimes sensitive to anesthetic agents. To minimize risk, light doses are recommended. If the teeth of a dog are to be cleaned, the animal should be very lightly anesthetized for the procedure. A desirable approach to dental hygiene is the daily application of hydrogen peroxide to the dog's gums. **Hip dysplasia, juvenile cataract, corneal dystrophy** and **bilateral cataract** [2,3,4] are documented in the breed.

Elbow joint malformation[6] is seen. This is bilateral malformation of articular surfaces of proximal radius and ulna. Afghans are reported to have an increased incidence of **hypothyroidism.**[7] Skin problems are rare in Afghans, although **demodectic mange** appears in a small percentage during the first two years.

Necrotic myelopathy is restricted to Afghans, and its occurrence in littermates suggests a genetic basis. The clinical course of this disease is characterized by **posterior paresis**, usually beginning at 3 to 6 months of age and progressing to **tetraplegia** and death from **respiratory paralysis** within 2 to 4 weeks. Histologically, the spinal cord shows malacia, necrosis and occasionally cavitation of the white matter, with typical sparing of a deep zone adjacent to the grey matter. The ventrolateral portions of the spinal cord from the midcervical to the anterior lumbar levels are most commonly involved. There is no known treatment for myelopathy in the Afghan.

The Afghan's testicles may migrate as late as 7 months of age. Young pups should not be given whole milk as many are allergic to it. They may also develop skin rashes from too much meat or fat; as well as an occasional grass allergy. They can also be sensitive to flea and tick dips and flea collars.

BEHAVIOR

In an unfamiliar setting, such as a veterinarian's office, a frightened Afghan should be approached slowly and touched without being spoken to. The owner should be in full view of the dog and have contact with it. A cornered Afghan should never be approached from the front.

The Afghan is not an effusive, face-licking breed that enjoys a romp with the children; he is a quiet, decorous and restrained companion.

OLD AGE

The breed enjoys good health. **Cancer** occurs in a small percentage. Afghans have an average life span of 14 years.

References
1. American Kennel Club *The Complete Dog Book*. 18th ed. (Howell Book House: New York, 1992).
2. Magrane, W.H. *Canine Ophthalmology* 2nd Ed. (Lea & Febiger: Philadelphia, 1971) 233.
3. Quinn, A.J. Personal Communications; 1994.
4. Roberts, S.R. and Helper, F.C., "Cataracts in Afghan Hounds," *JAVMA*; (160) 1972: 427-432.
5. Barnett, K.C. "The Diagnosis and Differential Diagnosis of Cataracts in the Dog.," *J. Sm. Anim. Prac;* 1985: 305-316. 20 ref.
6. Gondalen, J. "Malformation of the Elbow Joint in an Afghan Hound Litter," *J. Sm. Anim. Prac.* (14); 1973: 83-89.
7. Brignac, M.M. "Congenital and Breed Associated Skin Diseases in the Dog and Cat," *Kalkan Forum*; December, 1966: 9-16.

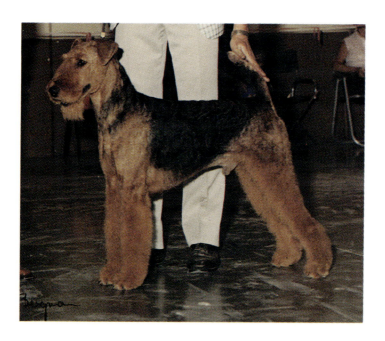

AIREDALE TERRIER

ORIGIN AND HISTORY

Airedale Terriers originated in the valley of the Aire River in the Yorkshire district of England. The breed is known for its love of children, its protectiveness of home and family and its companionship. Rarely do Airedales become self-willed because they are sensitive to their owners' wishes. They are generally even tempered and respond better to kindness than to domination.

DESCRIPTION

At birth, Airedale puppies look almost entirely black. Puppies likely to become show dogs should have tan markings above each eye, on the muzzle and the legs and on the underside. A white blaze on the chest is permissible. The mark may be more prominent in a puppy than in the mature dog. White toes or a half-white foot on a puppy will disappear with maturity, but more extensive white markings on the feet are likely to remain.

Airedales have a wiry outer coat and a softer undercoat. The best way to groom a wire-coated breed is to strip (pluck) the coat by hand or with a stripping tool, removing dead hair and making room for the new coat. If an Airedale is to be shown, the coat must be stripped.

Otherwise, it can be clipped. Clipping shortens the coat, allows the dead hair to remain and dulls the coat's color. Neither the whiskers nor the furnishings on an Airedale's legs or thighs should be removed. Airedales should be groomed because their coats can become shaggy and unkempt. Their coats do not shed, and a dog with a good coat may need little more than brushing and combing.

THE SHOW RING

A soft woolly coat is severely penalized in the show ring. Also penalized are yellow eyes, hound ears, white feet, over- or undersize, over- or undershot bite and poor movement.

BREEDING AND WHELPING

Onset of estrus may be as late as 13 to 15 months in the Airedale bitch. When estrus cycles begin, they are usually regular, occurring every six months.

A large, first litter is likely to be whelped early. The average size of a litter is eight to 12 puppies. Small litters sometimes cause problems in whelping, due to the lack of fetal bulk to respond to uterine contractions.

Puppy weight at birth averages 12 to 15 ounces. At 6 weeks, puppies weigh approximately 6 pounds and at 8 weeks, approximately 12 pounds. They grow at an even pace, achieving a weight of 50 pounds or more at maturity.

GROWTH

Dewclaws on the rear legs are rare and should be removed when they occur. The dewclaws on the front legs may be removed to prevent injury, but their removal is not required for the show ring. An Airedale's tail should be docked. On a grown dog the tip of the docked tail should be in line with the top of the head when the dog is on its toes with its neck extended. Generally this means cutting off about a third of a puppy's tail. A puppy's ears tend to fly when it is teething. Sometimes a dog's ears are too heavy and remain houndlike. This problem can often be alleviated by setting the ears.

To set the ears, attach them to the top front of the skull with liquid adhesive of the type used for applying false eyelashes or mending clothing. By this means the weight is taken off the ear and the muscle at the rear can work. The adhesive is applied to the tip of the ear, the ear is flipped over one finger, and the tip affixed to the top front of the skull. The space left by the finger provides room for the ear to work. Some ears must be set for a long time, but others correct immediately, especially ears that tend to break toward the rear while the puppy is teething.

RECOGNIZED PROBLEMS

Hip dysplasia is not a serious problem. **Umbilical hernias** have been reported.[1] **Malocclusion** is not unusual, and an undershot bite can develop in a pup up to a year of age. A collection of over 14,000 radiographs of the spine of ten breeds of dogs were examined for abnormal vertebrae in the lumbosacral region, which were manifestations of different types of fusion (**sacralisation and lumbalisation**). Such abnormalities were seen in 1.6% of 448 Airedales.[2]

Cerebellar hypoplasia is reported in the breed.[3,4] Puppies having this problem will be **ataxic** and show **hypermetria** at about 12 weeks of age.

Hot spots may develop on Airedales, and some bloodlines are predisposed to dry skin.

Airedales are one of a group of breeds at high risk for **canine lymphoma**.[5,6,7]

In one study over a two-year period, 56 dogs with signs of colonic disease were studied. Airedale Terriers appeared to be at increased risk of developing **colonic disease**. The presence of **watery stools**, **tenesmus**, **frank blood** and **mucus** were the most common clinical signs. No predisposing environmental factors were identified.[8]

A study in Germany demonstrated that feeding a milk replacer to Airedale puppies resulted in poor development and condition, impaired moving capacity, retarded change of teeth and pathological changes in the kidney (**renal calcification**, and **sclerosis, fibrosis of glomerula, dilatation of the tubuli**). Vitamin D3 concentration in the milk replacer was 3.45 million IU/kg feed. This concentration of Vitamin D3 was determined to result in intoxication in the Airedale puppies.[9]

Cushing's syndrome has been reported in the breed.[10] Airedales are one of several breeds with a significantly higher disposition for **malignant neoplasms** than the norm.[11]

In a Swedish study Airedales had a higher-than-average incidence of **primary hypothyroidism**.[12]

BEHAVIOR

It is important to note that Airedales accept pain and distress without complaining. Thus, an Airedale may be much sicker or in greater pain than outward appearance indicates.

A dominant dog can be deliberately disobedient toward people he considers submissive. Airedales easily become restless and bored. As a breed they are very playful, courageous and faithful.[13,14]

OLD AGE

Older bitches are subject to metritis and mammary tumors.

Older dogs remain playful and active, often despite muscular stiffness and arthritis.

They should be guarded against overexertion.

The life span of the Airedale ranges from 11 to 14 years.

References

1. Hayes, H.M. "Congenital Umbilical and Inguinal Hernias in Cattle, Horses, Swine, Dogs, and Cats: Risk by Breed and Sex Among Hospital Patients," *Am. J. Vet. Res.;* 35: 839-842.
2. Winkler, W. "Transitional Lumbosacral Vertebrae in the Dog," Dissertation, Fachbereich Veterinarmedizin der Freien Universitat Berlin. 1985: 143, 50 ref.
3. Erickson, F. et al, *Congenital Defects in Dogs. Canine Practice;* August 17, 1977: 58.
4. Cordy, D.R. and Snelbaker, H.A. "Cerebellar Hypoplasia and Degeneration in a Family of Airedale Dogs," *J. Neuropath. Exp. Neurol* (11); 1952: 324-328.
5. Madewell, Bruce R. "Canine Lymphoma," *Veterinarian Clinics of North America: Small Animal Practice;* Vol 15, No. 4, July, 1985.
6. McCraw, Dudley "Canine Lymphosarcoma," *AAHA's 56th Annual Meeting Proceedings;* 1989.
7. Rosenthal, Robert C. "The Treatment of Multicentric Canine Lymphoma," *Vet. Clinics of N. Amer. Sm. Anim. Prac.;* Vol 20., No. 4, July, 1990.
8. Houston, D.M. "An Integrated Study of Colonic Disease in the Dog," *Science and Engineering* (4); 1989: 1278-1279.
9. Kamphues, J., Meyer, H., Pohlenz J., and Wirth, W. "Vitamin D Intoxication in Airedale Puppies Fed with Milk Replacer," *Kleintierpraxis* (35); 1990: 9, 458-463.
10. Kramlich, C. "Airedale Column," *American Kennel Club Gazette;* December, 1992.
11. Kusch, S. "Incidence of Malignant Neoplasia in Dogs Based on PM Statistics of the Institute of Animal Pathology, Munich, 1970-1984," Inaugural Dissertation, Tierarztliche Fakultat, Ludwig Maximilians Universitat, Munchen, German Federal Republic.
12. Larsson, M. "The Breed, Sex and Age Distribution of Dogs with Primary Hypothyroidism," *Svensk-Veterinartidning* (38); 1986:15, 181-183, 3 ref.
13. Tortora, D.F. *The Right Dog for You* (Simon & Schuster, Inc., 1983).
14. Hart, B.L. and Hart, L.A. *The Perfect Puppy* (W.H. Freeman & Co., 1988).

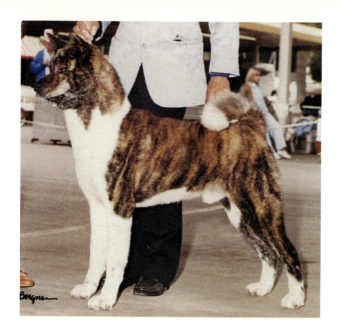

AKITA

ORIGIN AND HISTORY

The breed takes its name from Akita Prefecture on the main Japanese island of Honshu, where it was originally developed and bred. The original Akita was the result of breeding the Kari, the Tosa Fighting Dog, and other breeds imported from Europe. In the beginning, only royalty could own an Akita. Each dog was served by appointed attendants. Great ceremony surrounded such everyday action as training, eating and drinking.

Much spiritual significance has been attached to the Akita. In Japan the breed is so affectionately regarded as a protector of the home and a loyal companion and pet that it is a symbol of good health. The Japanese government has declared the breed a national monument of Japan and one of Japan's national treasures. Every champion dog is declared a National Art Treasure and made a ward of the government.

The breed dates back to 5000 B.C. when it was first brought to the Japanese Islands from the mainland of China. Bones of Akitas have been unearthed from shell burial grounds of this period and reconstructed. The written history of the Akita is about 100 years old. The earliest written information is in the records of directors of the Shogunate Hawk Chambers. These records tell of the care and training of dogs to work with hawks for hunting boar and deer.

DESCRIPTION

The Akita is the largest size of the ancient Nippon Inu, a purebred Japanese dog. The Nippon Inu consists of three sizes: Akita (large), Kari (medium) and Shiba (small).

In recent times the uses of the Akita have broadened beyond hunting. Akitas can pull a heavier load on a sled than most breeds of Alaskan dogs. They have also shown courage and intelligence as seeing-eye dogs, in police work and for beach patrol and life-saving. Akitas are natural hunters of deer, wild boar, bear, small game and fowl. They have keen noses, sight and hearing. Their feet can handle any type of terrain. When moving at full speed their hindquarters move in unison, enabling them to spring at their prey without breaking stride.

Akitas combine good nature, dignity, courage, alertness and docility. They are affectionate, sensitive to kindness and dependable. They thrive on human companionship and are unusually gentle and tolerant of teasing children and hazards of city life. They clean themselves like cats, by licking their paws and washing themselves. They are also odorless and need no clipping or cropping. They can be trained easily and respond willingly to verbal or signal commands. Akitas need little exercise and eat moderately. They bark only when thoroughly aroused and hunt silently.

Color and markings can change greatly until a puppy is one year old. Puppies dark at birth do not necessarily remain dark. In many cases a puppy that looks black becomes brown, or later, even fawn. Light colors generally lighten with age. Noses may be black at birth but are often mottled. Sometimes the black pigment does not fill in before 9 months of age. Pink noses are common on white puppies at birth and take longer to develop pigment than noses on darker-colored littermates. Albinos are not a problem in the breed.

Long coats are a problem in some lines. A puppy with a long coat can be recognized by 4 weeks. Tufts on the ears or hocks are the best indication. Some dogs with long coats also lack an undercoat. **Anemia** and **thyroid** problems have been found in the same lines that carry the gene for the long coat.

THE SHOW RING

Dewclaws, if present, should be removed from the hindlegs. They are often tiny and can be felt by rubbing against the grain.

Disqualifications: butterfly nose or total lack of pigmentation on nose; drop or broken ears; noticeably undershot or overshot; sickle or uncurled tail; dogs under 25 inches and bitches under 23 inches.

BREEDING AND WHELPING

Bitches come into estrus twice yearly. The first cycling occurs as early as 5 months of age. **False seasons**, in which ovulation does not occur but all other symptoms exist, are fairly common in young bitches.

Gestation usually requires 60 days. Akitas usually whelp easily but slowly. Often no signs of labor are apparent, and the puppies simply appear. The interval between whelps can be as long as four hours even with a female in excellent condition. Long intervals between whelps are common in the breed. Occasionally **umbilical hernias** occur. The size of a litter averages six, but 10 is not uncommon. Whelps generally weigh from 1 to 2 pounds. Birth defects, aside from hernias, are rare. Surveys conducted for Washington State University indicate that approximately 10% of all Akita puppies were stillborn or died shortly after birth.

GROWTH

Growth rates vary for different lines. Some Akitas reach full size by 1 year, but others do not reach full size until 4 years. Akitas are not fully mature before 3 years.

Any nutritious puppy food provides adequate nutrition. However, calcium and vitamin supplements are usually recommended from weaning until the ears are erect. In large animals with heavy ears, adhesive tape can support the ears if they are not erect by 4 or 5 months of age. The ears on some animals are not erect until the animal is 6 months old. Tails curve over the backs by 4 weeks. Selection or grading can begin at this age. Rears usually become narrower as the animals mature, so straight, wide ones are desirable. Long backs look longer at maturity, and slightly long and narrow muzzles look "snipy." Angulation decreases with age.

DENTITION

Bites are generally established by 6 months of age, but because of unequal growth of the lower and upper jaws, they can correct to a scissors bite as late as 1 year.

RECOGNIZED PROBLEMS

Hip dysplasia occurs in the breed, as well as **elbow dysplasia. Entropion** is fairly common. However, when entropion is diagnosed at an early age, it may not be truly entropion, but rather a condition due to small eyes. This condition corrects itself as the eyes grow, pushing the lid outward.

Progressive retinal atrophy has been described in the breed. **Multiple congenital ocular defects** have been reported in three Akita litters thought to have a common ancestor.[1]

Akitas are reported to have **congenital deafness and intussusception**.[2]

Some Akitas are very sensitive to anesthetics. A smaller than usual dose is often more than adequate.

As in other Japanese breeds, there is an inherited susceptibility to onion poisoning.[3]

Hypothyroid and hyperthyroid[4] are common in the breed.

Feeding a non-soy bean base food seems to eliminate skin problems, according to many breeders and veterinarians. **Sebaccous adenitis** is recognized in the breed.[5]

Several cases of **pseudohyperkalemia** have been reported. [6,7]

It was found that many Akitas have **high erythrocyte potassium content** relative to their plasma. Plasma from affected dogs has high potassium content after being refrigerated in contact with red cells for four hours or more.[8]

Researchers at Cornell University report a unique form of inherited **arthritis** in Akitas. The syndrome is referred to as "**juvenile-onset polyarthritis.**" Profound, incapacitating pain characterizes this disease, which is accompanied by a fever. A peculiar clinical feature of this disease is its cyclical occurrence.[9]

Harada's disease (**uveodermatological syndrome**) has been reported in Akitas. The disease is characterized by **uveitis**, **dermatitis** and CNS involvement.[10,11] Dogs often present with the initial complaint of anterior uveitis. Treatment with topical and oral corticosteroids and a combination of azathioprine and corticosteroids does not maintain remission. Treatment with cyclophosphamide resolves some clinical signs but may produce a persistent, sterile, hemorrhagic cystitis and predispose the dog to a subsequent **pseudomonas aeruginosa cystitis**.

Among 37 dogs with **pemphigus foliaceous** seen during nine years, Akitas were one of four breeds at significant elevated risk. The dorsal part of the muzzle was the most common site of initial involvement in over half of the dogs. **Scaling**, **crusting** and **alopecia** were seen in all the dogs. **Vesicles**, **pustules** and **bullae** were not seen commonly, but **target lesions** with **peripheral collarettes** were seen frequently. Most dogs had characteristic **footpad lesions** with **erythematous swelling** at the pad margins, **cracking** and **villous hypertrophy.** Generalized **exfoliative dermatitis** was seen in extensive disease. **Pruritus** was noted in less than half the dogs. Thirty-nine percent of the dogs responded to corticosteroid therapy alone, 50% to prednisone and cytotoxic drugs and 55% to prednisone with aurothioglucose. Aurothioglucose was successful alone in 27%. One-year survival was achieved in 53%.[12]

BEHAVIOR

The Akita makes an excellent house dog if he has a place to exercise. He is not destructive and he is not a barker. He does not like strange dogs, but is easily trained for obedience and does not resent children.

OLD AGE

Akitas usually live 15 years, and there are no aging problems peculiar to the breed.

References

1. Laratta, L.J., Riis, R.C., Kern, T.J., and Koch, S.A. "Multiple Congenital Ocular Defects in the Akita Dog," *Cornell Veterinarian* (75); 1985: 3, 381-392, 50 ref.
2. Strain, G.M. "Deafness in Dogs and Cats," *Proc. 10th ACVIM Forum*; May, 1992.
3. *Am. Journal of Vet. Research*, Vol. 53, No. 1; January, 1992.
4. Keffer, C. and McCulski, C. "Akita Thyroid Imbalance," *Akita Review*; Spring 1982: 51-55.
5. Griffin, C., Kwochka, K., and McDonald, J. *Current Veterinary Dermatology; the Science and Art of Therapy.* Mosby Yearbook, St. Louis, MO, 1993:171.
6. Veterinary Reference Laboratory et al, *Laboratory Communicator*; May & June, 1985.
7. Degen, M. "Pseudohyperkalemia in Akitas," *JAVMA* (190); 1987:5, 541-543, 6 ref.
8. Rich, L.J., Bernreuter D.C., and Cowell, P.L. "Elevated Serum Potassium Associated with Delayed Separation of Serum From Clotted Blood in Dogs of the Akita Breed," *Veterinary Clinical Pathology* (15); 1986: 2, 12-14; 2 ref.
9. "Juvenile Onset Arthritis," *American Kennel Club Gazette;* June, 1992.
10. Romatowski, J. "A Uveodermatological Syndrome in an Akita Dog," *Journal of the American Animal Hospital Association* (21); 1985: 6,777-780, 7 ref.
11. Cottrell B.D. and Barnett, K.C. "Harada's Disease in the Japanese Akita," *J. Sm. Anim. Prac.* (28); 1987: 6, 517-521, 11 ref.
12. Ihrke, P.J., Stannard,A.A., Ardans,A.A., and Griffin, C.E. "Pemphigus Foliaceous in Dogs: A Review of 37 Cases," *JAVMA* (186); 1985:1, 59-66, 58 ref.

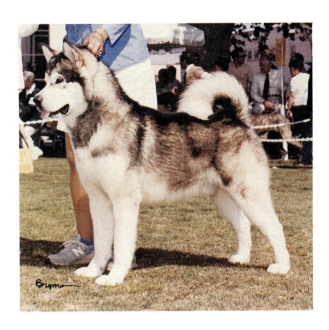

ALASKAN MALAMUTE

ORIGIN AND HISTORY

The Alaskan Malamute is the native Alaskan Arctic breed, cousin to the Samoyed of Russia, the Siberian Husky and the Eskimo dogs of Greenland and Labrador.

The two major foundation lines of the breed are M'Loot and Kotzebue. A third strain, Hinman or Hinman-Izwin, involving only a handful of dogs, made important contributions to breed quality. Today we have pure strains of both the M'Loot and Kotzebue, plus a desirable blending of the two.

DESCRIPTION

The Malamute is very affectionate and has an easygoing nature with human beings, but can be aggressive toward other animals or livestock. It is adaptable to southern climates with proper shelter.

THE SHOW RING

The breed Standard states, for desirable freighting: 25 inches, 85 pounds for dogs; 23 inches, 75 pounds for bitches. The subject has long been controversial among breeders, because there is such diversity in both size and weight. In the show ring if dogs are judged equal in type, proportion and functional attributes, the dog nearest the desirable freighting size is to be preferred.

The Malamute comes in a variety of colors but the most common are grey and white and black and white. The markings should be symmetrical; slight variation is acceptable, but no splashes, such as a half collar. Removal of front dewclaws is optional. The rear dewclaws, if any, must be removed. The Malamute as a sledge dog for heavy freighting is designed for strength and endurance and any characteristic of the individual specimen, including temperament, which interferes with the accomplishment of this purpose is to be considered the most serious of faults. Faults under this provision would be splayfootedness, any indication of unsoundness or weakness in legs, cowhocks, bad pasterns, straight shoulders, lack of angulation, stilted gait or any gait which isn't balanced, strong and steady, ranginess, shallowness, lightness of bone and poor overall proportion.

Blue eyes are a disqualifying fault.[1]

BREEDING AND WHELPING

The Alaskan Malamute seldom has any difficulty during gestation or whelping. The average litter size is seven puppies, although neither four nor 12 is unusual. Normal birth weight is from 12 to 22 ounces and generally doubles in two weeks.

RECOGNIZED PROBLEMS

Over 14,000 radiographs of the spine of ten breeds of dogs were examined for **abnormal vertebrae in the lumbosacral region**, manifested by different types of fusion. Abnormalities were seen in 4% of 90 Malamutes.[2]

The two main problems affecting the Malamute are **hip dysplasia**[3] and **chondrodysplasia**, more commonly called **dwarfism.** In chondrodysplasia, the Kotzebue strain is genetically uninvolved. The following is a summary of a paper published in the May-June 1975 issue of *AAHA*: The afflicted can be detected by x-ray of the front forefoot at 4 weeks of age or by observation in some cases at 8 to 12 weeks of age. Symptoms are those resembling rickets.

In the Alaskan Malamute dog, **hemolytic anemia** and chondrodysplasia are inherited as pleiotropic effects of a single gene.[4] Based on the clinical features, the mode of inheritance is autosomal recessive; test mating programs have been developed to eliminate the mutant from the breed base. When hematological parameters are more closely examined, however, heterozygoses are detectable and the mode of inheritance appears to be that of an incomplete dominant gene.

The skeletal disease results in the formation of a short-limbed dwarf because of **de-**

layed endochondral ossification.[5,6,7] Hematologically, red cell survival (51Cr) is decreased in affected dogs, with cross transfusion experiments indicating an intrinsic red cell defect. The **anemia**[8] is characterized by **stomatocytosis**, increased **erythrocyte** size (mean corpuscular volume-MCV), decreased mean **acorpuscular hemoglobin concentration** (MCHC), accompanied by the normal absolute amount of red cell hemoglobin (mean corpuscular hemoglobin-MCH). Thus the anemia, although hemolytic in nature, is distinguished from other regenerative anemias in the dog by the characteristic red cell indices. Serum iron, B12 and foliate levels are normal, and treatment of affected dogs with hematinics is inappropriate. A deficiency in the glycolytic enzymes has not been observed. Reduced glutathione (GSH) is diminished, but that which is present is stable.

The red cell sodium content is increased in affected dogs while the percent of solids is decreased. Flux studies (22Na) indicate transfer of sodium across the erythrocyte membrane rather than a defective ion transport mechanism.

The Alaskan Malamute anemia closely resembles some inherited human hemolytic disease with **stomatocytosis and altered red cell cation content**, and hence is expected to serve as a useful model in investigations of human erythrocyte membrane disorders. Study of the hyperactive red cell "pump" should also elucidate red cell electrolyte control in the canine. Identification of the red cell defect should supply additional information on the metabolic basis of the chondrodysplasia, and help eliminate much of the need for test-mating.

No simple means of detecting a producer of this defect exists. Suspect animals must be test-bred. An animal is considered suspect if known producers appear within a six-generation pedigree. A blood test developed by Dr. Fletch,[6] utilizing several parameters, should facilitate the eradication of this problem.

Test animals and further information may be supplied by the Alaskan Malamute Club of America's Master Plan Committee, 8014 Shallowford Rd., Chattanooga, Tn 37421.

Hemeralopia (day blindness) in dogs is characterized by inability to see in bright light, although ability to see in decreased illumination is retained.[9,10] This abnormality was discovered in 1960 in two breeds: Alaskan Malamutes and Poodles. Test breedings carried out by Rubin et al in 1966[11] proved that hemeralopia in Alaskan Malamutes is inherited as an autosomal recessive. **Corneal dystrophy** has been reported in the breed. Alaskan Malamutes have been seen with **Hemophilia B, Factor IX deficiency** which can cause severe bleeding disorder. It is inherited as a sex-linked recessive trait. They have also been reported with **Factor VII deficiency**, an autosomal incomplete dominant trait with subclinical to mild bleeding disorders.[12]

Another congenital dysfunction associated with Alaskan Malamutes is **renal cortical hypoplasia**.[13,14] The mode of inheritance is autosomal recessive, and the condition is characterized by polydipsia and polyuria. Alaskan breeds are more susceptible to **zinc responsive dermatosis**.[15] Researchers have also reported **castration-responsive dermatosis** in Alaskan Malamutes. [16]

Hereditary polyneuropathy has been reported in Malamutes. Eight dogs affected by progressive muscle weakness, ending in paresis, were examined and later autopsied. The affected dogs represented one third of the offspring from three matings of one male with three related bitches. The same male had previously produced six healthy offspring in matings with two different females. It was concluded that the condition is due to a single recessive autosomal factor.[17]

BEHAVIOR

The Malamute is not a barker; rather, he is a howler when left alone. He is not easily trained in obedience and can be destructive. He is fine with children in his own family but doesn't care much for strange children.

References

1. *The Complete Dog Book,* The American Kennel Club, 18th Ed.(Howell Book House: New York, 1992.)
2. Winkler, W. "Transitional Lumbosacral Vertebrae in the Dog," *Dissertation, Fachbereich Veterinarmedizin der Freien Universitat Berlin*; 1985: 143, 50 ref.
3. Erickson, F., et al, *Congenital Defects in Dogs,* Ralston Purina Co. (reprint from *Canine Pract.* Veterinary Practice Publ. Co.).
4. Dowdy, L.M. "Chondrodysplasia and the Veterinary Practitioner," *Alaskan Malamute Club of America Newsletter*; July 12, 1976.
5. Fletch, S.M., et al, "Clinical and Pathological Features of Chondrodysplasia in the Alaskan Malamute," *JAVMA* (162); 1973: 357-361.
6. Smart M.E. and Fletch, S.M. "A Hereditary Skeletal Growth Defect in Purebred Alaskan Malamutes," *Canad. Vet. J.* (12); 1972: 31-32.
7. Sublen, R.E., et al, "Genetics of the Alaskan Malamute Chondrodysplasia Syndrome," *J. Hered.* (63); 1972: 149-152.
8. Fletch, S.M. and Pinkerton, P.H. "An Inherited Anemia Associated with Hereditary Chondrodysplasia (Dwarfism) in the Alaskan Malamute," *JAVMA* (162); 1973: 357-361.
9. Rubin, L.F. "Clinical Features of Hemeralopia in the Adult Alaskan Malamute," *JAVMA* (158); 1971: 1696-1698.
10. Rubin, L.F. "Hemeralopia in Alaskan Malamute Pups," *JAVMA* (158); 1971: 1699-1701.
11. Rubin, L.F., et al: "Hemeralopia in Dogs," *Am. J. Res.* (28); 1967: 355-357.
12. Ettinger, S.J.; Textbook of Veterinary Internal Medicine. W.B. Saunders CO. Philadelphia, PA; 1989: 2259.
13. Kaufman, C.F., et al, "Renal Cortical Hypoplasia with Secondary Hyperparathyroidism in

the Dog," *JAVMA* (155); 1969: 1679-1685.

14. Kirk, R.W. and Bitner, S.I. *Handbook of Veterinary Procedures and Emergency Treatment: Hereditary Defects in Dogs;* Table 124. 1975: 661.

15. Samuelson, M. Personal Communication.

16. Griffin, C., Kwochka, K., McDonald, J. *Current Veterinary Dermatology, the Science and Art of Therapy.* Mosby Yearbook, St. Louis, MO. 1993; 171,299.

17. Moe, L., Bjerkas, I., Nostvold, S.O., and Offedal, S.I. "Herediteer Polyneuropathi Hos Alaskan Malamute," Proceedings, 14th Nordic Veterinary Congress, Copenhagen, 5-9 July, 1982: 171-174, 4 ref.

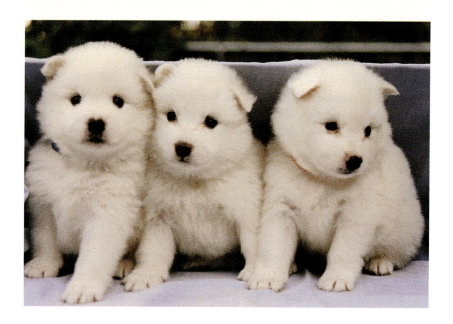

AMERICAN ESKIMO DOG

ORIGIN AND HISTORY

In 1992 the American Kennel Club asked that the name be officially changed to American Eskimo Dog from "Spitz," "Eskimo Spitz" or "American Eskimo Spitz." Some of the first AEDs seen in this country were seen in circuses. Ancestors of what is now called the American Eskimo Dog began arriving in America about 100 years ago.

The best estimate of informed breeders is that the AED included in its ancestry the white German Spitz (Weisser Grosspitz), white Keeshond, white Pomeranian, white Italian Spitz and possibly a bit of Japanese Spitz.

There is no evidence that canines living in Eskimo country were ancestors of the AED, or that Eskimos owned or bred them. There are many folkloric stories connecting the breed with Eskimos, none of which seems credible.

DESCRIPTION

The American Eskimo was admitted to registration in the American Kennel Club stud register on November 1, 1993. It can compete in the Miscellaneous class as of January 1, 1994. At a later date the American Eskimo will compete in the Non-Sporting Group.[1]

The Eskie is a loving companion dog, presenting a picture of strength and agility, alertness and beauty. It is a small to medium size Nordic type dog, always white or white with biscuit cream. It is a congenial breed that can be kept together and adapts to varied situations.

THE SHOW RING

There are three separate size varieties of the American Eskimo Dog (all measurements are heights at withers). The Eskie will be shown in the Open classes in three sizes: Toys are 9 inches to, and including, 12 inches; Miniatures are over 12 inches to, and including, 15 inches; and Standards are over 15 inches, to, and including, 19 inches. There is no preference in size within each variety. There is to be no trimming of the whiskers or body coat and such trimming will be severely penalized. The only permissible trimming is to neaten the feet and backs of the rear pasterns. The AED should trot, not pace, with good reach and drive and as speed increases will single track.

Disqualifications are: any color other than white or biscuit cream; blue eyes; oversize or undersize for its variety.

DENTITION

The breed must have full dentition, and the bite is level or scissors, with scissors preferred. Undershot mouths do occur.

BREEDING AND WHELPING

First estrus in the American Eskimo bitch is usually seen between 8 and 14 months, with the smaller varieties being earlier. The usual gestation time is 61 to 65 days. They are usually easy whelpers, although occasionally a Toy may require caesarean section. Toy whelps weigh about 6 ounces, Miniatures range from 6 to 8 ounces and Standards from 8 to 10 ounces. Occasional rear dewclaws are removed. Front dewclaw removal is optional.

GROWTH

Pink-pigmented whelps will begin to darken earlier if biscuit-marked. Black pigment can be complete as early as 2 weeks of age in the biscuit-marked puppy.

The pigment of solid white whelps is slower to develop, occasionally filling in as late as 6 months of age. Normally it completes between 8 and 16 weeks. Biscuit color often fades as the puppy matures. These dogs will have darker pigment. Dudley nose or incomplete pigment is faulted. Growth patterns vary by bloodlines or strains. Maturity is reached by 2 to 2 1/2 years.

Congenital abnormalities are rare in this breed.

RECOGNIZED PROBLEMS

Breeders report incidents of puppy **seizures**, which may prove to be low blood sugar as they seem to outgrow it. Hip dysplasia is seen, but the OFA has not had a sufficient number to estimate its prevalence.

BEHAVIOR

If not socialized and handled correctly as a puppy, the American Eskimo can be shy and diffident.

OLD AGE

Old age cataracts are seen in the American Eskimo Dog. Most live to be 16 to 18 years of age and succumb to the frailties common to all dogs.

References
1. *American Kennel Club Gazette*; May, 1993.

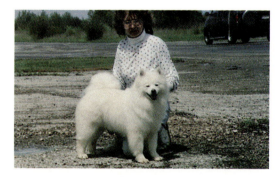

Standard

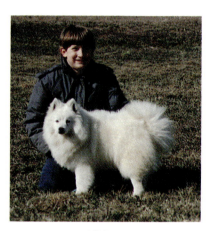

Miniature

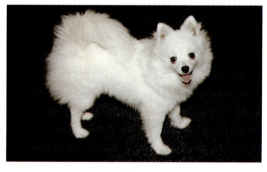

Toy

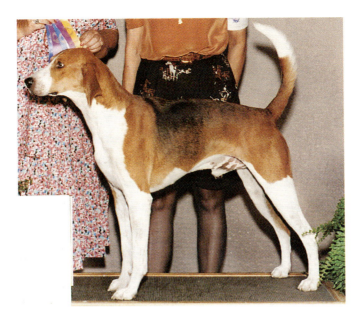

AMERICAN FOXHOUND

ORIGIN AND HISTORY

What is an American Foxhound? "The high type of the American Foxhound considered ideal by the American Foxhound Club has a physique and characteristics all his own, as marked in their way as those of the Thoroughbred horse. These characteristics have been developed through many generations of breeding to the fittest animals in the 'race' after the red fox in states where every other man owns foxhounds, and is willing to 'race' them for love and lucre on all occasions."

"Thus under American conditions of scent and going, a hound has been developed able to go for hours, under the roughest possible conditions of hill and dale, over rocks, sand and grass, through brush and briar, fording brooks, swimming rivers, able to follow scent in hot September and snowy January — in dusty roads and frozen fields with 'speed' and 'drive.'"

To meet these severe demands a certain type has demonstrated its ability — a type carrying as little superfluous weight as the high-class Thoroughbred or trotting horse, yet with sufficient bone, muscle and substance — of well knit mold to stand the wear and tear. In no sense a "weed," it is not so large and clumsy as to be unable to crawl through rail fences or woven wire or quickly walk or jump stone walls. Its fox-like foot carries it without lameness wherever the American red fox may lead. Its outward "quality" denotes the nervous energy within.

THE SHOW RING

Dogs should not be under 22 or over 25 inches at the shoulder. Bitches should not be under 21 or over 24 inches.

Considered as faults are: a flat skull; an excessively domed skull; small, sharp terrier-like eyes; prominent or protruding eyes; long or snipy muzzle; Roman or upturned nose; ears short or set on high. Also considered as faults are: thick, short neck; throatiness; long, swayed or roached back; straight shoulder; flat ribs; out at elbow; crooked legs; open feet; long hocks; straight hocks; long tail; rat tail, absence of brush; thin or soft coat.

There are no disqualifications in the Breed ring.

DESCRIPTION

The American Foxhound is a very distinct type: "It must not show Bloodhound characteristics nor those of English or other Foxhounds whether bred in this country or abroad. Such hounds as Bloodhounds, English Foxhounds, Welsh hounds, French hounds, Kerry Beagles or their crosses, although bred in America, are not American Foxhounds in characteristics or type."

In 1913, E. Lester Jones, secretary of the American Foxhound Club gave this definition,

1) The American Foxhound is not a house pet.
2) The American Foxhound is not a delicate physical specimen.
3) The American Foxhound is not a dog that requires special care, special diets and special treatments.
4) The American Foxhound has been produced for "the survival of the fittest."

The American Foxhound is a wonderful outdoor companion for boys and the family, but it is not a guard dog or a house dog. It should not be kept in heated kennels. A good, dry kennel, free from wind is all it needs. American Foxhounds can be successfully raised in outdoor kennels, provided the runs are a minimum of 10 feet by 50 feet. Both sexes do well kenneled together except during mating periods.

BREEDING AND WHELPING

There are practically no whelping problems with this breed. Sometimes mothers whelp more puppies than they can successfully feed.

Puppies weigh about 1 pound at birth. There are usually about six to eight puppies in a litter, and they gain 1 pound per week for the first five or six weeks. By the time they are 4 months old, they will weigh approximately 40 pounds and will measure 20 inches tall. At 6 months of age, they will weigh 50 pounds and measure 22 inches. By the time they are 1 year old, they will weigh about 65 pounds and measure 24 or 25 inches tall. Dewclaws on the front and back legs are usually removed. Grooming is the same as for a beagle.

RECOGNIZED PROBLEMS

Because of its strong physical body, the American Foxhound is not susceptible to very many diseases.

Hereditary deafness has been reported in a family of foxhounds by Adams[1] in 1956. In these cases the microscopic anatomy of the inner ear was unusual. The bone immediately surrounding the area in which the cochlea usually lies appeared to be made up of layers, which suggested new bone formation. The only resemblance to a normal cochlea was the cone-shaped case which normally contains the structures essential to hearing. The organ of corti, scala tympani, scala vestibuli and other structures usually found in the area were absent. The area was occupied by tissue which was histologically similar to skin, complete with sweat glands, hair follicles and sebaceous glands resting in a dense connective stroma.

Under the classification of Best and Taylor, this defect would be classified as a perceptive and transmission deafness. Mode of inheritance has not been determined.

Osteochondrosis of the spine in Foxhounds was described by Hime and Drake in 1965.[2] The evidence of familial or hereditary predisposition rests on the fact that all the affected hounds possessed the same sire. Victims of this condition have been described colloquially as "runners," a term in use for many years to describe hounds unable to gallop properly.

The mating of merle to merle (dapples) can result in **microphthalmia**.[3] The American Foxhound is one of the few breeds in which **thrombocytopathy (also thrombathemia, Glanzmann's disease, and thrombopathy)** is seen.[4] The condition manifests itself as moderate to severe bleeding diathesis, and it is inherited as an autosomal dominant or incomplete dominant trait.

BEHAVIOR

Foxhounds are very active, vigorous dogs. They are not territorial, are submissive and have stable temperaments.[5]

OLD AGE

A hearty breed, Foxhounds live an average of 13 years.

References
1. Adams, E.W. "Hereditary Deafness in a Family of Foxhounds," *JAVMA;* March 15, 1956: 302-303.
2. Hime, J.M. and Drake, J.C. "Osteochondrosis of the Spine in the Foxhound," *Vet. Rec.* (16); 1965: 445-449.
3. Sorsby, A. and Davey, J.B. "Ocular Association of Dappling (or Merling) in Coat Colors of Dogs: "Clinical and Genetic Data," *Journal Genetics* (52); 1954: 425-440.
4. Kirk, R.W., Ed. *Current Veterinary Therapy VI* (W.B. Saunders: Philadelphia).
5. Tortora, D.F. *The Right Dog for You* (Simon & Schuster: New York, 1983).

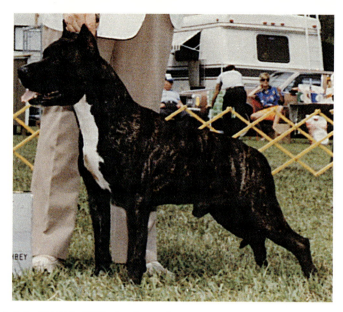

AMERICAN STAFFORDSHIRE TERRIER

ORIGIN AND HISTORY

The ancestors of the American Staffordshire Terrier were imported from the British Isles in the middle and late 19th century, and were used primarily, though not exclusively, for the purpose of pit fighting. They were known by various names, such as Bull and Terrier, Half and Half and Pit Bull.

DESCRIPTION

True dog lovers observed that American Staffordshire Terriers were more than capable fighters. They could dispatch rodents, serve as catch dogs in hunting parties, herd and guard farm animals, enjoy rough and tumble play of young children and protect home and family. The dogs' cheerful and affectionate nature, combined with strength and spirit, earned devoted fanciers, and the breed was recognized by the American Kennel Club in 1935 as Staffordshire Terrier. In 1974 the official name became American Staffordshire Terrier, although breeders commonly refer to them as Staffs or Amstaffs.

A mature Staff should show confidence and alertness. It is of medium size. The coat is short and comes in any color; solid, pied, brindle, with or without white markings. The tail is never docked. Because of its fighting heritage, the Staff requires a fenced area in which to play and should be exercised outside his fenced yard only on a leash. It should not be allowed to roam at large. This breed is well suited to obedience work, as it enjoys jumping, retrieving and generally doing things with its owner, but must be taught while young to give on command, as its instinct is to hold on.

THE SHOW RING

The American Staffordshire should give the impression of great strength for his size; muscular, yet agile and graceful. He should be stocky, not long-legged or racy in outline. The dogs should be about 18 to 19 inches at the shoulder and the bitches should be 17 to 18 inches at the shoulder. Height and weight should be in proportion. There are no breed disqualifications. Faults to be penalized are: Dudley nose, light or pink eyes, tail too long or badly carried, undershot or overshot mouths. Removal of dewclaws is optional, as is ear-cropping, although most seen in the show ring are cropped (See Appendix 1 for ear-cropping directions.)

BREEDING AND WHELPING

Onset of estrus occurs around 10 months of age. Intervals between 21-day estrous cycles vary from six to nine months. Ovulation and gestation time follow normal patterns and breeding partners are congenial provided the bitch has reached the receptive period of her cycle. She may seek human contact at whelping, but requires little or no assistance. She will demand privacy from other dogs, at least for the first week or two.

Average litter size is seven to eight puppies, with individuals weighing around 12 ounces. Noses and footpads are usually pink at birth, but darken to normal pigment, usually within two months. Testicles are usually in place by this time, although an apparent **monorchid** may drop the second testicle as late as 4 or 5 months. Gross defects such as **cleft palate** and **deformed limbs** have been observed.

GROWTH

A 12-ounce whelp may stand 18 inches high and weigh 50 pounds before 1 year. Its head and chest will widen and muscle mass increase in density throughout the second year, and with males, even into the third, resulting in a mature weight of 65 pounds or more. Females are less massive, and mature to 50 - 55 pounds by 2 years. The breed is active and performs better on two medium-sized meals per day, rather than one large one. Care should be taken with puppies to meet nutritional requirements without overfeeding, as excess weight may contribute to development of joint problems during the rapid growth period. An undershot bite in puppy teeth is not likely to improve with permanent teething. In selecting a puppy one should look for boundless energy, the air of confidence and trust typical of the breed, lively curiosity and normal scissors bite.

RECOGNIZED PROBLEMS

The American Staffordshire Terrier has an extremely high pain threshold when excited, and can injure itself with its own strength without realizing it. **Ruptured anterior cruciate** may be difficult to palpate, even under anesthesia, through the dense muscle mass. The injury is a common one.

Potential puppy buyers should be advised to seek breeders who use mature breeding stock that has been screened by X-ray for **hip dysplasia**. Universal screening in this breed has been delayed because of the absence of clinical symptoms, except in cases of severe dysplasia.

False pregnancy in the absence of breeding, occasionally accompanied by **metritis**, is a recurrent problem in the breed. **Patent ductus arteriosus**, and a predisposition to **cutaneous mast cell tumors** have been reported in the American Staffordshire Terrier.[1] **Congenital deafness** has also been reported.[2] Some individuals experience **allergic responses to grasses or insect bites**. **Bilateral cataract and clefts of lip and palate** are listed as hereditary defects.[3] **Distichiasis** and **progressive retinal atrophy** are seen in the breed.[4] Eight cases of **persistent hyperplastic primary vitreous**, apparently the first to be recorded in this breed, have been seen since May 1983. They ranged from mild, unilateral to severe, bilateral. A similar condition has been described in Bull Terriers. The mode of inheritance has not been investigated.[5]

The Staff does not bite and slash repeatedly in a fight, but grabs hold, hangs on and shakes. Its grip is so powerful that it can break its own teeth if the hold is through a fence. Breaking the hold safely is the primary consideration. Application of a stream of water from a garden hose directly into the nose and mouth is effective in breaking up a fence fight. If the dogs are loose, maximum pressure on the choke collar for several minutes may be required to force release of the hold. Owners should be advised to keep an ammonia ampule available as it can be held to the nose to help break a hold.

BEHAVIOR

The AmStaff is extremely courageous and full of vitality. It can be belligerent with strangers. It is a wonderful companion for children with whom it is raised.

OLD AGE

Life expectancy for the AmStaff is 12 to 14 years. **Arthritic changes** and **elbow calluses** may develop with aging.

References
1. "Veterinary News," *The American Kennel Club Gazette;* April, 1990: 44.
2. Strain, George M. "Deafness in Dogs and Cats," *Proc. 10th ACVIM Forum;* May, 1992.
3. Erickson, et al, "Congenital Defects of Dogs, Part I," *Canine Pract.* (4); 1977: 54-61.
4. Rubin, L.F. Inherited Eye Disorders in Purebred Dogs; 1989:13
5. Petrick, S.W. "Genetic Eye Diseases Diagnosed in Staffordshire Bull Terriers," *Journal of South African Veterinarian Association*; 1988: 59: 4, 177: 1 ref.

APPENDIX 1

The American Staffordshire Terrier

EAR CROPPING

About seven to 10 days after the ears have been cropped they will normally be healed enough to remove the stitches. The ears should then be rolled to help them shape and stand properly. Supplies used for rolling are: (1) foam rubber, (2) ether and (3) 1-inch cloth adhesive tape (not plaster).

Three people are required to place and hold the puppy in a steady position.

The specific steps in the procedure are as follows:

1. Cut two pieces of foam 4 1/2 to 5 inches long and 1 1/2 inches square.

2. Taper one end of the foam.

3. With a strip of gauze 8 x 4 inches roll the tapered foam into a tight and firm roll (about 1/2 inch diameter). Use 1/4-inch tape to hold roll tight.

4. With a strip of adhesive tape 10 x 1 inches, start about 1/2 inch from the tapered end of the gauze-covered roll and spiral wrap upward, leaving the sticky side of the tape out. Trying not to disturb the sticky surface of the tape, wrap tightly.

5. (a) Put the puppy on a suitable table in a sitting position. Two assistants are needed to hold the puppy gently but firmly and quietly in position, holding the head steady. Moisten cotton with ether and clean the inside and outside of the ear to remove the oil from the skin and hair and help ensure the tape sticking.

5. (b) Have an assistant grasp the tip of the ear, holding it steady and exerting a slight upward pressure. Grasp the ear at its base (opening) and pull slightly so as to admit the tapered end of the roll. With a twisting motion, gently and firmly insert the tapered end of the roll down into the ear as far as possible, 1/4 to 1 inch, making sure the puppy is held still. Hold the roll down in the ear by exerting slight downward pressure at the top of the roll with the fingers of one hand. With the other hand, grasp the top of the ear being held by the assistant. Exert slight upward pressure and shape the ear around the sticky roll, keeping the light downward pressure on the roll and the slight upward tension on the ear. When the ear has been shaped around the roll, have an assistant opposite you grasp the top of the ear and hold it in place around the roll. Continuing to exert slight upward pressure on the ear, take a strip of adhesive tape 8 x 1 inches and spiral wrap the ear from the base to the top. Always start the spiral on the inside and finish on the inside, cutting off any excess tape. When spiral wrapping the ear, lay the tape so it is snug but does not cut off circulation. (Practice on an older dog whose ears are healed and standing.) If the first strip does not go to within 1/2 inch of the top of the ear — use another strip.

Have an assistant grasp tape at the top of the ear and exert slight upward pressure. With a 6 x 1 inch strip of tape, start at the base of the ear on the inside and wrap around the ear twice at a downward angle, covering as much of the ear opening as possible. This keeps the bottom part of the roll from working up and out of the ear if the puppy scratches. Cut any excess part of the roll off just above the tip of the ear. Then take a strip of tape 2 x 1/4 inches and put it over the top and down each side of the rolled ear as far as it will reach, usually about 3/4 inch.

Leave the ears up in the rolls for six to seven days. Then use cotton saturated with ether to remove the tape. Remove the roll from the ear and clean off any sticky substance remaining on the ear. When removing the tape from the ear, find the end of the tape and lift slightly, pat with ether-saturated cotton while pulling gently on the tape. The tape will come off easily if plenty of ether is used. Discard the cotton when it becomes sticky and continue with a new piece.

Dust the ear lightly with a healing powder (Mexia, etc.). After the ear has been down six or seven days check it again. The ears usually shape and stand properly after being rolled one or two times. Continue the process as necessary (up six to seven days, then down six to seven days) until satisfied with the results.

This procedure requires practice. There will be three hands on the ear most of the time and the space is small. You and your assistants will need to learn how best to position the puppy while working in the small area around the ear and still keep the puppy quiet. A mild tranquilizer on the puppy about an hour before starting helps the puppy adjust to the new rolls on his head. The puppy usually doesn't mind the rolls, after the initial adjustment, but should be kept quiet and away from other dogs.

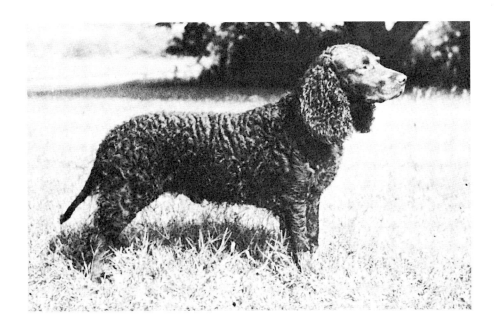

AMERICAN WATER SPANIEL

ORIGIN AND HISTORY

The exact origin of the American Water Spaniel is unknown. The Irish Water Spaniel and the Curly Coated Retriever are probably progenitors of this sporting breed, which evolved mainly in the Middle West. Sportsmen in many areas of the United States appreciated this excellent shooting dog and retriever long before its recognition as a breed by the American Kennel Club in 1940.

DESCRIPTION

American Water Spaniels are enthusiastic and eager to please. An excellent nose, strong swimming ability and versatility in the field also characterize this breed.

THE SHOW RING

As stated in the official Standard for the breed, height at the shoulder ranges from 15 to 18 inches. Males weigh from 28 to 45 pounds, females from 25 to 40 pounds. The coat color is solid liver or dark chocolate, a little white on the toes or chest being permissible. The closely curled but not coarse coat should be thick enough to protect against adverse weather, water and dense cover.[1]

Faults include: Long, slender or "snipy" muzzle, cowhocks, rat or shaved tail, and coats too straight, soft, fine or tightly kinked.

Yellow eyes are a disqualification in the breed.[1]

RECOGNIZED PROBLEMS

Anterior sutural lenticular opacities and **unilateral focal retinal dysplasias** have been reported to the Canine Eye Registration Foundation (CERF). [2]

Hermaphroditism has been reported by some breeders.

There are so few specimens of this breed tendencies cannot be determined.

BEHAVIOR

This breed is extremely responsive to training and is an enthusiastic worker. It makes an excellent companion and guard dog.

References
1. *The Complete Dog Book,* American Kennel Club, 18th ed. (Howell Book House: New York, 1992): 88-90.
2. Rubin, L.F., Inherited Eye Diseases in Purebred Dogs. Williams and Williams, 1989: 13.

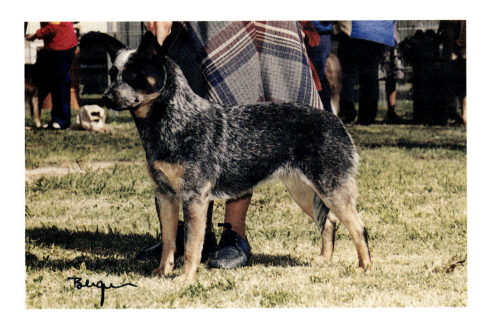

AUSTRALIAN CATTLE DOG

ORIGIN AND HISTORY

The Australian Cattle Dog was established as a pure breed in 1890 after a long period of experimentation by cattle owners and dog breeders to produce a type of dog suitable for Australian conditions. They needed a working dog with the stamina to travel and work in all weather, often through rough and inaccessible terrain. Because of the lack of fences and shortage of labor, cattle were often wild; thus, it was necessary to breed a dog that was not afraid to tackle savage bulls but would not frighten wild cattle by continuous barking. The dog needed to be tractable, intelligent and obedient.

In order to achieve this combination, a series of crosses was attempted, some unsuccessful, and others resulting in the present Australian Cattle Dog. The Cattle Dog originated basically from the crossing of the Blue Merle Collie and the wild Dingo, modified by introduction of the Dalmatian and later the black and tan Culpa.

Many of these dogs found their way to Queensland, where they proved invaluable for working cattle in the heat and harsh conditions.

They became known as Queensland Heelers. The name was later changed to Australian Heeler, then to Australian Cattle Dog, which is now accepted throughout Australia and overseas as the official name of the breed. The Standard for the breed was drawn up by Robert Coalesce in 1897 and was later adopted by the New South Wales Kennel Council. Adoptions by other states followed. In 1963 the present Standard for the breed was approved and adopted by the Australian National Kennel Club.

DESCRIPTION

The general appearance of the Australian Cattle Dog is that of a sturdy, compact, symmetrically-built working dog with the ability and willingness to carry out any task, however arduous. A combination of substance, power, balance and hard muscular condition convey the impression of great agility, strength and endurance. Soundness of movement is of paramount importance. Capability of quick and sudden movement is essential.

Since the main purpose of the breed is assistance in the control of cattle, the Australian Cattle Dog is ever alert, watchful, courageous and trustworthy, with an implicit devotion to duty. Its loyalty and protective instincts make it a self-appointed guardian over his herd and his property. Although suspicious of strangers, the Cattle Dog is required to be amenable to handling in the show ring.

THE SHOW RING

The desirable height at the withers for male dogs is 18 to 20 inches and for bitches, 17 to 19 inches. Those over or under these dimensions are considered undesirable. The ratio of height to length is 9 to 10. Length measurement is taken from breastbone to buttocks. Approximate weight for dogs and bitches is 45 to 55 pounds and 40 to 50 pounds, respectively.

The weather-resistant outer coat is moderately short, straight and of medium texture, with short, dense undercoat. The coat behind the quarters is longer, forming a slight breeching. Head, fore legs and hind legs below the hocks are coated with short hair.

Blue or blue mottle, with or without black marks on the head, evenly distributed is preferred. Black markings on the body are not desirable. Tan on legs, head, breast, throat and inside of thighs is desirable. The richer the better. Tan undercoat is permissible, if it does not show through the blue of the outer coat.

The red Cattle Dog should be a good, even, red speckle all over, including the undercoat, with or without darker red markings on the head. Even head markings are desirable. Red markings on the body are permissible, but not desirable. White or cream on outer or undercoat are not permitted.[1]

Any tendency to grossness or weediness is a serious fault. Stilted movement, loaded or slack shoulders, straight shoulder placement, weakness at elbows, pasterns or feet, straight stifles, cow or bow hocks must be regarded as serious faults.

Other faults include undershot or overshot jaws; walleyes, or white blemishes in eyes; curly coat, or wavy coat; "snipy" muzzle; lop ears (after 9 months); spoon or bat ears; dewclaws on hind legs; stumpy tail, pronounced hook or curl in tail, or tail carried above the line of the back; sway back or roached back.

50

BREEDING AND WHELPING

The pups are born white, except for undesirable black marks. The blue or red speckle gradually appears at about two weeks after birth. This is believed to spring from their Dalmatian inheritance.

The pups are usually born with dewclaws on front legs only, and these are not removed. EARS ARE NOT CROPPED AND TAILS ARE NOT DOCKED.

The bitches are usually easy whelpers and very good mothers. Pups are generally hardy and vigorous; they thrive well and grow fast.

DENTITION

Dentition should be sound, strong and regularly spaced. Jaws should grip with a scissors-like action, the lower incisors close behind and just touching the upper.

RECOGNIZED PROBLEMS

Occasionally **eczema** arises, especially in the croup area, usually related to a lack of grooming of the thick undercoat and/or to flea infestation. Dogs and bitches exhibit a tendency to obesity, which can be controlled by proper diet management.

Dr. George M. Strain reports that of 63 Australian Cattle Dogs tested for hearing problems eight (12.7%) showed either **unilateral or bilateral deafness**.

A **lysosomal storage disease (ceroid lipofuscinosis)**[2] was diagnosed in two siblings. Both dogs developed clinical signs of the disease at about 1 year of age. Vision and motor function deteriorated over several months and by 2 years of age, the dogs were blind and had **progressive ataxia**. **Cytoplasmic inclusions** with ultrastructural patterns characteristic of **ceroid lipofuscin** were observed in most neurons examined and in the cells of several other parenchymatous tissues.

Biochemical studies, including determination of lysosomal enzyme activities, excluded several other lysosomal storage diseases. In these dogs, the clinical and pathological features of the disease were similar to those of the juvenile subtype of ceroid lipofuscinosis (Batten Disease) in human beings.[2] The case records of 21 dogs with **congenital portosystemic encephalopathy** show the disorder most common in Australian Cattle Dogs. **Extra-hepatic shunts** occurred in small breeds, while **infra-hepatic shunts** occurred in the medium to large breeds.[3] Recognized ophthalmic problems are **cataracts, lens luxations** and **progressive retinal atrophy**.[4]

BEHAVIOR

The breed tends toward a possessive nature, leading to aggression if encouraged. The breed is extremely intelligent and they are outstanding workers. The breed has an atavistic habit of biting at the heels of cattle and people.

OLD AGE

Australian Cattle Dogs, a hearty breed selected for health and working ability, live an average of 13 years.

References

1. American Kennel Club, *The Complete Dog Book;* (Howell Book House, New York, 1992.)
2. Bask, D.B., Levesque, D.C., Wood, P.A., and Sayer, E.L. "Clinical and Pathologic Features of Ceroid Lipofuscinosis in Two Australian Cattle Dogs," *JAVMA* (197); 1990: 3, 361-364, 22 ref.
3. Addison, "Canine Congenital Portosystemic Encephalopathy," *Australian VALET. Journal* (65); 1988:8, 245-249, 30 ref.
4. Quinn, Arthur DVM; *Personal Communication.* January 1994.

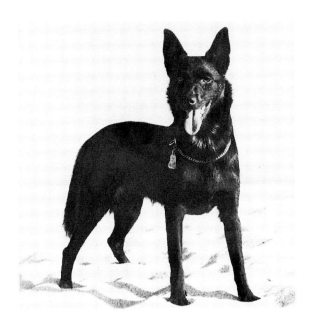

AUSTRALIAN KELPIE

ORIGIN AND HISTORY

The Australian Kelpie or Barb is said to have originated as late as 1870 and is every bit as indispensable to the Australian rancher as his relative, the Heeler. Just as the Heeler tends cattle, the Kelpie herds sheep. It was bred according to ability to work sheep in Australia's pasturelands.

DESCRIPTION

Kelpies are enthusiastic and intelligent working dogs with natural ability and aptitude to work sheep and respond to human commands. They have an excellent temperament but become restless if kept as city pets and have a tendency to wander.

THE SHOW RING

The Kelpie is medium sized, dogs measuring between 18 and 20 inches at the withers and weighing about 30 pounds: bitches measure between 17 and 19 inches and weigh slightly less. The coat is fairly short, flat and straight with a short, dense overcoat. The hair is short on the head, ears, feet and legs, but around the neck it is longer, showing a fair amount of ruff, and at the rear of the thighs forms a mild breeching.

The tail is bushy and not docked.

Coat colors are black, black and tan, red, red and tan, fawn chocolate and smoke blue.[1] The ears are naturally pricked.[2]

The Kelpie is strong and athletic, and any tendency to cow hocks, stiltiness or restricted movement, weaving or plaiting are serious faults.

BREEDING AND WHELPING

Reproductive problems in Kelpies are uncommon, as the original line developed largely by natural selection. The average litter size is five to six pups. Congenital or hereditary problems are rare.

Selection of a puppy for a working dog should be based on the ability of the pup's parents, the breeder's reputation and previous record, the pup's temperament and physical development.

The dogs are intelligent and rapidly learn sheep work. Initial training should begin at 4 months, yet a dog may not reach its peak of herding ability until about 3 years old.

Good nutrition is important and intake should be increased during periods of hard work. The working dogs are strong and athletic, with a resting heart beat of about 70 beats per minute.

RECOGNIZED PROBLEMS

Although rare, **hip dysplasia** has been encountered. Working dogs occasionally develop **heat exhaustion**. Adequate rest, shade and water must be provided.

Hereditary cerebellar abiotrophy has been diagnosed in Kelpies. In a test breeding the mode of inheritance was not fully identified but a single recessive autosomal gene may be involved.[3]

BEHAVIOR

The Kelpie is active, intelligent and difficult to control. He is accustomed to wide open spaces and does not tolerate confinement.

OLD AGE

Arthritis is the most common problem associated with the older dogs. They usually live to be about 10 to 12 years but have been known to live to 21.

References
1. The American Kennel Club, *Miscellaneous Breed Standards;* June, 1993.
2. Royal Agricultural Society (Australia), *Breed Standards.*
3. Thomas, J.B. and Robertson, B. "Hereditary Cerebellar Abiotrophy in Australian Kelpie Dogs," *Australian Veterinary Journal* (66); 1989: 9, 301-302, 10 ref.

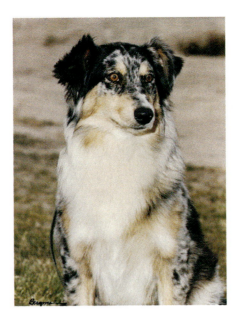

AUSTRALIAN SHEPHERD

ORIGIN AND HISTORY

The Australian Shepherd has an uncertain origin. The most widely accepted theory places the origin of the breed in the Spanish Pyrenees with the Basque sheepherders, who found this breed a valuable asset in assisting with the flocks. It is believed the Australian Shepherd found its way to Australia in the early 19th century, when many sheep were imported to that country from Spain.

The Basques who went to Australia to serve as herdsmen were accompanied by their canine partners. Around the time of the California Gold Rush, large numbers of Australian sheep were imported to the western United States, again accompanied by the Basque herders and their dogs. The Americans, unfamiliar with this merled breed, coined the name "Australian Shepherd," indicating the association of the breed with the imported sheep.

DESCRIPTION

The Australian Shepherd is an amalgamation of traits from across the seas: intelligence, loyalty and unique beauty combined with a physical agility for ease in doing the job it enjoys so much. It is so sound-minded that it easily adapts to various situations.

Today the Aussie serves humanity in every imaginable way: as working ranch dogs, seeing-eye dogs, hearing-ear dogs, pet therapy participants, drug detectors and search-and-rescue dogs. A loyal companion, with strong guarding and herding instincts, it has the stamina to work all day. The Australian Shepherd is a hardy breed, very resistant to weather and adaptable to a variety of climates.

THE SHOW RING

The "Aussie" is slightly longer than tall, of medium size and bone, with a docked or naturally bobbed tail (should not exceed 4 inches as an adult). He comes in four acceptable colors: black, blue merle, red and red merle. White body splashes of any size are a disqualification. The male is 20 to 23 inches tall at the withers; the female is 18 to 21 inches. The eyes are almond shaped and can be brown, amber, blue or any combination or shade of these colors, and can include flecks or marbling.

Pendulous, low-set ears or prick ears are severe faults. The nose should always be completely pigmented of the same color that surrounds the eye, given the different colors.

Any degree of undershot in the jaw is a disqualifying fault, as is an overshot greater than 1/8 of an inch. Aggression or shyness are severe faults.[1]

BREEDING AND WHELPING

Puberty starts from 6 to 18 months with the first estrus occurring at an average of 10 months. Estrus occurs twice a year, approximately every six months. The period of gestation is 60-65 days, ending with a normal and easy delivery. The bitch exhibits an intense mothering instinct and strong milking ability. Weaning is followed by extreme shedding of the dam's coat. Males tend to be exceptionally accepting of the puppies.

Litter size ranges from five to 10, with the newborn pups weighing from 1/2 to 1 pound each. The flesh-colored noses seen at birth rapidly darken and are usually completely pigmented at 1 year. Copper trim, if present, increases in intensity within a few days following birth for merles, a few weeks for solid-colored dogs. Merles tend to darken with age. Shortly after birth, tails are docked to the fourth or fifth coccygeal vertebra, and dewclaws are removed. Removal of the front dewclaws, while optional in the Standard, is recommended for aesthetic purposes on show stock and as they tend to be predisposed to injury in the working dog.

Litters from two merled (heterozygous) parents will produce an average of 25% homozygous merles. They are mostly white in color and are euthanized at birth because of a recessive trait of defective eye and ear development apparently associated with the merling gene.[2] Instances of **spina bifida (open spine)** have been observed in lines intensely bred for natural bobtails. Other defects observed at birth are **cleft palate** and **malocclusions of bite**.

GROWTH

Rate of growth varies with the strain, the larger strains exhibiting faster growth rates. Rapid skeletal growth is accompanied by slower muscular development, with the dog reaching full maturity at 3 years. Puppies exhibiting the homozygous merle trait and other obvious defects should be eliminated, with selection made on the basis of overall soundness and outgoing personality. Temperament is good; however, temperament does vary within the breed, and the prospective owner is encouraged to observe the temperament of the parents prior to selection.

DENTITION

Permanent teeth begin to erupt at 4 months. Bite is usually determinable by 6 months. Malocclusions are strongly penalized in this working breed. In some strains permanent dentition may not be complete until 2 years.

RECOGNIZED PROBLEMS

Mild **umbilical hernias**, **hip dysplasia**, ocular anomalies including **microphthalmia,**[3] **cataracts**, **retinal detachment** and **progressive retinal atrophy** and, in rare instances, **dwarfing syndrome** have been observed in the breed. Most prominent breeders obtain OFA certification and eye certification on their breeding stock.

Multiple ocular colobomas have been reported and have been described as an inherited syndrome.[4] **Collie eye anomaly** has been described in the Australian Shepherd. Test breedings have indicated an autosomal recessive mode of inheritance.[5]

A **syndrome of multiple defects** lethal to males, including **cleft palates, polydactyly, syndactyly, shortened tibia-fibula, brachygnathism** and **scoliosis**, is described in a family of Australian Shepherd dogs. Female pups lack the cleft palates and survive, but may exhibit the other defects to a lesser degree than males. Litter data suggest that the trait is inherited as an x-linked lethal gene, but the possibility of a sex-influenced autosomal allele cannot be ruled out. The syndrome may have arisen in conjunction with instability of the merle locus.[6]

Hereditary deafness is associated with the presence of the merle, piebald or extreme piebald genes. It is often reported as a syndrome that includes **piebaldism or partial albinism, heterochromia iritis, absence of retinal pigment and cochlear stria, vascularis pigment** and **various facial defects**. The syndrome is usually inherited as an autosomal dominant trait with incomplete penetrance so that affected individuals may not display all components. Typical examples are blue-eyed cats, Dalmatians, English Setters and Australian Shepherds.[7] The diagnosis and treatment of suspected **ivermectin** and **piperazine toxicosis** are reviewed with Illinois Animal Poison Information Center data. Data indicate that (1) the Collie and Australian Shepherd were the only dog breeds in which more than one suspected ivermectin toxicosis occurred after estimated dosages of 100 to > 500 mg/kg, and (2) piperazine neurotoxicity in dogs and cats was usually manifested by muscle tremors, ataxia and behavioral disturbances within 24 hours after estimated dose(s) between ≥ 20 and < 110 mg/kg.[8]

Australian Shepherds have the highest incidence of **nasal solar dermatitis**.[9] Lesions begin either at the junction of the haired and nonhaired planum nasals or on the planum itself.

The early erythema most closely resembles a true sunburn. With chronic sun exposure the affected sites may have an ulcerated crust. Veterinarians must be careful to rule out discoid lupus erythematosis and other autoimmune diseases.

BEHAVIOR

The Australian Shepherd can adapt to family life and is loyal, affectionate and playful.

OLD AGE

The Australian Shepherd may be expected to live for 10 to 15 years.

References
1. Little, C. *The Inheritance of Coat Color in Dogs.*
2. *The American Kennel Club Gazette;* January, 1993.
3. Gelate, K.N. and McGill, L.D. "Clinical Characteristics of Microphthalmia with Colobomas of the Australian Shepherd Dog," *JAVMA* (162); 393-396.
4. Cook, C.S., Burling K. and Nelson, E.J. "Embryogenesis of Posterior Segment Colobomas in the Australian Shepherd," *Progress in Veterinary and Comparative Ophthalmology* (1); 1991: 3, 163-170, 20 ref.
5. Rubin, L.F., Nelson, E.J. and Sharp, C.A. "Collie Eye Anomaly in Australian Shepherds," *Progress in Veterinary and Comparative Ophthalmology* (1); 1991: 2, 105-108, 23 ref.
6. Sponenberg, D.P. and Bowling, A.P. "Heritable Syndrome of Skeletal Defects in a Family of Australian Shepherds," *Journal of Heredity* (76); 1985: 5, 393-394, 6 ref.
7. Strain, G.M. "Congenital Deafness in Dogs and Cats," *Compendium on Continuing Education for the Practicing Veterinarian* (12); 1991: 2, 245-250, 252-253, 42 ref.
8. Lovell, R.A. "Ivermectin and Piperazine Toxicosis in Dogs and Cats," *Veterinary Clinics of North America, Small Animal Practice* (20); 1990: 2, 453-468, 108 ref.
9. Griffin, C., Kwochka K., and MacDonald, J. "Current Veterinary Dermatology," *Mosby;* 1993: 225.

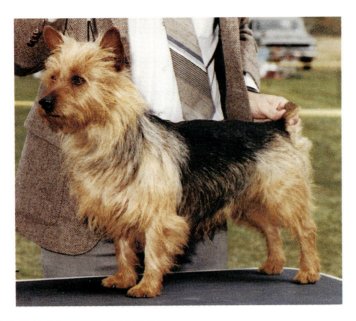

AUSTRALIAN TERRIER

ORIGIN AND HISTORY

The Australian Terrier appeared in 1885 as a hunter in the bushland. The breed traces its origin to several terriers, including the Cairn, Dandie Dinmont and Skye. It was recognized by the AKC in 1960.

DESCRIPTION

Australian Terriers (Aussies) are unusually responsive, and some are also quite sensitive. They perform better than most terriers in obedience work because of their intense desire to please their owners. Although they seem independent, no breed depends more on understanding and affection.

A healthy, normal Aussie is interested, observant and active. Some can climb like a monkey, jump like a horse and dig like a fox. They are not nasty or aggressive, although they possess the general terrier trait of keen interest in people, other dogs and other animals. Aussies flourish when living close to their families.

Australian Terriers are excellent watch dogs. Normally they can hold their own when attacked or faced with a need to protect loved ones, especially against strangers that appear aggressive. Aussies are also known to ward off snakes and guard against them.

Aussies are good companions both for the elderly and for children.

If an Aussie becomes whiney or snappy, the cause is probably improper treatment or a physical disorder. The breed responds well to any of the acknowledged training methods. Every Aussie has a distinct personality and for this reason requires individual treatment.

Australian Terriers are usually good travelers; they seldom need tranquilizers.

Dogs with blue-tan coats are much darker at birth than at maturity. Normally if a puppy has definite bright or deep tan markings at the edge of its ears, it will have a good color as an adult. Tan markings on newborn dogs should conform to markings characteristic of the breed. Australian Terriers with sandy red coats sometimes have deeply toned coats at birth. The presence of scattered black hairs (smut) in a sandy-red coat is undesirable. Frequently the black hairs disappear with age. If they remain, they can be hand plucked. Undesirable small white patches on puppies usually lessen or disappear as the animal grows. Aussies have a hairless, V-shaped area on the top of the nose.

THE SHOW RING

Faults include all black body coat in the adult dog, white markings on chest or feet, light colored or protruding eyes, **cryptorchidism**, **monorchidism**. Undesirable are overly shy, nasty or snappy temperaments and tails that are not docked.

Serious, but not disqualifying faults are prominent or light eyes, incorrect set or shape of ears, over- or undershot bites, crooked front legs (sometimes known as cabriole legs), and rear legs set too close. Tail sets are often too low. The level, straight backline and long neck and good lay-back of shoulder are desired. The coat should be about 2 1/2 inches long. A top-knot is essential to meet AKC Standards for the breed.[1]

Other faults include white or light colored toenails and white markings on the chest or legs. The coat should not be too soft or too wavy.[2]

BREEDING AND WHELPING

Aussie bitches should be bred about the tenth to the sixteenth day of estrus. Aussies generally whelp easily, often a couple days before they are due, suggesting a gestation of 59 to 61 days. Six- and 7-year-old bitches deliver healthy litters, although sometimes their litters are fewer in number than those of younger bitches. Dogs are still excellent studs at 10 to 12 years old. A dog should not serve at stud before it is a year old. Litters normally are four to five puppies, but there can be as few as one puppy or as many as nine. Puppies range in weight from 5 to 7 ounces. Congenital abnormalities or birth defects are rarely seen.

GROWTH

Front dewclaws should be removed as should rear dewclaws if present. Tails should be docked when puppies are 3 to 10 days old, leaving a generous 2/5 of the tail. Ten days is usually too long to wait, but if the litter is large and the pups seem frail, the delay may seem advisable. Australian Terriers with blue-tan coats have a V-shaped line of tan under their tails.

The proper distance for docking is estimated by holding a dime upright and cutting at a point about the width of the dime beyond the tan line. An estimate of a generous 2/5 of the tail must serve as a guide for docking the tails of sandy-red Australian Terriers. A male with heavy bones should have more tail left after docking than a small, light-boned female puppy.

Ears should not be cropped. They should stand erect by the time the pup reaches 3 to 4 months of age. Massaging and constant cleaning may help a drooping ear to stand. If ears are not erect within 4 months, they may be taped. Poor health, teething, worms, ear mites, coughs and psychological problems can cause drooping ears.

After the pups are 6 months old, they may gain slightly and become more compact. Although Australian Terriers mature at 12 to 15 months, some individuals do not reach their best stature as show dogs until they are 3 years old. Adults average 12 to 14 pounds in weight and 10 inches in height. Puppies should be watched carefully during the growth period. Failure of an individual to develop and behave like other members of a litter can indicate a health problem. Sometimes a bully in the litter can deprive other pups of food and adversely affect the personalities of the other pups. The problem can be overcome by separating the puppies at feeding time and disciplining overly aggressive individuals. Such discipline can begin when the pups are 5 weeks old.

Australian Terriers respond to early training. A prospective show specimen should be taught to stand on table and become accustomed to a fine leash as soon as possible. Affectionate handling by human beings improves the physical and emotional growth of puppies, but they should not be separated from the dam too soon. Separation should be achieved gradually until the dam shows no interest in the puppies or snaps at them. Occasionally this lack of maternal interest begins when the pups are less than 5 weeks old. In those cases, the dam should be carefully disciplined. Some Australian Terrier puppies may begin self-weaning by eating from the dam's dish when they are 2 to 3 weeks old.

DENTITION

An Australian Terrier's bite should be even to scissors; the latter is more common. Aussies seldom lack any teeth, and incorrect bites occur only occasionally.

Puppy teeth should be removed if they do not fall out normally by the time the second teeth appear. With proper cleaning, diet and care, the teeth usually last well into old age.

RECOGNIZED PROBLEMS

Australian Terriers are not subject to serious disturbances of growth and development. The breed is considered hardy. **Hip dysplasia** is not common to the breed. **Legg-Perthes disease** occurs rarely, but **diabetes mellitus** does occur in the breed.[3] Aussies have a keen sense of sight and hearing. No specific form of eye trouble is common to the breed.

Australian Terriers should not be tied outside. Strong sun fades their coats and harms their temperaments. Although the breed originated in Australia, excessive heat is as hard on them as on any other breed, as is excessive cold, dampness or wind.

Hot spots, **allergies** and similar conditions appear in some strains more often than in others. This breed is reported to be predisposed to **malassezia dermatitis**.[4] They exhibit no unusual reaction to any drug. Because of their conformation, Australian Terriers are not subject to **back or heart problems**, **asthma** or **eye or ear conditions**. Sometimes a narrow, dark mark appears inside an Aussie's ear tip. This normally disappears slowly with application of a topical steroid antibiotic. **Cryptorchidism** is reported in the breed.[5]

A V-shaped leathering on the top of the nose is characteristic of the breed. It is not **alopecia**, as persons unfamiliar with Aussies have believed.

BEHAVIOR

The Aussie is a lively, spirited and affectionate companion. He is playful, loyal and needs little grooming.

OLD AGE

Old Aussies bear their years gracefully, although their keen sight and hearing often diminish. Older Aussies generally sleep more. Some get too fat, but frequently males become too thin; thus, special attention should be given to diet. Spayed bitches do not gain more weight than intact bitches. Care should be taken to see that their skin does not become too dry. Frequent brushing and bathing are recommended.

The life span of Australian Terriers ranges from 14 to 17 years.

References
1. American Kennel Club, *The Complete Dog Book*, 18th ed. (Howell Book House: New York).
2. Royal Agricultural Society, *Australian Breed Standards*.
3. Kirk, R.W. *Current Veterinary Therapy VI* (W.B. Saunders: Philadelphia, 1977).
4. Griffen, C., Kwochka, K., McDonald, J. *Current Veterinary Dermatology, the Art and Science of Therapy*. Mosby Yearbook, St. Louis, Mo. 1993: 44
5. Copen, C.C., et al, *Veterinary Internal Medicine* (W. B. Saunders, Philadelphia, Pa.).

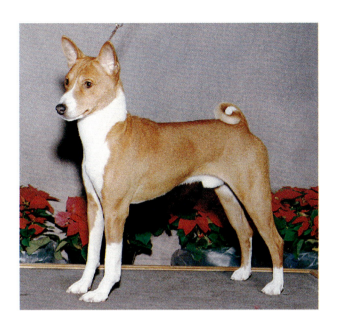

BASENJI

ORIGIN AND HISTORY
The Basenji, popularly known as the barkless dog, was brought to America from Africa in 1937.

DESCRIPTION
Basenjis have a keen scenting ability. They are fastidious dogs of dainty habits and clean themselves all over, like cats. No dog is more ideally suited to the demands of an immaculate housekeeper.

Gentle and tireless at play, the breed is alert, independent and aloof. Basenjis like to make the first overtures of friendship. They should not be assumed friendly unless such overtures have been displayed.

THE SHOW RING
Ideal height for dogs is 17 inches and for bitches it is 16 inches. The weight for dogs is 24 pounds and for bitches 22 pounds. They should be lightly built within this height-to-weight ratio.

Wrinkles appear on the forehead when the ears are erect, and are fine and profuse. Side wrinkles are desirable but should never be exaggerated into dewlap.

Colors are chestnut red, pure black, tricolor or brindle, all with white feet, chest and tail tip. White legs, blaze or collar are optional. There are no disqualifications in the breed.

BREEDING AND WHELPING

Basenji bitches come into estrus once a year, in the fall, in the northern hemisphere. The estrus period may last four weeks. Breeders report bitches may accept as early as five days and as late as fifteen. Bitches whelp easily and are excellent mothers. Litter size averages five or six, with puppies weighing from 6 to 8 ounces.

Umbilical hernias are common. Some breeders claim that if the hernia is reduced by gently pushing it back into the abdomen during puppyhood, the opening usually closes, leaving only a fatty deposit.

Puppies that are dark brown at birth will be red as adults. In tricolored puppies (black, tan and white), the tan is discernible when the puppies are dry. The pink noses fill in with black and the raspberry colored footpads darken.

Removal of both front and back dewclaws is recommended.

Level or undershot bites in puppies tend to become more pronounced.

RECOGNIZED PROBLEMS

Persistent pupillary membrane is a common problem.[1,2] The degree of severity varies. It may be extensive enough to obscure vision, or discernible only with a slit lamp. The condition is hereditary, but the mode of inheritance is uncertain.

Erythrocyte pyruvate kinase deficiency (PK), a genetically transmitted deficiency of the red cells that causes a hemolytic anemia, is a problem among Basenjis.[3,4,5,6] PK deficiency causes symptoms only in individuals with two genes for the defect. Thus, carriers with one defective gene and one normal gene show no clinical signs and may go unidentified. Tests are available to diagnose affected and carrier dogs.

Dogs with the pyruvate kinase deficiency sleep a great deal and tire easily. Seriously affected dogs may faint. **Orange stool, pale mucous membranes, tachycardia** and **splenomegaly** are the most common clinical findings. Hematologic examination reveals moderate to severe **anemia** with a regenerative response. Packed cell volume ranges from 15 to 30 percent, and hemoglobin concentration from 5 to 9 gm/100 milliliters. Mean corpuscular hemoglobin concentration increases because of incomplete hemoglobin synthesis in the immature cell. Extensive polychromasia, anisocytosis, large numbers of metarubricytes and markedly elevated reticulocyte counts reflect the intense erythropoietic response of the bone marrow.

64

A fundamental determination in evaluating the pathogenesis of regenerative anemia is whether the animal is experiencing hemorrhage or hemolysis. Hyperbilirubinemia is rare in affected dogs, but orange stools indicate increased excretion of bile.

Markedly elevated reticulocyte counts are more likely to indicate hemolysis than hemorrhage. If parasitic infections, toxic results, or antibody-induced hemolysis can be eliminated from the differential diagnosis, congenital hemolytic anemia must be considered. This diagnosis can be confirmed only by erythrocyte pyruvate kinase analysis. Hematologically, normal carriers of this defect can also be detected by pyruvate kinase assay.

No effective treatment exists for congenital hemolytic anemia in Basenjis. Owners should be informed that the average life span of affected dogs is 3 to 4 years. Supportive care includes a nutritious diet. Blood transfusions are the only specific therapy, but their beneficial effects are limited because of isoimmunization. Iron therapy, as in most hemolytic anemias, is unnecessary and may be contraindicated because of the development of hemosiderosis.

The incidence of **colibacillosis (coliform enteritis)** among Basenjis is reported to be abnormally high.[7] There is a heritable disease in Basenjis called **immunoproliferative enteropathy**. It may have a gradual or a sudden onset and may exhibit signs of occasional inappetence or intermittent vomiting.

Diarrhea may appear in puppyhood or may wait until the dog is a little older. Studies have shown that diet — particularly the protein source — may influence the onset and progression of this inherited diarrheal disease.[8]

Intestinal digestive and absorptive function and the gross and histological appearance of the gastrointestinal tract were investigated in Basenji dogs with chronic diarrhea (8), asymptomatic Basenji dogs (9) and healthy control dogs (9). Hypertrophy of the gastric rugae, lymphocytic gastritis and gastric mucosal atrophy occurred in asymptomatic and affected Basenji dogs. All affected dogs had moderate or severe intestinal lesions characterized by villous clubbing and fusion, increased tortuosity of intestinal crypts and diffuse infiltration of mononuclear inflammatory cells.

Intestinal lesions in asymptomatic Basenji dogs invariably were less severe than those in affected dogs, but the small intestinal lamina propria of asymptomatic Basenji dogs consistently contained greater numbers of mononuclear inflammatory cells than did that of controls. As compared to healthy Beagle controls, intestinal function was abnormal in both affected and asymptomatic Basenji dogs in combined N-benzoyl-L-tyrosyl-p-aminobenzoic acid and d-xylose tests, but malabsorption and maldigestion were most severe in affected Basenji dogs.[9]

Immunological isotypes in serum and intestinal secretions of Basenji dogs with diarrhea, asymptomatic Basenji dogs and healthy control dogs were measured, and their molecular sizes characterized to detect alpha-chain, beta-chain or H-chain fragments. Measurements of immunoglobulin isotypes in serum showed that affected Basenjis have significantly increased serum Ia values as compared to asymptomatic Basenjis and normal control dogs. However, Ia concentrations in intestinal wash fluids were not significantly different for the three groups. Immunoelectrophoresis (IEP) and polyacrylamide gel electrophoresis (PAGE) demonstrated that virtually all Ia was in the dimeric form.

Using IEP and immunoselection, it was possible to detect evidence for the presence of alpha chain or other heavy (H) chain fragments. Hyperimmune serum obtained from rabbits immunized with serum or a globulin fraction of affected Basenjis also failed to detect H-chain fragments.

It is concluded that immunoproliferative enteropathy of Basenjis resembles closely the nonsecretor form of human immunoproliferative small intestine disease.[10]

In 1993 the Basenji Club of America announced the formation of a long-awaited health research endowment fund, called the Founders Health Endowment. Beneficiaries must be tax-exempt and be engaged in research directly related to Basenji health, including such issues as **hemolytic anemia**, **persistent pupillary membrane**, **progressive retinal atrophy**, **Fanconi syndrome**,[11] **immunoproliferative small intestinal disease** and **breeding problems.**

Both inguinal and umbilical **hernias** are a problem in the breed.[12,13] **Uveodermatologic syndrome** has been recognized in the breed. [14]

Intestinal malabsorption in the Basenji has been described. Allergic responses to insecticide dips, grass, detergents and fleas seem to be a common problem.

Renal tubular dysfunction[11,15,16] (Fanconi syndrome) has been reported in the Basenji. History usually includes polydipsia and polyuria, persistent weight loss with normal appetite and progressive deterioration of the coat; the hair is extremely dry and brittle and epilated easily. Laboratory findings include glucosuria, proteinuria and isosthenuria. Blood glucose is within normal range.

Corneal leukoma has been described in the Basenji.

BEHAVIOR

The Basenji is cheerful, affectionate and usually good with children. He is an extremely clean dog with little odor and is called barkless although he can make a characteristic yodeling noise when happy and a screaming sound when unhappy.

OLD AGE

The normal life expectancy of the Basenji is 10 to 13 years.

References

1. Kirk, R.W. and Bistner, S.L. *Handbook of Veterinary Procedures and Emergency Treatment: Hereditary Defects of Dogs*; Table 124, 1975: 661.

2. Barnet, K.C. "Persistent Pupillary Membrane and Associated Defects in the Basenji," *Vet. Rec.* (85); 1962: 242-249.

3. Ewing, G.O. "Familial Anemia in the Basenji Dog," *JAVMA* (154); 1962: 503-507.

4. Searcy, G.P., et al, "Congenital Hemolytic Anemia in the Basenji Dog Due to Erythrocyte Pyruvate Kinase Deficiency," *Canad. J. Comp. Med. V.* (33); 1970: 67-70.

5. Tasker, J.B., et al, "Familial Anemia in the Basenji Dog," *JAVMA* (154); 158-165.

6. *JAVMA;* Vol. 198, No. 10, May 15, 1991.

7. Fox, M.W., et al, "The Epidemiology, Pathogenicity, and Breed Susceptibility of Endemic Coliform Enteritis in the Dog," *J. Lab. Anim. Care* (15); 1965: 194-200.

8. *American Journal of Vet. Res.;* Vol 53, No. 2, February 1992

9. MacLachlan, N.J., Breitschwerdt, E.B., Chambers, J.M., Argensio R.A., and De Buysscher, E.V. "Gastroenteritis of Basenji Dogs," *Veterinary Pathology* (25); 1988: 1, 36-41, 15 ref.

10. De Buysscher, E.V., Breitschwerdt, E.B., and MacLachlan, N.J. "Elevated Serum Ia Associated with Immunoproliferative Enteropathy of Basenji Dogs: Lack of Evidence for Alpha Heavy-Chain Disease of Enhanced Intestinal Ia Secretion."

11. Noonan, C.H.B. and Kay, J.M. "Prevalence and Geographic Distribution of Fanconi Syndrome in Basenjis in the United States," *JAVMA* (197); 1990: 3, 345-349, 10 ref.

12. Fox, M.W. "Inherited Inguinal Hernia and Midline Defects in the Dog," *JAVMA* (143); 1963: 602-604.

13. Fox, M.W. "Developments in Veterinary Science: Inherited Structures and Functional Abnormalities in the Dog," *Canad. Vet. J.* (11); 1970: 5-12.

14. Griffin, C., Kwochka, K., and McDonald, J. *Current Veterinary Dermatology: The Art and Science of Terapy*. (Mosby Yearbook: St. Louis) 1993: 218.

15. Easley, J.R. and Breitschwerdt, E.B. "Glucosuria Associated with Renal Tubular Dysfunction in Three Basenji Dogs," *JAVMA* (10); 1976: 938-943.

16. Picut, C.A. and Lewis, R.M. "Comparative Pathology of Canine Hereditary Nephropathies: An Interpretive Review," *Vet. Res. Comm.* (11); 1987: 6, 561-581, 91 ref.

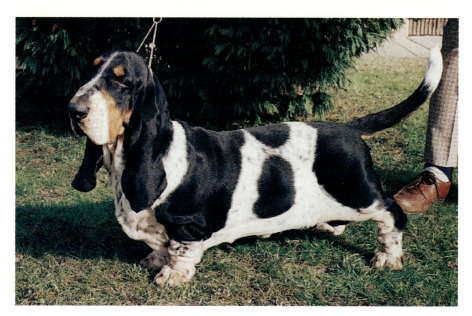

BASSET HOUND

ORIGIN AND HISTORY

Basset Hounds are descended from the old St. Hubert hounds. Used to trail and drive game away, the Basset has had such famous admirers as King Edward VII and Shakespeare. His thorough, unhurried conduct in the fields moves game to gun without startling the game into flight.

DESCRIPTION

The Basset Hound is a very gentle, sweet, and affectionate breed, quite stubborn at times, but very loyal. An extremely shy or aggressive Basset should not be tolerated.

Red and white puppies are pale in markings at birth, the red or lemon growing deeper in color with age. The tricolor puppies are normally black and white with light tan markings which grow lighter, the tan becoming more noticeable with age.

THE SHOW RING

Hounds with **distinctly long coats, knuckled over front legs or hounds over 15 inches at the shoulder are disqualified under the breed Standard.** Under 14 inches is the ideal height. The breed does not have hind dewclaws. The front dewclaws may be removed if desired.

BREEDING AND WHELPING

Given good care, adequate feeding, and proper exercise, Bassets are normal whelpers and good mothers. In the final weeks the food may be increased and divided into two feedings. Bassets should be walked regularly and kept as active as possible.

Bassets can be slow whelpers and generally have large litters. Breeders and veterinarians may have trouble determining when a Basset has completed whelping and radiography may be necessary. Cesarean sections are routinely performed in the breed.

The Basset is a prolific breed having up to 16 in a litter, the average being eight to 10.

GROWTH

Given proper care with good mother's milk, puppies will grow rapidly. At 8 weeks they will weigh between 10 and 15 pounds depending on the amount of bone carried. If the dam has a large litter, the puppies should be given supplementary feedings three times a day and should be weaned early. The diet of a puppy should be balanced. Never overload the diet with calcium and extras which will cause abnormal growth. A Basset puppy should never be given too much exercise because of the "man made front" on the breed.

It is best to check the bites shortly after whelping, making sure the gums meet and that there are no bad mouths in the litter.

RECOGNIZED PROBLEMS

The Basset breed is placed in the chondrodystrophoid group of dogs. The conformation of the breeds in this category leads to many inherent problems. The most common problem in the Basset is the high incidence of **shoulder and foreleg lameness**. There appears to be a high incidence of **osteochondritis dessicans**. **Deformities of the distal radius, ulna and carpal joint** are frequently seen. Radiographic diagnosis is essential to delineate the type of deformity. Most commonly seen are deformities due to **premature closure of the distal epiphysis or growth plate** due to trauma. Subsequent lack of growth of the ulna and continual growth of the radius produce marked bowing of the legs with deviation of the carpal joints. **Osteodystrophies** also occur in the radial carpal joints and may be due to poor mineralization, poor nutrition or excess mineralization. **Patellar luxation** is also seen.

The long, drooping ear predisposes to **otitis externa**. Inversion of the eyelids (**entropion**) and excess drooping of the eyelids (**ectropion**)[1,2] are common. Basset hounds are troubled with both primary and secondary **glaucoma**.[3,4] A study has concluded that there are eight breeds at a higher risk of developing glaucoma than mixed-breed dogs. Bassets are one of these breeds.[5] Symptoms are increased intraocular pressure associated with lens luxation. **Mesodesmol dysgenesis** leading to glaucoma has been reported.

Torsion of the lung has also been reported in the breed. **Gastric dilatation with**

torsion of the stomach and/or torsion of the spleen, and intussusception of the small intestine (ileum) into the colon or cecum occurs.

Achondroplasia is common, as it is in all chondrodystrophoid dogs.[2] Inter-vertebral disc disease is seen due to their short legs and long bodies. Basset hounds appear to have a higher incidence of brucellosis than most other breeds. Interdigital inclusion cysts, abscesses and fungus infections between the digits are relatively frequent due to the Basset's large paws. Clearly defined inherited defects are achondroplasia of the limbs (Stockard, 1941), and cervical vertebral deformities, producing wobbler syndrome (Palmer & Wallace, 1967, Wright et al 1973).

Many veterinarians feel the Basset has a much higher incidence of foreign object obstruction than the average breed. Also, Bassets suffer a higher incidence of pseudocyesis, pyometra and mammary gland tumors.

Lafora's disease (progressive myoclonus epilepsy) has been described as hereditary in Basset hounds. Clinically, dogs develop a progressive central nervous system disease culminating in epileptic seizures. Histologically, Lafora bodies are found in neurones in the middle and deeper cerebral cortex and midbrain, in Purkinje cells and their processes and in glial cells of the molecular layer of the cerebellum. Many are also observed free in the neutrophile.[6,7]

Immunodeficiency has been reported and studied in the Basset Hound. Five of 12 male Basset Hound puppies, born in two litters to the same affected parents, were studied. The disease was characterized by retarded growth, superficial pyoderma and susceptibility to bacterial and viral infections. All affected puppies died or were euthanized by 5 months of age with signs of distemper, infectious hepatitis or bacterial pneumonia. Circulating B lymphocyte counts and serum IgM were normal; IgA and IgG were low or absent, indicating a defect in differentiation of IgG and IgA B cells into immunoglobulin-secreting plasma cells. This was supported by the lack of induction of IgG or IgA plaque-forming cells and by the lack of lymphocytes. Circulating T-cell counts were normal to low but response to mitogens was severely depressed. PM signs included thymic dysplasia and hyperplasia of lymphoid tissue. Pedigree and breeding experiments suggested an x-linked mode of inheritance.[8]

Inguinal hernias are considered a high risk to the breed.[9]

Bassets are subject to a platelet disorder, an inherited condition transmitted as a dominant or dominant with incomplete expression trait.[10,11] Signs are moderately severe bleeding and prolonged bleeding time. There is also abnormal platelet aggregation and adhesiveness.

Bassets have been identified as one of a group of breeds having a higher risk for canine lymphoma.[12,13,14]

70

Bassets are one of the breeds that have reported **urinary calculi**.[15] The incidence of **urolithiasis** in dogs is about 0.5-1%.

BEHAVIOR

The Basset is mild, friendly toward children, very affectionate, stubborn and difficult to housebreak if not trained at an early age.

OLD AGE

Given good care, the Basset can run in the field at 12 years of age and be active as a stud dog. It enjoys its food in old age and, if allowed, becomes fat and lazy. The Basset is an easy keeper and a steady hound in the field and usually lives 8 to 12 years.

References
1. Magrane, W.G. *Canine Ophthalmology*. 3rd ed. (Lea & Febiger, Phil., Pa.,1977) 305.
2. Kirk, R.W. and Bistner, S.J. *Handbook of Veterinary Procedures and Emergency Treatment: Hereditary Defects in Dogs*. Table 124, 1975: 661.
3. Barnett, K.C. "Primary Glaucoma in Dogs," *JAVMA;* 1962: 145:1081-1091.
4. Martin, C.L. and Wyman, M. "Glaucoma in The Basset Hound," *JAVMA;* 1968: 1320-1327
5. Slater, M.R. and Erb, H.N. "Effects of Risk Factors and Prophylactic Treatment on Primary Glaucoma in the Dog," *JAVMA;* 1986: 188: 9, 1028-1030; 7 ref.
6. Jian, Z., Alley, M.R., Cayzer, J., and Swinney, G.R. "Lafora's Disease in an Epileptic Basset Hound," *New Zealand Vet. Journal;* 1990: 38: 2, 75-79; 14 ref.
7. Kaiser, E., Krauser, K., and Schwartz-Porsche, D. "Lafora's Disease (Progressive Myoclonus Epilepsy) in the Basset Hound: Early Diagnosis by Muscle Biopsy," *Tierarztliche-Praxis;* 1991: 19: 3, 290-295; 26 ref.
8. Jezyk, P.F., Felsburg, P.J., Haskins, M.E., and Patterson, D.F. "X-Linked Severe Combined Immunodeficiency in the Dog," *Clinical Immunology and Immunopathology;* 1989: 52: 2, 173-189; 43 ref.
9. Fox, M.W. "Inherited Inguinal Hernia and Midline Defects," *JAVMA;* 143: 602-604.
10. Dodds, W.J. "Inherited Hemorrhagic Disorders," *JAAHA;* 1975: 11; 366-373.
11. Erickson, F., et al, *Congenital Defects in Dogs: A Special Reference for Practitioners.* Ralston Purina (reprint from *Canine Prac.*), Veterinary Practice Publ.; 1978.
12. Madewell, Bruce R., VMD, MS., "Canine Lymphoma," *Veterinarian Clinics of North America Small Animal Practice*; July, 1985: Vol. 15, #4.
13. McCaw, Dudley, DVM., "Canine Lymphosarcoma," AAHA's 56th Annual Meeting Proceedings, 1989.
14. Rosenthal, Robert C., DVM, MS, PhD., "The Treatment of Multicentric Canine Lymphoma," *Vet Clinics of N. Amer: Sm. Anim. Prac.*; July, 1990: Vol.20, #4.
15. Hesse, A. and Bruhl, M. "Urolithiasis in Dogs, Epidemiological Data and Analysis of Urinary Calculi," *Kleintierpraxis*; 1990: 35:10, 505-512; 18 ref.

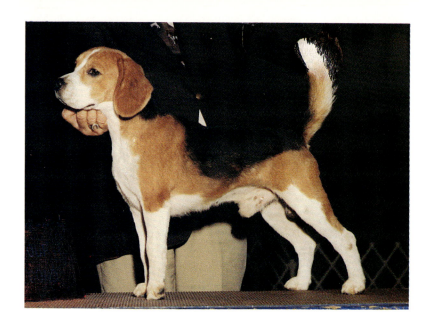

BEAGLE

ORIGIN AND HISTORY

The exact origin of today's Beagle is not known, but its probable ancestors were the hounds that hunted by scent in ancient Rome and also in early England. The distinction was made early between the large hounds (probably our Bloodhounds) called "Buck Hounds" and the small hounds called "Beagles," which hunted hare.

The modern Beagle dates back to the middle of the 19th century, to the pack of Parson Honeywell of England. The Beagle was brought to the United States seriously in the 1880s and 1890s and the National Beagle Club was formed in 1888. The AKC now sanctions many general and specialty shows for the Beagle because of their great popularity.[1]

DESCRIPTION

The Beagle is relatively small in stature but large in heart and desire. There are two sizes of Beagles: under 13 inches in height at the shoulder, and over 13 inches but under 15 inches in height at the shoulder. These two sizes are considered two separate varieties by the American Kennel Club.[1] Few breeders attempt to breed either variety exclusively so that eventually they would breed true to size. Most breeders interbreed the two varieties.

There is a question whether a true breed size should be attempted since, when such an attempt is made, the substance and quality of the 13-inch variety is lost.

THE SHOW RING

The Beagle gives the appearance of a miniature Foxhound, and the faults for both are the same. Any true hound color is acceptable for Beagles.

Any Beagle measuring over 15 inches shall be disqualified.

BREEDING AND WHELPING

Whelping in Beagles sometimes presents problems. The 15-inch variety is normally a free whelper and, if left alone, will deliver the litter with no problems. Once the first puppy has arrived the others present few problems and follow with regularity.

Since the two varieties are often interbred, the small 13-inch bitch usually carries some traits of the larger variety and also some large puppies. She often has trouble whelping and requires a cesarean delivery in many cases.

Beagles are normally black and white at birth. The tan and brown come in at approximately 3 weeks. Lemon and whites or golden and whites are normally all white at birth. Color, however, is irrelevant, since there is not a color standard for the breed. The choice is simply a matter of personal preference.

Dewclaws may be removed three to five days after birth. Some puppies have dewclaws on the front legs only and others have them on all four legs. All should be removed.

DENTITION

Beagles often have poor occlusion but the breed rarely fails to have full dentition. The Standard calls for a scissor bite. If there is evidence of a bad bite, the dog should not be used for breeding.

RECOGNIZED PROBLEMS

Abnormalities at birth normally consist of **broken and short tails, missing toes, short toes, clefts of the lip and palate,**[2,3] **umbilical hernias and hypospadia.**[4]

Hip dysplasia, which is common in larger breeds, is remarkably unknown in Beagles. Eye problems sometimes seen in Beagles include **primary glaucoma,**[5] **prolapse of the third eyelid gland,**[9] **unilateral cataract, cataract with microphthalmia**[6,7,8] **ectasia syndrome,**[9] **progressive retinal atrophy**[10] **and hereditary tapetal degeneration.**[11] Inherited tapetal degeneration is associated with a lightly pigmented eye.[10] The development of pigmentation was followed morphologically from seven days after birth to 9 years of age. The melanin deposition was usually patchy and irregular. With time, many of these granules appeared to condense into residual bodies. The retinal pigmented epithelium in peripheral and inferior posterior regions of affected animals never contained normal-appearing melanin granules at any state of postnatal development. It is proposed that a defect in synthesis of the matrix component of two melanosomes could result in absent or abnormal deposition of melanin and initiate a process of autophagy of these organelles.[10] **Primary glaucoma,** associated with **lens luxation,** is known to be a hereditary condition transmitted as a recessive trait. In a study comparing purebred dogs with mixed-breed dogs there were eight breeds at higher risk of developing glaucoma, one of which was the Beagle.[12] A unilateral cataract is most likely to develop in the posterior portion of the left lens. Ectasia syndrome is evident in increased tortuosity of the retinal vessels and may be associated with retinal detachment.

Beagles are also reported victims of several blood disorders. A recessively transmitted **Factor VII deficiency** is reported by several studies, but there are unfortunately no clinical signs of the condition.[13,14] **Hemophilia A (Factor VIII deficiency)** is a sex-linked recessive trait found in the breed.[15] This classic hemophilia is characterized by prolonged breeding, hemorrhaging, prolonged PPT and reduced Factor VIII.[16]

Beagles are particularly subject to **intervertebral disc disease.**[17,18,19,20] The breed conformation is a probable cause of this crippling condition. **Hypochondrodysplasia** characterized by limb shortening and a normal skull occurs in Beagles. Major problems associated with these changes include elbow dysplasia and intervertebral disc disease.[21]

Unilateral kidney aplasia[22] and **renal hypoplasia** are problems that have been reported in the breed. **Mononephrosis**[23] is a cystic degeneration of one kidney. **Agenesis** is reviewed in a Cornell study of hereditary nephropathies.[24]

Amyloidosis, a chronic fatal renal disease, may be heritable.[25]

Lymphocytic thyroiditis[26,27] is a nonprogressive disease with clinical signs of glandular enlargement and is sometimes seen in Beagles. The mode of inheritance has not been determined.

Epilepsy is also a problem in the Beagle; the first signs of seizures usually do not begin until after one year of age, but an EEG may detect the condition at an earlier age.[28,29]

Multiple epiphyseal dysplasia[30,31] in Beagle puppies is a recessively passed condition in which the hind leg joints sag, causing a noticeable swaying gait of the hindquarters. The cause is a "stippling" from defective ossification.

Beagles are among the breeds reported with **congenital deafness.**[32]

The Beagle has an increased risk of developing **generalized demodectic mange.**[33]

Other problems thought to be hereditary in Beagles include **atopic dermatitis, panosteitis, otocephalic syndrome, pulmonic stenosis, hypercholesterolemia, pyruvate kinase deficiency, PRA** and **cerebellar cortical degeneration.**[34]

Hereditary XX sex reversal has been described in the Beagle.[35]

BEHAVIOR

Beagles are not fighters and two to three may be kept in the same pen. Beagles have been known to "bark at the moon." However, Beagles, as all other breeds, will do whatever they are permitted to do. Bad habits result from improper obedience training or neglect by the owner.

The Beagle is a very nice companion dog. He is clean, cheerful and affectionate. He may roam away from home on a hunting expedition, so he should always wear proper identification.

OLD AGE

The Beagle's life expectancy is somewhere between 12 and 15 years. Beagles, of course, become less active as they get older, but they are always ready and willing to give a tail wag to show their happiness with companionship.

References

1. American Kennel Club, *The Complete Dog Book*. 18th ed. (Howell Book House, Inc., New York, 1992) 152-156.
2. Kirk, R.W. and Bistner, S.I. *Handbook of Veterinary Procedures and Emergency Treatment: Hereditary Defects of Dogs*; Table 24, 1975: 661.
3. Horowitz, S.L. and Chase, H.B. "A Microform of Cleft Palate in the Dog," *Journal Dent. Res.*; 1970: 49:892.
4. Ettinger, S.J.: Textbook of Veterinary Internal Medicine. W.B. Saunders, Philadelphia, PA. 1989: 1884.
5. Gelatt, K.N. "Familial Glaucoma in the Beagle Dog," *JAAHA;* 1972: 8: 23-28.
6. Heyward, R. "Juvenile Cataracts in the Beagle Dog," *J. Sm. Anim. Prac.*; 1971: 8:171-177.
7. Anderson, A.C. and Schult, F.J. "Inherited (Congenital) Cataract in the Dog," *Am. J.Path.* 1958: 34:965-975.
8. Barnett, K.C. "Types of Cataract in the Dog," *JAAHA;* 1972: 8: 2-9.
9. Priester, W.A. "Congenital Defects in Cattle, Horses, Dogs and Cats," *JAVMA*; 1972: 160:1504-1511.
10. Magrane, W.G. *Canine Ophthalmology* 3rd Ed.(Lea & Febiger, Philadelphia, PA. 305; 1977).
11. Burns, M.S., Tyler, N.K., and Bellhorn, R.W. "Melanosome Abnormalities of Ocular Pigmented Epithelial Cells in Beagle Dogs with Hereditary Tapetal Degeneration," *Current Eye Research*; 1988: 7:2, 115-122, 10 ref.
12. Slater, M.R., Erb, H.N., and Bellhorn, R.W. "Effects of Risk Factors and Prophylactic Treatment on Primary Glaucoma in the Dog," *JAVMA*; 1986: 188:9, 1028-1030; 7 ref.
13. Mustard, J.F., et al, "Canine Factor VII Deficiency," *Brit. J. Haemat.*; 1962: 8:43-47.
14. Spurling, H.W., et al, "Hereditary Factor VII Deficiency in the Beagle," *Brit. J. Haemat.*;

1971: 23:59-67.

15. Brock, W.E. et al: "Canine Hemophilia," *Arch. Patha.*; 76:464-469; 1963.

16. Erickson, F., et al, "Congenital Defects in Dogs: A Special Reference for Practitioners," Ralston Purina Co. (reprint from *Canine Prac.*, Veterinary Practice Publication Co.) 1978.

17. Burns, M. and Fraser, M.N. *Genetics of the Dog;* Oliver and Boyd, London; 1966

18. Goggins, et al, "Canine Intervertebral Disk Disease Characterization by Age, Sex, Breed and Anatomic Site of Involvement," *Am. J.Vet. Res*; 1970: 11:1687-1692.

19. Hanson, H. "A Pathological-Anatomical Study of Disk Degeneration in the Dog," *Orthop. Scand. Suppl.*; 1952: 11:1-117.

20. Hanson, H. "The Body Constitution of Dogs and Its Importance for the Occurrence of Disease," *Nord.Vet. Med; 1964:* 16:977-987.

21. Ettinger, S.J.; *Textbook of Veterinary Internal Medicine.* W.B. Saunders Co., Philadelphia, PA. 1989: 2383.

22. Vymetral, F. "Renal Aplasia in Beagles," *Vet. Rec.*; 1965: 77:1344-1345.

23. Fox, M.W. "Inherited Polystic Mononephrosis in the Dog," *J. Hered.*; 1964: 55:29-30.

24. Picut, C.A. and Lewis, R.M. "Comparative Pathology of Canine Hereditary Nephropathies," *An Interpretive Review*; 1987: 11:6, 561-581; 91 ref.

25. *JAVMA*; August 15, 1992: Vol. #4.

26. Tritz, T.E., et al, "Pathology and Familial Incidence of Thyroiditis in a Closed Beagle Colony," *Exper. and Molec. Path*; 1970: 12:14-30.

27. Mandesky-Thomas, L.E. "Lymphatic Thyroiditis in the Dog," *J. Sm. Anim. Prac.*; 9:539-550.

28. Biefelt, S.W., et al, "Sire and Sex-Related Differences in Rates of Epileptiform Seizures in a Purebred Beagle Dog Colony," *Am. J. Vet. Res;* 1971: 32:2039-2048.

29. Palmer, A.C. "Pathological Changes in the Brain Associated with Fits in Dogs," *Vet. Res.;* 1972: 90:167-172.

30. Rasmussen, P.G. and Redmann, I. "Multiple Epiphyseal Dysplasia with Special Reference to Histological Findings," *ACTA Path. Microbio. Scand.*; 1971: 81:381-389.

31. Rasmussen, P.G. "Multiple Epiphyseal Dysplasia in a Litter of Beagle Puppies," *J. Sm. Anim. Prac.*; 1972, 12:91-96.

32. Strain, George M. "Deafness in Dogs and Cats," *Proc. 10th ACVIM Forum*; May, 1992.

33. Griffin, C., Kwochka, K., McDonald, J.: *Current Veterinary Dermatology, the Art and Science of Therapy.* Mosby Yearbook, St. Louis, MO. 1993: p 74.

34. Yasuba, M., Okimoto, K., Lida, M., and Itakura, C. "Cerebellar Cortical Degenerations in Beagle Dogs," *Vet. Path.*; 1988: 25:4, 315-317; 10 ref.

35. Bell, Jerold S. DVM: "Sex Related Genetic Disorders: Did Mama Cause Them?" *American Kennel Club Gazette*, Feb. 1994; 76.

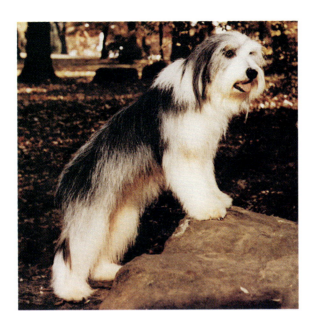

BEARDED COLLIE

ORIGIN AND HISTORY

The Bearded Collie originated in Scotland and Northern England, where it has been found in recognizable form since the early 1900s. It is believed to be descended from three Lowland Polish Sheepdogs traded to Scottish shepherds and has been traced to the Kommondor of the Magyars. The breed has been called the Highland Sheepdog, Highland Collie and Hairy Moued Collie. There were originally two varieties: the Lowland type, which was slate-colored with a harsh straight, long coat and measured around 25 inches in height; and the Highland type, a brown dog of much smaller stature with a shorter, softer, curlier coat. These have been interbred to form the present breed. All colors are now similar in characteristics, with size and straighter coats being standard.

The Bearded Collie is an ancestor to both the modern Old English Sheepdog and Border Collie breeds. It gained full recognition with the AKC in 1976. The Bearded Collie was nearly lost because it was strictly a worker and was kept reasonably pure in lineage by shepherds. As the sheep ranchers became fewer, so did the Bearded Collie. Mrs. Willison, an English breeder, acquired a brown Bearded Collie bitch and was instrumental in saving the breed from extinction. In 1959 she gained recognition for the Bearded Collie as a show breed in England. It has since spread throughout the world, with all registered stock tracing to a few original working dogs, most having at least one cross to Mrs. Willison's bitch, Jeannie of Boathkennar.

DESCRIPTION

The Bearded Collie is an active dog with a good herding instinct. It is highly intelligent, adaptable, responsive and trainable, yet it can be independent in nature. It makes a good family dog and is friendly. It needs an owner who exerts enough dominance to control its exuberance. With proper upbringing, the Bearded Collie is a gentleman and delightful companion; without it, the dog can become strong-willed.

The eyes are large and will tone with coat color. The coat is black, blue, brown or fawn at birth, but grays anywhere from silver to black or from sandy fawn to chocolate with maturity. The coat often lightens to pale silver or cream color at a year of age before darkening to its adult shade. It will continue to change color slightly with each new coat. Pigmentation of the nose, eye rims, lips, etc. follows the birth color of the coat. Pigmentation may be lacking at birth, but should fill in within a few weeks. The puppy coat is either wooly and made up of undercoat or sparse and wiry. This coat sheds at 1 year and the intermediate coat is much shorter on the forequarters than on the hindquarters. The adult coat is moderately long, harsh and straight (a slight wave is permissible) and is predominantly outer coat, with the soft, insulating undercoat evident near the skin. The adult coat is achieved by the third year.

Dewclaws appear only on the front legs and removal is recommended, especially on pets, as the long hair on the legs of an adult covers the nail and often results in neglect of the nail.

THE SHOW RING

The Bearded Collie is a medium-sized, long bodied, moderately built, shaggy dog with a long tail and a moderately long, harsh coat. It has a long, flat rib cage which accounts for its body length. Its croup is fairly flat, and it has good angulation front and rear, with extremely low-set or short hocks. Its head should be broad, flat and rectangular in shape. Its bearing should denote grace: the dog should be left natural in every respect, never trimmed.

The ideal size for adult Bearded Collies is 21 to 22 inches at the withers for dogs and 20 to 21 inches for bitches. They are found from 18 to 23 inches in height, with bitches usually being considerably smaller than dogs. Heights over or under the ideal are to be penalized. The express objective of this criterion is to insure that the Bearded Collie remains a medium sized dog.

A very long, curly, silky or single coat is faulted, as are snipiness, flat croup or steep croup, trimmed or sculptured coat. There are no disqualifications in the breed.

BREEDING AND WHELPING

Most bitches start their first heat cycle from 6 to 8 months of age and cycle regularly every six months thereafter. A few do not show signs of estrus until past a year of age. Bitches can cycle anywhere from four to eight months between heats. Once a cycle is determined, it is usually consistent for that individual.

Gestation can be from 56 to 63 days, with a significant number of bitches whelping by the 57th day.

Because the Bearded Collie is a slow-maturing breed, bitches should be at least 18 months of age before being bred, with some breeders recommending 2 years. Bearded Collie bitches are good mothers, generally easy to breed, and are efficient, trouble-free whelpers. Puppies, even the early ones, appear healthy and vigorous with no signs of being premature. It is recommended that puppies be kept on carpet or other surfaces with adequate footing as **swimmers** may develop if they are kept on a slick, hard surface such as newspaper. Hair should be clipped around the bitch's nipples so it cannot wrap around and sever the nipple.

Litters range from four to 12 in number, the average being seven puppies. Birth weight varies with litter size but averages about 8 to 10 ounces. There are few birth defects other than an occasional severe overbite, **cleft palate** or color deviation. Puppies with these defects should be euthanized.

The puppies receive early weaning because they are precocious and can run down the dam's health if allowed to nurse longer than necessary. Once the puppies are weaned the dam should return to help with their psychological development.

GROWTH

Puppies should be very outgoing and self-confident, with the temporary display of typical avoidance behavior seen in most breeds at 3 months of age. Some individuals, especially males, are prone to adolescent trauma. If not stressed during this period, puppies will outgrow the symptoms by 18 months. Overactive dogs may be showing signs of neglect and usually settle down if given more attention. If neglected to the point of frustration, Bearded Collies can become mildly destructive.

Growth rate is fast, with puppies reaching most of their adult height by 7 months.

Generous feeding from 2 to 6 months may be beneficial, but over-supplementation may be harmful.

Puppies should be selected first on temperament and health, then on structure and balance; and finally on head and coat markings. For show purposes, individuals are selected with good overall balance, strong pigmentation and outstanding gait and structure.

Testicles are usually descended by 8 weeks of age. Males that remain **cryptorchid** (either unilateral or bilateral) by 5 months will probably remain so permanently and castration is recommended to avoid testicular tumors.

DENTITION

Bites are peculiar in the breed. A scissors bite with full dentition is desirable in an adult and should be evident at 1 week of age. Between 6 weeks and 11 months of age the jaws can grow randomly. Some bites remain perfect, but many develop severe overbites (some as much as 3/4 inches) or other deviations during growth periods. Those which were satisfactory at birth will usually correct by 1 year of age. Pulling the lower canines may enable the dog to lead a normal life as a pet. An undershot jaw is serious and probably will not correct.

RECOGNIZED PROBLEMS

The Bearded Collie has a low incidence of hereditary and congenital defects. For this reason it is important that breeding stock be examined to prevent problems before they become widespread. The following problems have been diagnosed in a small number of Bearded Collies: **hip dysplasia**, **subvalvular aortic stenosis**, **progressive retinal atrophy, persistent pupillary membrane, corneal dystrophy, cataracts, retinal dysplasia, Cushing's Disease** and **Von Willebrands**.

Fading pigmentation is sometimes a problem with this breed. This condition causes a fully pigmented adult dog to develop spots of pink skin around the eyes, lips and eventually the nose. Some lose pigment entirely on these parts. The condition, if not attributed to allergies, is believed to be hereditary, but no mode of inheritance has been determined. Tattooing the area may be beneficial if pigment loss is not too extensive.

Certain bloodlines report dogs with **seizures** resembling the idiopathic (probably hereditary) form of **epilepsy.** Although the numbers of affected individuals is small, research specific to Bearded Collies is being conducted by Dr.Clive Eger, Dept. of Animal Studies, Ontario Veterinary College, University of Guelph, Ontario N1G 2W1, Canada.

Beardies have been listed as one of several breeds with an increased risk of developing **colonic disease.**[1] It has been reported that Bearded Collies are one of four breeds reported at significant risk for **pemphigus foliaceous** (see Akita).

Some puppies are normal in all respects except coat, which can be decidedly smooth with no long guard hairs. Smooths should not be registered and can be detected by 8 weeks of age and positively identified by 3 months of age.

Beardies are usually stoic in outlook and may have a slow heartbeat, as low as 60 when resting.

SPECIAL CARE

Adult Bearded Collies require daily exercise and a good maintenance diet. Avoid feeds with arsenic or hormone additives. Grooming should be done once a week (or more often if warranted by the dog's environment). In dry climates, addition of a coat oil in the grooming spray is beneficial. Dampen the coat before grooming and then linebrush over the entire body with a good bristle or combination pin brush. Hair should be plucked from the ear canal to avoid infection. Teeth, anal glands and toenails require periodic attention. Hair may be plucked at the inside corner of each eye if it obscures the eye or causes irritation.

BEHAVIOR

The Beardie has a pleasing personality and is joyous and affectionate. He is attentive to his work and his coat makes him "weather resistant." He makes an excellent companion dog, but loves to be outside.

OLD AGE

Older dogs are susceptible to **kidney disease**, **skin problems** and **tumors** (including **sebaceous cysts**). Most Bearded Collies age gracefully because they are functionally constructed and slow to mature. Life span averages 15 years with some individuals reproducing at 12 years or older. Some live to 17 or 18 years with good care.

References
1. Houston, DM, "An Integrated Study of Colonic Disease in the Dog," Dissertation-Abstracts-International.B, Sciences and Engineering; 1989: 50:4, 1278-1279.

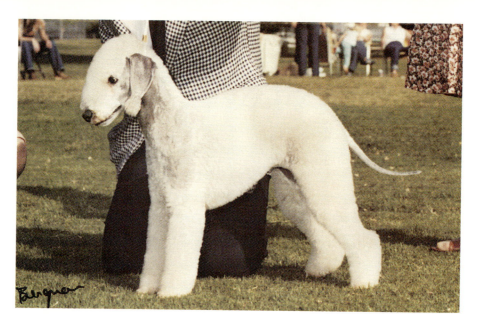

BEDLINGTON TERRIER

ORIGIN AND HISTORY

The common description of the Bedlington Terrier is "it looks like a little lamb." They may look like lambs, but they are independent, stout-hearted dogs with minds of their own. The Bedlington was first known in the 1820s in the town of Bedlington, England. The chief industry there was coal mining, and the Bedlington was used by the miners to kill rats, badgers and other small vermin in the pits.

Because these terriers were quick, fearless and had large teeth, they were quite successful. Since then, the Bedlington has been sought as a different type of pet and companion. They are very affectionate family dogs, but, if trained, can be protective. They are very alert.

DESCRIPTION

The Bedlington has a distinctive coat, thick and linty, not wiry like most terriers. Also, the coat does not lie flat on the body. It should be brushed up to stand away from the body. A carefully trimmed top-knot makes the skull appear high and the head Roman-nosed.

In show trim the coat should not exceed 1 inch on the body and legs. It can be slightly longer on the head.

THE SHOW RING

The preferred height is 16 1/2 inches at the withers for dogs and 15 1/2 inches for bitches. Under 16 inches or over 17 1/2 inches for dogs and under 15 inches or over 16 1/2 inches for bitches are faults. Weight is proportionate to height in the range of 17 to 23 pounds.

82

Colors are blue, sandy, liver, blue and tan, sandy and tan and liver and tan. In bi-colors, the tan markings are found on the legs, chest, under the tail, inside the hindquarters and over each eye. Blues and Blue and Tan have black noses. The others have brown noses. Darker skin pigmentation is encouraged with all coat colors. The top-knot and legs are a lighter color than the rest of the body in adults. The patches of dark hair from an injury are not faults, as they are only temporary.

The head is narrow, deep and rounded with the muzzle longer than the skull. There is no stop. The eyes are almond shaped, small, bright and well sunk. The Blues have dark eyes; Blue and Tans' eyes are less dark with amber lights; Sandies and Sandy and Tans have light hazel eyes. Liver and Liver and Tans have slightly darker hazel eyes. The eye rims are black in Blues and Blue and Tans and brown in all other solid and bi-colors. The ears are not trimmed and are triangular in shape with round tips, set low with the tips reaching the corner of the mouth. Thin and velvety in texture, they form a tassel at the tip.

The neck is long and tapering with no throatiness. Shoulders are flat and sloping. The forelegs are straight, being wider at the chest than at the feet. The hindlegs are well angulated and the hocks are strong, turning neither in nor out. The feet are long hare feet with thick, smooth pads. Dewclaws should be removed. The body is muscular. The chest, deep and flat ribbed, should reach to the elbows. The back has a natural arch over the loins and a definite tuck up of the underline. The body is slightly greater in length than height. The tail is not docked. It is set low, scimitar-shaped, tapering to a point which reaches the hock. The tail should not be carried high over the back nor tight to the underbody.

There are no disqualifications for this breed.

BREEDING AND WHELPING

Breeding and whelping of litters in Bedlingtons are similar to other terriers. They do not have any particular problems, although in whelping, the bitch sometimes can injure a whelp's tail in removing it from the sac. This injury can cause a knot to form. Litters average four to six whelps.

DENTITION

The Bedlington should have a level or scissors bite. The lower canines clasp the outer surface of the upper gum just in front of the upper canines. Missing canines are not uncommon. The lips should be close fitting with no flews.

RECOGNIZED PROBLEMS

Three principal hereditary defects have been reported in the Bedlington Terrier.

Retinal dysplasia[1,2] and **renal cortical hypoplasia**[3] have been reported and are accurately described in texts. A chronic progressive **hepatitis**[4] in the breed has been reported. The syndrome occurs in young dogs, but chronic cases have been reported. The dogs are asymptomatic until the appearance of a frequently fatal hepatic failure syndrome, characterized by elevated transanimase values and other common signs of hepatic disease. A markedly elevated copper concentration has been found in the lines of affected dogs, and other causes of hepatic degeneration have been ruled out. The syndrome is considered similar to **Wilson's disease. Coppertoxicosis** is a recessively inherited autosomal liver disease. Research is underway to find a method to identify carrier dogs.[5] Scientists are exploring the efficacy of zinc acetate as treatment.[6]

Other problems reported in the breed are **osteogenesis imperfecta**,[7] **distichiasis**[8] and **lacrimal duct atresia**.

BEHAVIOR

The Bedlington of today is considered affectionate, devoted and intelligent. In the past he was a dog who would snap when irritated. He is a barking watch dog, happy in an apartment.

OLD AGE

Bedlingtons usually live to be 12 to 14 years of age. Though they slow down with age, they carry their dignity to the end. They make endearing pets.

References
1. Rubin, L.F. "Heredity of Retinal Dysplasia in Bedlington Terriers," *JAVMA;* 1968:152:260-262.
2. Wikstrom, B. "Retinal Dysplasia," *Svensk-Veterinartidning*; 1986: 38:15, 129-130; 10 ref.
3. Oksaner, A. and Sittaekow, K. "Familjar Nefropati med Sekundar Hyperparathyroidism hos tre Unghunder," *Nor. Vet. Med.*; 1972: 24:278-280.
4. Hardy, R.M., et al, "Chronic Progressive Hepatitis in Bedlington (Bedlington Liver Disease)" *Current Veterinary Therapy VI*; (R.W. Kirk, Ed., W.B Saunders, Philadelphia, PA.,1977) 995-998.
5. *Journal of Vet. Int. Med.*; January-February 1992; Vol.6, No.1.
6. Veterinary News, *The American Kennel Club Gazette*; March, 1993.
7. Kirk, R.W. and Bistner, S.J. *Handbook of Veterinary Procedures and Emergency Treatment: Hereditary Defects of Dogs.* 1975: Table 124, 661.
8. Magrane, W.G. *Canine Ophthalmology.* 3rd Ed. (Lea & Febiger, Philadelphia, Pa.,1977) 305.

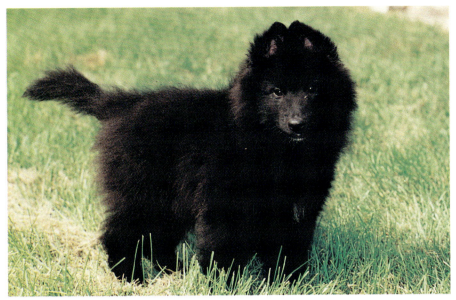

Belgian Sheepdog Puppy

BELGIAN SHEEPDOG
BELGIAN MALINOIS

ORIGIN AND HISTORY

Originally the Belgian Sheepdog, the Belgian Malinois, and the Belgian Tervuren were shown in the United States as one breed. However, since 1959 the three coats of Belgians have been recognized as three distinct breeds. All three (Belgian Sheepdog, Malinois and Tervuren) are still registered in Belgium and France under the name Chien de Berger Belge.[1]

There were originally six varieties (according to the Belgian records) of Belgian Sheepdog; however, the distinctions never were made official and there remains only the one "breed."[1] The Belgian Sheepdog (dog with black hair) was developed in the Groenendad region of Belgium by M. Rose, who first bred a long-haired black to another in 1893.

DESCRIPTION

The Belgian Malinois is a shorter-haired, denser-coated dog, ranging in color from rich fawn to mahogany. A black mask and black ears are required. The underparts of the body, tail and breeches are lighter fawn, but a faded fawn color on the body is a fault.

Belgian Sheepdogs excel as herding animals. They are intelligent, alert guardians of the property and person of their masters.

In appearance, they are well-balanced, square animals with proud carriage of head and neck. They are agile dogs giving the impression of solidity without bulkiness.

THE SHOW RING

In both breeds, the ideal dog should be 24 to 26 inches in height and bitches 22 to 24 inches. There is no standard weight, but bone structure is moderately heavy, so it is important that there is good balance of weight, not too heavy in the chest.[1]

Although front dewclaws may be removed, rear dewclaws should always be removed.

Often confused with the German Shepherd, a side view shows where the Belgians differ. The Belgian stands squarely on all fours without extreme rear angulation.

Breed ring disqualifications for the Belgian Sheepdog are: males under 22 1/2 or over 27 1/2 inches in height and females under 20 1/2 or over 25 1/2 inches; ears hanging; cropped or stumped tail; any color other than black; viciousness.

Disqualifications for the Belgian Malinois are: males under 23 inches or over 27 inches in height and females under 21 inches or over 25 inches; ears hanging; prick ears; and undershot bite in which two or more of the upper incisors lose contact with two or more of the lower incisors; cropped or stumped tail.

BREEDING AND WHELPING

Sheepdog and Malinois bitches may have their first estrus as early as 6 months or as late as 18 months. Most bitches whelp on the 63rd day and are easy whelpers.

Litters range from eight to 11 whelps and normal birth weight is 16 ounces.

Puppies born with solid white chests and white extending down the inside of the front legs and/or with solid white feet should be considered mismarked. The "frost," or whitening which is allowable on the muzzle, can sometimes be seen on the newborn and is not the greying of age.

DENTITION

Full dentition is called for in the Standard. More undershot mouths are seen than overshot.

RECOGNIZED PROBLEMS

Hip dysplasia is seen in the breeds, but it is not a statistically overwhelming problem.

Epilepsy has been reported by some breeders.[2,3] An EEG may detect the condition at an early age. These breeds are known to have had fatal reactions to routine immunizations. Currently, breeders are reporting sensitivity to tranquilizers and to anesthetics such as Acepromazine. During the shedding season, **dermatitis** may be a problem; brisk brushing is necessary. **Vertiligo** has been recognized in Belgian Sheepdogs.[4]

Breeders are reporting a high incidence of **neoplasia**.

86

BEHAVIOR

The Malinois has an instinctive aggressiveness that makes him a good watchdog if trained properly and carefully. The Belgian Sheepdog breeders are working to eliminate an innate shyness and timidity in a breed that is a good watch dog and good with children within the family, to which he is devoted.

OLD AGE

Belgian Sheepdogs and Malinois live an active life until about 12 years and some live several years longer.

References
1. American Kennel Club, *The Complete Dog Book*. 18th ed. (Howell Book House, New York, 1992) 67-69.
2. Van derVelden, N.A. "Fits in Tervuren Shepherd Dogs: A Presumed Hereditary Trait," *J. Sm. Anim. Prac.*; 1968: 9:63-70.
3. Kirk, R.W., Ed., *Current Veterinary Therapy VI.* (Lea & Febiger, Philadelphia, Pa. 1971).
4. Griffin, C., Kwochka, K., McDonald, J. *Current Veterinary Dermatology: the Art and Science of Therapy*. Mosby Yearbook, St. Louis, MO. 1993: 231.

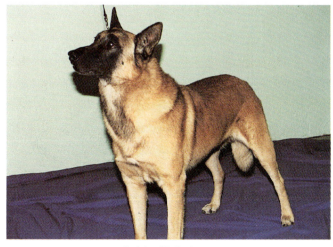

Belgian Malinois

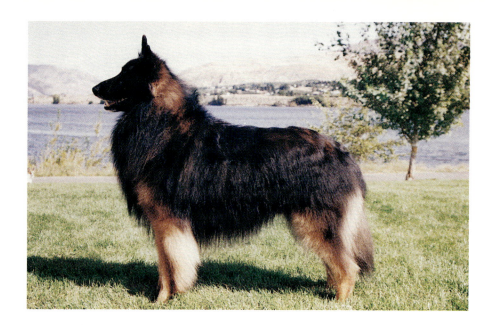

BELGIAN TERVUREN

ORIGIN AND HISTORY

The American Kennel Club recognized the Belgian Tervuren as a breed separate from the Belgian Sheepdog in 1959. Before 1959, the three coats of Belgians were shown in the United States as one breed. All three (Belgian Sheepdog, Malinois and Tervuren) are still registered in Belgium and France under the name Chien de Berger Belge.[1]

Originally used as hunting dogs, their intelligence makes them ideally suited for obedience.

DESCRIPTION

The Belgian Tervuren has a coat of long, straight, abundant hair, which is neither too silky nor too wiry in texture. The color is rich fawn to russet mahogany, with the tip of each fawn ear blackened and/or the mask and ears black.

Tervurens need human contact and socialization from birth. They do not thrive well in kennels. Belgian Tervurens are active, graceful and quick. Sensitive, they try to please. They also learn quickly, and retain active herding instincts. These are rugged dogs with general good health and boundless energy. They make excellent watch dogs and family companions. Like all herding dogs, they are suspicious of strangers, but they are not shy. Tervurens have keen noses and many of them receive tracking degrees each year.

THE SHOW RING

Dogs are medium sized; males are 24 to 26 inches in height and weigh 55 to 70 pounds; bitches measure 22 to 24 inches and weigh 45 to 55 pounds. The typical body conformation is square, not bulky or spindly. Bitches have slightly longer bodies than dogs.

Disqualifications in the breed standard are hanging ears, as on a hound; males under 23 inches or over 26.5 inches or females under 21 inches or over 24.5 inches; undershot teeth such that contact with the upper incisors is lost by two or more of the lower incisors; a cropped or stumped tail; solid black, solid liver or any area of white except as specified on the chest, tips of the toes, chin and muzzle.

Faults are lack of shoulder angulation, uneven backline, tail too short (last vertebra not reaching the level of the hock), shallow chest (not reaching to the elbow), neck too short, shyness or unstable temperament and missing teeth.

Dewclaws on the hind legs should be removed.[1]

BREEDING AND WHELPING

Belgian Tervuren bitches usually come into first estrus when they are 10 to 12 months old, but estrus begins later in some individuals. After estrus begins, it occurs regularly. Bitches should usually be bred around the 10th day. Belgian Tervurens that receive adequate care and proper nutrition during gestation have no trouble delivering their litters. The gestation period is usually 60 days. Newborn puppies are very dark, ranging from almost black to dark seal-brown, with black heads, legs, tails and streaks down the back. They have black pigment on their noses, foot pads and eyelids. The puppies lighten in color as they mature.

The puppies' eyes open in 12 to 14 days, but even before their eyes open they are on their feet trying to walk. Dogs and bitches have similar growth rates, usually gaining about 1 pound a week. Their height increases approximately 1 inch a month until they are about 7 months old. Growth slows down to 1/2 inch or less until they are 12 months old. Most Belgian Tervurens have attained their adult height by one year, but some grow a bit until they are 18 months old. They are considered mature at 3 years and have usually attained their adult weight by that time.

DENTITION

Undershot or wry bites are common faults in the breed. These bites are difficult to predict in puppies. The bite and alignment of the teeth can be correct until the pup is about 8 months old and then can become undershot. Sometimes these bites become even again. Alignment of teeth can change even after a dog has reached 2 years. The two lower central incisors on many Tervurens are smaller than the other incisors. Some dogs lack premolars.

RECOGNIZED PROBLEMS

Hypothyroid has been found to occur more commonly in the Belgian Tervuren than was previously realized. Attempts to raise the level of thyroid hormone by medication is thought to prevent **seizure-like attacks** in some dogs.

Vertiligo has been recognized in this breed.[2]

Some breeders have encountered **pancreatic problems** in the breed. A possible cause of this condition is high fat diet.

Belgian Tervuren breeders have been very conscientious about using radiography to check their dogs for **hip dysplasia**. The breed is relatively free of the condition, but it does occur in some individuals.

Epilepsy in Belgian Tervurens has been reported.[3,4] **Clonic-tonic convulsions** in Tervurens in the Netherlands have also been reported. Results of a survey of dog owners indicate that this is a severe problem in the breed. The mode of inheritance is unknown.

Tervurens between 1 and 2 years old are generally poor eaters, especially the males. Thus, conditioning them for showing is difficult. After they are 2 years, Tervurens begin to gain weight and look better for showing.

BEHAVIOR

The "Terv" is prized for his quick intelligence. He is easily trained and a devoted family protector. He demands affection and is possessive of his owner.

OLD AGE

The average life expectancy of the Belgian Tervuren is about 12 years, although some live to 16.

References

1. American Kennel Club, *The Complete Dog Book*. 18th ed. (Howell Book House, New York, N.Y., 1992) 561-565.
2. Griffin, C., Kwochka, K., McDonald, J. *Current Veterinary Dermatology: the Art and Science of Therapy*. Mosby Yearbook, St. Louis, MO. 1993: 231.
3. Van derVelden, "Fits in Tervuren Shepherd Dogs: A Presumed Hereditary Trait," *J. Sm. Anim. Prac.*; 1968: 9:63-70.
4. Graves, T.K., DVM., "Seizures in Dogs," *The American Kennel Club Gazette*; March, 1992.

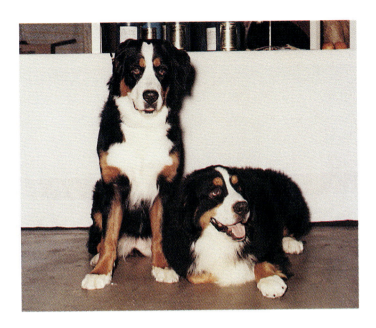

BERNESE MOUNTAIN DOG

ORIGIN AND HISTORY

The Bernese Mountain Dog is a very old breed. Skulls and dog skeletons closely resembling the Bernese Mountain dog dated 800 to 400 B.C. were found in Germany and in ruins near Berne, Switzerland.

The dog was commonly used as a cow herding dog. Later it was also used as a draft dog, pulling milk carts and basket carts for weavers from the rural areas to the city of Berne.

The Bernese Mountain Dog was introduced to the United States in 1936. From this time until the late 1960s it was difficult to find suitable mates for the dogs and bitches. Breeders began to communicate, and the Bernese Mountain Dog Club of America was formed. Serious breeders have since been developing the dogs to the Standard recognized in 1937 by the American Kennel Club.

DESCRIPTION

The Bernese Mountain Dog is a well balanced dog, active and possessing a combination of shrewdness, loyalty and utility. The long, wavy hair is predominantly black with russet-brown on all four legs and white feet. The brown should be located between the black and white on the forelegs, on each side of the white chest marking and with a spot over each eye. The tip of the tail should be pure white and a blaze marks the foreface. A white star-shaped mark on the chest is common. A few white hairs on the back of the neck are acceptable.

Dewclaws on the hind feet should be removed, but may be left on the front feet. Sur-

91

gery should be performed at 3 to 5 days of age. Many puppies have five or six toes on each hind foot or five toes and one dewclaw. Whatever the combination, all extra toes and dewclaws should be removed to leave four toes on each hind foot. Removal of the extra toes requires suturing to close the defect.

THE SHOW RING

Physically the dog has a flat skull with a defined stop. It has a short body, compact and well-ribbed. A broad chest and a good depth of brisket are important, as are muscular loins.

Weighing 80-110 pounds, the dogs are from 25 to 27 1/2 inches at the shoulders. The bitches should be 23 to 26 inches at the shoulders.

Breed disqualifications are blue eye color and any ground color other than black.[1]

BREEDING AND WHELPING

Estrus begins between 9 and 12 months. The estrus cycle is every 6 months.

Males have been reported to be **"lazy breeders,"** and an artificial insemination may be necessary.[1] Gestation is 62 to 63 days.

Quite often a cesarean section is required. Litter size averages eight to 10 puppies and the weight of the pups can vary from 1 to 1 1/2 pounds. No unusual defects are common at birth.

When first whelped, only markings, dewclaws, extra toes and **cleft palates** can be noted. Between 3 weeks and 6 weeks, temperament can be determined. Puppies should be kept in their litter until they are at least 8 weeks old. Larger puppies are often found in smaller bitches. However, the smallest puppies in a litter can become the large adults.

For show quality dogs, the most positive selection of quality, type, temperament and soundness is made from 12 to 18 months. If considering a dog for a pet only, selection can be made any time after the 8-week growth period.

GROWTH

Each breeder has favorite diets, but essentially a well balanced commercial puppy feed should be fed four times a day. When a good, steady growth rate is achieved feedings should be reduced to three times a day. At 1 year of age one feeding per day is acceptable. The large puppies should be kept on the thin side as fat puppies tend to have joint trouble. Joint problems (**osteochondritis dessicans** and **hip dysplasia**) are normally first seen during the 4- to 8-month growth period.

Bad bites in puppies can become good as their jaws develop. Conversely, bites good in puppies can become bad later.

RECOGNIZED PROBLEMS

Hip dysplasia is common, but seems to be radiologic in incidence rather than clinical in appearance. In a study of 4,489 dysplastic dogs, prevalence of dysplasia in Bernese was 25.3%.[2] In a Norwegian study 26% of x-rayed Bernese were dysplastic.[3] Puppies should be x-rayed at 6 months, at 1 year and at 2 years. Progression of the abnormality can be observed quite accurately. **Elbow dysplasia** has been reported by OFA.[4]

Osteochondritis dessicans of the humeral head has a low incidence and is handled the same as with other large breeds.

Umbilical hernias are common but are small and have posed no serious problems.

Blue eyes or a blue eye or even flecks of blue pigment on the iris is considered a disqualification.[5]

Cerebellar degeneration with a genetic basis has been documented in the breed.[6]

Fragmented coronoid process[7] is seen in Bernese Mountain Dogs. In 33 dogs surveyed, 15 animals were affected. No sex predisposition was found.

A **hypomyelinating** condition has been reported in the Bernese Mountain dog, resulting in a tremor of the limbs and head. The tremor becomes more intense with excitement or stress and disappears with sleep. It is first noticeable between 2 and 8 weeks old, and may persist throughout life but decline in severity. Post-mortem examination of affected dogs showed hypomyelination of the spinal cord. This condition may be inherited as an autosomal recessive trait.[8]

Three Bernese Mountain Dog littermates were presented with **fever and cervical pain**. Clinical findings were suggestive of **aseptic suppurative meningitis**. **Necrotizing vasculitis of the pachyleptomeningeal arteries** was found in two dogs examined after euthanasia. The third dog is normal clinically nine months after discontinuing long-term corticosteroid therapy. An immunological etiology is suspected.[9] **Malignant histiocytosis** has been diagnosed in the Bernese Mountain Dog.[10,11]

BEHAVIOR

Bernese Mountain dogs are devoted and easily trained. They have remarkable memories and superior intelligence. They are excellent guardians and companion dogs.

OLD AGE

Older dogs require reduction of caloric intake. The life span of the Bernese Mountain Dog is from 10 to 12 years.

References

1. Walkowicz, Chris "The Mechanics of Breeding," *American Kennel Club Gazette*; May 1990:68.
2. Keller, G.G and Corley, E.A. "Canine Hip Dysplasia: Investigating the Sex Predilection and the Frequency of Unilateral CHD," *Vet-Med.* 1989: 84:12, 1162, 1164-1166; 13 ref.
3. Lingaas, F. and Heim, P. "A Genetic Investigation on the Incidence of Hip Dysplasia in Norwegian Dog Breeds," *Norsk-Veterinaertidsskrift*; 1987: 99:9, 617-623; 22 ref.
4. Bodner, Elizabeth, DVM, "Genetic Status Symbols," *The American Kennel Club Gazette*; September, 1992.
5. American Kennel Club, *The Complete Dog Book.* 18th ed. (Howell Book House, New York) 1992.
6. de la Hunta, et al, "Hereditary Cerebellar Cortical Abiotrophy in the Gordon Setter," *JAVMA; 1980:* 177:538-541.
7. Wind, A.P. "Incidence and Radiographic Appearance of Coronoid Process," *Calif. Vet.* 1982: 6:19-25.
8. Palmer, A.C., Blakemore, W.F., Wallace, M.E., Wilkes, M.K., Heritage, M.E., and Matic, S.E. "Recognition of a 'Trembler', a Hypomyelinating Condition in a Bernese Mountain Dog," *Veterinary Record*; 1987: 120: 26, 609-612; 13 ref.
9. Meric, S.M., Child, G., and Higgins, R.J. "Necrotizing Vasculitis of the Spinal Pachyleptomeningeal Arteries in Three Bernese Mountain Dog Littermates," *AAHA Journal*; 1986: 22: 4, 459-465; 34 ref.
10. Tisdall, C.J., Thornton, R.N., and Veal, B.M. "Malignant Histiocytosis in a Bernese Mountain Dog," *New Zealand Vet. Journal*; 1988: 36: 1, 43; 3 ref.
11. Lord, F.F. and Dubielzig, R.R. "Radiographic Diagnosis: Histiocytosis in a Bernese Mountain Dog," *Veterinary Radiology*; 1991: 32: 1, 17-18; 9 ref.

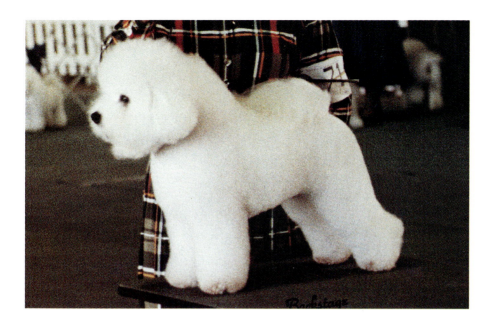

BICHON FRISE

ORIGIN AND HISTORY

The Bichon Frise is a gay, happy dog of good temperament.

It was introduced into the United States from France in 1958, tracing its origin to the Mediterranean area around 1300.

The Bichon is a relatively new breed in the United States. It was admitted to Miscellaneous Class competition of the American Kennel Club in 1971, and to regular competition in 1973.

The French Standard was written in 1923.

DESCRIPTION

Bichons are white with tan or light cream color on the ears. The color shows up at 2 weeks and usually fades by adulthood. The pink nose should fill with black pigment by 3 months.

The coat should be curly with a thick undercoat. The coat is trimmed to reveal the natural outline of the body.

Eyes should be dark brown or black with ringed lids.

THE SHOW RING

Bichon dogs and bitches should be from 9 1/2 to 11 1/2 inches tall at the shoulder.

Faults are cowhocks, "snipy" nose, undershot or overshot bite, corkscrew tail or black hairs in the coat.[1] **There are no disqualifications in this breed.**

BREEDING AND WHELPING

Bichon Frise go into estrus first at 8 to 9 months and normally follow a six-month cycle. Estrus cycles tend to be irregular in some families. This breed is prone to silent heat, and some families have an annular ring of the vagina that has to be cut prior to breeding. They are also sensitive to pain and often need assistance at delivery, either naturally or by cesarean section. The normal litter size is four to five with puppies weighing 3 1/2 to 4 ounces. Puppies are slow in cutting teeth and should have a scissors bite. They do not reach maturity until 1 to 1 1/2 years.

RECOGNIZED PROBLEMS

Patellar luxation is a common structural problem. Breeding animals should be selected to try to eliminate this defect.

Epilepsy is a problem in this breed. Prophylactic dental care is a must for the Bichon, as the animals have a tendency toward **heavy tartar formation which in time leads to pyorrhea, septicemia** and organic disorders. Regular grooming is also a must. Their fine hair tends to mat, causing multiple skin problems when the dirt is held tightly to the skin. The whole skin is sensitive to contact irritants,[2] but does not seem to be particularly subject to allergic inhalant dermatitis. **Pemphigus**, a chronic ulceration disease involving the oral mucosa, can be a problem.

Ciliary dyskenesia has been documented in Bichon Frise. Puppies with this disorder are presented with a moist productive cough, rhinitis, and recurrent pneumonia.[3]

BEHAVIOR

The Bichon is a charming, lively dog with a stubborn streak. It needs frequent grooming and can become hand-shy if groomed painfully.

OLD AGE

There are no particular problems peculiar to this breed in the geriatric individual. They often live to be 16 to 17 years of age.

References
1. *The Complete Dog Book,* The American Kennel Club. 18th Edition, (Howell Book House, New York) 1992.
2. Muller and Kirk, *Small Animal Dermatology.* 2nd Ed. 704.
3. King, L.G. DVM "Respiratory Congenital Disorders" Western Veterinary Conference, Feb. 1994.

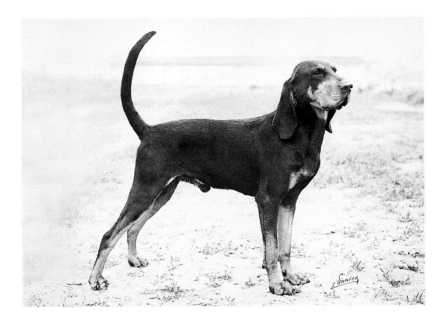

BLACK AND TAN COONHOUND

ORIGIN AND HISTORY

The Black and Tan Coonhound is a descendant of the Talbot Hound found in England during the 11th century. Ancestry includes the Bloodhound and Foxhound, specifically the Virginia Foxhound of the 1700s, often referred to as the "Black and Tan," predecessor of the modern American Foxhound.[1]

The Black and Tan Coonhound was admitted to AKC registry in 1945, although UKC has the largest registry. This working dog, an easily trained specialist in coon and opossum, has a natural instinct for night hunting.

It trails entirely by scent, holding its nose to the trail and signaling with a deep musical voice when the quarry is treed.[2] It works the trail with skill and determination, but without a fast pace. Deer, mountain lion and bear are among its quarry.

DESCRIPTION

This breed is considered superior to similar breeds in tracking quarry in the most efficient manner.[1] Emphasis is placed on stamina to work well in any climate over difficult terrain. It gives the impression of power, agility and alertness with a powerful, rhythmic stride.

THE SHOW RING

The head is cleanly modeled, the medium stop occurring midway between the occiput bone and the nose. The headskin has no folds or excess dewlap. The black nostrils are well open; flews are well developed with typical hound appearance.[3] The skull tends toward an oval

97

outline.[4]

Eyes show an alert, friendly, eager expression. They are hazel to dark brown, almost round and not deeply set. The ears are low-set and well back, hanging in graceful folds for a majestic appearance and extending well beyond the tip of the nose. The teeth fit evenly with a slight scissors bite. The neck is muscular, sloping and of medium length.

This breed has powerful shoulders, a deep chest, well-sprung ribs and a level back sloping from withers to rump. The tail is set below the level of the back line and is carried free, in a right angle to the back when it is in action. It has straight forelegs with elbows well let down, compact cat-like feet with well arched toes and thick, strong pads. Hindquarters are well boned and muscled, long and sinewy from hip to hock with hock to pad short and strong. They have an easy, graceful stride with considerable reach in front and drive behind.

The short, dense coat is coal black with tan above the eyes, sides of the muzzle, chest, legs and breeching with black pencil markings on the toes. Dogs are 25 to 27 inches at the shoulder; bitches are 23 to 25 inches.

A solid patch of white which extends more than one inch in any direction is a breed disqualification.

Undesirable traits include undersize, elbows out at the shoulder, lack of hindquarter angulation, splay feet, sway or roach back, flat-sided ribs, lack of chest depth, yellow or light eyes and shyness or nervousness.[4]

RECOGNIZED PROBLEMS

The breed has a high incidence of **hip dysplasia**.

Ectropion is an eye problem reported by breeders to occur often in Black and Tans.

Hemophilia B (Factor IX deficiency) is a sex-linked recessive hereditary trait found in Black and Tan Coonhounds.[5,6] The condition is characterized by prolonged bleeding, abnormal prothrombin consumption and thromboplastin generation. Homozygotes bleed more than Heterozygotes with Hemophilia A.

Polyneuritis (coonhound paralysis) is primarily an occupational hazard of coonhounds, although it can occur in any dog that encounters raccoons. A raccoon bite or scratch precedes the onset by seven to 14 days. The onset is marked by weakness in the pelvis. In the incipient stage, this syndrome can be confused with muscular-skeletal disorder. Spinal reflexes are reduced or absent. Hypotonicity of limb musculature is manifested by reduced resistance to passive manipulation. Paralysis usually reaches a peak within 10 days. The animal's condition remains stable for a variable period before paralysis abates. Its clinical and pathological features closely resemble the idiopathic polyneuritis of Guillain-Barrè in man.

Treatment is directed at supporting the patient through paralysis and the subsequent dystrophic effects. Affected dogs maintain a normal appetite, but those with cervical paresis require assistance in order to eat and drink. Enemas and bladder catheterization may be necessary to relieve fecal and urine retention.

Animals should be maintained on a straw bed and turned hourly to prevent ulcers. Once afflicted, dogs are prone to redevelop the syndrome on subsequent encounters with raccoons.

BEHAVIOR

This dog is intelligent, alert, obedient and a dedicated worker.

References

1. Jones, A.F. and Hamilton, F., Eds., *World Encyclopedia of Dogs*. (New York, N.Y. 1971) 335.
2. *New Dog Encyclopedia*. (Harrisburg, PA,1970) 519-521.
3. American Kennel Club, *Complete Dog Book*. (Howell Book House. New York, N.Y. 1979) 171-172.
4. *American Kennel Club Breed Standard*; Approved December 11, 1990.
5. Erickson, F., et al, *Congenital Defects in Dogs: A Special Reference for Practitioners*; Ralston Purina Co. (reprint from *Canine Practice*,Vet. Prac. Publ. Co.)
6. Dodds, J.W. and Kaneko, J.J. *Hemostasis and Blood Coagulation.* In *Clinical Biochemistry of Domestic Animals 22*. J.J.Kaneko and C.E.Cornelius, Eds. (Academic Press, New York, N.Y. 1971).

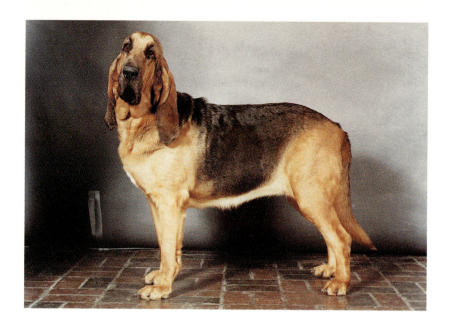

BLOODHOUND

ORIGIN AND HISTORY

Bloodhounds possess dogdom's keenest noses. The breed was nurtured by monks in Europe and developed further in America for their skill in tracking.

DESCRIPTION

The Bloodhound is an excellent house pet. It has an even disposition and thoroughly enjoys a home environment. The adult temperament develops between 12 and 16 months. Removal of dewclaws is recommended at 2 to 3 days of age but is not required.

THE SHOW RING

An average dog weighs 90 pounds and measures 25 to 27 inches in height. The bitch averages 80 pounds and measures 23 to 25 inches.[1] Dogs attain the weight of 110 pounds, bitches 100 pounds. The greater heights and weights are to be preferred provided that character, quality and proportion are also combined.

The ideal bite or closure is not specified in the Bloodhound Standard. Many Bloodhounds develop undershot bites between the ages of 3 and 13 months.

There are no disqualifying faults in Bloodhounds.

BREEDING AND WHELPING

The bitch matures late, often not coming into estrus until 12 months or older. Breeding is not recommended until the female is at least 18 to 20 months old. Bitches in good physical

100

condition have been bred and successfully whelped at 9 years of age. Ovulation may occur from 9 to 12 days after onset of estrus. If a bitch is not bred or fails to conceive, false pregnancy is common. Pregnancy is difficult to diagnose until late in the gestation period. Resorption of fetuses occurs frequently. Litter size varies from one to 14, averaging eight.

Length of time of delivery between puppies tends to be longer for Bloodhound bitches than for those of smaller breeds. A two-hour interval is usual. If the interval approaches three hours, professional help should be sought.

GROWTH

Black and tan adults are nearly all black at birth. Red adults are born red.

Puppies grow rapidly and require a balanced diet. The appetite of a poor eater can be stimulated by substituting cat food for the meat in the ration.

RECOGNIZED PROBLEMS

Bloodhounds are relatively free from congenital abnormalities, although **elbow and hip dysplasia** are seen. **Malformed eyelids** are the most common problem.[2] The lower lid tends to open as a pouch **(ectropion)** and to gather debris. The resultant **conjunctivitis** and **keratitis** cause **prolapse of the third eyelid**, thus severely restricting vision. Surgical repair of the eyelid, when indicated, is usually successful. Removal of the third eyelid is rarely necessary. **Entropion** is common in Bloodhounds.[3]

Bloodhounds are predisposed to the **gastric torsion-bloat syndrome,**[4] a leading cause of death in the breed. A regular exercise program, twice daily feedings and an ample supply of water have helped reduce the incidence.

Disturbances of bone growth resulting from surpluses of calcium and other vitamin supplements have been reported.

External ear infections are frequent, due to the drooping ears of the Bloodhound. As with other hound breeds, **hematoma of the ear** is often encountered.

Skin problems are less troublesome for the Bloodhound, with its short hair and dark skin pigment, than for dogs with light skins and heavy coats. Because of the large amount of loose skin and heavy folds around the throat and neck, that area is predisposed to **moist dermatitis**. Patchy hair loss and bald spots are also common in the bitch after nursing or after estrus without breeding.

Bloodhound puppies have been diagnosed as having **toxoplasmosis**.

Bloodhounds generally require a smaller dose of sedating drugs in relationship to their large size.

BEHAVIOR

The Bloodhound is a large, solid, dignified dog. He has the keenest sense of smell of any domestic animal. He is meek, silent, good-natured and rather timid. He makes a good companion dog, but is not temperamentally suited to be a watch dog.

OLD AGE

The life span of the Bloodhound is approximately 10 years.

References
1. American Kennel Club, *The Complete Dog Book*. 18th ed. (Howell Book House,Inc., New York, NY,1979); 160-163.
2. Magrane, W.H. *Canine Ophthalmology*. 3rd Ed. (Lea & Febiger. Phila., Pa 1979) 305.
3. Bloodhound Column, *The American Kennel Club Gazette;* May, 1990.
4. Andrews, A.H. "A Study of Ten Cases of Gastric Torsion in the Bloodhound," *Vet. Rec.*1970: 86: 689-693.

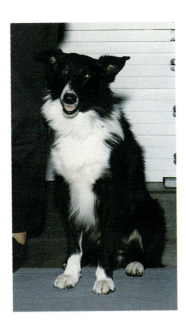

BORDER COLLIE

ORIGIN AND HISTORY

The Border Collie derives its name from its origin near the border of Scotland and England. For 200 years the Border Collie has been bred for its intelligence, athletic ability and herding instinct. During the last 60 years, the Border Collie has become recognized as among the best of all breeds at its craft.[1]

Shepherds have been proud of this breed for many years. In 1973, the first sheep dog trials and shows were organized and held in Baia. These trials have become quite popular, giving the breeders a chance to show off their dogs, and also providing a valuable pool of information on the breed.

In 1906 the International Sheep Dog Society was formed,[2] and since then, other organizations, such as the American International Border Collie Registry and the North American Sheep Dog Society,[3] have been created. These organizations have kept stud books and provided regulations for trials, thereby standardizing the show of this truly international animal.

DESCRIPTION

Border Collies are known as intelligent, outgoing and friendly dogs. They are very good with children and protective of them. Border Collies make great pets as well as outstanding working dogs.

In his book, *The Intelligence of Dogs*, Stanley Conen ranks Border Collies as number one in the ability to learn owner-pleasing behavior.

Dewclaw removal is optional. They should be removed when the Border Collie will be in rough terrain where they tend to get snagged on brush and become inflamed. Ears are not trimmed and tails are not docked.

THE SHOW RING

The Border Collie Standard is very liberal, because breeders want an intelligent dog with herding instincts, regardless of individual characteristics. However, breeders do not ignore conformational hereditary defects. Although the AKC now classifies the Border Collie as a miscellaneous breed,[4] some breeders are fighting for AKC recognition.

The Standard requires a Collie-type head, fairly broad in skull, slightly blunt in muzzle; moderate stop; level bite; large teeth; medium broad ears, tapering to tip, carried prick or semipricked. Eyes are fairly large, dark and set wide apart.

The body should be slightly longer than high with back straight from withers to loin; forelegs straight, forearms muscular, hindlegs long and underset; feet, oval with heavy pads.

The dense coat may be rough or smooth, wavy or slightly curly.

Most individuals will be black with white markings, but gray or blue merle with white points or black with white and tan are acceptable.

Dogs average 18 inches at the shoulder, bitches 17 inches. Weight is 30 to 45 pounds.[5]

BREEDING AND WHELPING

Border Collie bitches may have first estrus between 6 and 8 months of age, but average around 10 months of age. Gestation is the usual 63 days, and most bitches have no trouble whelping. Litter size varies greatly, but the average is five to eight puppies. Whelps average 16 ounces at birth.

RECOGNIZED PROBLEMS

Central progressive retinal atrophy[6,7,8] has been a severe problem in the Border Collie.[9,10,11,12] Incidence in the breed has been as high as 7%, but has dropped to below 1% through careful screening. This problem has been more severe in Great Britain than in the United States. The mode of inheritance is unknown, but it is suggested to be dominant. **Corneal dystrophy, lens luxation, progressive retinal atrophy** and the **Collie eye syndrome** are also seen in the breed.

Patent ductus arteriosus (PDA) was diagnosed by thoracotomy examination in five related female Border Collies. It is suggested that PDA is genetically transmitted in Australian Border Collies.[13]

Hip dysplasia is rare, but **osteochondritis dessicans**[14] is becoming more widespread

104

in the larger dog and tends to be familial. Males tend to be more affected because of their faster rate of growth. The genetics of the disease is unknown, but nutrition seems to be a factor in its development.

Ceroid lipofuscinosis was diagnosed by histopathological and histochemical findings in related Border Collies and by clinical signs in six of their litter mates. Behavioral changes, first hyperactivity and later aggression, commenced at 16 to 23 months of age. Motor abnormalities and blindness were observed at the mean ages of 20.8 and 21.2 months, respectively. All dogs were euthanized one to six months after the onset of clinical signs, mean age 23.1 months. Pedigree data supported an autosomal recessive mode of inheritance.[15]

Cerebellar degeneration has been described in Border Collies and is believed to be familial. There is a loss of granule and purkinje cells from the anterior solia of the cerebellar vermis. Clinical signs appear in 6- to 8-week-old puppies. They are ataxic, hyperkinetic and have head tremors. Prognosis is poor. Clinical signs worsen with age.[16]

Cryptorchidism is fairly common in the breed. As this is thought to be a recessive trait, dogs with the condition should not be used for breeding.

Strain reports that **congenital deafness** does occur in Border Collies.[17]

Bad bites have been reported as common occurrence by several breeders.

BEHAVIOR

This is a very sensitive breed that thrives on praise. The border Collie is intelligent, stable, willing and easily trainable.

OLD AGE

Well cared for, the Border Collie will live a long life. Ages of 10 to 14 years are not uncommon.[3]

References
1. Stewart-Gordon, J. "The Border Collie: Herder of the World's Sheep," (*Reader's Digest* reprint). March, 1961.
2. Longton, T. and Hart, E. *The Sheep Dog, Its Work and Training*. (David and Charles Publishing) 1976: 112.
3. North American Sheepdog Society, 210 E. Main, McLeansboro, IL.,62859
4. American Kennel Club, *The Complete Dog Book*. (Howell Book House, New York, NY. 1992) 610.
5. *Miscellaneous Class Breeds.*(Published by The American Kennel Club, June 1993).
6. Magrane, W.G. *Canine Ophthalmology*. (Lea & Febiger, Philadelphia,PA.,1977) 266.
7. Barnett, K.C. "Abnormalities and Defects in Pedigree Dogs, IV; Progressive Retinal Atrophy," *J. Sm. Anim. Prac.*; 1963: 4:465-467.

8. Barnett, K.C. "Canine Retinopathies, III, The Other Breeds," *J. Sm. Anim. Prac.*; 1965: 6:185-196.

9. Barnett, K.C. "Primary Retinal Dystrophies in the Dog," *JAVMA*; 1968: 154:804-808.

10. Barnett, K.C. "Genetic Anomalies of the Posterior Segment of the Canine Eye," *J. Sm. Anim. Prac.*; 1969: 10: 451-455.

11. Quinn, A.J. Ophthalmology Lecture Notes, OSU; College of Veterinary Medicine; 1980.

12. Patterson, D.F. *Current Veterinary Therapy.* R.W. Kirk, Ed. (W.B. Saunders, Philadelphia, PA., 1977) 84.

13. Malik, R., Turnbull, G.R., and Black, A.P. "Patent-Ductus Arteriosus in Five Related Female Border Collies," *Australian Veterinary Practitioner*; 1991: 21: 1, 2-4; 10 ref.

14. Olson, Stein-Erik, *Current Veterinary Therapy.* R.W. Kirk, Ed.(W.B. Saunders, Philadelphia, PA., 1977) 881.

15. Taylor, R.M. and Farrow, B.R.H. "Ceroid Lipofuscinosis in Border Collie Dogs," *Acta-Neuropathologica*; 1988: 75: 6, 627-631; 10 ref.

16. Ettinger, S.J.; *Textbook of Veterinary Internal Medicine.* W.B. Saunders Co., Philadelphia, PA. 1989: p 598.

17. Strain, George M. "Deafness in Dogs and Cats," *Proc. 10th ACVIM Forum*; May, 1992.

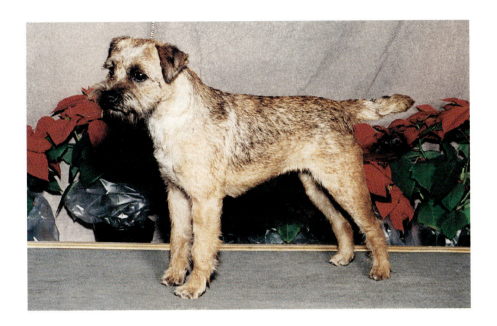

BORDER TERRIER

ORIGIN AND HISTORY

Border Terriers were bred to "bolt" foxes – that is to drive foxes from their hiding places – and kill them. This was no easy feat for a dog weighing only about 14 pounds. The breed is valuable to farmers and shepherds of the border country between England and Scotland but is not often seen in the United States.

DESCRIPTION

Though small, Border Terriers are hardy and have the personality of a large dog. They make excellent family pets, adapting well to new owners or living situations.

Border Terriers are not overly aggressive. They seldom spar in the show ring or fight among themselves as puppies. Adults may be kenneled in pairs or small groups including up to three bitches. Adult males used for stud purposes should not be kenneled together, but other adult males often live happily together. Bitches in season may become quarrelsome. For exercise or hunting, large groups of Border Terriers can be run together under supervision.

Puppies of this breed are usually dark seal-brown. Dogs with blue-and-tan coats are born black, with small tan points. Dogs that will have rich red or dark, grizzled coats at maturity are often black at birth, with a tan sheen to the head. Eventually these dogs show tan under-coats. Dogs with blue-and-tan coats retain black undercoats on the back. The tan spreads gradually, and the black becomes blue as silver and silver-based hairs appear. The silvering usually starts when the pup is 4 to 6 months old, but it can start as late as 10 months. A solid

107

black-and-tan adult Border Terrier without this silvering is undesirable. White spots on the chest are common at birth, as are white hairs on the chin and toes. The latter usually disappear as the dog matures. Chest spots become less obvious and are acceptable; however, any other white is a cause for penalty in the show ring. Rear dewclaws, if present, should be removed. Removal of front dewclaws is recommended but not required.

Tails are naturally short, usually about 1/2 to 3/4 as long as the tails of dogs of similar size. Abnormally short tails and wry or kinked tails have been reported. Puppies with abnormal tails should be neutered and placed as pets. The Border Terrier's tail should not be docked nor its ears cropped.

THE SHOW RING

The characteristic "otter head" with its keen eye, combined with a body poise which is "at the alert," gives a look of fearless and implacable determination, characteristic of the breed.

Dogs should average 13-15 1/2 pounds, bitches 11 1/2-14 pounds. The proportions should be that the height at the withers is slightly greater than the distance from the withers to the tail.

There are no disqualifying faults in this breed.

BREEDING AND WHELPING

Estrus in Border Terrier bitches occurs at regular intervals, but silent heats do occur. Some bitches show neither vaginal discharge nor swelling of the vulva, but they can be bred to whelp normal litters. Others may show no obvious discharge, but show behavioral evidence of estrus. Occasionally a bitch does not dilate during estrus.

Gestation is normal. Most Border Terriers are free whelpers. Cesarean section is sometimes necessary because of a large litter, improper presentation, or uterine inertia.[1,2] Occasionally a bitch strongly resents any aid or interference during whelping. The size of a litter is commonly four to seven puppies, but litters of 9 to 10 have been reported.

GROWTH

The puppies weigh 8 to 12 ounces at birth. Puppies may mature slowly, often not reaching adult size until they are 14 to 18 months old. As early as 12 weeks of age many Border Terriers go through a phase in which their legs are short in proportion to body length. The mature Border Terrier should be up on leg and racy in outline. A balanced body at 8 weeks of age usually means the dog will have a balanced body as an adult. Puppies with short legs at 8 weeks usually have short legs as adults. Some individuals do not attain mature depth of chest, breadth of head and length of leg until they are 18 months old. Other puppies may mature as early as 10 months, but their heads continue to broaden until they are 2 years old.

Ears should break below the topline of the skull, and should not reach forward beyond the outer corner of the eye. The tail should be short and carrot shaped.

The skin should be thick and very loose. The proper harsh outer coat can first be detected at the base of the tail when the pup is between 8 and 9 weeks old.

Testicles may be slow to descend and may not be present in the scrotum until a dog is 5 to 7 months old. **Cryptorchidism** is seen.

Socialization is extremely important for Border Terrier puppies. They should be exposed to human contact and handling as soon as their eyes are open and they can walk. Frequent socialization, both with their littermates and individually, is necessary. Older puppies should be exposed to new environments. Socialization should continue if a Border Terrier enters a period of shyness, but new people and situations should not be forced on it. With proper early socialization, a Border Terrier puppy will outgrow a shy phase.

DENTITION

The teeth should be large, with a scissors bite. Correct dentition and bite cannot be determined until after the permanent teeth arrive. Full dentition is usual; however, occasionally an upper lateral incisor may be missing. A deciduous incisor, recognizable by its shape and small size may have been retained if the permanent incisor is missing. Improper undershot bites also occur. A bite that is undershot after the permanent teeth have arrived remains undershot. In most instances the bite stabilizes by the time the puppy is 6 1/2 months old. A level or tight scissors bite should be suspect until that time because such bites can become undershot. A slight overshot bite usually is self-correcting within 6 1/2 months.

RECOGNIZED PROBLEMS

Congenital ventricular septal defects have been identified in puppies from seven litters. The hereditary nature of the defect is now established but the mode of inheritance is still unknown. It is important that all puppies with congenital heart murmurs be watched, the nature of the defect established by a cardiologist or autopsy, and the results and pedigree sent to the Genetics and Research Committee of the Border Terrier Club of America.

Hip dysplasia is found in this breed. Some breeders report an unusual incidence of **cesarean sections**.

Progressive retinal atrophy has been confirmed in one individual. PRA symptoms were not noticed by the owner until the dog was 3 1/2 years old. Eye examinations by a veterinary ophthalmologist are recommended for all breeding stock. The Genetics and Research Committee is interested in receiving copies of all Border Terrier eye examinations.

BEHAVIOR

The Border Terrier is an excellent companion dog. His size is ideal for an inside dog. He is game, agile and agreeably social. He is especially affectionate with children.

OLD AGE

Border Terriers usually live 14 to 15 years. They are affected by the usual diseases of old age.

References
1. Freak, M.J. "The Whelping Bitch," *Vet. Rec*; 1948: 60:295-301.
2. Freak, M.J. "Abnormal Conditions Associated with Pregnancy and Parturition in the Bitch," *Vet. Rec*; 1962: 74;1323-1335.

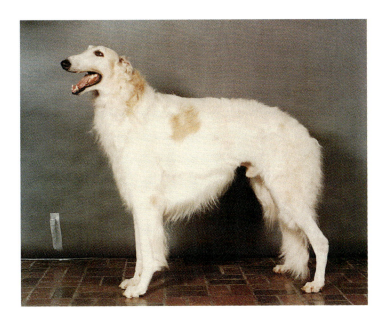

BORZOI

ORIGIN AND HISTORY

The Borzoi (known as the Russian Wolfhound before 1936) has been used since the 17th century for hunting wolves, coursing hare and other game.

DESCRIPTION

The Borzoi is generally even-tempered and adjusts well to any situation. Lack of stability of temperament is a fault.

The standard specifies that "special emphasis is placed on sound running gear, strong neck and jaws, courage and agility, combined with proper condition. The Borzoi should always display unmistakable elegance with flowing lines, graceful in motion or repose...The overall appearance in motion should be that of effortless power, endurance, speed, agility, smoothness and grace."

A unique feature of the breed is its slightly convex topline. This arch in the back should not be extreme, nor should its apex be too far forward. The Standard (as of 1992) states, "Back – rising a little at the loin in a graceful curve."

Any color is permissible. Colors at birth may vary, and the color may change considerably as the dog matures. Silver spots usually turn lemon or cream. Mahogany may lighten to apricot, and black spots may turn to red. Pigmentation in fleshy parts may be lacking at birth, but begins to appear in a few days and is generally complete in a few weeks. The Borzoi is not plagued with unique malformations, but any of the usual anomalies may be encountered.

111

THE SHOW RING

The Borzoi Standard does not list any specific disqualifying faults.

The mature dog should be at least 28 inches at the withers, the mature bitch at least 26 inches at the withers. The weight of the dog ranges from 75 to 105 pounds; bitches weigh 15 to 20 pounds less. Most mature Borzoi dogs now being shown are 31 to 33 inches at the shoulder; most bitches measure 28 to 30 inches at the shoulder.

BREEDING AND WHELPING

Onset of estrus may occur as early as nine months, but 15 to 18 months is more common. In some individuals first estrus may be delayed until 24 months or longer. Once established, however, the estrus cycle is usually regular. Some bitches will accept the dog during only a short time, perhaps 12 hours. Usually the breedings are successful if the bitch is serviced two or three times at 36- to 48-hour intervals. Because the breed matures slowly, bitches should not be bred before they are 2 years old.

Only the more precocious dogs can be used as studs before their second birthday. Because of the size of the dogs, at least two persons should supervise the breeding. Bitches may yelp and protest when the tie is made, and unless they are restrained, serious injury to one or both may result.

Just before whelping, the long hair should be clipped from the bitch's thighs and tail to improve sanitation and prevent puppies from becoming entangled. Newborn puppies have been strangled by the long hair. Clipping does not harm the appearance of the bitch since bitches normally shed several weeks after whelping. Both dogs and bitches shed seasonally, but the extent of shedding is greater in bitches, who also shed heavily after estrus.

Borzoi bitches usually do well throughout pregnancy and do not require special attention beyond that given any other pregnant bitch.

Whelping generally proceeds without difficulty, although some bitches, after a long labor, may have difficulty presenting the last puppy. The Borzoi's large, deep chest makes uterine palpation difficult. In order to determine that all pups have been delivered, radiography should be a regular postpartum procedure.

At birth, healthy puppies weigh about 1 pound, but a variance of 4 ounces is acceptable. Puppies should be weighed and show a gain each day. Occasionally, some puppies do not gain; they may even lose weight during the first 24 hours, but thereafter gain should be dramatic. The birth weight of especially robust puppies should double within one week; that of normal healthy puppies should double within 10 days. Failure to double birth weight within two weeks may indicate health problems. Generally, older puppies weigh about 10 pounds for each month of age.

GROWTH

Rapidly growing puppies normally go through a period of unsoundness and awkwardness. Since male puppies usually are larger than females, this ungainliness tends to be more pronounced in males. Epiphyses of the long bones enlarge greatly at this time, as do the costochondral junctions. Unless the pup shows evidence of pain, such enlargements should be considered normal and not an indication of metabolic bone disease.

Most puppies have passed the stage of rapid growth by the time they are 9 to 12 months old, when their genetic potential for soundness has been realized. No amount of dietary manipulation will correct the defects of genetically unsound dogs. Of course, any large, rapidly growing puppy requires ample and properly balanced nutrients. Diets should be carefully assessed to ensure no nutritional deficiencies develop. In the case of **calcium or phosphorus imbalances**, the most prominent signs are splayed feet and breaking down at the pasterns.

Two- and 3-month-old puppies often carry their tails high. However, if the tail-set is correct (i.e. low) the tail usually will be held down properly as the dog ages and tail feathering develops. Borzoi puppies are nearly full grown at 9 to 12 months, but they sometimes grow another inch during the second year. Despite its size, the Borzoi is not fully mature until it is at least 3 years old. The Borzoi eats only a small amount of food, often requiring no more than many medium-sized dogs. The Borzoi's calm temperament and lack of nervous activity may account for this small intake of food. Although not required, removal of dewclaws when the pup is 2 to 3 days old is recommended.

DENTITION

Either an even or scissors bite is acceptable. Occasionally an adult Borzoi lacks one or more teeth, usually upper or lower premolars. Although the dog suffers no ill effects, a penalty for missing teeth is imposed in the show ring. A dog with missing teeth probably should not be used for breeding.

RECOGNIZED PROBLEMS

Hip dysplasia rarely occurs in the Borzoi, but it has been reported. Any dog used for breeding should be certified free of hip dysplasia.

Gastric bloat and torsion are dreaded by all Borzoi owners. Empirical evidence suggests this idiopathic condition may be most prevalent in 4- to 6-year-old dogs.

Aspermatogenesis sometimes associated with **hypothyroidism** has been reported in this breed.[1] Familial **lymphocytic thyroiditis** has been recognized in the Borzoi.[2] As with any large breed, **hygromas** may develop over bony prominences or joints if soft bedding is not provided.

Calcinosis circumspecta is seen in the Borzoi.

Like other sight hounds, the Borzoi seems especially sensitive to cholinesterase inhibitors. If a flea collar is used, it should be exposed to the air for several days before being put on the dog, and should be removed several days before any elective treatment or surgery.

The response of the Borzoi to all barbiturates is unpredictable; violent recovery, extremely long sleeping time or death frequently occurs. The thiobarbiturates (e.g., thiamylal sodium) should be avoided. Barbiturates should not be administered without a preanesthetic and they should always be given to effect. Whenever possible, general anesthesia should be avoided, but if it is necessary, the best approach is a minimal dose of a preanesthetic, such as Acepromazine Maleate (Ayerst) followed by a volatile anesthetic. Even this approach is not without risk. **Persistent pupillary membrane, cataracts, progressive retinal atrophy, Borzoi retinopathy**, and **microphthalmia** have been recognized in the breed.[3]

BEHAVIOR

The Borzoi has adapted to in-home living, but does need exercise. He is silent, docile, reserved and, like many hounds, has a stubborn streak. He is very loyal.

OLD AGE

If a Borzoi passes the age of 4 to 6 years in good health, a life span of 12 to 15 years is not uncommon.

References
1. Johnston, S.D. "The Effect of Maternal Illness on Perinatal Health," *Vet. Cl. of N. Amer.* 1987: Vol.17:555-556.
2. Griffin, C., Kwochka, K., McDonald, J.; *A Current Veterinary Dermatology, the Art and Science of Therapy.* Mosby Yearbook, St. Louis, MO. 1993: 266.
3. Rubin, L.F.; *Inherited Eye Diseases in Purebred Dogs.* Williams and Williams, Baltimore, MD, 1989: 44.

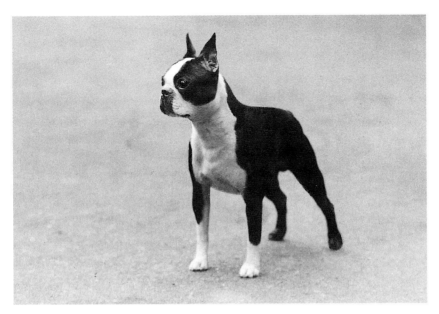

BOSTON TERRIER

ORIGIN AND HISTORY

First mentioned in New England in 1865, the Boston Terrier was cross-bred from an English Bulldog and a terrier, probably a Bull Terrier or an English Terrier. Later, the French Bulldog was bred into the breed for size and color. By 1891 records were kept and in 1893 the breed was registered as Boston Terrier.

DESCRIPTION

Boston Terriers became popular because of their expressive round eyes, alert and pleasant expression, intelligence, square "snitch" nose, square face and terrier body. Originally nearly-white markings, splashes of white and off-white markings were accepted. Occasionally these markings still appear, but the brindle, seal and white markings have become the norm. These classic markings, which give the dog the appearance of wearing a tuxedo, combined with its position as the first breed developed in America, led to its designation as the Little American Gentleman. Boston Terriers do poorly when kenneled, but flourish with human contact. Mistreatment and teasing ruin them. Usually they are clean dogs, and when understood and respected, are intelligent, protective companions.

THE SHOW RING

Boston Terriers have been bred down in size. Weight is divided by classes: under 15 pounds, 15 pounds and under 20 pounds; 20 pounds and not to exceed 25 pounds. No minimum weight is specified; good Boston Terriers as light as 6 or 8 pounds are sometimes seen.

Disqualifying faults are: eyes blue in color, or any trace of blue; Dudley nose; docked tail; solid black; solid brindle, or solid seal without required markings; gray or liver colors.

BREEDING AND WHELPING

Bitches of the brachycephalic breeds experience more reproductive problems — especially **dystocia —** than do those of other breeds. The same **pituitary deficiencies** that produce the square head, short muzzle and shortening or absence of coccygeal vertebrae also cause malfunctioning in other endocrine glands. The result is a lack of the hormones that initiate and control labor.

Cesarean section is frequently necessary. Reducing the allowable weight range for the breed from 10 to 25 to 10 to 18 pounds can help eliminate the dystocia problem. Labor is often prolonged in the Boston Terrier bitch, and **uterine inertia** is too often mistaken for absence of labor. Males are often **"lazy breeders"** and an AI is required.[1]

GROWTH

Puppies during the first week of life often show their adult characteristics. Some grow consistently, others develop unevenly. These ungainly phases may occur until the puppy is 8 months to more than a year old.

In Boston Terrier puppies, front dewclaws should be removed within five days of birth, not only for appearance but also to protect their very vulnerable eyes.

Usually the ears of a Boston Terrier stand without trimming, but they may drop during teething. Ear trimming, a matter of preference, is done less often than in the past. Owners of Boston Terriers should be encouraged to leave the ears natural if the ears are small, erect, have pointed tips and are well-placed on the head.

If trimming is necessary it should not be done until the head is fully formed, when the dog is at least 6 months old. Most of the length should be left; removing the burr or triangle of cartilage anterior to the lateral attachment of the ear and suturing it gives a much cleaner attachment of the ear to the head and also makes the skin on the neck appear tighter. After trimming, the ear should be long, slender and straight with the side of the head to accentuate the square look of the head.

If the tail is carried gaily, tail docking can greatly improve a appearance. The tail may be either screw type or a spike. The length of the tail becomes less obvious as the animal ages.

RECOGNIZED PROBLEMS

Congenital defects, many of them hereditary, that afflict the breed include hydrocephalus, cleft palate and lip,[2] heart defects (especially patent ductus arteriosus), deafness, juvenile cataracts,[3,4] and esophageal achalasia.

Partial or total deafness is a congenital problem in the breed. An ophthalmic anomaly is an off-colored iris: either a "watch" eye or blue pigment in a brown eye (heterochromia irides). Also, eyes may be deviated laterally (cocked eyes). Other eye problems include endothelial dystrophy, prolapse of the nictitans gland and distichiasis.[5] In a recent study, compared with mixed-breed dogs, there were eight breeds at higher risk of developing glaucoma, among them the Boston Terrier.[6] Animals with any of these faults should not be bred. Bostons are susceptible to inhalant allergies,[7] and are at increased risk for generalized demodectic mange.[8]

Boston Terriers sometimes have stenotic nostrils, which may interfere with respiration. Surgical correction of such defects is possible but eliminates the animal as a show dog. The problem may be self-correcting after the puppy reaches 4 months of age. Surgery should be postponed until formation of the muzzle is complete.

A puppy's abdomen should be checked for umbilical hernias, another heritable defect. Some umbilical hernias do not require surgical repair because the animals outgrow them. Scrotal or inguinal hernias may also be present; surprisingly, many of these disappear with maturity. The Boston Terrier is one of the breeds listed as having Hypospadia.[9] Some Boston puppies are viable at birth but look like walruses. They have huge edematous heads, depressions instead of muzzles and swollen bodies and limbs. This is the walrus syndrome, due perhaps to dysplasia of the lymphatic system or to multiple heart defects that are considered hereditary.

Vascular ring anomaly (persistent right aortic arch) is suspected to have a genetic cause, although the exact mode of inheritance is unclear.[10]

The "swimmer" puppy syndrome may also be encountered. It is characterized by inability of the puppies to use their hindquarters at 4 to 6 weeks. The puppies move by dragging themselves on flattened chests, with their legs widely abducted. The problem is not as serious as it appears and affected puppies will do as well as their littermates if properly handled. Usually the puppies are the larger puppies from a small litter without access to a floor surface providing traction. The hind legs should be taped together back to back below the hocks or the puppies should be exercised on a track. Either remedy will soon have the puppy walking as well as its littermates. If the condition is ignored, damaged ligaments of the hip joint and a permanently flattened thorax will result.

Stifles should be checked for excessive straightness and flexed with one hand over the patella and the other at the foot to check for luxation of the patella.[11,12,13] Luxated patella is frequently accompanied by a **lateral curvature of the femur**, which increases the possibility of **medial patella luxation**. **Hemivertebra** is another skeletal problem found in Bostons.[14,15] Signs of the condition are asymmetric development of vertebrae which may result in neonatal death. Vertebrae become wedge-shaped. Kinked tails or crowded ribs may result. Often this is a result of **achondroplasia**, an incomplete dominant autosomal trait. Achondroplasia manifests itself as limb shortening, flared metaphyses, depressed nasal bridge, shortened maxilla and wedge or hemivertebrae. Elbow luxations and medial patella luxation can result from increased joint laxity.[16]

The bite should be even or sufficiently undershot to square the muzzle. The breed has a history of **craniomandibular osteopathy**.

Boston Terriers share with other basicranial chondrodystrophic dwarfs various **hormonal imbalances** that influence their development in utero, their birth, reproduction, reaction to extreme temperatures and even digestion and longevity.

The active brachycephalic Boston Terrier is prone to **heat stroke,** so it should be kept quiet in air conditioned quarters during hot, humid weather. Tranquilization should be employed if necessary. Owners must guard against strenuously exercising their dogs in hot, humid weather. A Boston Terrier must never be left alone in a car on a warm day.

Owners of Boston Terriers frequently complain that their pets vomit or eat feces. Some of these dogs may lack proper **digestive enzymes**, both proteolytic and amylolytic. Vitamin B complex, papain (meat tenderizer) and pancreatin therapy may be needed. The Boston Terrier must be intubated whenever given general anesthetic. Failure to do so may result in a malpractice suit. It has been reported that Bostons are predisposed to **cutaneous mast cell tumors,**[17] and pituitary dependent **hyperadrenocorticism**.[18]

BEHAVIOR

The Boston is well-behaved, likeable, clean, alert and lively. He is exceptionally affectionate. He loves to play and is very patient with children.

OLD AGE

Cushing's disease is encountered more often in older Boston Terriers than in dogs in other breeds. The disease results from **hyperplasia, adenoma or carcinoma of the adrenal cortex**. The disease manifests in many ways: enlargement of the abdomen, **alopecia** (especially of the extremities), muscular weakness, **polyuria** and **polydipsia**. The presence of lymphopenia, eosinopenia and an increase in 17-ketosteroids and 17-hydroxicorticoids confirm the diagnosis.

Because of the breed's pigmented skin, older Boston Terriers are subject to the development of **melanomas**. They also are predisposed to **mastocytomas**, which start as thickenings of the skin, often on the hind legs, followed by alopecia and development of a round nodule fixed to the skin. Over a period of time ranging from months to years, the nodule may begin to grow rapidly, invading the surrounding skin and subcutaneous tissue. Any small skin growth should be removed and submitted to histopathology. Other neoplasms that commonly affect aging Boston Terriers are **pituitary tumors** and **aortic and carotid body tumors**.

Rather than follow the whims of the public or the fads of judges, owners of Boston Terriers are advised to study and apply the American Kennel Club Standard to the breed.

References
1. Walkowicz, Chris *The American Kennel Club Gazette*; June: 1990: 68.
2. Erickson, F., et al, *Congenital Defects in Dogs: A Special Reference for Practitioners*; Ralston Purina Co.(reprint from *Canine Practice*. Veterinary Practice Publishing Co. 1978).
3. Barnett, K.C. "Types of Cataract in the Dog," *JAAHA;* 1972: 8:2-9.
4. Barnett, K.C. "The Diagnosis and Differential Diagnosis of Cataract in the Dog," *J. Sm. Anim. Prac.*;1985: 26:6, 305-316; 20 ref.
5. Magrane, W.C. *Canine Ophthalmology*. 3rd ed. (Lea & Febiger, Philadelphia, PA 1977) 305.
6. Slater, M.R. and Erb, H.N. "Effects of Risk Factors and Prophylactic Treatment on Primary Glaucoma in the Dog," *JAVMA*; 1986: 188:9, 1028-1030; 7 ref.
7. Ackerman, Lowell, DVM, "Allergic Skin Diseases," *American Kennel Club Gazette*; 1990.
8. Griffin, C., Kwochka, K., McDonald, J.; *Current Veterinary Dermatology, the Art and Science of Therapy*. Mosby Yearbook, St. Louis, MO. 1993: 74,274.
9. Ettinger, S.J.; *Textbook of Veterinary Internal Medicine*. W.B. Saunders, Philadelphia, PA. 1989: 1883-1884.
10. Kern, Maryanne, DVM, "Diseases of the Esophagus," *The American Kennel Club*; 1993.
11. Knight, K.C. "Abnormalities and Defects in Pedigree Dogs,III,Tibio-Femoral Joint Deformity and Patella Luxation," *J. Sm. Anim. Prac.*; 1963: 4:463-464.
12. Kodituwakku, C.F. "Luxation of the Patella in the Dog," *Vet. Rec.*; 1962: 74:1499-1507.
13. Pearson H. and Gibbs, C. "Abnormal Vertebral Development in Bulldogs," *Vet. Rec.*; 1974: 95:27-28.
14. Done, S.H., et al, "Hemivertebra in the Dog: Clinical and Pathological Observations," *Vet. Rec.*; 1975: 96:313-317.
15. Drew, R.A. "Possible Association Between Vertebral Development and Neonatal Mortality in Bulldogs," *Vet. Rec.*; 1974: 94:480-481.
16. Ettinger, S.J.; *Textbook of Veterinary Internal Medicine*. W.B. Saunders, Philadelphia, PA. 1989: 2383.
17. Veterinary News. *The American Kennel Club Gazette*; 1990: 44.
18. Griffin, C., Kwochka, K., McDonald, J.; *Current Veterinary Dermatology, the Art and Science of Therapy*. Mosby Yearbook, St. Louis, MO. 1993: 74,274.

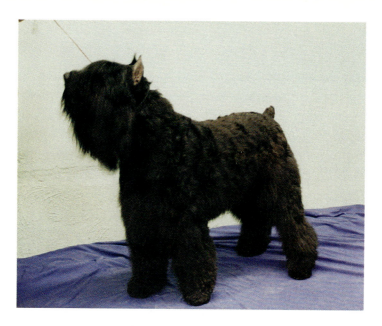

BOUVIER DES FLANDRES

ORIGIN AND HISTORY

It is almost impossible to trace the origin of the Bouvier des Flandres. During the last decade of the nineteenth century a program of selective breeding of the dogs native to Belgium was begun under the guidance of Professor Ad. Reul, a veterinary surgeon and author of "Les Races de Chiens" (1894). The Bouvier is mentioned, "for the most part, a shepherd dog or a dog that resembles him in general make-up but who is bigger, fiercer, more aggressive and has a bolder look." Breeding emphasis has always been placed on performance in Europe. The breed has a long history of excellence as a herd and guard dog. A Bouvier cannot complete his championship in Belgium without demonstrating his ability in working trials.

DESCRIPTION

The adult Bouvier is alert, active and playful, although the breed can be very stubborn and emotional. Bouviers are natural guard dogs, protective of family and property. They are very trustworthy with children and make excellent companions and house dogs. In recent years they have served the police as patrol dogs and have demonstrated exceptional olfactory capabilities in searching for narcotics. The training should be started early as the breed displays above-average intelligence.

Coat color of the puppies can run from fawn to black, including all shades of gray and brown-tipped coats which later turn gray. Faulty variations include large white areas of coat, the totally brown coat and pink noses in combination with white toenails.

Bouviers should be bred with dark coat color and good pigmentation in mind. Repeated fawn to fawn generations can produce a loss of color intensity, light bone development and sensitive skin problems.

THE SHOW RING

Dogs should measure 24 1/2 to 27 1/2 inches at the withers, bitches from 231/2 to 26 1/2 inches. Deviation from the minimum or maximum limits mentioned should be severely penalized. There are no disqualifications for this breed in the show ring.

BREEDING AND WHELPING

There is considerable size variation in both sexes which may present a problem to the bitch in whelp. Despite the general ruggedness of the breed, there is an inordinate number of distocias including uterine inertia, associated with large litters and the single- or two-puppy pregnancy. Litters vary from one to 15 puppies. The whelps weigh from 8 ounces to 1 1/2 pounds at birth. Those weighing more than a pound may be over the Standard size as adults.

GROWTH

Dewclaws should be removed and tails docked to 5/8 inch by ventral measurement at 3 days of age.

The ears should be cropped at 7 weeks in a wide triangle shape. The initial cut for length should be made from a point even with the point where the ear reaches the lateral canthus of the eye.

The cut should be made in a relatively straight line with little bell. The ear should be wider than a Doberman ear, with less bell than that of a Dane or a Boxer.

Care should be taken that the litter is well socialized. The breeder should try to place the puppies between 9 and 11 weeks of age; Bouvier puppies develop guarding tendencies by 12 weeks.

DENTITION

Occlusion problems exist; many undershot and some overshot bites are seen. It is difficult to breed away from the overshot bite. The breed can become undershot as late as a year of age.

RECOGNIZED PROBLEMS

Umbilical hernias and **cleft palates** may be expected from some bloodlines.

The breed has major **reproductive difficulties**, possibly the result of its recent development from a very few individuals remaining after World War II. **Cystic ovaries, pseudopregnancies** and **endometritis** are frequently seen. Estral irregularities make determination of a breeding date difficult. Vaginal smears and progesterone testing help to achieve conception.

Congenital **phimosis** is seen in the Bouvier Des Flandres.[1]

There is a significant incidence of **lymphosarcoma** in this breed, surfacing in the middle and later years. **Torsion** of the stomach and spleen are also seen. **Gastrointestinal disturbances**, possibly emotionally based, are a problem in some bloodlines. These syndromes respond well to the use of antacids, tranquilizers and well-formulated diets.

In contrast to other large breeds, the Bouvier experiences little trouble with hip dysplasia. The probable explanation is the excellent musculature in the pelvic region, as well as the lack of genetic potential for hip dysplasia. OFA reports **elbow dysplasia** in the breed.[2]

Recently, there has been a significant increase in **hypothyroidism. Laryngeal spasm** has been encountered with dogs that have excessive soft palates. Some hereditary and congenital **cardiac defects** have been noted.

BEHAVIOR

The Bouvier is extremely intelligent. He is good-natured and adapts readily to being a family dog and watch dog.

OLD AGE

Coat color will gradually deepen as the dog grows older. Light to medium gray dogs turn black after 7 years of age.

Fawn dogs tend to have the coat color pale to almost white in old age. In general, the Bouvier enjoys a relatively healthy lifespan with very few chronic ailments.

The breed remains playful and active into old age. The life expectancy falls within 10 to 12 years of age, with the dogs usually outliving the bitches.

References
1. Ettinger, S.J.: *Textbook of Veterinary Internal Medicine*. W.B. Saunders, Philadelphia, PA 1989: 1884.
2. Bodner, Elizabeth, DVM, "Genetic Status Symbols," *The American Kennel Club Gazette*; September, 1992.

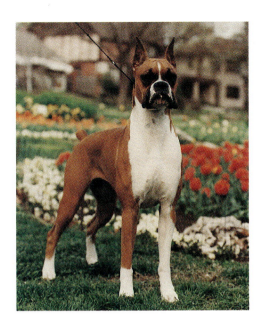

BOXER

ORIGIN AND HISTORY

The Boxer owes its type to many years of diligent breeding of bulldogs and terriers in Germany. The breed derives its name from the tendency of these dogs to begin combat by rising on the hind legs and striking out with their forepaws.

DESCRIPTION

The Boxer is a great family dog, fearless and loyal, but also determined and stubborn under force. Consistent, quietly enforced commands are most effective, for the Boxer is happy to please when guided. Dogs of this breed are stoic when subjected to pain, thus being excellent patients.

Although white or check puppies may result from any breeding, a higher incidence results from the mating of two flashy individuals. This is a risk taken by breeders to retain the desirable white markings (flash).

Discounting the whites and checks, which are always possible, fawn to fawn breeding results in only fawn puppies. If a brindle results from such a breeding, one of the parents probably has imperceptible brindling on some part of the anatomy. Fawn to brindle or brindle to brindle breedings may produce both fawn and brindle puppies, although there are some homozygote brindles which, mated with either fawn or brindle animals, can produce only brindles.

The muddier the coat of the newborn puppy, the redder the fawn will be in the adult. A dark streak on the spinal column and any dark hairs throughout the fawn portions of the coat will clear with the shedding of the puppy coat by the time the puppy is 2 weeks old. White markings on the neck and face may become less prominent as the animal grows. Narrow blazes between the eyes may disappear within 8 to 10 weeks.

The leather on the nose of white-muzzled puppies obtains pigment very slowly, occasionally taking as long as a year to develop.

The pattern of white markings is progressive. Even the plainer puppies have a few white hairs on the tip of the un-docked tail and some white on the chest. The chest and feet (or legs) usually have an appreciable amount of white before white will occur on the face or the back of the neck.

Unpigmented haws (third eyelids) are no longer listed in the breed Standard as a fault. They are a hazard of the often desirable white face markings. A Boxer is penalized for haws only if they detract from the dog's general appearance. Undiseased, unpigmented haws should never be removed, as they are necessary protection for the eye.

THE SHOW RING

Adult dogs average 22 1/2 to 25 inches at the withers; bitches average 21 to 23 1/2 inches. Dogs should not measure less than the minimum, nor bitches more than the maximum. Both dogs and bitches fare best in the show ring when their size is within the stated range, although they will not be disqualified on the basis of size.

Removal of dewclaws is optional; however, it is preferable that dewclaws be removed when the tail is docked. A Boxer with front dewclaws is rarely seen in the ring.

Boxers of any color other than fawn or brindle, and Boxers with a total of white markings exceeding one-third of the entire coat are disqualified by the Breed Standard. The Standard says, "White markings on fawn or brindle dogs are not to be rejected and are often very attractive." Although plainer dogs may win more class placements, a Boxer without extensive white markings on at least its chest and legs would have difficulty reaching its championship. Solid white or more than one-third white puppies are euthanized at birth by serious breeders. Boxers more than one-third white are called "checks." Boxers with white on the legs, face, chest and collar are probably not checks if no patching appears elsewhere.

Chief faults of the Boxer are an atypical head; unserviceable bite; teeth or tongue showing with mouth closed; poor ear carriage; light (bird of prey) eyes and poor temperament.

BREEDING AND WHELPING

Eight months to 2 years of age is not unusual for first estrus, nor is a regular interval of 8 to 11 months between estrus periods.

Although Boxer bitches seldom have problems during gestation, the incidence of cesarean sections among Boxers is higher than that for other working breeds.

In normal whelpings the dam should be assisted in severing umbilical cords.

Boxer bitches often carry puppies tucked up in the rib-cage. For this reason, a radiograph may be advisable after delivery of what is believed to be the last pup.

The average weight of newborn puppies is 10 to 16 ounces; however, small puppies may thrive, and large ones are whelped without difficulty. The newborn puppies should be checked for harelip and cleft palate although these defects occur only rarely in the modern Boxer.

GROWTH

Growth rate varies radically among Boxers. Some bloodlines have an early growth spurt; others a longer, steadier pattern of growth. It is most important that the dog have good bone for its size.

Boxers have a long puppyhood and should be guarded from temptation until they are mature and trained. During puppyhood and adolescence a Boxer's freedom should be restricted when the animal is unsupervised. The Boxer is usually 18 months to 2 years old before it matures and emerges as a family protector. The mature dog thinks before acting, enhancing its desirability as a watchdog.

Tails should be docked when the puppies are 5 to 7 days old. A good rule of thumb for assuring proper tail length is to measure, on the underside of the tail, a distance of 3/4 inch from the rectum. The end of the tail must be padded so that the dog can comfortably carry the tail erect. To ensure proper padding, the skin in the tail is drawn back toward the dog as the tail is docked. Docking should include trimming out a bit of the protruding bone. The tip is then covered with the excess skin and joined by two sutures. Non-absorbable sutures are recommended, because reaction to absorbable suture material is unfavorable in some Boxers, and the sutures will not hold until healing occurs.

Because both advance preparation and post-treatment are imperative in ear-clipping of Boxers, only a skilled veterinarian is competent to conduct the procedure. The veterinarian should immunize the puppies and determine the proper age for cropping their ears. The ears of puppies that have been properly prepared are usually cropped when the puppies are approximately 8 weeks old. The objective is to have the ears standing before the puppies are teething.

When the ears are cropped, care must be taken to remove the protruding tip of cartilage at the base of the ear. Without removal, the ear appears to jut suddenly from the head, giving the skull a broadened appearance. Ears are cut long and tapering and should be sutured. The size and bone structure of each puppy are evaluated to determine the puppy's ultimate size and build, and the ears are cropped accordingly. Because the puppy's adult stature has been anticipated, newly cropped ears always appear too long.

Puppies should be separated from others for the 10 days the ears are sutured. During healing, the ears may either lie flat over the head or be stretched straight upward. Either way, they should be stretched from base to tip to eliminate curling.

When sutures are removed at the end of 10 days, the ear should be stretched upward, either on a splint or by reinforcing. One procedure is to cone or round-roll the ear from the base to the tip. Masking tape, rather than adhesive tape, is used because it removes less hair. Tape should be changed every three or four days; between tapings, vigorous upward stretching is imperative.

DENTITION

The Boxer's bite is normally undershot; however, the tongue and teeth must not be exposed when the jaws are closed. Although a Boxer can occasionally snag a canine tooth, no discomfort results. If the bite is excessively undershot or the upper jaw does not fit tightly to the mandible behind the lower teeth, the tongue may show at the front of the mouth. A wry mouth can allow the tongue to escape at the front of the mouth or, rarely, the tongue may protrude because it is too long.

Extra incisors are more common than missing teeth in Boxers.[1] The extra teeth are desirable because the added incisors give the lower jaw greater width.

Because the bite of Boxers is so important, tug-of-war play is not recommended.

RECOGNIZED PROBLEMS

The incidence of **hip dysplasia** in the Boxer breed is not known, since some breeders do not routinely radiograph their stock.

A collection of over 14,000 radiographs of the spines of 10 breeds of dogs were examined for abnormal vertebrae in the lumbosacral region, which were manifested by different types of fusion. There was some link between these abnormalities and hip dysplasia. Such abnormalities were seen in 5% of 3300 Boxers.[2]

Male boxers have a higher incidence of **unilateral cryptorchidism** than the canine norm. This is probably because the Boxer Standard formerly allowed cryptorchids to be exhibited, and many were used for breeding. As a rule, the testicle is evident in the channel but not fully descended, due either to shortness of the attached cord or to an obstructed scrotum. If the testicle is retained inside the abdominal cavity, it should be removed while the animal is young. Retained testicles seem predisposed to development of Sertoli cell tumor.

Esophageal dilatation in the Boxer breed has been reported.[3]

Ulcerative keratitis (Boxer ulcer or corneal erosion),[4] is peculiar to Boxers. No

126

causative bacterium or virus has been identified. The ulceration of the cornea may affect one eye or both. The lesion is small, superficial and has no tendency to spread. With fluorescein staining, the lesion appears to be surrounded by an overhanging border. In the early state, no associated discharge, corneal opacity or vascularization occurs. In the later stages, profuse lacrimation develops and may resist treatment. More than 80% of these ulcers occur in spayed bitches over 5 years of age. Estrogen therapy reportedly helps prevent recurrence.[4] Another eye problem of Boxers is **distichiasis**.

The Boxer in mid-to-late life is frequently bothered by a **hyperplasia of the gingiva.**[5] Although this epulis is often mistaken for an oral tumor, it is a fibrous overgrowth of the gingiva. When an animal's mastication is impaired, the fibrous tissue should be surgically removed. **Congenital deafness has been reported in Boxers.**[6]

The incidence of **tumors** in Boxers is high.[7,8] The breed is prone to **mastocytoma**, **histiocytoma, lymphosarcoma**[9,10,11,] **osteosarcoma**, **aortic body tumors**, **glioma**, **hemangioma**, **dermoid cysts,**[12] and **thyroid, lung** and **testicular tumors**.[13] Adnexal and mammary tumors rarely occur and are usually benign.[8]

The Boxer, being large and deep-chested, is subject to **gastric torsion**. The condition usually occurs shortly after the dog has exercised just after eating. Signs consist of pain in the area of the stomach, unproductive attempts to vomit and salivation. The animal may die as a result of cardiovascular collapse.

Granulomatous colitis affects Boxers 2 months to 2 years old. It is characterized by soft, bloody stools. The cause is not known; however, an immunologic basis is most likely. At the onset, the dog may not appear to be ill, except for the bloody stools. The course of the disease, usually slow, is accompanied by progressive debilitation. Even persistent treatment may be unsuccessful.

Boxers have a predisposition to **intervertebral disc degeneration**. The vertebral column of 324 Boxers were radiographed.[13] Spondylitic signs were localized and classified into five degrees of intensity and statistically evaluated according to various criteria. A typical section site for spondylitic changes in the German Boxer was found at T_{12}/T_{13} because of the typical shape of the body.

Earliest signs of **spondylosis** were observed at the age of 9 months. With one exception, regardless of sex, all the dogs over 4 years old were affected by spondylosis. Forty percent of all affected dogs showed clinical symptoms of varying degrees. Examination concerning consanguinity among the dogs confirm that in **spondylosis deformans**, and even more in **syndesmitis ossificans**, genetic influences are present.[14]

Subaortic stenosis, **pulmonic stenosis**, [15,16] **atrial septal defect** and **mast cell tu-**

mors also occur in the Boxer breed. In Arizona the breed seems to be especially susceptible to **coccidioidomycosis** (Valley fever). There is also a report of multiple **cardiac defects** in one litter. **Dilated cardiomyopathy** has been reported.[17] Some recent studies have suggested that cardiomyopathy may be in part the result of an L-carnitine deficiency.[18] A blood deficiency reported in Boxers is **Factor II deficiency (hypothrombinemia)**.[19] The condition is characterized by severe **epistaxis**.

Endocardial fibroelastosis is described in the Boxer,[10] as is **vaginal hyperplasia**.

Cystine urea and **cystine stones** occur more commonly in male Boxers.

A retrospective study of 412 spayed bitches showed an incidence of **urinary incontinence** in 20.1 percent. There appears to be a strong correlation between body weight and incontinence. Of bitches with a body weight of less than 20 kilograms. only 9.3% were incontinent, whereas in bitches with a body weight of more than 20 kilograms. the incidence was 30.9%. Boxers showed the highest incidence with 65%. Alpha-adrenergic drugs (phenylpropanolamine or ephedrine) are the most appropriate treatment for sphincter incompetence (good results 73.7%). Stimulation of the alpha receptors in the uretal wall increases urethral closure pressure. Alternatively, estrogens can be used (good results 64.7%).[20]

Sinus arrhythmia is the usual cardiac rhythm in the healthy resting dog (Detweiler,1968) and this can be pronounced in the brachycephalic breeds (Fisher,1967). In Boxers, **fainting at rest occurs**, also described by owners as collapsing. In extreme cases, the clinical condition is similar to the Adams-Stokes syndrome described in humans.[21] Difficulty may arise in attempting to explain the faint since the dogs appear healthy, have not shown soft palate abnormalities, and when examined, show neither sinus tachycardia (due to excitement) or sinus arrhythmia.[22,23,24,25]

Examination of seven Boxers that had fainted revealed, under the quietest resting conditions, sinus arrhythmia extending into a sinoatrial block. The vagal origin was suggested by its abolition with atropine and by the production of complete syncope for as long as 11 seconds with a vagal stimulant. This syncope was accompanied by a disastrous lowering of blood pressure, collapse, loss of consciousness, somatic tremor and micturition. Fainting might be explained by the natural occurrence of vaso-vagal syncope, since there seems to be an excessive vagal tone. Boxers have increased breed incidence of both **hyperadrenalcorticism** and **hypothyroidism**.[26] **Congenital hypothyroidism**, referred to as cretinism in human children occurs in the Boxer. The dogs have short, wide limbs and broad skulls, and are dull and lethargic. Thyroid supplement helps their lethargy and attitude, but usually not their growth deformities.[27] They also have an increased risk of getting generalized **demodectic mange**.[28]

In a survey of skin disorders, **atopy** was reported in Boxers.[29] Boxer **neuropathy** is an autosomal recessive disorder of peripheral and central neuronal axons that has been described in three families of dogs in The United Kingdom. Clinical signs are pelvis and limb ataxia in dogs under 6 months of age along with bilaterally depressed patellar reflexes.

Boxers are one of several breeds reported with significantly higher disposition for **malignant neoplasms.**[30]

Idiopathic epilepsy has been detected in the Boxer.[31]

BEHAVIOR

The Boxer is a good-natured, lively and amiable companion. He is especially affectionate with children. He is easily trained with a gentle but no-nonsense manner. He is a good watch dog, being loyal and a little suspicious of strangers.

OLD AGE

Boxers do not lose their tolerance and good nature with age. When a Boxer begins to age, all the organs usually begin to deteriorate rapidly. Life expectancy is not long. Eight to nine years is average, although some Boxers live longer.

References
1. Aitchinson, J. "Incisor Dentition in Short Muzzled Dogs," *Vet. Rec.*; 1964: 76:165-169.
2. Winkler, W. "Transitional Lumbosacral Vertebrae of the Dog," Dissertation, Fachbereich Veterinarmedizin der Freien Universitat Berlin. 1985: 143; 50 ref.
3. Osborne, C.A. "Hereditary Esophageal Achalasia in Dogs," *JAVMA*; 1967: 151:572-578.
4. Roberts, S.R. "Superficial Indolent Ulcer of the Cornea in Boxer Dogs," *J. Sm. Anim. Prac.*; 1965: 6:111-115.
5. Burnstone, M.S., et al "Familial Gingival Hypertrophy in the Dog," *Arch. Path.*; 1952: 54:208-212.
6. Strain, George M. "Deafness in Dogs and Cats," *Proc. ACVIM*; May, 1992.
7. Kirk, R.W. and Bistner, S.I. *Handbook of Vet. Proc. and Emergency Treatment: Hereditary Defects of Dogs.* Table 124, 1975: 661.
8. Erickson, F., et al. "Congenital Defects of Dogs, Part III," *Canine Prac.*; 1977: 4:48.
9. Madewell, Bruce R., VMD, MS. "Canine Lymphoma," *Vet. Clinics of N. Amer: Sm. Anim. Prac.*; July, 1985: Vol.15, #4.
10. McCaw, Dudley, DVM, "Canine Lymphosarcoma," AAHA's 56th Annual Meeting Proceedings, 1989.
11. Rosenthal, Robert C., DVM, MS, PhD, "The Treatment of Canine Lymphoma," *Vet Clinics of N. Amer.*; July, 1990: Vol 20, #4.
12. Burgisser H. and Sinterman, J. "Kystes Dermoides de la Tate chez la Boxer," *Schweiz. Arch. Tierheilk.* 1961: 103:309-312.
13. Monlux, A.W. Personal Communication. Pathology Dept., Oklahoma State University, Stillwater, OK.

14. Muhlebach, Von R., Freudiger: "Rontgenologische Untersuchungen uber die Erkrankungsformen ded Spondylose beim Deutschen Boxer," *Schweiz. Arch. Tierheilk.* 1973: V.15: 539-558.

15. Welgelius, O. and von Edden, R. "Endocardial Fibroelastosis in Dogs," *Act. Pact. Micro. Scan* 1969: 77: 69-72.

16. Pyle, R.L. and Patterson, D.F. "Multiple Cardiovascular Malformations in a Family of Boxer Dogs," *JAVMA*; 1972: 160:965-976.

17. "All About Cardiomyopathy," *American Kennel Club Gazette*; June, 1989.

18. Harpster, Neil, DVM., "Bulldog Column," *American Kennel Club Gazette*; December, 1990: 107.

19. Dodds, W.J. "Inherited Hematologic Defects," In *Canine Vet. Therapy*; R.W. Kirk, Ed. (W.B Saunders, Philadelphia,PA. 1977) 438-445.

20. Arnold, S., Arnold, P., and Hebler, M., et al. "Incontinentia Urinae bei der Kfastrierten Hunden: Haufigheit und Rossedisposition," *Schweiz. Arch. Tierheilk.*; 1989: 131: 259.

21. Fisher, E.W. "Fainting in Boxers: The Possibility of Vaso-Vagal Syncope," (Adams-Stokes Attacks) *J. Sm. Anim. Prac.*; 1971: 12: 347-349.

22. Quinn, A.J. Personal Communication. Oklahoma State Univ., Stillwater, OK.

23. Detweiler, D.K. In *Canine Medicine*. (Am. Vet. Publ. Santa Barbara, CA;1968).

24. Fisher, E.W. *J. Sm. Anim. Prac.*; 1967: 8: 151.

25. Friedberg, C.K. *Diseases of the Heart*. (W.B. Saunders. Philadelphia, PA;1966).

26. Brignac, Michele M. "Congenital and Breed Associated Skin Diseases in the Dog and Cat," *KalKan Forum*; December, 1989: 9-16.

27. Ettinger, S.J.: *Textbook of Veterinary Internal Medicine*. W.B. Saunders Co., Philadelphia, PA. 1989: 2385.

28. Griffin, C., Kwochka, K., McDonald, J. *Current Veterinary Dermatology, the Art and Science of Therapy*. Mosly Yearbook, St. Louis, MO 1993: 74, 274, 171.

29. Scott, D.W. and Paradis, M. "A Survey of Canine and Feline Skin Disorders Seen in a University Practice," Small Animal Clinic, University of Montreal, Saint-Hyacinthe, Quebec, (1987-1988) *Can. Vet. Jour.*; 1990: 31: 12, 830-835; 50 ref.

30. Kusch, S. "Incidence of Malignant Neoplasia in Dogs Based on PM Statistics of the Institute of Animal Pathology," Munich, 1970-1984. Inaugural Dissertation, Tierarztliche Fakultat, Ludwig Maximilians Universitat, Munchen, German Federal Republic. 1985: 21 pp. ref.

31. Bell, Jerold S. DVM: "Sex Related Genetic Disorders: Did Mama Cause This?" *American Kennel Club Gazette*, Feb. 1994; 76.

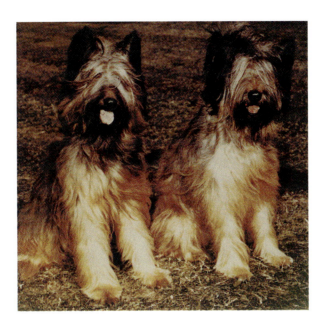

BRIARD

ORIGIN AND HISTORY

The Briard has for centuries been the preeminent sheep dog of France. The breed can be trained to herd, guard and perform obedience tasks, and makes an excellent family companion. Characteristically, these dogs do not wander and remain near their owners.

DESCRIPTION

Briards are instinctively protective and are generally good watch dogs. They are devoted, loyal, highly intelligent companions with a stoic nature.

Dewclaws on the front legs are usually single and may be removed or retained. When double or triple dewclaws are present on the front legs, it is advisable to remove them when the puppy is 2 to 5 days old, assuring a neater appearance in the adult dog. However, individuals with multiple dewclaws on the front legs seldom produce puppies lacking proper rear dewclaws. For this reason they are often preferred for breeding stock.

THE SHOW RING

Briards range from 22 to 27 inches at the shoulders. Their long, stiff, slightly wavy coats occur in all colors. The puppies are either tawny (dark fawn) or black. The nose and footpads of newborn puppies may be pink but change to black at approximately 1 week of age.

Double Dewclaws on the hind legs are prominent at birth and must never be removed. The Briard Standard requires rear dewclaws because they are a centuries-old characteristic of the breed. They should be set low on the leg, almost like two additional toes, and be well separated. Each nail should emerge from its own pad. A single pad with two nails is unacceptable in an animal to be shown or used for breeding.

The Briard Standard disqualifies the following: 1) nose of any color but black; 2) yellow or spotted eyes; 3) tail nonexistent or docked; 4) fewer than two dewclaws on each rear leg; 5) white or spotted coats, or a white spot on the chest exceeding one inch in diameter; 6) failure to meet standard size (23 to 27 inches at the withers for dogs; 22 to 25 1/2 inches for bitches.)

BREEDING AND WHELPING

The most common cause of puppy deaths in the first two weeks is smothering by the bitch. This problem can be avoided by installing a raised bumper in the whelping box and dividing the puppies into small groups.

Puppies should be fed at two- to four-hour intervals and rotated for feeding so that the bitch nurses only four to seven at a time. Most bitches are content if puppies not being nursed are put in a cardboard box in the corner of the whelping box. If the puppies are not crying, the bitch will not disturb them. Despite the size of the litter, supplementary feeding is rarely necessary because the Briard bitches are excellent milk producers.

BRIARD EAR CROP

Crop ears at 5 to 6 weeks of age, before fatty tissue develops between the skin and cartilage.

1. Shave ear on outside just around the edge in a triangular fashion; shave entire ear on the inside.
2. Make a notch 1/8 to 1/4 inch from top of the ear on the front edge.
3. Lay umbilical hemostat along a line running from the notch to the "V" in the lobe of the ear; lock hemostat in place.
4. Make cut with a scalpel starting from the center and cutting toward either end.
5. Cut a triangular piece off 1/8 inch from the top of the cropped edge, rounding points off. No sutures needed.
6. Use gas.

GROWTH

The puppies grow rapidly. They weigh 20 to 25 pounds at 3 months and approximately 50 pounds at 6 months. A mature Briard bitch weighs 60 to 75 pounds and a dog weighs 70 to 90 pounds. Briards do not attain full maturity until they are 3 years old.

To develop properly, the puppies require extensive socialization beginning when they are 3 weeks old and continuing through the first year. Pups with minimal human contact may become shy or aggressive. The mature Briard is characteristically aloof to strangers but should not be vicious. Briards are poor kennel dogs because they have a strong need for human companionship and when placed in a kennel for prolonged periods may decline physically and mentally.

Tails should never be docked.

The ears of Briard puppies should be cropped when the puppies are between 5 and 6 weeks. If the ears are cropped when a puppy is too young, the growth of the ear cannot be accurately foreseen. The ideally cropped ear is full and long (Appendix I). The narrow or pointed crop of the Bouvier breed should never be adapted to the Briard.

The long coat of the Briard requires regular care. By the time puppies reach 1 year of age, weekly grooming is necessary to keep the coat free of mats. This routine grooming also reveals skin problems before they become serious. The incidence of dermatitis is higher when the coat becomes matted, trapping moisture and reducing air circulation.

DENTITION

Incomplete dentition is rare in Briards. The bite of the young puppy is sometimes slightly overshot but generally corrects with the second teething. A scissors bite is desired, though the even bite typical of the sheepherding breeds is often seen. Occasionally the teeth cannot meet in front, causing an open bite. This condition will not become evident until the eruption of the permanent teeth.

RECOGNIZED PROBLEMS

The Briard, though usually a remarkably strong and healthy dog, is subject to a few inherent weaknesses. **Hip dysplasia** remains a problem in the breed, although its crippling effects are observed less frequently because of careful breeding.

Gastric torsion is a serious problem in the Briard and is a significant cause of death among adults. Any dog showing abdominal distention and discomfort, with or without retching, should receive immediate attention. Factors thought to contribute to torsion are ingestion of a large meal and copious amounts of water, followed by vigorous exercise. As a precaution, rather than one large feeding, the adult Briard should be fed smaller amounts twice daily. Water should be available at all times, and exercise should not be permitted for two hours after feeding. A higher incidence of gastric torsion has been noticed following boarding; therefore, special care should be taken at that time.

Hypothyroidism appears fairly often in the Briard. Testing should be done at 18 months of age, as a low T_3 or T_4 can be readily corrected with medication. Symptoms of hypothyroidism

133

include hair loss, itchy skin and low fertility.

PRA (progressive retinal atrophy) has been diagnosed in Briards bred and raised in England. **Night-blindness** and **loss of peripheral vision** has appeared in older dogs. Though few American specimens have tested positive, the Briard Club of America[1] is conducting extensive research. All Briards should be tested for PRA annually.

An unusual form of **renal dysplasia** has been reported in a single litter of Briards.[2]

BEHAVIOR

The Briard is very sensitive and with loving attention and training can become a devoted family member. Some, bred as companions, may be timid with strangers.

OLD AGE

Cysts are common in older Briards and must be watched carefully for signs of malignancy. Bloat is a major cause of adult death, and the usual geriatric conditions such as heart disease and cancer are observed.

The usual life expectancy of the Briard is about 10 years; however, some live longer and remain active until they are 12 to 13 years of age.

References
1. Briard Club of America
2. Gysling, C. and Hagen, A. "Renal Dysplasia in the Briard in Comparison to Other Kidney Diseases in the Dog," *Kleintierpraxis*; 1986: 31:1, 3-4, 6-8; 27.

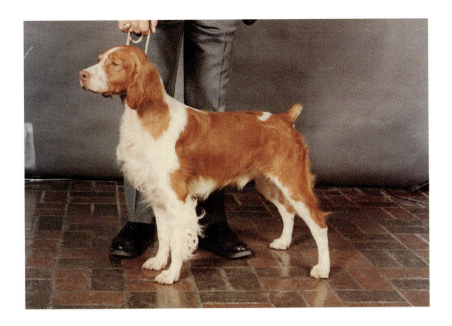

BRITTANY

ORIGIN AND HISTORY

The first tailless ancestor of the modern Brittany was bred a century ago at Pontov, a little town situated in the Valley of Dovron. The modern history of the breed dates back only to the beginning of the present century. Although known on the Continent for centuries, the breed had degenerated until Arthur Enaud, a French sportsman with a biological turn of mind, endeavored to improve its appearance. Brittanys were first imported to America in 1931. They are capable gun dogs and are easily trained as retrievers.

DESCRIPTION

The Brittany is an alert, obedient and inquisitive dog. It is a "natural" breed, requiring little cosmetic care. It should be compactly built, but leggy, giving the appearance of being able to cover a lot of ground. Ruggedness, without clumsiness, is characteristic of the breed. It has no tail, or at most, a tail of not more than 4 inches.

THE SHOW RING

Brittanys should weigh between 30 and 40 pounds, and should stand from 17 1/2 to 20 1/2 inches. The coat should be dense, flat or wiry, not curly. It should be dark orange and white or liver and white. Tricolor (liver and white with some orange) dogs are faulted. Disqualifications in the breed: height under 17 1/2 inches or over 20 1/2 inches, black in the coat or a black nose.

BREEDING AND WHELPING

A Brittany bitch should have first estrus between 9 and 12 months of age. Gestation period is 62 to 63 days. These dogs are free whelpers having an average litter size of seven.

Umbilical hernias are occasionally found. Tails should be docked, leaving one finger's width (3/4 inch) on a 2-day-old dog. Front dewclaws are removed, but removal is not required for show.

RECOGNIZED PROBLEMS

Hip dysplasia is a problem in the breed, as is **unilateral cryptorchidism**. In Norway 33% of 265 Brittany Spaniels x-rayed were dysplastic.[1] **Luxating patellas** have been reported as a problem in this breed.[2] **Epilepsy** is a functional disorder characterized by recurrent seizures or convulsions that are sudden in onset and brief in duration. The condition usually appears at about one year of age and is believed to be hereditary.

Lipfold dermatitis occurs because of the pendulous upper lip in Spaniels. Treatment consists of clipping, cleaning and drying of involved area. Occasional **overshot** and **undershot** bites are found. **Hemophilia A (Factor VIII deficiency)**[3] is a blood disease reported in Brittanys. This is a classic hemophilia, with the familiar signs of prolonged bleeding and reduced, but not absent, Factor VIII. The condition is a sex-linked recessive hereditary trait.

BEHAVIOR

The Brittany adapts easily to apartment life. He is sweet, playful, easily trained and well-mannered. He can be timid if treated harshly.

OLD AGE

The average life span of the Brittany is 12 to 13 years. Some can be hunted as late as 12 years of age, and one Champion was still on the field-trial circuit at 9 years of age.

References
1. Lingaas, F. and Heim, P. "A Genetic Investigation on the Incidence of Hip Dysplasia in Norwegian Dog Breeds," *Norsk-Veterinaertidsskrift*; 1987: 99: 9, 617-623; 22 ref.
2. BRITTANY column, *American Kennel Club Gazette*; July, 1990.
3. Brock, W.E., et al "Canine Hemophilia," *Arch. Path.*; 1963: 76: 464-469.

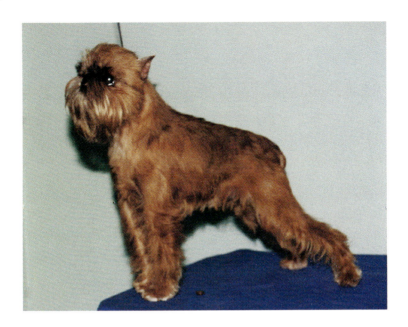

BRUSSELS GRIFFON

ORIGIN AND HISTORY

From the backstreets of Brussels and a somewhat shaded ancestry comes the little Brussels Griffon. Possessing a high intelligence with an almost human expression, the Brussels Griffon has been fondly tagged the "street urchin of Belgium." History recounts that the cabbies of Brussels bred these little stable dogs for use as ratters.

Opinion is divided among breed authorities as to the origin of the breed. Some claim the Griffon to be very old, documenting this claim by a van Eyck painting dated 1434, "The Marriage of Giovanni Arnolfinia."

Others claim the breed to be of a more recent vintage when in the 1880s the Belgian breeders took interest and crossed the little stable dog with a succession of toy breeds — including the Toy Spaniel, Pug, Affenpinscher and Yorkshire Terrier. These crossings resulted in the Brussels Griffon recognized today.

DESCRIPTION

The most influential of these crosses came from the Pug. We can attribute the large head, big eyes, cobby body and deep chest to the Pug. It is an interesting note that many Griffons are born with the Pug "trace" (a dark stripe running down the center of the back); very rarely will one be born with a screw tail. The Pug was also responsible for the smooth-coated Griffon, correctly called the Brabancon. The dark red color, turned-up jaw and rounded forehead comes from the Ruby Spaniel cross.

137

THE SHOW RING

Griffons come in two coat varieties, rough and smooth, and in four colors: red, beige (red and black mixed), black and black and tan. Before 1990 the black smooth was disqualified by the American Standard. The rough coat is similar to a terrier, a non-shedding coat which must be stripped. A hard and wiry coat is preferred. Since coat textures vary greatly it is difficult to predict the exact length of time for a coat to grow or when it will "blow." The whiskers of a rough are never stripped. It is the whiskered face of the rough that makes it so appealing.

The smooth variety is identical to the rough in all respects except for its coat, which resembles the texture of a Pug's. The smooth lacks the adornment of whiskers and, generally, is much more reserved in temperament than its rough brother. This variety does not do as well in the show ring. They make excellent house dogs because grooming is minimal. **The disqualifications include Dudley or butterfly nose, white spot or blaze anywhere on the coat, hanging tongue or overshot bite.**

BREEDING AND WHELPING

Generally the bitch comes into season with a 6-month cycle. It is not rare, however, to find bitches coming into their first heat at 13 to 18 months.

Whelping problems occur most often in small bitches weighing less than 7 pounds. The ideal size of a brood bitch would be in the 8- to 10-pound range. As with many large-headed toy breeds, there may be whelping difficulties. This seems to be the paramount problem within the breed. Litters of six puppies are not rare, but three to four are more normal.

Cleft palates, with or without **hare lips**, are also common.

GROWTH

Most puppies are born with dewclaws on the front legs and rarely on the hind legs. It has become customary to remove all dewclaws when the tail is docked on about the fifth day. The Standard calls for the tail to be docked to one-third.

Whether to crop the ear is a personal choice. Generally speaking, the natural ears fare poorly in the show ring. Poor ears can always be cropped, but to breed beautiful ears should be recognized and rewarded. The ear lends itself to ear cropping very well. The cartilage is adequate to support the ear erect after cropping without external support after surgery. It is advisable to wait until at least 3 months of age before surgery is performed. The usual method of measuring the ear is to fold it down over the eye; the cropped ear should almost, but not quite, touch the lateral canthus of the eye. This will vary depending on the individual dog. The full ear should be cut with an adequate, graceful bell to insure enough cartilage for support.

138

DENTITION

The undershot bite in the breed (an overshot being a breed disqualification) makes dental maintenance extremely important from puppyhood through old age. In puppies, the milk teeth are sometimes slow to fall and must be pulled to allow the permanent teeth to drop normally. It is usually the canine teeth that require extraction, but total dentition should be watched during the teething period.

RECOGNIZED PROBLEMS

Some abnormalities are reported from time to time. The **hydrocephalic puppy** is generally discernible at 6 weeks if not at birth.

A chocolate and even a blue puppy will occasionally occur. The chocolate puppy can be identified by its complete lack of black pigment. The pads are pink or red, the stomach is a deep pink, and the nose is always pink or liver. Some puppies are born with pink noses that turn black within a few days. **Leaker puppies** make their appearance in certain family lines. The severe case can be determined in the nest where the puppy is always wet. These puppies should be euthanized. Puppies with less severe cases will dribble urine constantly, causing problems throughout their lives.

Dislocation of the shoulder has been documented in the breed.[1] **Short skull** has been described as occurring in the breed,[2] as has **distichiasis**. The Brussels Griffon is relatively clear from breed-specific diseases. It is a hearty dog and far removed from the nomenclature tagged to most toys, that of "lap dog."

BEHAVIOR

The Brussels is inquisitive, ever watchful, affectionate and intelligent. He is a barker.

References
1. Campbell, J.R. "Shoulder Lameness in the Dog," *J. Sm. Anim. Prac.*; 1968: 9: 189-198.
2. Stockard, C.R. "The Genetic and Endocrine Basis for Difference in Form and Behavior as Elucidated by Studies of Contrasted Pure Line Dog Breeds and Hybrids," *American Anatomical Memoirs*; Winston Institute of Anatomy and Biology, Philadelphia PA., 1941.

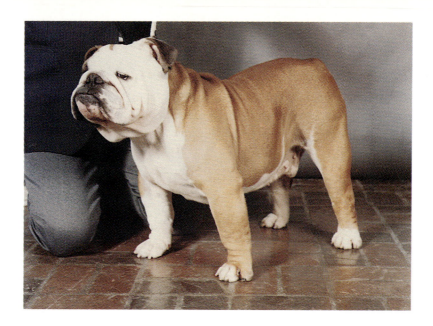

BULLDOG

ORIGIN AND HISTORY

The evolutionary history of the Bulldog has been lost. Long ago the breed became a pet and its original function as a bull-baiter was ended.

The ferocious appearance of the Bulldog belies its calm, friendly temperament. This breed is especially friendly with children.

DESCRIPTION

Today's Bulldogs are shorter, more compact and have more massive heads than their ancestors.

THE SHOW RING

According to the breed Standard, 50 pounds is the ideal weight for males, 40 pounds for bitches. The Bulldogs seen in the show ring are usually slightly heavier.

The breed Standard allows all colors and mixtures of colors except black. The nose and rims of the eyes should be dark and well-pigmented.

The only breed disqualification is a brown or liver-colored nose.

BREEDING AND WHELPING

Because of the short, massive, compact body, accomplishing a tie during breeding is difficult, and frequently the dog and bitch must be held together during mating or artificial insemination must be used.

The gestation period for the Bulldogs is usually 60 days, although in extremely small litters, gestation may exceed 63 days. The average litter size is five.

Bulldog bitches have an unusually hard time whelping.[1,2] Routine cesarean section is recommended for two reasons. First, the dogs have been bred to have large heads and small pelvises, making whelping difficult, and second, since they are a quiescent breed, their muscle tone is poor. Although many bitches can expel one or more puppies, they can rarely sustain the muscle contractions necessary to empty the uterus. An exhausted bitch is a poorer surgical risk for a cesarean section than a bitch that has not been in labor for many hours.

The birth of 160 litters of Bulldogs was supervised from 1954 to 1957. A bitch that successfully whelped an entire litter without assistance was considered a natural whelper. Only 6% of the observed bitches whelped naturally. This small incidence of natural whelpers is further reason for routine cesarean section.

For cesarean section in the Bulldog a flank incision on the lateral aspect of the abdomen is preferable to a ventral midline incision. The characteristic barrel-shaped abdomen of the breed results in more weight per square inch of viscera on the floor of the abdomen than occurs in any other breed. This heavy visceral weight, in conjunction with the abdominal fluids that accompany cesarean section, tends to keep ventral incisions too moist for quick healing. Because the mammary glands of Bulldogs tend to be pendulous during lactation, they also keep a ventral incision moist and resistant to healing. The flank incision avoids areas where abdominal fluids accumulate. Also, excessive visceral weight in this breed tends to help close the flank incision.

RECOGNIZED PROBLEMS

Bulldogs are subject to a number of birth defects. One of these is **cleft palate**.[3,4,5] At birth, the cleft appears to be about the same size in each puppy affected. The cleft originates approximately 0.5 centimeters posterior to the incisor ridge and continues posteriorly through the hard and soft palates. The cleft is 0.2 to 0.3 centimeters wide at birth. The bony palate is always completely open, exposing the medial nasal septum. As the puppies mature, the development of the cleft varies. At 3 months of age, some puppies have a cleft 0.5 centimeters wide while others have one 2 centimeters wide. In mature dogs, the medial nasal septum may grow ventrally until it meets one of the plates of the maxilla's palatine process, thus closing off one side of the nasal passage from the mouth cavity.

If one of these cleft palate puppies is to be raised, it should be removed from its mother and fed via stomach tube. When allowed to nurse, affected puppies invariably aspirate milk and either die from inhalation pneumonia or are stunted and in poor physical condition when they reach the age for corrective surgery.

Records show that of 707 puppies delivered in 150 cesarean sections, 37 had cleft palates. This is approximately 5%, a rather significant percentage of occurrence.

There is a higher incidence of **cryptorchidism** reported in the Bulldog.[6]

Vaginal hyperplasia is seen in this breed.

Another common anomaly in Bulldogs is the **walrus (anasarca) syndrome**.[7] It occurs more often than cleft palates. However, in recent years the incidence has declined. Records of 150 cesarean sections performed on Bulldogs show that 58 of the 707 (8.2%) puppies delivered exhibited the syndrome. All 58 of these puppies were so edematous that they died shortly after birth. In addition, more than 58 puppies showed evidence of mild subcutaneous edema in the regions of the neck and the thorax.[8] Many of these puppies survived.

The heaviest walrus puppy weighs 3 1/4 pounds, whereas the average birth weight of a normal Bulldog puppy is 14 ounces. Usually only one walrus is found in a single litter. In 1959 a litter of six puppies were all walruses. The same bitch subsequently had a litter of four normal, healthy puppies.

Affected puppies are positioned normally in utero, but a much greater quantity of fetal fluid is inside the fetal membranes containing a walrus puppy. A puppy that develops beside a walrus in utero is often normal, although the amount of fluid in the placenta is abnormally large. When a walrus is born, hydramnion is commonly found in all the placenta membranes, although only one puppy is a walrus.

The mode of inheritance is unknown; therefore, the cause of the walrus syndrome is unknown. It has been noted that walrus puppies are born to bitches susceptible to **hydramnion**. Diuretics administered during pregnancy do not eliminate hydramnion or prevent walrus puppies.

Pathology work done by Ladds et al[6] found generalized subcutaneous edema and fluid accumulation in the abdominal and thoracic cavities. The livers consistently had foci of necrosis and subcapsular calcification. Congestion of blood vessels and dilation of lymph vessels were other findings.

Other anomalies seen in the 707 puppies delivered by cesarean section were: **schistosomus reflexus** (6); **cranial bifida** (3); **open urethra** (1); **spinal bifida**[9](1); and **arrested uterine development** (8).

Ectopic ureter was diagnosed in 228 dogs; female to male ratio was 217:11. Six breeds represented more than half of the total cases. The strength of association in certain purebred dogs suggests a familial relationship.[10]

In proper conformation of the Bulldog's skull, the lower jaw protrudes beyond the upper

142

jaw. The lips must cover the teeth. A **wry jaw** is a major fault. In adult dogs, wry jaws develop due to malocclusion. An extra incisor is often present.[11]

Muzzle pyoderma is common in the Bulldog, as well as the Boxer and the Bullmastiff. The condition is evidenced by pustules that develop in the pigmented part of the muzzle. It responds well to antibiotic therapy.

Wrinkle dermatitis is common in the facial and nasal folds and under the tail. It is characterized by mild pruritus and weeping. Dogs afflicted under the tail scoot on the floor, as with an anal gland disorder. The screw tail is especially susceptible to this problem. An affected tail must be cleaned, dried and treated with an antibiotic powder every day. **Facial fold dermatitis** is treated the same way. Bulldogs also have an increased risk for **generalized demodectic mange** and are predisposed to **inhalant allergies**.[12]

Ectropion, **entropion** and **distichiasis** are also common in this breed. These problems must be corrected before chronic conjunctivitis adversely affects the cornea.[13] **Keratitis sicca** is a common sequel to neglected entropion and distichiasis. **Keratoconjunctivitis sicca** is probably seen in Bulldogs more than any other breed.[14] **Membrana nictitans (gland prolapse — haws)** and **chronic follicular conjunctivitis** are also seen in Bulldogs and should be treated surgically.

As in other brachycephalic breeds, **stenotic nares** occur frequently, and when severe, may cause stunted growth. This defect should be corrected while the animal is young. Also seen in these breeds is **oligodendraglioma**.[15]

Bulldogs have been identified as one of a group of breeds with a high risk for **canine lymphoma**.[16,17,18] It has been reported that Bulldogs are predisposed to **cutaneous mast cell tumors**.[19]

The proper ear carriage for a Bulldog is the rose ear. This ear folds upon itself at the posterior aspect. Often a puppy at 8 weeks of age or older has an ear that does not fall into a fold, but falls flat against the face. This can usually be corrected if remedial action is taken early. The fold should be glued into place at the posterior border with a good surgical adhesive. If the dog disturbs this fixation, the ear is sutured in place for a month with stay sutures.

Bulldogs often have an **elongated soft palate**. Unless it is corrected, many affected dogs suffer respiratory failure after strenuous exercise or when overheated. When an affected dog pants, the constant movement of the soft palate can cause the palate to swell and occlude the larynx, usually leading to death by suffocation. Resecting the soft palate can alleviate this condition. When this surgery is performed, the proximal palate should not be clamped, since this may produce sufficient postsurgical swelling in the pharynx and cause further restriction of the airway. The technique of cut and suture, cut and suture with a continuous pattern of absorbable suture using a swaged-on-needle is employed. A tonsillectomy is also performed when hypertrophy of the tonsil tissues is visible.

Everted laryngeal ventricles are another common condition. These saccules of mucous membrane usually return to normal or near-normal after the soft palate is resected. **Hypoplasia of the trachea** has been described in the breed.[20]

Reflex regurgitation immediately after drinking or eating is often encountered in Bulldogs. In most cases the problem is caused by an elongated soft palate, and resecting of the soft palate usually corrects the condition. Reflex regurgitation may persist after the soft palate has been resected. In such cases, **pyloric stenosis** is the cause. Surgical correction of the restricted pylorus relieves the condition. Good surgical technique calls for tracheal intubation of all breeds; however, due to their restricted airways, Bulldogs MUST BE intubated whenever general anesthesia is induced.

Hip dysplasia is common in English Bulldogs as it is in many large breeds. Because of their high pain thresholds, English Bulldogs usually exhibit no clinical signs. Severe hip dysplasia is often found in routine radiographs of champion dogs that have never had an abnormal gait.

One of the most devastating conditions found in the Bulldog is **foreleg lameness** caused by **flaccid shoulder joints**. When loose shoulders are detected in the examination of a new puppy, the owner should be informed that this condition can cause severe chronic strain on the shoulder and elbow joints, which results in a debilitating foreleg **arthritis**. **Elbow dysplasia** has been reported by OFA,[21] and should be ruled out.

Swimmer puppies are common in the Bulldog breed, as they are among puppies of other heavy-bodied, inactive breeds. Affected puppies have flat chests and spraddle legs. Since they cannot stand, the pressure of their body weight flattens the cartilaginous portion of the ribs, decreasing chest space and causing labored breathing. Unlike normal puppies, these fat little pups cannot stand when they are 4 weeks old. They often lie in the corner of the whelping box with their heads elevated and hyperventilate. These pups can be saved by placing "O" rings on their rear legs, above the hocks, and fastening the rings together to force the legs into a 90° angle to the plane of the pelvis. The treatment allows the puppies to draw their legs under them and use them. Also, the owners are instructed to tack down carpeting or burlap in the whelping box so the pups will have secure footing. Newspapers, though convenient, are detrimental to swimmer pups.

Typical signs of **urethral prolapse** are a history of dribbling urine with frank blood, frequent urination, sexual excitement, intermittent erections and the small "red pea" mass at the tip of the penis. Sexual excitement and/or urethral infections are causes of this condition. The

144

condition has occurred primarily in young Bulldogs between 9 and 13 months of age, indicating a predisposing congenital or genetic defect.[22]

Achondroplasia occurs in the Bulldog as an incompletely dominant autosomal trait causing limb shortening and flared metaphyses. Depressed nasal bridge, shortened maxialla and wedge or hemi-vertebrae also occur. Elbow luxations and medial patella luxation can occur due to joint laxity.[23]

Other conditions common in Bulldogs are **brachyury (short tail)**, **valvular pulmonic stenosis**, **hydrocephalus**, **hemivertebra**,[24,25] and **circulatory problems** such as **mitral valve defects** and **arteriovenous fistula**.[26,27,28]

Bulldogs have an increased breed incidence for **hypothyroidism**.[29] This breed is listed as having a slight incidence of **deafness**.[30]

BEHAVIOR

The Bulldog is treasured as a family dog. He is good-natured, conservative, dignified and loyal. He is clean but he is a drooler.

OLD AGE

The average life span of this breed is from 8 to 10 years, although some dogs live to 14 years of age.

References
1. Freak, M.J. "The Whelping Bitch," *Vet. Rec*; 1947: 60: 295-301.
2. Freak, M.J. "Abnormal Conditions Associated with Pregnancy and Parturition in the Bitch," *Vet. Rec*; 1962: 74: 1323-1335.
3. Kirk, R.W. and Bistner, S.I. *Handbook of Veterinary Procedures and Emergency Treatment: Hereditary Defects of Dogs*; 1975: Table 124; 661.
4. Hutt, F.B. "Inherited Lethal Characteristics in Domestic Animals," *Cornell Vet*; 1934: 2. 1-25.
5. Pearce, R.C. "Anomalies of the English Bulldog," *Southwest Vet J.*; 1969: 22:218-220.
6. Bell, Jerold S. DVM "Sex Related Genetic Disorders: Did Mama Cause Them?" American Kennel Club Gazette, Feb. 1994; 76.
7. Ladds, P.W., et al, "Lethal Congenital Edema in Bulldog Pups," *JAVMA*; 1971: 159:81-86.
8. Stockard, C.R. "The Genetic and Endocrine Basis for Differences in Form and Behavior As Elucidated by Studies of Contrasted Pure-Line Dog Breeds and Hybrids," *Am. Anat. Mem.;* Wistar Institute of Anatomy and Biology.
9. Curtis, R.L., et al, "Spinal Bifida in a Stub Dog Stock: Selectively Bred for Short Tails," *Anat. Rec*; 1964: 148:365.
10. Hayes, H.M., Jr., "Breed Association of Canine Ectopic Ureter: A Study of 217 Female

Cases," *J. Sm. Anim. Prac.*; 1984: 25:8, 501-504; 12 ref.

11. Aitchison, J. "Incisor Dentition in Short Muzzled Dogs," *Vet. Rec*; 1964: 76:165-169.

12. Griffin, C., Kowchka, K., McDonald, J.; Current Veterinary Dermatology, the Science and Art of Therapy. Mosby Yearbook, St. Louis, MO 1993: 74, 101.

13. Magrane, W.G. *Canine Ophthalmology*; (3rd ed. Lea & Febiger, Philadelphia, PA 1977) 305.

14. Pearce, Richard C. DVM, Bulldog Column, *American Kennel Club Gazette*; 119, December, 1991.

15. Erickson, F., et al, "Congenital Defects of Dogs III," *Canine Practice*; 1977: 4(6): 48.

16. Madewell, Bruce R., VMD, MS., "Canine Lymphoma," *Veterinarian Clinics of North American Small Animal Practice*; July, 1985: Vol. 15, #4.

17. McCaw, Dudley, DVM, "Canine Lymphosarcoma," AAHA's 56th Annual Meeting Proceedings, 1989.

18. Rosenthal, Robert C., DVM, MS, PhD., "The Treatment of Multicentric Canine Lymphoma," *Veterinarian Clinics of North America Small Animal Practice*; July, 1990: Vol 20, #4.

19. Veterinary News, *The American Kennel Club Gazette*; April, 1990: 44.

20. Suter, P.F., et al, "Congenital Hypoplasia of the Canine Trachea," *JAAHA;* 1972: 8:120-127.

21. Bodner, Elizabeth, DVM., "Genetic Status Symbols," *The American Kennel Club Gazette*; September, 1992.

22. Sinibaldi, K.R. and Green, R.W. "Surgical Correction of Prolapse of the Male Urethra in Three English Bulldogs," *JAAHA;* 1973: 9: 450-453.

23. Ettinger, S.J.; Textbook of Veterinary Internal Medicine. W.B. Saunders, Philadelphia, PA. 1989: 2283.

24. Done, S.H., et al, "Hemivertebra in the Dog: Clinical and Pathological Observations," *Vet. Rec.*; 1975: 96: 313-317.

25. Drew, R.A. "Possible Association Between Vertebral Development and Neonatal Mortality in Bulldogs," *Vet. Rec.*; 1974: 94: 480-481.

26. Mulvihill, J.J. and Priester, W.A. "Congenital Heart Disease in Dogs, Epidemiologic Similarities in Man," *Teratology*; 1973: 7: 73-78.

27. Patterson, D.F. "Epidemiologic and Genetic Studies of Congenital Heart Disease in the Dog," *Circulation Research*; 1968: 23: 171-202.

28. Patterson, D.F. "Canine Congenital Heart Disease, Epidemiological Hypotheses," *J. Sm. Anim. Prac.*; 1971: 12:263-287.

29. Brignac, Michele M. "Congenital and Breed Associated Skin Diseases in the Dog and Cat," *KalKan Forum;* December, 1989: 9-16.

30. Strain, George M. "Deafness in Dogs and Cats," *Proc. 10th ACVIM;* May, 1992.

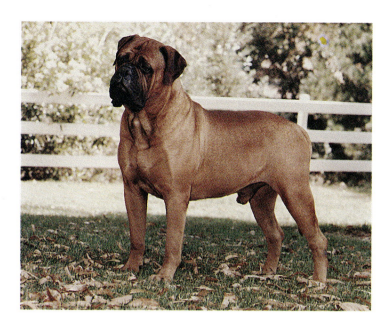

BULLMASTIFF

ORIGIN AND HISTORY

The Bullmastiff is entirely British. It is a man-made breed, approximately 40% Bulldog and 60% Mastiff. Lacking an official breed name, it was called Gamekeeper's Nightdog or Holding Dog.

The hybrid was fearless and would attack on command. The poacher was to be thrown and held, but not mauled. The gamekeeper's life was made much safer by the Bullmastiff, for the poacher faced the death penalty and had nothing to lose.

Recognition was given the Bullmastiff by the English Kennel Club in 1924.

DESCRIPTION

The temperament of the Bullmastiff combines high spirits, reliability, activity, endurance and alertness. It has just enough aggressiveness to be an efficient watch dog.

Members of the breed love children and are protective of the household. They often exhibit this guard-dog instinct as puppies. However, breeders might keep in mind that dogs tend to be more aggressive than bitches.

Dewclaws, if any, are removed. Tails are not docked and ears are not cropped.

THE SHOW RING

Dogs should be 25 to 27 inches at the shoulder. Bitches should be 24 to 26 inches.

Dogs should weigh from 110 pounds to 130 pounds; bitches, 100 to 120 pounds. Within the size limit, the dogs should display proportion and balance.

The coloring should be entirely brindle, fawn or red, without preference. The black muzzle fades toward the eye, and darker ears are required for all colors. Except for a small white spot on the chest, white markings are a serious fault. The coat is short and dense, giving good weather protection. A long, coarse or shaggy coat is a serious fault.

The head is of major importance to Bullmastiff judges. The skull is large and square, broad and deep with a fair amount of wrinkle. This breed often has an extra incisor.[1]

Serious faults include the following: shyness or viciousness, crossing over, stilted or restricted movement, short striding or vertical pitching motion of the rump, rolling of the body or side-to-side movement. Other serious faults are a head lacking wrinkling, a long or narrow muzzle, teeth not covered, light or self-colored eyes, very large ears or rose ears, liver blue or gray nose and an overshot bite. The body should never be shallow in the chest or flat in the ribs. Splay feet, white nails, elbows turned out or in, bowed legs and narrow hips are also faults in the body conformation. Any washed-out or bleached colors are unacceptable.

There are no breed disqualifications.

BREEDING AND WHELPING

The first heat cycle may occur anytime from 6 to 16 months of age and still be considered normal.

Some males are **"lazy breeders"** and an artificial insemination is required.[2] According to Bullmastiff Bulletin, June 1970,[3] 70% of whelpings are normal deliveries; litters average seven puppies.

RECOGNIZED PROBLEMS

Short tails, **screw tails** and **cleft palates** are listed as birth anomalies.

Contact dermatitis, **alopecia** and **eczema** are common complaints in the breed. **Vitiligo** has been recognized in the Bullmastiff.[4]

Other defects are **progressive retinal atrophy**, **glaucoma**, **retinal dysplasia** and **entropion**.[5] **Vaginal hyperplasia** occurs in Bullmastiffs. **Bloat** and **cancer** are the most frequent causes of death in the breed. **Hip dysplasia** is found in this breed, as is **elbow dysplasia.**

Cervical vertebral malformation[6] is a reportedly hereditary problem in Bullmastiffs. The malformation is evidenced in any one of several ways, including **subluxation, malformation of articular facets**, **stenosis of the cranial orifice of the vertebral foramen** and **hyperplasia of the ligamentum flavum.** Age of onset of signs varies from 3 months to 5 years. Signs range from minimal **ataxia** of the hind limbs to **paresis** of both fore and hind limbs, with corresponding gait abnormalities.

      Cerebellar degeneration is believed to be an autosomal recessive cerebellar disease affecting Bullmastiff puppies usually between four and nine weeks of age. Clinical signs include ataxia, most obvious in pelvic limbs, hypermetria, proprioceptive deficits and head tremor which is accentuated as puppies attempt to eat. Prognosis is guarded. There is no treatment.[7]

BEHAVIOR

      Because of his size, this breed needs careful training at an early age. The Bullmastiff needs obedience training to control its natural exuberance. He is an affectionate household pet and can be surprisingly patient with children.

References
1. Aitchison, J. "Incisor Dentition in Short-Muzzled Dogs," *Vet. Rec.* 1964: 76:165-169.
2. Walkowicz, Chris "The Mechanics of Breeding," *American Kennel Club Gazette*; June, 1990: 68.
3. Report of the Health Committee. Reprinted from the Bullmastiff Bulletin, May 1972: 19.
4. Griffin, C., Kowcha, K., McDonnald, J. *Current Veterinary Dermatology, the Art and Science of Therapy.* Mosby Yearbook, St. Louis, MO 1993: 231.
5. Magrane, W.G. *Canine Ophthalmology.* 3rd ed. (Lea & Febiger, Philadelphia, PA.; 1977) 305.
6. Raffe, M.R. and Knecht, C.D. "Cervical Vertebral Malformation in Bullmastiffs," *VM/SAC*; 1978: 14: 593.
7. Ettinger, S.J. *Textbook of Internal Medicine: Diseases of the Dog and Cat.* W.B. Saunders Co., Philadelphia, PA. 1989: 598.

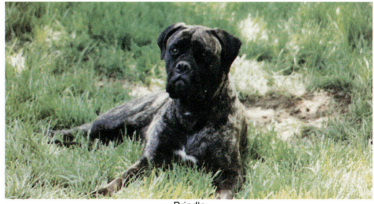

Brindle

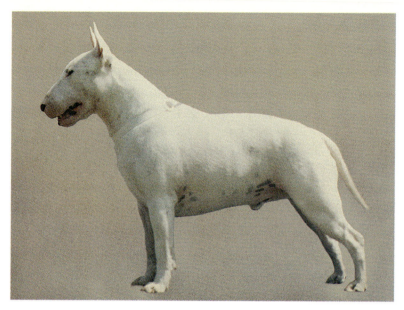
White Bull Terrier

BULL TERRIER (WHITE AND COLORED)

ORIGIN AND HISTORY

The Bull Terrier originated in England by crossing a now extinct white Manchester Terrier and a Bulldog (not necessarily the English Bulldog of today). This cross developed what was then called the Bull and Terrier, a small dog of less than 30 pounds. White was bred to animals with the most white, until the pure white was developed. At about the same period the Dalmatian was introduced to increase the size. The resulting white animal was called the White Cavalier. Later the name Bull Terrier was adopted for the all-white breed. Problems developed in many lines — blue eyes, deafness and slightness of substance. About 1900, the Staffordshire Bull Terrier was introduced, helping to eliminate many of the problems in the animals but presenting the problem of color. The acceptance of the Colored has been a long-running struggle. Presently, England and Canada show Colored and White Bull Terriers together; in the United States they are shown as one breed, with two varieties — White and Colored.

DESCRIPTION

Bull Terriers are unique; they are the gladiators of the canine race. Strongly built and muscular with a determined, intelligent expression, they are full of fire, courageous and amenable to discipline. They think they are human, and they love to please. Usually they are loving companions to their families and adapt well to most environments. They are possessive of their families and distrustful of other dogs. Average weight for a bitch is 40 to 45 pounds and 50 to 56 pounds for a dog, although the size may range from a bitch weighing only 30 pounds to a dog

150

weighing more than 70 pounds.

White Bull Terriers are all white but may have colored markings on the head. Colored Bull Terriers must be predominantly colored — usually with some white. Brindle is the preferred color, although they can also be red or fawn. It is difficult to breed a perfectly marked Colored Bull Terrier with a beautiful full white collar, white feet and white tip on the tail. The coat should be harsh to the touch and have a shine or luster. In the White Bull Terrier, blue eyes are a disqualification; in the colored Bull Terrier blue eyes and a coat predominantly colored constitute a disqualification.

BREEDING AND WHELPING

A bitch usually comes into her first estrus at about 7 months, but she may go as long as 11 months. Usually the bitches come into heat every 6 to 7 months, but some have only one season a year. It is advisable not to breed until the bitch is mature (her second or third season).

Gestation is usually 62 to 63 days. Bull Terriers have a higher incidence of cesareans than the average breed.

Bull Terriers sometimes develop eclampsia. The bitch pants excessively, appears anxious, sometimes carries puppies in her mouth, loses track of her surroundings and may destroy the litter. The commonly accepted treatment is 10 cc of calcium gluconate administered intravenously. A second dose may be administered as needed. The bitch and litter should be watched for several days as hysteria may be prolonged.

Litter size may vary from one to 11, although average litters are five to seven puppies. The pups range in size from 9 to 16 ounces, averaging 11 to 13 ounces. The number of puppies cannot always be predicted by the bitch's size.

White bred to White will always produce white or white with colored head markings. White bred to Colored with white markings can produce all white, white with head markings or colored with white markings. Colored with white markings bred to Colored with white markings can produce all white, white with head markings or colored with white markings.

GROWTH

Dewclaws may or may not be removed. If not removed, they should be clipped to avoid tearing. Tails are never docked. A short tail is desirable — heavy at the croup and tapering to the tip. The hair growing beyond the tip of the tail should be clipped and tapered to give the tail a clean look. Ears on Bull Terriers are never cropped; they should stand by themselves, usually at about 8 to 12 weeks. At least one breeder helps achieve erectness by placing a cone-shaped piece of moleskin on the inside of the ear at 6 weeks. Usually the ears are up within a week; occasionally the ears need additional taping.

DENTITION

Bite should be scissors or over as a pup's level bite sometimes goes under. Underbite is a serious fault. Sometimes the adult teeth come in while the baby teeth are still retained. These must be removed to prevent problems with the normal bite pattern.

RECOGNIZED PROBLEMS

Bull Terriers are usually vigorous animals with few health problems. **Umbilical and inguinal hernias** are listed as genetic disorders by several researchers.[1,2,3]

Owners should give only large knuckle bones to bull Terriers, as they are inclined to swallow small bones whole; they also like to chew leather.

A bald spot sometimes appears on the center top side of the tail. This is called **"stud tail"** and is caused by excessive secretion of the sebaceous glands in the area. It is best treated by alcohol and/or bathing with shampoo designed for oily skin. The **"spinning syndrome"** is seen in Bull Terriers and is believed to be a form of epilepsy.[4]

Photo-induced folliculitis/furunculosis of Bull Terriers primarily affects the flank and abdomen. At first, regular sunburning occurs and the affected areas are erythematous and scaly. Running a hand over affected areas of skin may produce a bumpy feeling, as the white areas of skin are thickened, while pigmented areas are normal. At this stage, biopsy reveals variable degrees of superficial perivascular dermatitis with necrotic keratinocytes. Superficial dermal fibrosis may be prominent. Solar elastosis may be seen. After two or more summers, the sunburned areas become thicker and develop erosion, ulceration, crusting and comedomes, and they occasionally develop necrosis, fistulae and scarring. At this stage, a skin biopsy may reveal follicular cysts, pyogranulomatous inflammation and premalignant actinic keratosis. Finally, a squamous cell carcinoma can develop, especially if the dog continues to be exposed to direct sunlight. Such squamous cell carcinomas should be removed surgically, and the procedure should be repeated if necessary. There is always a danger of metastasis.

Puppies that are born **deaf** should be put to sleep. Deafness is not limited to one breeding line.[5,6,7] A 1992 study by Dr. George M. Strain found that of 238 white Bull Terriers, 19.3% were unilaterally or bilaterally deaf. In 213 colored Bull Terriers, 2.3% were unilaterally deaf.[8]

Acrodermatitis is an inherited autosomal recessive trait causing a **lethal condition** in Bull Terriers. Puppies show **retardation**, severe skin disease. They get ulcerated crusty lesions on their feet, ears, muzzle and body orifices. The condition may improve temporarily with antibiotic therapy but resists all treatment. Retarded growth is the most chronic characteristic. By 10 weeks of age affected pups weigh 1/2 as much as normal littermates. Skin lesions occur by the 6th week along with loss of facial hair. Diarrhea and respiratory infections develop.

152

They usually die at about 7 months of age of severe bronchopneumonia.[9] **Acrodermatitis** has been reported as a problem of defective zinc metabolism, but the affected dogs did not respond to oral zinc supplements.[10]

OLD AGE

Bull Terriers usually live to be 12 years or older. The adult dog is easy to live with, still requiring love, but not so demanding of play time as when younger. It likes its own private place to sleep and eat, regular feeding and exercise.

The teeth of the older dog should be regularly checked to ensure proper chewing and eating. Any cysts on the body should be removed before a serious condition develops.

References

1. Phillips, J.M. and Felton, T.M. "Hereditary Umbilical Hernias in Dogs," *J.Hered.*; 1939:30:433-435.
2. Kirk, R.W. and Bister, S.I. *Handbook of Veterinary Procedures and Emergency Treatment:Hereditary Defects of Dogs.* 1975: Table 124, 661.
3. Erickson, F., et al., *Congenital Defects in Dogs: A Special Reference for Practitioners.* Ralston Purina (reprint from *Canine Practice,*Veterinary Practice Publishing Co.)
4. Bull Terrier Column, *American Kennel Club Gazette;* January, 1992.
5. Burns, M. and Fraser, M.N. *Genetics of the Dog.* (Oliver and Boyd, London, England, 1966).
6. Hirschfield, W.K. Fokkerji op Genotype. Gene en Phoenen 3:1-5;1956.
7. Young, G.B. "Inherited Defects of Dogs," *Vet. Rec.* 1955: 67:15-19.
8. Strain, George M. "Deafness in Dogs and Cats," *Proc. 10th Forum ACVIM;* May, 1992.
9. Brignac, Michele M. "Congenital and Breed Associated Skin Diseases in the Dog and Cat," *KalKan Forum;* December, 1989.
10. Smits, B., Croft, D.L., and Abrams, G.G. & C.G. "Lethal Acrodermatitis in Bull Terriers: A Problem of Defective Zinc Metabolism," *Veterinary Dermatology;* 1991: 2:91-96.

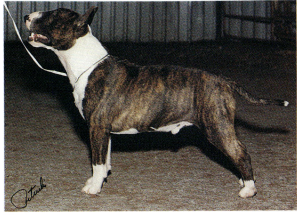
Colored Bull Terrier

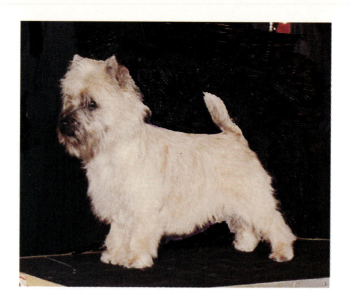

CAIRN TERRIER

ORIGIN AND HISTORY

The modern Cairn Terrier is the result of trying to preserve the oldtime working terrier of the Isle of Skye. The latter were working terriers with courage for bolting otter, foxes and other vermin from among rocks, cliffs, and ledges of the wild shores on the misty isle.

DESCRIPTION

Equally adaptable to country or city living, the Cairn has a cheeky, sometimes exasperating character. He is restless and curious about any disturbance. Unlike most terriers, he won't start a fight but he will respond if attacked. He is affectionate and totally devoted to his owners. The tail is not docked. Back dewclaws should be removed. Front dewclaws may be removed, but it is not required.

THE SHOW RING

The Cairn's typical coat has a harsh, hard, outer jacket and a soft, furry undercoat. Any color except white is acceptable. Dark muzzle, ears, and tail tip are desirable. Cairns are not trimmed except for minor "touch ups."

The ideal dog weighs 14 pounds and is 10 inches tall; the bitch weighs 13 pounds and is 9 1/2 inches tall. Their length should be 14 1/2 to 15 inches. **There are no breed disqualifications.**

RECOGNIZED PROBLEMS

Cairns suffer from **globoid cell leukodystrophy, (Krabbe type)**.[1,2,3] In man, Krabbes disease is under the broad category of demyelinating diseases, a group of nervous diseases characterized primarily by destruction of myelin sheaths and subsequent glial capacity to nurture or maintain myelin or to degradate myelin breakdown products to the fatty acid state. It also implies that the demyelination is inherited and progressive.

This disease has been seen in this country and Europe, predominantly in Cairn Terriers and West Highland White Terriers. Most cases have been attributed to heredity. The signs are seen in puppies a few weeks to a few months of age; coordination and locomotion are primarily affected. Motor defects may progress to paralysis. Visual deficiency may be seen. Tremors and loss of spinal and postural reflexes are common.

The diagnosis should be differentiated from other progressive CNS diseases such as **distemper syringomyelia**, **toxoplasmosis**, and **spinal anomalies**. **Hip dysplasia** and **myasthenia gravis** might be considered. Histological examination must establish the absolute diagnosis.

Cranial mandibular osteopathy[4] occurs in the breed. Other syndromes are **hemophilia A**[5] and **hemophilia B**,[6] **inguinal hernia**,[7] and **cystinuria**.

Inhalant allergies tend to be a significant problem in Cairn Terriers.[8]

Two eye problems of Cairn Terriers are **secondary glaucoma** and **aberrant cilia**.[9]

Cerebellar hypoplasia is most commonly observed in cats as a result of prenatal infection with panleukopenia virus. It has also been observed in Cairn Terriers. A specific etiology has not been established. Heredity has been suggested in progressive ataxia in smooth-hair terriers and in cerebellar abiotrophy in Kerry Blue Terriers. In the latter, the clinical signs were progressive; two of the animals reported by Knecht (1979)[10] showed nonprogressive signs, and one affected dog became clinically normal with age.

Some microscopic features were found in all the dogs necropsied. Marked gliosis and demyelination of the cerebellum were not observed. Focal diminution of granular cells was occasionally seen. Degenerative changes of the Purkinje cells were not present and the deep cerebellar and olivary nuclei were normal.

In recessive transmission, consanguinity of the parents is expected when a litter from normal parents contains approximately one affected progeny in four animals. Examination of the five-generation pedigree of one affected dog revealed no ancestor common to both paternal and maternal lineage. Thus, if the transmission of cerebellar hypoplasia is recessive, it occurs in more than one bloodline and may even be widespread in the breed. **Primary cystic disease** has been reviewed in a Cornell study of hereditary nephropathies.[11] **Pyruvate kinase deficiency** has been reported in Cairn Terriers (see Basenji).

There is a higher than usual incidence of **crytorchidism** in the Cairn Terrier.[12]

Bronchial esophageal fistula has been reported in this breed.[13] Dogs with this condition develop chronic pneumonia or even a pyothorax.

BEHAVIOR

The Cairn is adaptable, but restless, having to investigate each disturbance. He won't start a fight but will be happy to finish it if attacked. He is affectionate and can be jealous of his owners' attention to someone else. The Cairn leash trains the easiest of all terriers.

OLD AGE

Cairn Terriers live long lives if not afflicted by one of the above mentioned anomalies.

References

1. Kirk, R.W.; Bistner, S.I.: *Handbook of Veterinary Procedures and Emergency Treatment: Hereditary Defects of Dogs.* 1975; Table 124, 661.
2. Fletcher; et al; "Globoid cell leukodystrophy (Krabbe Types) in the Dog." *JAVMA* 149:165-172; 1966.
3. Hirth, R.S.; Nielson, S.W.: "A Familial Canine Globoid Cell Leukodystrophy (Krabbe Type)." *J. Sm. Anim. Prac.* 8:569-575; 1967.
4. Riser, W.H. et al: "Canine Craniomandibular Osteopathy." *J. Am. Vet. Rad. Soc.* 8:23-20; 1967.
5. Hoving, T. et al: "Experimental Hemostasis in Normal Dogs with Congenital Disorders of Blood Coagulation." Blood. 30:636; 1967.
6. Roswell, H.C. et al: "A Disorder Resembling Hemophilia (Christmas Disease) in Dogs." *JAVMA*, 137:247-250; 1960.
7. Hayes, H.M.: "Congenital Umbilical and Inguinal Hernia in Cattle, Horses, Swine, Dogs and Cats: Risk by Breed and Sex Among Hospital Patients." *Am. J. Vet. Res.* 35:839-842; 1974.
8. Griffin, C., Kwochka, K., McDonald, J. *Current Veterinary Dermatology, the Art and Science of Therapy.* Mosby Yearbook, St. Louis, MO 1993: 101.
9. Magrane, W.G.: *Canine Ophthalmology*, 3rd ed. Lea & Febiger, Philadelphia, Pa., 1977; 305.
10. Knecht, C.D., et al: Cerebellar Hypoplasia in Chow Chow. *JAAJA.* 15(1):pp 51-52; 1979.
11. Picut, CA; Lewis, RM. "Comparative Pathology of Canine Hereditary Nephropathies: An Interpretive Review." Vet. Res. Comm. 1987, 11:6, 561-581; 91 ref.
12. Bell, Jerold S. DVM "Sex Related Genetic Disorders: Did Mama Cause Them?" *American Kennel Club Gazette*, Feb. 1994; 76.
13. King, L.G., DVM "Respiratory Congenital Disorders" Western Veterinary Conference, Feb. 1994.

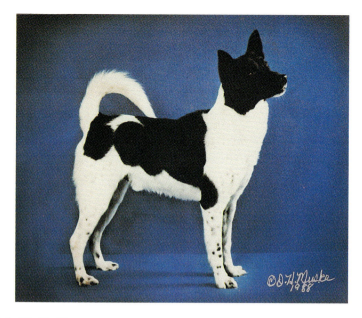

CANAAN DOG

ORIGIN AND HISTORY

This breed is indigenous to Israel, dating back many centuries. Formerly known only in the Middle East, it has in recent years also found favor in Europe and the United States. It is primarily used as a watch dog for herds or houses, and as a guide dog for the blind. During the conflicts in Israel, these dogs were used as mine detectors (where they proved superior to the mechanical devices) and to carry messages over the rocky desert and to find the wounded.[1]

DESCRIPTION

The Canaan is a lively, elegant, medium sized dog. The Canaan also has an extremely high capacity for learning and is an outstanding companion dog.[2]

THE SHOW RING

Dogs should be 20 to 24 inches tall, and weigh from 45 to 55 pounds. Bitches should be 19 to 23 inches tall, and weigh from 35 to 45 pounds. The head should be well proportioned with a deep muzzle and a dark nose. Eyes are almond-shaped, ears are erect, and the tail is of medium length with a slight plume. The front legs should be perfectly straight with a light bone structure. The body is robust but not massive. The coat is of medium length, coarse, with a good undercoat. These dogs have a pronounced semi-annual shed. Colors are: predominantly white with marking(s) of color, or solid colored with or without white trim; black, all shades of brown, sandy to reddish or liver are allowed. Shadings of brown, tan or rust, on a black dog, or black on a brown or tan dog are frequently seen. The solid colored white dog without a mask is not allowed. The mask is a desired and distinguishing feature of the predominantly white dog. The mask is the same color as the body markings on the dog. The mask is basically symmetrical and must cover from the rear base of the ears to at least the start of the muzzle and extend down onto the cheeks so that the eyes and ears are completely covered. The only allowed white in the mask is a white blaze and/or white on the muzzle below the mask.

Major faults: Absence of mask, half-mask or grossly asymmetrical mask on predominantly white dogs and other than prick ears in adult dogs. **Disqualification: gray color and/or brindle color as in tiger striped.**

BREEDING AND WHELPING

The Canaan bitch often has her first estrus as early as 6 months of age, but most are 8 or 9 months old. Gestation is the normal 60 to 63 days. The average litter is of four to six puppies that weigh from 13 to 16 ounces.

RECOGNIZED PROBLEMS

Hip dysplasia has been seen in the breed, but the percentage (.2%) is among the lowest. **PRA** was seen in early stock, but the Parent Club maintains a health chart where reported genetic problems are recorded, and the information is available to anyone breeding a litter. This has helped in eliminating such problems. **Thyroid imbalance** is rare, as is **diabetes**, having been reported only once. **Epilepsy** is seen in the breed and an occasional **unilateral cryptorchid** is seen.

BEHAVIOR

Pugnacious, devoted, gentle, home-loving and extremely clever, the Canaan is highly trainable and an exceptional companion dog.

OLD AGE

The Canaan will live to be 15 to 17 years old. Death is from the usual geriatric debilities.

References
1. *Illustrated Book of Dogs*, Reader's Digest, 1989
2. *Guide to Dogs*, Simon and Schuster. 1980

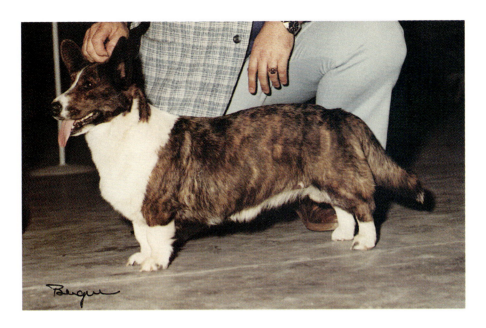

CARDIGAN WELSH CORGI

ORIGIN AND HISTORY

The Corgi is a descendant of the same family that produced the Dachshund, but has been bred separately since being introduced to Wales by the Celts 3,000 years ago. The breed's original use was as a cattle and game working dog, but it has largely been a pet in recent years.

DESCRIPTION

These dogs have a good, even-tempered and friendly nature. The Cardigans are large and more robust than the Pembroke Corgis. Corgis make excellent house pets. They are amusing, intelligent, loyal, affectionate and good with children. They are suspicious of strangers.

THE SHOW RING

Corgis are small and stocky, being only 10 1/2 inches to 12 1/2 inches at the highest point of the shoulder and usually between 36 and 43 inches from the nose to tail tip. Length to tail base should be height plus 50 percent. The coat color should be red, sable, red-brindle, black-brindle, black, tricolor, or blue merle (other merles not allowable). They often have white flashings on chest, neck, face, feet or tail. The coat is medium length and harsh in texture.

The ears are large and rounded but should be held erect. The tail is not docked but should be long and have a moderate brush (like a fox). The tail is set low on the body line and carried low. Hind dewclaws, if any, are removed. **Disqualifications are drop ears, blue eyes, or partially blue eyes in any coat color other than blue merle, nose other than solid black,** except in blue merles, any color other than specified, body color predominantly white.

BREEDING AND WHELPING

Breeding problems are infrequent. Litter size is usually 5 or 6, with 8 pups not being uncommon and 13 reported. Birth weight is usually 8 to 16 ounces. Not many defects are noticed at birth; some lines have curly tails occasionally, and **cleft palates** are seen.

RECOGNIZED PROBLEMS

Corgis have been reported to be at a high risk for **urolithiasis** compared to other breeds.[1] Congenital problems of the Corgi are **progressive retinal atrophy**[2] and **secondary glaucoma**.[3] **Orthopedic problems** are occasionally encountered in these chondrodysplastic dogs. Rapidly growing pups will sometimes develop **sprain of the shoulder joint capsule**[4] if allowed to descend stairs frequently. This problem will respond to confinement and gradual physical therapy and return to exercise. Ramps will help prevent the problem. The Cardigan is less susceptible to **epilepsy** than Pembrokes.

The **carpus**, which are crooked laterally up to 45 degrees, will sometimes cause problems in individuals with excessive deviation. **Back problems** occur in older dogs, particularly if they are overweight and poorly exercised. **Luxated intervertebral lumbar discs** and **posterior paresis** are not uncommon. **Neck pain** may occur due to **calcified cervical discs**.

BEHAVIOR

The Corgi is a pleasant companion dog. He is lively, affectionate and easily trained. The Cardigan Corgi is suspicious of strangers.

OLD AGE

Average life span is 10 to 12 years. When treating these dogs it should be remembered that they are moderately sized dogs with short legs.

References
1. Bovee, KC, McGuire, T. "Qualitative and Quantitative Analysis of Uroliths in Dogs: Definitive Determination of Chemical Type." *JAVMA*. 1984: 185: 9, 983-987 18 ref.
2. Keep, J.M.: "Clinical Aspects of Progressive Retinal Atrophy in the Cardigan Corgi." *Aust. Vet. J.* 48:197; 1972.
3. Magrane, W.G.: *Canine Ophthalmology*, 3rd ed. Lea & Febiger, Philadelphia, Pa., 1977.
4. Miller, C.O.: "Glenjoy," Dent Road, Churchton, Maryland — Personal Communication.

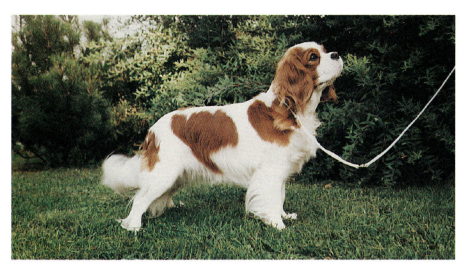

CAVALIER KING CHARLES SPANIEL

ORIGIN AND HISTORY

The Cavalier King Charles Spaniel of today is recognized in many European paintings of the 17th, 18th and 19th centuries in works by Van Dyke, Titian, Goya and de Hoch. During the latter half of the 19th century the breed became virtually extinct, having been bred down to the short-faced, apple-headed variety now known as the English Toy Spaniel (King Charles in the United Kingdom).

In 1926, Roswell Eldridge, an American visiting England, was shocked to find none of the "nosey little Van Dyke spaniels" in existence. He offered a cash prize for three consecutive years at the Crufts Show to the dog most resembling the old type.

Breeders, with this incentive, achieved a rebirth of the Cavalier by using long-faced culls from the short-faced litters, introducing the larger Blenheim and Marlborough Spaniels and also the drop-eared Papillon. In 1945, the breed was considered established enough to be granted registry by the English Kennel Club.

Relatively rare in the United States, the breed is fast becoming too popular in Britain, where more than 10,000 Cavaliers are registered annually.

Known as "Comforters" and "Spaniells Gentell" in the 17th century, Cavaliers remainpretty, happy, "pet" dogs. Today's Cavalier, however, is blessed with a sporting instinct doubtless inherited from its larger spaniel ancestors and should be considered a sporting toy dog rather than a lap dog.

It needs both physical and mental exercise as well as the constant companionship of its owner to fulfill its potential as an affectionate, natural, well-adjusted companion.

DESCRIPTION

An active, graceful, well-balanced dog, the Cavalier King Charles is very gay and free in action. It is fearless and sporting in character yet gentle and affectionate.

THE SHOW RING

Head: Skull appears flat because of the high placement of the ears. Eyes are large, round, set well apart and very dark. Stop is shallow, nose at least 1 1/2 inches long. Muzzle tapered but generous, scissors bite (level bite acceptable), nostrils well-developed and black.

Neck: Fairly long with muscle at the crest to form a graceful arch. Set smoothly into well laid back shoulders.

Body: Short-coupled, well-sprung ribs, moderate chest with plenty of heart room. Level top-line. Strong, well-muscled hindquarters. Tail set so as to be carried level with the back. Docking is optional, and no more than one-third should ever be removed; one-quarter is usually enough. Tails of broken colors must have a white tip; in some cases, this may preclude docking. All dewclaws should be removed at two to four days.

Legs and Feet: Forelegs straight, bone moderate, elbows close to the sides. Hindlegs moderately muscled, stifles well turned, hocks well let down. Pasterns strong, feet compact with well-cushioned pads. The dog stands level on all four feet.

Coat and Colors: The coat is long, silky and free from curl.

Only four colors are permitted:

1. Blenheim: Rich chestnut well broken up on a pearly white ground. The "Blenheim spot" or lozenge in the center of the head is desirable but not required.

2. Tricolor: Jet black markings well broken up on a pearly white ground, with rich chestnut over the eyes, on cheeks, inside ears and around the vent.

3. Ruby: Whole-colored rich red.

4. Black-and-Tan: Jet black with rich red over eyes, on cheeks, inside ears, on chest, legs, and underside of tail.

There should be no white hairs on whole-colored dogs, and heavy freckling or ticking on broken-colored dogs is to be discouraged.

Size: Height 12 to 13 inches at the withers; weight in proportion, from 13 to 18 pounds. Slight variation is permitted, and an undersized weedy specimen should be penalized just as heavily as an oversized one.

Faults: Light eyes, undershot mouths, crooked jaws, pale noses, weak pasterns, cowhocks, gay tails. **Bad temper, nervousness or meanness are not to be tolerated and are considered disqualifying faults.**

BREEDING AND WHELPING

The Cavalier comes into estrus from 6 to 9 months of age, with 7 months being average. Normally a bitch's season lasts three weeks and repeats at six-month intervals, though intervals of both five and seven months are not uncommon. Dogs attain puberty at 7 to 8 months, and can be successfully used at stud at 10 months.

Matings are usually accomplished easily, but should always be supervised. It is recommended that a bitch intended for breeding be examined prior to her season to be sure a natural mating is possible. Pregnancy and whelping seldom present any problems. Cavaliers are natural whelpers and exceptionally devoted mothers. The average litter numbers four or five, although litters of eight and nine do occur. When litters consist of only one or two whelps, breeders should not be alarmed if the puppies are very slow to walk. (One breeder was advised to destroy a litter of three because they were not walking at 5 weeks. At 7 weeks the litter started to walk; at 11 weeks none showed any abnormality of gait or construction.) Whelps weigh from 5 to 8 ounces, though some of 3 and 14 ounces have survived without later difficulty. No consistent birth defects have been noted, but whelps should be checked for **cleft palate** if any problem occurs in nursing. **Umbilical hernias** occur with some frequency in young puppies (6 to 12 weeks). These seldom require medical attention as by 4 to 6 months they become small, fatty deposits with no possibility of strangulation. There seems to be no hereditary factor, nor are such hernias found to be the result of rough treatment by the dam at whelping. There is no aesthetic problem, as the hernias are completely hidden when the dog grows its full coat.

Puppies of the Blenheim variety can be whelped almost completely ivory colored; in a few days the red markings become obvious. Other Blenheims are whelped with a rich red already defined. Mismarks (clown-faces, broken colors with heavy smudges, solids with white areas) make fine pets but not good breeding stock. However, a few white hairs on solids will probably disappear by the time the puppy is 6 months.

GROWTH

Puppy growth is quite rapid, with pups of 2 months weighing about 4 pounds. The size of a puppy at whelping is seldom indicative of its full-grown size, except that puppies of a very small litter tend to start and finish considerably larger than those of a litter of six or more. Dams are reluctant to wean before 7 weeks, at which time they effectively refuse to nurse and puppies usually adapt to dry puppy kibble with no difficulty.

Diet is vitally important. Cavaliers should be maintained on sensible, dry food with a minimum of owner's additives! Obesity is their greatest enemy, and they should be fed as a small sporting dog, never as a lap dog.

The Cavalier coat requires no trimming, except for the hair between the pads under the foot — any other trimming is expressly forbidden in the Standard. The Cavalier should only be shampooed when absolutely necessary. The use of a brush and comb three or four times a week makes bathing unnecessary, and, except for regular nail trimming, is all the grooming a Cavalier requires.

Cavaliers are easily handled, amenable and unusually stoic. However, they must be handled properly — firmly held and supported both front and rear — when picked up. When removed from a crate or cage, they should never be pulled by the forelegs or lifted by the scruff of the neck. They should be brought out with one hand under the tail and one under the chest.

Annual veterinary checkups are imperative, with special attention given to the skin, eyes and ears. Cavaliers are better-than-average patients and can be nursed at home to great advantage provided the owner follows instructions.

DENTITION

Undershot mouths can, and frequently do, correct up to 18 months of age; this is a very common occurrence. Overshot mouths are far less common, and less likely to correct, although they can finish as scissors bites.

After Cavaliers are 6 years old they should have their teeth cleaned annually.

RECOGNIZED PROBLEMS

Luxated patella occurs in this breed. Affected stock should not be used for breeding. **Monorchidism** and **cryptorchidism** occur infrequently; dog puppies should ideally have both testicles descended by 8 weeks. Puppies that have been slower, up to 4 months, have not subsequently been found to sire males that were slow to descend. A dog that does not have both testicles normally descended by 6 months should not be used for breeding even if they descend later.

Cardiovascular problems are reported in some families and there may be a hereditary factor. A **murmur** developing at 7 to 9 years often seems to be asymptomatic, with those affected living to 14 and 15 years without medication.

The association between breed, sex and **canine heart valve incompetence** was investigated by an observational study of a veterinary hospital population. Odds ratio estimations from 370 affected dogs and 9028 controls of 15 breeds revealed significant positive associations between some small and medium-sized breeds, including the Cavalier King Charles Spaniel, and heart valve incompetence and significant negative associations between some large breeds and heart valve incompetence. The log odds, determined for each breed and sex, indicated that males were more susceptible.[1]

Hallucinatory behavior, also called Fly-catching, is recorded in English publications.

Onset of symptoms ranges from 8 to 18 months; post-mortem evaluation of two cases studied revealed no pathology, except slight enlargement of the kidneys in one. Some consider it a manifestation of **epilepsy**.

Corneal dystrophy has been noted in several cases. The condition has usually cleared itself without medication within a period of 6 to 18 months, leaving no scars.

Hereditary cataract has been seen in the breed.[2]

Skin irritation in the form of dandruff is frequently reported in puppies from 4 to 10 months. Careful checks and scrapings should be made because in several instances scurf blamed on "puppy coat changing" or "change of diet" has been found to be due to cheyletiella mite. Ear mites can be a problem if left unchecked, particularly since leathers are fairly long and thick, preventing adequate circulation.

The King Charles Spaniel has become a very popular breed recently, an event that has focused attention on a special problem with **episodic weakness** and **episodic collapse** in some members of the breed. Wayne L. Berry of the University of Pretoria, South Africa, says that the condition, which has been known for about the last 20 years, develops after exercise. The dog walks with a stiff and stilted stalking gait, holding its head close to the ground and its rump raised. The animal collapses to one side but retains consciousness. After recovery, the dog appears to be normal. Equally puzzling is the fact that both blood tests and electromyographic examinations are normal. Although muscle lesions have been identified in affected dogs, the significance of the lesions is not known. The best that can be said at this time is that the episodic collapse appears to be a rare inherited disorder but is not caused by the same events that cause myasthenia gravis.

BEHAVIOR

The Cavalier is an excellent companion dog. He has outstanding senses of vision and smell. He is lively and outgoing.

OLD AGE

The Cavalier is a natural dog whose Breed Standard was drawn up to avoid any potential health hazards resulting from any exaggerations. They should live a medically uneventful life with an expectancy of 13 to 15 years.

References
1. Thrusfield, M.V., Aitken, C.G.G. "Observations on Breed and Sex in Relation to Canine Heart Valve Incompetence," *J. Sm. Anim. Prac.*; 1985: 709-717; 14 ref.
2. Barnett, K.C. "The Diagnosis and Differential Diagnosis of Cataract in the Dog," *J. Sm. Anim. Prac.*; 1985: 26:6, 305-316; 20 ref.

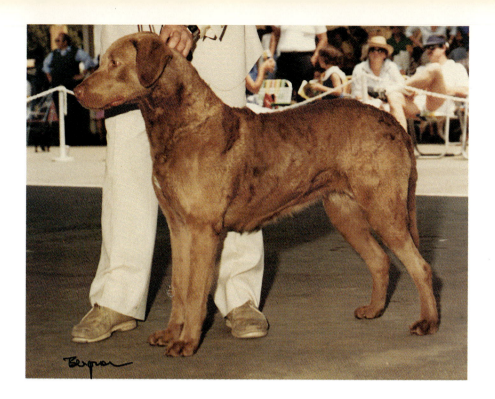

CHESAPEAKE BAY RETRIEVER

ORIGIN AND HISTORY

In the year 1807 an English brig was wrecked off the coast of Maryland, and the crew and cargo were rescued by the American ship Canton. Also rescued were two Newfoundland puppies, a dingy red dog named Sailor and a black bitch named Canton, after the rescuing ship. Presented to the gentleman who gave hospitality to the sailors of the wrecked brig, the two dogs were found to possess wonderful qualities as retrievers. They were mated with many nondescript dogs, then used for retrieving and probably crossed with the flat-coated or curly-coated retrievers. By 1885 a definite type of dog had developed, a breed known for its prowess in the rough, icy waters of Chesapeake Bay, where dogs were often called upon to retrieve 200 to 300 ducks per day.[1]

DESCRIPTION

Chesapeakes stand higher than or as high in the rear as they do in the shoulder. Some observers erroneously judge this to be swayback.

Back dewclaws should be removed; front dewclaws are optional. Litters average seven to 10, and puppies weigh from 10 to 16 ounces.

166

THE SHOW RING

Males should stand 23 to 26 inches and weigh **65 to 80** pounds. Females should stand 21 to 24 inches and weigh **55 to 70** pounds.

They may vary in color from dark brown to a faded tan or deadgrass. Deadgrass varies from a tan to a dull straw. A white spot on the chest and/or toes is permitted but solid is preferred.

Disqualifications include back dewclaws, black color, white on any part of the body other than feet, breast or belly. Dogs are also disqualified with feathers on the tail or legs more than 1 3/4 inches long, with undershot or overshot mouth, with coat curly or tendency to curl all over body and specimens unworthy or lacking in breed characteristics.

RECOGNIZED PROBLEMS

Reported abnormalities include **progressive retinal atrophy** and **entropion**.[2] OFA reports a decrease in frequency of **hip dysplasia** from 1974 to 1984.[3] **Cerebellar abiotrophy** has been reported by breeders as occurring in the breed.

BEHAVIOR

The Chessie has no peer when it comes to guarding its family, especially the children. There are many stories of drowning children being rescued by the family Chesapeake Bay Retriever. He is lively, cheerful and trainable.

OLD AGE

They are a hearty breed and average life span covers 10 to 13 years.

References
1. American Kennel Club, *Complete Dog Book*. 18th ed. (Howell Book House,New York, N.Y. 1992) 54-57.
2. Magrane, W.G. *Canine Ophthalmology.* (Lea & Febiger, Philadelphia, PA.,1968).
3. Corley, E.A. and Hogan, P.M. "Trends in Hip Dysplasia Control: Analysis of Radiographs Submitted to the Orthopedic Foundation for Animals," *JAVMA*; 1985: 187:8, 805-809; 8 ref.

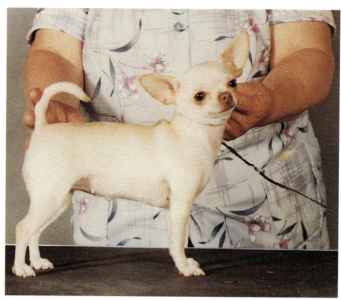
Smooth Coat Chihuahua

CHIHUAHUA

ORIGIN AND HISTORY

The diminutive Chihuahua, a native of the Americas, was described by Christopher Columbus.

Chihuahuas are remarkably clannish. They thrive together but will adjust to other breeds.

DESCRIPTION

The Chihuahua breed includes two varieties; smooth-coat and the less familiar long-coat. The latter type is distinguished by its full, fluffy ruff, bushy "culottes" on the rear legs, fringes on the legs and ears and a plumed tail. As a neonate, the long-coat Chihuahua has a soft, wavy coat similar to that of a newborn Poodle or Cocker Spaniel.

Color varies greatly among Chihuahuas, both at birth and at maturity. Because of their wide range of coloring and multiple patterning genes, they are unusually difficult to breed for color.

Chihuahuas should be carefully protected from sharp blows on the head because an open fontanel is not unusual in this breed. The opening may be quite large in relationship to the size of the dog. The breed Standard calls for a well-rounded, apple-domed skull, with or without molera (open fontanel). Some uninformed veterinarians have alarmed new owners of a Chihuahua by referring to the fontanel as a deformity.

THE SHOW RING

Breed disqualifications include cropped or bobbed tails and broken down or

cropped ears, or a dog weighing more than 6 pounds. A coat so thin that the dog looks bare will disqualify a long-coated Chihuahua. Listed as serious faults are undershot or overshot bites and any distortion of the mouth.

Rear dewclaws, prevalent in some bloodlines, should be removed. Removal of front dewclaws is optional.

BREEDING AND WHELPING

Chihuahua puppies often suffer from **hypoglycemia** from the time they are weaned until they reach maturity. Episodes of low blood sugar seem to be precipitated by stress resulting from a change of home, change in pen-mates, etc. Any normally healthy puppy found in a dazed condition should immediately be given syrup or honey thinned with warm water, administered with an eye dropper or spoon if the puppy will not drink. Even a semiconscious animal will usually respond to this treatment within a few minutes. If response does not follow, glucose should be given subcutaneously or intravenously.

The rate of growth and maturation varies among different bloodlines. However, the weight of a Chihuahua at 3 months is usually doubled at maturity.

DENTITION

Chihuahuas normally lose their baby teeth and erupt permanent teeth at 5 or 6 months. Often the baby teeth do not loosen voluntarily and must be extracted. Full dentition is usual, but the absence of canine teeth is not rare. Undershot or overshot bites, as well as wry mouths, are common orthodontic faults of the breed. Dogs with these faults should not be bred.

RECOGNIZED PROBLEMS

Skull measurements were taken on 66 dogs of 7 breeds. Using mostly data from breeders' studbooks, breed differences in reproduction were also examined. Litter size averaged 2.45±1.28 for Chihuahuas. Pup mortality averaged 16.59% for Chihuahuas.[1]

Some bloodlines are prone to **patellar luxation**.[2,3] **Cleft palate** is also a genetic defect in some bloodlines.

Health problems to which the breed is susceptible include **hemophilia A**[4] and **valvular pulmonic steriosis**.[4] Eye problems include **corneal edema** and **iris atrophy, keratitis sicca**[5] and **secondary glaucoma**.[3]

Chihuahuas are reported to be predisposed to **yeast skin infections** caused by **Malassezia** and are also at increased risk for **generalized demodectic mange**.[6]

Circulatory defects reported in the breed are **pulmonic stenosis**[7,8,9] and **mitral valve defects**.

The association between breed, sex and canine **heart valve incompetence** were investigated by an observational study of a veterinary clinic population. Odds ratio estimations from 370 affected dogs and 9028 controls of 15 breeds revealed significant positive associations between some small and medium-sized breeds, including the Chihuahua, and heart valve incompetence, and significant negative associations between some large breeds and heart valve incompetence. The log odds, determined for each breed and sex, indicated that males were more susceptible.[10]

Other sources report the following problems in some bloodlines of Chihuahuas: **dislocation of the shoulder**,[11] **collapsed trachea**,[12,13,14,15,16] and **hypoplasia of dens (odontoid process)**.[17,18, 19,20]

Fatty liver syndrome has been reported in several toy breeds.[21]

There is a higher incidence of **cryptorchidism** reported in Chihuahuas than in most other breeds.[22]

BEHAVIOR

The Chihuahua is loyal, lively and easily trainable. He is not totally comfortable with strangers. He should not be cooped up, because of his size. He needs and enjoys exercise.

OLD AGE

The average life span of a Chihuahua is approximately 12 years, but some have lived as long as 20 years.

References
1. Hahn, S. "Variation of Skull Traits and Reproduction in Breeds of Small Dogs," Thesis, Tierarztliche Hochschule Hannover, Ger. Fed. Rep. 1988: 130; 111 ref.
2. Knight, G.C. "Abnormalities and Defects in Pedigree Dogs, III, Tibio-Femoral Joint Deformity and Patella Luxation," *J. Sm. Anim. Prac.*; 1963: 4: 463-464.
3. Koditawakku, G.E. "Luxation of the Patella in the Dog," *Vet. Rec.*; 1962: 74:1499-1507.
4. Patterson, D.F. "A Catalogue of Hereditary Diseases of the Dog. In *Current Veterinary Therapy* V, Kirk, R.W., Ed. (W.B. Saunders, Philadelphia, Pa.,1974).
5. Magrane, W.G., *Canine Ophthalmology.* 2nd ed. (Lea & Febiger, Philadelphia, PA.,1971) 269.
6. Griffin, C, Kwockhka, K., McDonald, J. *Current Veterinary Dermatology: The Art and Science of Therapy.* Mosby Yearbook, St. Louis, MO 1993: 45, 74.
7. Mulvihill, J.J. and Priester, W.A. "Congenital Heart Disease in Dogs: Epidemiologic Similarities to Man," *Teratology*; 1963: 7: 73-78.
8. Patterson, D.F. "Epidemiologic and Genetic Studies of Congenital Heart Disease in the Dog," *Circ. Res.*; 1968: 23: 171-202.

9.   Patterson, D.F. "Canine Congenital Heart Disease: Epidemiological Hypotheses," *J. Sm. Anim. Prac.*; 12:263-297.

10. Thrusfield, M.V., Aitken, C.G.G., and Darke, P.G.G. "Observations on Breed and Sex in Relation to Canine Heart Valve Incompetence," *J. Sm. Anim. Prac.*; 1985: 26:12, 709-717; 14 ref.

11. Campbell, J.R. "Shoulder Lameness in the Dog," *J. Sm. Anim. Prac.*; 9: 129-198.

12. Done, S.H., et al, "Tracheal Collapse in the Dog: A Review of the Literature and Report of Two New Cases," *J. Sm. Anim. Prac.*; 1970: 11: 743-750.

13. Vaughan, L.C. and Jones, D.G.C. "Congenital Dislocation of the Shoulder Joint in the Dog," *J. Sm. Anim. Prac.*; 1969: 10: 1-3.

14. Leonard, H.C. "Collapse of the Larynx and Adjacent Structures in the Dog," *JAVMA;* 137: 350-360.

15. Leonard, H.C. "Surgical Correction of Collapsed Trachea in Dogs," *JAVMA*; 1971: 560-598.

16. O'Brien, J.A., et al, "Tracheal Collapse in the Dog," *J. Amer. Vet. Rad. Soc.*; 1966: 7: 12-19.

17. Downey, R.S. "An Unusual Cause of Tetraplegia in a Dog," *Canad. Vet. J.*; 1967: 8: 216-217.

18. Geary, et al, "Atlanto-Axial Subluxation in the Canine," *J. Sm. Anim. Prac.*; 1967: 8: 577-587.

19. Ladds, et al, "Congenital Odontoid Process Separation in Two Dogs," *J. Sm. Anim. Prac.*; 1970: 12:463-471.

20. Parker, A.J. and Park, R.D. "Atlanto-Axial Subluxation in Small Breeds of Dogs: Diagnosis and Pathogenesis," *VM/SAC;* 1973: 68: 1133-1137.

21. J.S. Van-der-Linde-Sipman and Van-den-Ingh, TSGAm; Van Toor, AJ. "Fatty Liver Syndrome in Toy Breeds," *Tijdschrift-voor-Diergeneeskunde*; 1988: 113:Suppl.1, 102S-103S.

22. Bell, Jerold S. DVM "Sex Related Genetic Disorders: Did Mama Cause Them?" *American Kennel Club Gazette*, Feb. 1994; 76.

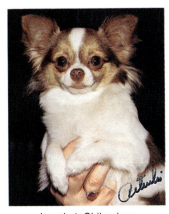

Longhair Chihuahua

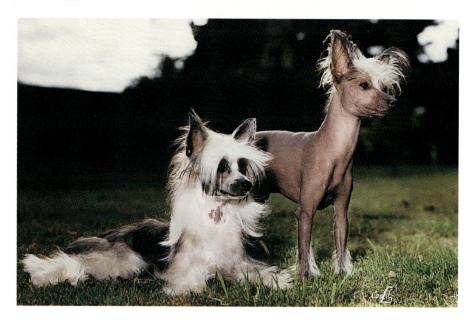

CHINESE CRESTED

ORIGIN AND HISTORY

This dog is said to have existed as far back as 1000 B.C. Common in China in the mid-1800s, the breed has been extinct there for nearly half a century.

DESCRIPTION

The Chinese Crested is active, affectionate, clean, odorless and does not shed. It is a splendid pet for adults. It is finely boned and graceful. At first sight the two types of Chinese Crested — Hairless and Powderpuff — may appear to be two separate breeds. However, they are almost exactly the same; the amount of hair is the only difference.

The Hairless should have hair on its head, feet and tail — the Powderpuff is born fully coated.

A unique feature of hairless dogs is that they have sweat glands.[1,2] Rather than panting to release body heat as coated dogs do, they simply sweat.

Properly cared for, the skin of the Hairless remains soft to the touch, yet it is thicker and tougher than that of a coated dog and it heals very quickly if scratched or cut.

The Chinese Crested has a hare foot, and its elongated toes grip like human hands.

THE SHOW RING

The Chinese Crested, ideally, is 11 to 13 inches high and rectangularly proportioned. It can be any color or combination of colors. Excessively heavy, kinky or curly coat is to be penalized. Missing teeth in the Powderpuff are to be faulted. The Hairless variety is not to be faulted for absence of full dentition.[1]

BREEDING AND WHELPING

Chinese Crested are usually free whelpers of three to five puppies per litter. Breeding a Hairless to a Hairless, or a Hairless to a Powderpuff may produce either or both in the same litter. Breeding Powderpuff to Powderpuff will produce only Powderpuffs.[3]

RECOGNIZED PROBLEMS

Blackheads can be a problem; frequent bathing helps. **Sunburn** can be a real problem to the Hairless variety. Sunscreen can be used if the dog is to be outdoors for any length of time in strong sunlight. Many are **allergic** to wool and products containing lanolin.[2]

The Hairless has a **primitive mouth**, meaning there are teeth extending forward, missing pre-molars, and, occasionally, missing teeth. The teeth in the Hairless have less enamel and therefore they lose their teeth early.[2]

Skull measurements were taken on 66 dogs of seven breeds. Using mostly data from breeders' studbooks, breed differences in reproduction were also examined. Litter size averaged 2.36±1.22 for Chinese Crested. It was concluded that **dwarfism** results in small litters and, in combination with extremely domed heads, tends to increase the incidence of **dystocia.**[4]

BEHAVIOR

This is a companion dog that needs a warm atmosphere. He is lively, intelligent and cheerful. He is never aggressive or noisy.

References
1. *The Complete Dog Book*. The American Kennel Club, 18th ed. 1992: 433
2. *Readers Digest Illustrated Book of Dogs*. 1989: 209.
3. Information provided by: *The American Chinese Crested Club, Inc.* at a 1991 seminar in New York.
4. Hahn, S. "Variation of Skull Traits and Reproduction in Breeds of Small Dogs," Thesis, Tierarztliche Hochschule Hannover, Ger. Fed. Rep., 1988: 130; 111 ref.

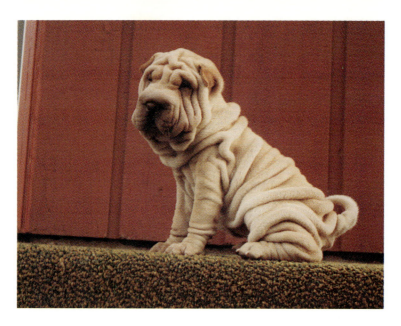

CHINESE SHAR PEI

ORIGIN AND HISTORY

At one time the *Guinness Book of World Records* stated that the Shar Pei was the rarest dog in the world.[1] This heavily wrinkled dog, once called a "creature badly in need of a good ironing," is depicted in Chinese statuettes dating from the Han dynasty (202 BC-220 AD). The name Shar Pei is generally accepted to mean "dog with a sandy coat." The coat was developed for the purpose of protection when fighting.

The breed became almost extinct in the late forties when the Communist Party took power in China, and dogs were considered a nonessential luxury but a staple food source. The Shar Pei had another problem; its hide made excellent coats for humans.

By the fifties, the breed had dwindled to a few scattered specimens. Through the efforts of a Hong Kong breeder who published a letter in an American magazine, dogs were shipped to homes in America and the breed was reestablished.

DESCRIPTION

In China, the Shar Pei was used to hunt bears and wolves and to fight. The short-haired Shar Pei originated in southern China. The long-haired type is from northern China.

Shar Peis can have two different coat textures: the "horse," which is less than 1/2 inch long and very harsh, and the "brush," which is over 1/2 inch long but less than 1 inch. Some American breeders are breeding away from the long-haired variety because they feel these dogs too closely resemble the Chow. Most Shar Peis are easy to work with, but some, especially bitches, can be pugnacious.

THE SHOW RING

The Chinese Shar Pei Club of America breed standard calls for a dog that stands from 18 to 20 inches at the withers and weighs 40 to 55 pounds. The dog is usually larger and more square bodied than the bitch,[2] but both should appear well proportioned.

Predominant coat colors are fawn, cream, red and black, although all solid colors are allowed. A solid blue-black tongue is preferred, except in dilute colors, where solid lavender pigmentation is acceptable. A spotted tongue is a major fault. Disqualifications include pink tongue, prick ears, albinoism and coat colors which are brindled, particolor, spotted and tan-pointed pattern. **A "bear" coat is unacceptable in the ring.** The "bear" coat displays length in excess of 1 inch.

BREEDING AND WHELPING

Shar Pei bitches have a typical estrous cycle, but may show no color, very minimal swelling and the accompanying odor of estrus may be missing. Many breedings are by artificial insemination after careful observation. A gestation period of 58 to 59 days is normal for the breed.

Shar Peis are excellent mothers and experience no remarkable deviations from the norm. Shar Pei puppies should be fed a diet meeting the nutritional needs of a giant breed, as they have an unusually fast rate of growth. Breeders report infant puppies gaining as much as 4 ounces per day. Front dewclaw removal is optional; rear dewclaws must be removed.

DENTITION

The Standard calls for a scissors bite, deviation from which is a major fault. Undershot mouths are seen.

RECOGNIZED PROBLEMS

All anesthetic should be administered with caution, as this breed has abnormal responses. Excessive folds of skin and fluid-filled subcutaneous tissue present medical and surgical problems for veterinarians. **Stenotic nares, fluid-filled palate** and **pharyngeal tissues** sometimes interfere with normal respiration, usually in puppies. Surgery is seldom necessary because the respiratory problems are mitigated as the puppies grow.

The large muzzle should not be confused with an allergic reaction. It has been treated as such by some veterinarians.

A hereditary defect, **parrot mouth**, has been identified in the Shar Pei, but breeders appear to be preventing propagation of affected animals. Another problem, **otitis externa**, often occurs because the ears are held tightly to the head. Excessive skin around the eyes presents one of the more severe problems. **Entropion**[3] frequently occurs, resulting in ulceration of the corneas. If not treated, loss of sight may result. **Photophobia** and **blepharospasm** may manifest soon after the puppy first opens its eyes at 2 to 3 weeks.

Various techniques have been used to try to correct entropion in Shar Pei puppies. The most satisfactory method has been properly placed nonabsorbable sutures. The procedure can be performed on puppies as early as 2 to 3 weeks of age. This technique everts the eyelids thus relieving the entropion and blepharospasm without the sutures being in contact with the cornea.

The sutures are left for 3 weeks if possible, however replacing or repositioning the sutures may be necessary. During this time the wrinkles partially regress as the puppy grow as into the skin. Dogs older than 4 months sometimes respond to this method.

Because blinking is still possible, **keratitis sicca** is avoided. If ulceration is present, application of an ophthalmic antibiotic drop or ointment without corticosteroid onto the eyes aids healing. If the sutures are anchored too far from the lid margins, or if the ends are too long, the sutures may be torn out by the puppy or its littermates.

Blepharospasm associated with **conjunctivitis** in adults may result in entropion. If ulceration is not present, systemic corticosteroids will often alleviate the blepharospasms, thereby correcting the entropion. Radical techniques often result in scarring and/or deformities. Surgical correction for entropion is a **disqualification**.

Bowed forelegs have been observed in some litters. Supplementing the diet with calcium and placing the affected legs in casts will help correct this condition. In one case, when the dog was a puppy, its forepaws extended laterally from the carpi and it walked seal-like on its carpi. To treat the condition, the legs were placed in casts, the flexor tendons were shortened, and wire ligaments were constructed. As an adult, the dog walked almost normally. This dog sired one litter. The puppies had no severe deformities of the forelegs, but did have a rickets-like bowing. A probable cause of this defect is heredity. Puppies exhibiting these signs should not be bred. Radiographs have not been definitive.

Medial and lateral luxations of the patella often occur in the Shar Pei. The trochlear groove is generally shallow. Deepening the groove, reconstructing collateral ligaments, and imbricating the retinaculum have been used successfully to correct these luxations. **Hip dysplasia** is common in Shar Peis, though lameness caused by the condition is rare. **Elbow dysplasia** has been reported by OFA.[4]

A jelly-like subcutaneous tissue lies under the Shar Pei's thin epidermis. The dogs inflict wounds when they fight. After a wound is sutured, it heals rapidly without complications.

The stress of whelping, heat or other changes seem to precipitate **patchy loss of hair**. A generalized shedding without skin changes, which gives the dog a moth-eaten appearance, is normal. **Interdigital erythema** and **pruritus** associated with skinfolds are common. Some-times the skin, particularly on the ventral cervical area, becomes thickened, resembling that of the elephant.

Generalized dermatitis is common in Shar Peis. **Staphylococcus** organisms have been isolated as a primary cause. Antibiotic-steroid therapy will often alleviate symptoms. In a few dogs, **demodectic mange** causes severe dermatitis. Skin scraping should be done to differentiate the conditions. Shar Peis are highly susceptible to **inhalant allergies,**[5] and they may be predisposed to food allergy.[6]

Dr. William H. Miller, Jr. of Cornell, computer-searched Shar Pei treatment records of that institution for 1981-1989. Fifty percent of the animals treated exhibited skin disease, sup-porting the conclusion of increased incidence of skin disorders.[7]

In a study being completed in conjunction with Michigan State University on thyroid function in 100 Shar Peis, many were found to be **hypothyroid**. This condition makes the dog susceptible to skin problems. Hypothyroidism also affects the libido of many males, making artificial insemination common.

Inguinal hernias, usually bilateral, have been frequently observed, particularly in bitches. This condition is hereditary. **Umbilical hernias** are also seen, but may not be hereditary. **Hiatal hernias** are uncommon, but may appear more frequently in Chinese Shar Peis. **Primary megaesophagus** has been recently reported in the breed.[9]

Idiopathic mucinosis of Chinese Shar Peis is a poorly understood condition usually seen in young Shar Peis of either sex. Affected dogs present with generalized pitting "edema," variable pruritis (concurrent allergies?), alopecia, hyperpigmentation and often severe puffiness and wrinkling of the head and extremities. Vesicles may be present which, when ruptured, drain a clear, viscous, stringy substance. Biopsies reveal severe, diffuse, full-thickness dermal mucinosis. A sticky mucinous material may be discernible grossly at biopsy. The so-called "mucin prick test" may also confirm diagnosis. This is performed by pricking the skin with a 25 gauge needle. If excessive mucin is present, a strand of mucinous material will be attached to the needle. Some cases may spontaneously resolve as the dogs mature, and others appear to benefit from glucocorticoid therapy, perhaps because of the drug's effect on fibroblasts.

FUO (fevers of unknown origin) has become a problem for Shar Pei breeders. It is frequently accompanied by **SHS** (swollen hock syndrome). When these two conditions appear together the animal is considered to be at high risk for **renal amyloidosis**.[10]

The Chinese Shar Pei is one of a few breeds in which **ciliary dyskenesia** has been documented. They are presented with recurrent pneumonia, rhinitis and moist productive cough.[11] Some owners are allergic to Shar Peis. These people exhibit an erythematous, pruritic contact reaction when handling the dogs.

BEHAVIOR

Some Shar Pei are wary of strangers. Most live happily in the house and are devoted, loyal companions. They are particularly good with children.

OLD AGE

Life expectancy for the Shar Pei is 8 to 10 years.

References
1. McWhirter, N. *Guinness Book of World Records*; (New York, NY: Sterling Publishing Company, Inc., 1972).
2. American Kennel Club, *The Complete Dog Book*; (Howell Book House. 18th ed. 1992).
3. Barnett, K.C. "Inherited Eye Disease in the Dog and Cat," *J. Sm. Anim. Prac.*; 1988: 29:7, 462-475; 33 ref.
4. Bodner, Elizabeth, DVM, "Genetic Status Symbols," *The American Kennel Club Gazette*; September, 1992.
5. Ackerman, Lowell, DVM. "Allergic Skin Diseases," *American Kennel Club Gazette*; September, 1990.
6. Werner, A. "Aspects of Food and Food Supplements in Skin Disease," *Pedigree Breeder Forum*; 1993: Vol. 2 # 1.
7. Werner, A. "Aspects of Food and Food Supplements in Skin Disease," *Pedigree Breeding Forum*; 1993: Vol. 2 #1.
8. Cornell University Newsletter.
9. Kern, Maryanne, DVM, "Diseases of the Esophagus," *The American Kennel Club Gazette*; January, 1993.
10. Chinese Shar-Pei Column, *The American Kennel Club Gazette*; February, 1992.
11. King, L.G. DVM; "Respiratory Congenital Disorders," Western Veterinary Conference, Feb. 1994.

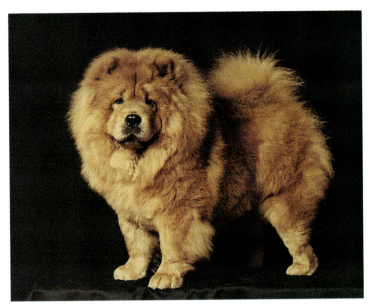

CHOW CHOW

ORIGIN AND HISTORY

The Chow Chow is the product of 2,000 years of breeding in China. This ancient guard dog is set apart from other breeds, not only by aloof temperament, but also by the blue-black color of its tongue and the roof of its mouth. The modern Chow is intensely devoted to its owner, tolerant of children, immaculate and extremely alert to strange noises and situations.

DESCRIPTION

A great improvement has been made in the Chow's temperament during the past two decades, but distrust of strangers is an inherent trait. Chows therefore require more understanding in the initial approach. The Chow should be approached initially from under the chin and simultaneously addressed in a soft, reassuring voice.

Because of its characteristic deep-set eyes, the Chow has poor peripheral vision and distrusts anyone who approaches from the rear. If possible, an owner should be in attendance while a Chow is at a veterinary hospital.

The Chow is lighter in color at birth than at maturity. In dogs with red or cinnamon coats, the more dark hairs at birth the darker the mature coat will be. Frequently it is difficult to distinguish between blue and cinnamon at birth. A cinnamon puppy will have some obviously pink hairs on the stomach and feet, but a blue puppy will be solid blue-grey, with perhaps some lighter silvery tips.

THE SHOW RING

The average height of the adult is 17 to 20 inches at the withers, but consideration of type and proportions should take preference over size. The average weight for dogs is 55 to 70 pounds and for bitches 45 to 60 pounds. A unique feature of the breed is the **desired straight hind leg**, which has little angulation of hock or stifle. The breed Standard states: "Gait — completely individual. Short and stilted because of straight hocks." This straight hind leg predisposes Chows to **subluxation of the patella**. Loose kneecaps are often found in puppies.

Another distinctive trait of the Chow is the pigmentation of the tongue and mouth. The Standard says: "Tongue — blue-black. The tissues of the mouth should approximate black." The tongue is pink at birth, but the characteristic color develops rapidly. Usually the tongue is completely blue-black by the time the puppy is 6 weeks old. A tongue that does not change within 8 weeks is cause for concern, although some tongues may not turn for as long as 9 months.

Disqualifications listed in the breed standard are nose spotted or distinctly other than black, except in blue Chows, which may have solid blue or slate noses; tongue red, pink or obviously spotted with red or pink; and drop ear or ears.

BREEDING AND WHELPING

Bitches usually have normal estrous cycles, although some have estrus at intervals of less than six months. The time of ovulation varies, and vaginal smears are not entirely reliable. Conception can result from breedings as early as the third day and as late as the 22nd day after onset of vaginal bleeding. Genital-tract infections are common in the breed. Chow bitches are notoriously difficult to settle; research is needed as to the causes. Progesterone testing has been a big help in determining ovulation.

Pregnancy may be difficult to diagnose. A "barrel-bodied" female may carry one or two puppies undetected, especially after one pregnancy. The duration of gestation is usually normal. The need of **cesarean section** is common to the breed and is often associated with an unusually large or small number of puppies. The average litter size is four to six puppies. The weight of puppies varies from 10 to 20 ounces. The extreme variability of adult size in Chows is reflected in the size and growth rate of the puppies.

RECOGNIZED PROBLEMS

Elongated soft palates and **cleft palates** are sometimes found in neonates. **Bronchial dysplasia** has been reported in Chows.[1] Abnormally **short tails** are also encountered.

Lack of full dentition in the Chow is rare. Overshot and undershot bites occur in specific bloodlines. Some of these bites will correct with the appearance of mature teeth. Also, a correct scissors bite may become undershot as the adult teeth appear.

Hip dysplasia is common. It is estimated that as many as 40% of the breed show some deviation from normal. In a Norwegian study of 103 dogs X-rayed, 22% were dysplastic.[2] **Elbow dysplasia** has also been reported.

Skin problems characterized by **alopecia,**[3] **skin thickening** and **hyperpigmentation** are seen. Hormonal disturbances other than hypothyroidism are thought to cause these problems. Also seen is **alopecia**, associated with the genes for dilution, which produce blue-colored dogs.[4]

Tyrosinase Deficiency, a variant of a metabolic disease comparable to **idiopathic vitiligo**, has been observed in Chow Chows that were normal at birth but developed **hypopigmentation** affecting the nares and tongue as well as **leukotrichia**. A deficiency of Tyrosinase prevents the formation of melanin. This metabolic defect is not amenable to treatment. **Uveodermatologic syndrome** has been reported in Chow Chows.[5]

Congenital entropion[6] is a problem in the breed and has been seen in puppies as young as 4 weeks of age. **Entropion** may also develop in the adult dog and **secondary entropion** may be encountered due to **keratoconjunctivitis** or corneal injury. There is evidence for occurrence of familial or inherited cataracts in the Chow Chow.[7] It has also been reported that **distichiasis** is a problem[8] as well as **persistent pupillary membrane, nystagmus, retinal folds** and **microphthalmia.**[9] **Narrowed palpebral fissure** has also been observed.

Cerebellar hypoplasia has been reported by Knecht, et al (1979).[10] The condition is most commonly observed in cats as a result of prenatal infection with feline panleukopenia virus. Two of the Chows reported by Knecht showed nonprogressive signs and one became clinically normal with age.

Some microscopic features were found in all dogs necropsied. Marked gliosis and demyelination of the cerebellum were not observed. Focal diminution of granular cells was occasionally seen. Degenerative changes of the Purkinje cells may be absent and the deep cerebellar and olivary nuclei were normal. The occurrence in six out of 14 dogs born to clinically normal parents indicates an autosomal recessive mode of transmission. A genetic basis is further supported by previous observation of ataxia and shaking in a distant female relative of the Small Animal Clinic at Ohio State University.

In recessive transmission, consanguinity of the parents is expected when a litter from normal parents contains approximately one affected progeny in four animals. Examination of the five-generation pedigree of one affected dog revealed no ancestor common to both paternal and maternal lineage. Thus, if the transmission of cerebellar hypoplasia is recessive, it occurs in more than one bloodline and may even be widespread in the breed.[3] A familial **myotonia** has been described in Chow Chow dogs. An autosomal recessive mode of inheritance has been suggested but not proven. Clinical signs usually appear at 2-3 months but sometimes not until 5-9 months. These puppies have stiffness especially in the pelvic limbs resulting in a bunny-hopping gait. Occasionally dogs will have great difficulty walking. Exercise tends to help the clinical signs. There can be muscle hypertrophy. Serum creatine kinase is elevated. Muscle biopsy reveals variation of muscle fiber sizes, central nuclei, increased subsascolemnal nuclei, fiber necrosis and fiber splitting. Both fiber types are affected. These changes are considered "dystrophic." Treatment with membrane-stabilizing drugs such as phenytoin, quinidine and procainamide sometimes helps.[11] **Bloat** occurs and is often fatal unless quickly relieved with medical or surgical treatment.

The desired head structure of the Chow is brachycephalic. Therefore, anesthesia should be approached with extreme care as in all brachycephalic breeds. Because Chows are often sensitive to morphine and meperidine, these drugs should not be used routinely. **Laryngospasm** following administration of intravenous barbiturates is common. Anesthesia in the Chow Chow is further complicated by the blue-black pigment of the tongue, which makes impossible the detection of early signs of cyanosis by observing the color of the mouth and tongue. Chow Chows with normal thyroid, adrenal and gonadal function have developed a characteristic **alopecia** and **hyperpigmentation** that has shown a favorable response to growth hormone therapy.[12] The authors state that "treatment of the disease would appear to be impractical until growth hormone becomes more readily available to the medical profession." Breeder observations suggest this condition is hereditary. **Castration responsive dermatosis** has been reported commonly in just a few breeds. Chow Chows are one of these breeds.[4] The Chow Chow has an increased breed incidence for **hypothyroidism**[13] and for **melanomas**.[4] **Idiopathic epilepsy** has been detected in the Chow Chow.[14]

BEHAVIOR

The Chow Chow is a one-owner dog and it is loyal and devoted to those it likes. It does not take easily to strangers and is sometimes aggressive and unfriendly towards them.

OLD AGE

The average life span of the Chow is 12 years. Blindness is common in the older dogs. Death is generally attributed to heart or kidney failure.

References

1. King, L.G. DVM "Respiratory Congenital Disorders"; Western Veterinary Conference, Feb. 1994.
2. Lingaas, F. and Heim, P. "A Genetic Investigation on the Incidence of Hip Dysplasia in

Norwegian Dog Breeds," *Norsk-Veterinaertidsskrift.* 1987: 99:9, 617-623; 22 ref.

3. Scott, D.W. and Paradis, M. "A Survey of Canine and Feline Skin Disorders Seen in a University Practice," Small Animal Clinic, University of Montreal, Saint Hyacinthe, Quebec, 1987-88.

4. Griffin, C., Kwochka, K., McDonald, J.; *Textbook of Veterinary Dermatology, the Art and Science of Therapy.* Mosby Yearbook, St. Louis, MO 1993: 218, 239, 289, 299.

5. The Whippet column, *The American Kennel Club Gazette*; September, 1992.

6. Erickson, F., et al, "Congenital Defects of Dogs, III," *Canine Prac.* 4: 48, Table 18; 1977.

7. Veterinary News. *The American Kennel Club Gazette*; February, 1991.

8. Magrane, W.C. *Canine Ophthalmology.* 3rd ed. (Lea & Febiger, Philadelphia, PA., 1977) 305.

9. *JAVMA*; Vol. 200, #10, May 15, 1992.

10. Knecht, C.D., et al "Cerebellar Hypoplasia in Chow Chows," *JAAHA*; 15:1, 51-53;1979.

11. Ettinger, S.J. *Textbook of Veterinary Internal Medicine.* W.B. Saunders Co., Philadelphia, PA, 1989: 738.

12. Parker, W.M. and Scott, D.W. "Growth Hormone Responsive Alopecia in the Mature Dog: A Discussion of 13 Cases," *JAAHA;* 16(6);1980.

13. Brignac, Michele M. "Congenital and Breed Associated Skin Diseases in the Dog and Cat," *KalKan Forum*; December, 1989.

14. Bell, Jerold S. DVM; "Sex Related Genetic Disorders: Did Mama Cause Them?"; *American Kennel Club Gazette*, Feb. 1994: 76.

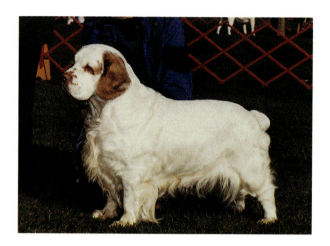

CLUMBER SPANIEL

ORIGIN AND HISTORY

The popular notion that the Clumber came from a Basset and an Alpine Spaniel cross cannot be proved. Others theorize that it came from the ancient Blenheim Spaniel. Probable origin was England in ancient times.

The Clumber has been in America since Colonial days and was one of the first breeds to be registered with the AKC.

It was bred in England by the Duke of Newcastle; King George V also had a large kennel of field Clumbers. They lost their popularity in England with the decline of the large estates where they adeptly hunted game in the dense underbrush. The breed has gained increased recognition in the United States in recent years.

DESCRIPTION

Breed books often portray the Clumber as a clumsy, inactive dog. It is actually very active, plays fetch for hours and though it can be independent, responds to affection with great loyalty. Some may be suspicious of strangers. They are quite stoic at the veterinarian's office, but often urinate when frightened or excited.

THE SHOW RING

Bitches average 55 pounds, dogs 70 pounds. They should be white with lemon or orange markings on the head and ears, and ticking on muzzle and forelegs; the fewer body markings, the better. Dewclaws should be removed. Tails should be docked at the taper, similar to English Springer Spaniels. Tails are docked quite long in England, but should not have a pump handle appearance. Too short a tail also destroys balance. Four inches is about right for the adult depending on its size.

There are no disqualifying faults in this breed.

BREEDING AND WHELPING

Difficulties in breeding are often encountered because of the structure of the dogs and lack of enthusiasm on the male's part. Some breeders utilize artificial insemination.

Clumber bitches may have uneven heat cycles. It is not uncommon for a bitch to have her first estrus as late as 2 years. A few cases have had uterine inertia necessitating cesarean sections. Road work helps prepare the bitch for a fast, efficient delivery. Whelps are often from 12 to 16 ounces; average litter size is four to six.

GROWTH

Clumbers tend to be overzealous mothers and often mutilate newly docked tails.

Pups grow rapidly, though not so rapidly as the giant breeds. They need exercise and should not be allowed to become fat. They appear to be slow maturers like the giant breeds. Over-supplementation is definitely not recommended.

RECOGNIZED PROBLEMS

Undershot and **wry mouths** and **missing adult teeth** are reported. **Hip dysplasia** is sometimes encountered as are the **disc problems** anticipated in a long, low, heavy dog. **Entropion** is the most common hereditary defect. **Ectropion or "diamond eye"** is also a health problem.

Clumbers should be kept lean and will function best when walked two to three miles a day. Actual work in the field is even better.

BEHAVIOR

The Clumber is a playful, calm and quiet companion. They are intelligent and always pleasant.

OLD AGE

Life span is about 12 years, but older Clumbers are not uncommon.

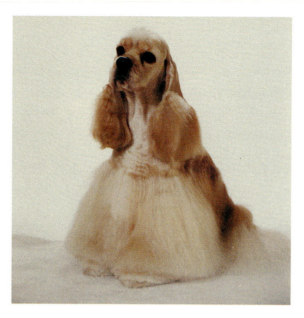

COCKER SPANIEL

ORIGIN AND HISTORY

The word "Spaniells" is mentioned as early as 1386 in Spain, where the forebears of all Spaniels had their roots. Until the middle of the 19th century, Spaniels were classified simply according to size. In England the "Cocking" Spaniels, named for their use in hunting wood-chuck, were bred down in size to make them manageable. During the last quarter of the 19th century, the Cocker fell into disrepute as a working Spaniel. The long, low-set structure was responsible for the inefficiency of the Cocker in the field. Obo, the great foundation Cocker, was only 10 inches tall and weighed 22 pounds.

In the 1920s interest again increased in the hunting Cocker, which at this time was becoming taller and shorter-backed. The onset of World War II virtually ended the Cocker field trials. The Cocker's beauty and quality as a pet and show dog ended his popularity as a field dog. In 1977 Cockers were again permitted to compete in field trials, with many dogs now holding WD and WDX titles.

DESCRIPTION

The Cocker is a merry, busy, light-hearted, intelligent breed. For 17 years (1938-1955) the Cocker was the most popular breed in America. As often occurs to meet current popularity, indiscriminate breeding resulted in poor dispositions, frequent bowel-control problems and mani-festations of hereditary problems. Recent breeder efforts have returned the breed to the merry little Cocker everyone loved as a child. The breed's popularity is again on the rise.[1,2] Consider-ation of disposition is of paramount importance in the breeding of any Cocker Spaniel to avoid

186

destroying the trait that made them famous. Behavior problems still exist and need to be eliminated.

THE SHOW RING

The Standard for the Cocker Spaniel calls for dogs to be 15 inches at the withers and bitches to be 14 inches. Height may vary 1/2 inch above or below without disqualification, but **dogs over 15 1/2 inches and bitches over 14 1/2 inches will be disqualified.** The Cocker is divided into three varieties according to color: Blacks, ASCOBs and Parti-colors. The Black variety consists of solid black dogs and black dogs with tan points. A small amount of white is allowed but penalized on the throat and chest; **white in any other location disqualifies.** Puppies may be born with small amounts of white on the chin, chest and feet which disappear with age.

The second variety, termed ASCOB (any solid color other than black), includes many shades of silver, buff, red, chocolate (liver) and chocolate and tan. The tan points in the black and tans and chocolate and tans must be located over each eye, on the muzzle and cheeks, on the underside of the ears, on feet and legs and under the tail. **Tan markings in excess of 10% is a disqualification. Absence of tan markings in any of the specified locations in an otherwise tan-pointed dog is a disqualification. A small amount of white on the throat or chest is allowed, although penalized. White in any other location shall disqualify.**

The third variety, Parti-colors, must have two or more distinct colors with the primary color not exceeding 90%. **If the primary color exceeds 90%, the dog will be disqualified.** Parti-colors may appear in black and white, black and white with tan points (tricolor), red or buff and white, liver and white, liver and white with tan points, sable and whites, and roans.

Texture of the coat is important. The coat should be silky, flat or slightly wavy but never curly or cottony. According to the Standard both front and rear dewclaws may be removed. Tail docking is extremely important to the show breeder, as the correct length of tail lends much to the overall balance of the showdog.

BREEDING AND WHELPING

It is not unusual for Cocker bitches to whelp before the 63rd day. Some breeders report that Parti-colors tend to whelp early and the solid colors most frequently whelp on time or a day late. Cockers are generally free-whelpers. Litters average five puppies with birth weights averaging six ounces.

Dock tails and remove dewclaws at 3 to 5 days of age. Leave about 1/4 inch of the tail.

Cleft palates and **harelips** are the most frequently reported **birth defects**.[3] **Umbilical hernias, inguinal hernias,** and **reverse rear legs** are also reported by breeders as being frequent in occurrence.

Other problems which may be noted at birth include **pseudohermaphrodites, anasarca (edematous puppies), swimmer puppies (flattened ribcage), anury (tailless)** and **brachyury (short tail)**.[4,5,6]

GROWTH

Height is generally reached by 8 to 9 months of age with some variation in time of development and maturation within different blood lines. Breeders usually make the first evaluation of a litter at 8 weeks of age. At this time they most resemble their adult appearance.

DENTITION

The standard calls for a scissors bite. **Malocclusion** in all of its forms exists frequently in the breed. Bites can change at any time in the growing puppy with some not going "off" until 8 to 9 months of age.

RECOGNIZED PROBLEMS

The most perplexing problem within the breed at the present time is the incidence of **cataracts**.[7] Cataracts have been acknowledged in the breed for at least 35 to 40 years. Within the last 10 to 15 years slit-lamp examinations have enabled the early diagnosis of cataracts in the breeding stock. A clear hereditary pattern has not been established, but research by Yakely indicates a recessive mode of transmission. In the early 1950s the prevailing opinion was that cataracts were color-linked and appeared only in the black Cocker. By the late 1950s, this theory was disproved, as cataracts began appearing in the buffs and parti-colors. Cataracts may make their appearance at any age. The American Spaniel Club in "Guidelines for Breeding and Purchasing Cocker Spaniels" recommends never breeding an individual who has cataracts regardless of the age of onset of cataracts or the state of development. It also recommends that sons and daughters of a dog with cataracts never be bred.[8]

Cocker Spaniels are listed as having **congenital deafness**.[9]

There exists in the Cocker Spaniel a hereditary **blood coagulation disorder** identical to the Factor X deficiency in man. This disorder has been found mainly in certain buff lines as an autosomal incomplete dominant genetic factor. It may be characterized by neonatal mortality, severe bleeding in the young or minor bleeding in the adult.

Factor IX deficiency (hemophilia B) is a sex-linked recessive trait that has been reported in the Cocker Spaniel and several other breeds. The severity of the disease in dogs depends on the degree of deficiency of Factor IX and on the size of the animal. **Autoimmune hemolytic anemia** has a familial tendency in Cocker Spaniels with a reported higher incidence

188

in females.[10,11] Pale mucous membranes are the most prominent physical finding but **jaundice**, **hepatomegaly** and **splenomegaly** are frequent findings.

Cockers also have a hereditary predisposition to **primary glaucoma**, which seems to have a frequency of acute attacks varying seasonally, being most prevalent from October to May. The left eye is most commonly affected first with the second eye becoming involved generally within a year. A recent study compared mixed-breed dogs with purebred dogs. The study concludes eight breeds are at higher risk of developing glaucoma; one of these is the Cocker.[12] Within the last few years, a condition called **retinal dysplasia** has been diagnosed in the Cocker Spaniel. It is a recessive trait that causes no blindness in this breed though it may in other breeds. Other problems affecting the Cocker's eyes and eyelids include **progressive retinal atrophy**, **distichiasis**, **ectropion** and **entropion**. **Keratitis sicca** and **pigmentary keratitis** are two problems within the breed that can cause considerable discomfort and even blindness. Cockers are also predisposed to **prolapse of the gland of the nictitating membrane (cherry eye)**. The Cocker is also one of dogs most commonly affected with **lens-induced uveitis.**[13]

Luxated patellas (slipped stifles) exist quite commonly and may involve one or both legs. The patellas may luxate either medially or laterally. Luxations may occur only on occasion causing some discomfort, or the patellas may slip in and out quite freely, causing no apparent discomfort to the dog until arthritis and lameness occur in later years. Owners may notice the dog stretching the rear leg out straight to "pop" the patella back in place. A simple autosomal recessive has been suggested, but the exact mode of inheritance is not known. **Hip dysplasia** should also be a concern among Cocker breeders. It would be wise to radiograph all breeding stock before the problem becomes more serious. **Disproportionate dwarfism (achondroplasia)**[14] has been reported in the Cocker Spaniel. These dogs have a normal sized body and disproportionately short limbs resulting in a Cocker that resembles a Dachshund. This condition appears to be transmitted as an autosomal recessive trait. The Cocker is also predisposed to **intervertebral disc disease,** and cases of **elbow dysplasia** have been reported.

A collection of over 14,000 radiographs of the spine of 10 breeds of dogs were examined for abnormal vertebrae in the lumbosacral region, which included different types of fusion. There was some link between these abnormalities and hip dysplasia. Such abnormalities were seen in 4% of 1315 Cockers.[15]

Allergies, **seborrhea**, **hypothyroidism**[16], **epidermal cysts** and **lip fold pyodermas** are common problems involving the skin of the Cocker. Cockers also have a higher incidence of food allergies than many other breeds.[17] **Allergic inhalent dermatitis (atopy)** results in a foot-chewing, face-rubbing, underarm-scratching dog. Skin lesions may be the result of primary or secondary **seborrhea, hypothyroidism** or **staph hypersensitivities**. Cockers are also at increased risk for **generalized demodectic mange**.[17] Hypothyroidism may or may not manifest itself in the form of skin problems and has been diagnosed in dogs less than a year old. Seborrheic conditions occur most frequently in the buff Cocker. In the show dogs, the parti-colors and chocolates seem to have skin problems more frequently. **Otitis externa** is very common and is often found as part of the seborrheic complex. Otitis externa can result in proliferation of tissue within the external ear canal and the ossification of the lateral ear cartilage. **Vitamin A responsive dermatosis** has been identified in the Cocker Spaniel.[17] They also occasionally develop nasodigital hyperkeratosis.[17]

A study in Sweden analyzed 218 dogs with **primary hypothyroidism**. One of the breeds with higher-than-average incidence of the disorder was the Cocker Spaniel.[18]

Renal cortical hypoplasia[19,20] has been reported in young Cocker Spaniels between the ages of 6 months and 2 years. The first clinical symptom is **proteinuria** which persists and increases in intensity. It is probably an inherited syndrome.

Cockers are one of many breeds reporting **urinary calculi**.[21] Male dogs suffer from urinary calculi twice as frequently as bitches, whereas the latter have urinary tract infections. Twenty-nine percent of all dogs with urinary calculi were classified as overweight.

In a recent study of 839 **uroliths** submitted by veterinarians for analysis, 562 (67%) were composed of at least 70% magnesium ammonium phosphate, and 57 (6.8%) at least 70% calcium oxalate. Most were found in the bladder.

Uroliths occurred more frequently in males than in females, but there was little difference in prevalence between dogs aged 1 to 12 years. The uroliths were found in 60 known breeds of dogs; 3% of the uroliths were from Cockers.[22]

In a Swedish study the high incidence of **chronic liver disease** and **liver cirrhosis** in Cockers indicated that hereditary factors might be of importance in the development of **chronic hepatitis** and liver cirrhosis.[23]

Cocker Spaniels have a predilection for **melanomas**.[17]

Other problems that may be found in the breed include **tonsil enlargement, epilepsy, hydrocephalus, cranioschisis (skull fissures), esophageal achalasia, patent ductus arteriosus, undescended testicles** and **persistent penile frenulum. Cerebellar degeneration** with a genetic basis has been documented in the breed as well.[24] **Hermaphroditism** and **nasolacrimal puncta atresia** has been described in the breed.

Phosphofructokinase (PFK) deficiency has been diagnosed in a Cocker Spaniel.[25]

BEHAVIOR

The proper Cocker is cheerful, sweet and a wonderful child's companion. He is respectful of his master's authority. He is essentially a companion dog now, but still has hunting instincts. However, data was obtained on 245 cases of **aggressive behavior** in 55 breeds. One of the breeds with the greatest incidences of possessive aggression and fear-elicited aggression was the Cocker Spaniel.[26]

OLD AGE

Cocker Spaniels can be expected to live from 14 to 15 years of age. As they age, they are more susceptible to skin and ear problems and bad teeth. Cockers are easy keepers and tend to put on excessive weight as they get older.

References

1. Grossman, A. *Breeding Better Cocker Spaniels.* (Denlinger's Publishers, Ltd., Fairfax, Va; 1977).
2. Hart, E.H. *The Cocker Spaniel Handbook.* (T.F.H. Publications, Inc., Jersey City, N.J.; 1968).
3. Kirk, R.W., Ed. *Current Veterinary Therapy IV.* (W.B. Saunders, Philadelphia, Pa., 1971).
4. Kraeuchi, R. *The Cocker Spaniel.* (Judy Publishing Co., Chicago, Ill; 1956).
5. Liepold, H.W. "Nature and Causes of Congenital Defects of Dogs," *The Vet Clinics of N. America;* 1978: 8(1):47-78.
6. Moffit, E.B. *The Cocker Spaniel.* (Orange Judd Publ. Co., Inc. New York, NY; 1953).
7. Yakely, W.L. "A Study of Hereditability of Cataracts in the American Cocker Spaniel," *Am. Cocker Review;* July, 1978: 23-25.
8. Barnett, K.C. "The Diagnosis and Differential Diagnosis of Cataract in the Dog," *J. Sm. Anim. Practice;* 1985: 26:6, 305-316; 20 ref.
9. Strain, Geroge M. "Deafness in Dogs and Cats," *Proc. 10th ACVIM Forum*; May, 1992.
10. Switzer, H.W. and Jain, N.C. "Autoimmune Hemolytic Anemia in Dogs and Cats," *Vet. Clin. N. America;* 1981: 11 (2): 405-418.
11. Johnstone, J.B. "Inherited Defects of Hemostasis," *Comp. Cont. Ed.* 1982: 4(6): 483-487.
12. Slater, M.R. and Erb, H.N. "Effects of Risk Factors and Prophylactic Treatment on Primary Glaucoma," *JAVMA*; 1986: 188:9, 1028-1-30; 7 ref.
13. Van der Woerdt, A., Nasisse, M.P., and Davidson, M.G. "Lens-Induced Uveitis in Dogs:151 Cases," *JAVMA*; 1992: 201:6, 921-926; 46 ref.
14. Beachley, M.C. and Graham, F.H., Jr., "Hypochondroplastic Dwarfism in a Dog," *JAVMA;* 1973: 163:283-284.
15. Winkler, W. "Transitional Lumbosacral Vertebrae in the Dog," Dissertation, Fachbereich Veterinarmedizin der Freien Universitat Berlin. 1985: 143pp.; 50 ref.
16. Larsson, M. "The Breed, Sex and Age Distribution of Dogs with Primary Hypothyroidism," *Svensk-Veterinartidning.* 1986: 38:15, 181-183; 3 ref.
17. Griffin, C., Kowchka, K., McDonald, J.; <u>Current Veterinary Dermatology, the Science and Art</u>

of Therapy. Mosby Yearbook, St. Louis, MO. 1993: 74, 123, 171, 239.

18. Larsson, M.; "The Breed, Sex and Age Distribution of Dogs with Primary Hypothyroidism." *Svensk-Veterinartidning.* 1986, 38:15, 181-183; 3 ref.

19. Johnson, M.E., et al, "Renal Cortical Hypoplasia in a Litter of Cocker Spaniels," *JAAHA;* 1972: 8:268-274.

20. Picut, C.A. and Lewis, R.M. "Comparative Pathology of Canine Hereditary Nephropathies: An Interpretive Review," *Vet. Res. Comm.*; 1987: 11:6, 561-581; 91 ref.

21. Hesse, A. and Bruhl, M. "Urolithiasis in Dogs, Epidemiological Data and Analysis of Urinary Calculi," *Kleintierpraxis.* 1990: 35:10, 505-512; 18 ref.

22. Osborne, C.A., Clinton, C.W., Bamann, L.K., Moran, H.C., Coston, B.R., and Frost, A.P. "Prevalence of Canine Uroliths: Minnesota Urolith Center," *Vet. Clinics of N. Amer., Sm. Anim. Prac.;* 1986: 16:1, 27-44; 6 ref.

23. Anderson, M. and Sevelius, E. "Breed, Sex and Age Distribution in Dogs with Chronic Liver Disease: A Demographic Study," *J.Sm. Anim. Prac.;* 1991: 32:1, 1-5; 20 ref.

24. de La Honta, A. "Comparative Cerebellar Disease in Domestic Animals," *Comp. Vet.* 1980: Ed. II: 8-19.

25. Wilford, Christine, DVM, "Veterinary News," *American Kennel Club Gazette;* December, 1993: 34.

26. Borchelt, P.L. "Aggressive Behavior of Dogs Kept as Companion Animals: Classification and Influence of Sex, Reproductive Status and Breed," *Applied Animal Ethology.* 1983: 10:1, 45-61; 24 ref.

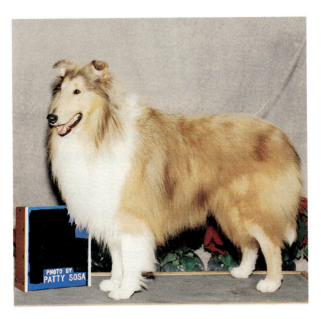

COLLIE (ROUGH)

ORIGIN AND HISTORY

The earliest Collies carried a lot of black in their coat and became known as "Coally dogs." From this origin has come the modern name of "Collie." It is thought that the rough Collie originated in the colder climate of Scotland, where the finer quality of wool was raised.

DESCRIPTION

The rough Collie is a thoroughly enjoyable and relatively easy dog to raise as a pet or to breed. The Collie is generally an intelligent, fun-loving dog with a great capacity for tolerating and accommodating many types of owners. The breed is excellent with children, and dogs with little or no experience with young humans will often show great perspicacity in dealing with them. Though some lines and individuals may be more reserved than others, a vicious Collie is unnatural, and the cause should be sought in either the dog's health or his treatment or training.

The Collie personality thrives on human companionship. A Collie left extensively to his own devices may grow up to be charming, but his major goal in life will be to please himself rather than his owner. A quiet puppy needs more attention in order to become a satisfactory adult dog. Obedience training is useful and enjoyable for both dog and owner and usually results in a close bond between the two. However, with the Collie, harsh measures should be shunned, as they are not necessary and most often produce negative rather than positive results.

While Collies usually do not change color from birth, dark sables may take up to three years to reach maximum pigmentation. White face blazes usually narrow within the first few

193

weeks of life; sable merles usually lose most of their merle spots. Sables are sometimes born with face markings which resemble the tricolor mask, though these markings change to the traditional sable mask within the first few months of life. **"Grey Collies"** are those which are homozygous for a lethal gene which dilutes the basic coat color of the dog. The primary defect in these dogs is in the **immune system (cyclic neutropenia)** and inevitably results in the death of the puppy.[1] This condition should not be confused with **merling** or a condition that appears nutritional. These Collie pups mature with full pigmentation. If the entire litter is affected, the latter condition should be suspected, as true "grays" usually occur one or two to a litter. In a few strains, pups may be born with dewclaws on their hind legs. These should be removed when the pup is about 3 days old. Front dewclaws may be removed at the option of the owner.

THE SHOW RING

Dogs are from 24 to 26 inches at the shoulder and weigh from 60 to 75 pounds. Bitches are from 22 to 24 inches at the shoulder, weighing from 50 to 65 pounds.

The major emphasis of the Standard is on head type, expression and overall balance. Special attention should be paid to these characteristics, though unsoundness has received an increasing measure of attention in the show ring in recent years. **There are no breed disqualifications.**

BREEDING AND WHELPING

The bitches are usually easy breeders, easy whelpers and good mothers. Difficulties with breeding can often be attributed to unbroken **vaginal strictures** or **season related polyps**. The former occasionally require veterinary attention while the latter sometimes require the bitch to be serviced later in her season as the size of these polyps generally reduce as the vulvar swelling subsides. If the bitch can be normally bred, neither of these conditions appears to interfere with the whelping process. Bitches require a minimum of special care during pregnancy. Many breeders augment the diet with appropriate levels of vitamin and calcium supplements and extra food during the last four weeks of pregnancy.

GROWTH

A typical growth rate is difficult to establish, as there are wide variations within lines. Generally, the puppy should be well-covered with flesh but not inclined to fatness. Since the Collie, especially the male, is a fast-growing animal, a well-balanced diet should be provided to keep the pup trim but in good flesh. Once a male becomes overly thin, it is difficult to bring him back to proper weight.

DENTITION

The correct bite is the scissors bite. However, it is not unusual for puppies to go overshot between 8 and 12 weeks of age. The majority recover from this condition over a period of months. Bites may continue to improve up to 18 months of age with the major changes taking place before 9 months. Pups which show this condition before 8 weeks will often not correct completely. A slight degree of overshot in an adult is not a handicap. In some lines with very strong muzzle and/or underjaw, the undershot condition may be seen. This is more serious in a show puppy, as the condition usually continues to worsen with age. Pups with a minimal degree of this condition have been known to correct. The same holds true for even bites. Collies with a narrow bottom jaw may show a condition involving the two lower middle incisors. These two teeth are pushed out of line and are even with the matching upper teeth. This is a relatively minor fault compared to the fully even or undershot mouth; it is often associated with a "v"-shaped lower palate rather than a broad, flat one.

RECOGNIZED PROBLEMS

In some lines of Collies, an infrequent genetically transmitted condition results in **dwarfing**. Usually only one or two puppies in a litter are affected. Without vigorous attempts to salvage them, these pups will die in the nest. They are born the same size as their littermates, but do not grow well and often do not open their eyes until five to seven days after the normal pups in the litter. Characteristically they have small eyes (sometimes to the extent of having **micropthalmia**[1,2] and occasionally **neurological disorders**), straight head profiles, tiny high-set pricked ears and very heavy coats. If raised to maturity these pups are usually under standard size and are usually sterile.

The eye condition currently labeled **"Collie Eye Problem" (ectasis syndrome)**,[3,4,5,6,7,8] is shared by other breeds and can be diagnosed in puppies. Accurate readings can be taken when the pup is between 6 and 8 weeks old. For a definite diagnosis, the eyes must be dilated and an indirect ophthalmoscope used. Older pups or adults with minimal lesions sometimes appear normal though they will breed as affected dogs. Although the fine genetic distinctions have not been definitely made, this syndrome can be treated as simple Mendelian recessive. Puppies with **tortuous vessels** and/or **chorioretinal dysplasia** do not show any clinical signs of visual deficiency and are often used in breeding programs. They make excellent pets. A concentrated breed-improvement program by informed Collie breeders has resulted in an increase in the number of normal-eyed dogs. The more serious forms of this syndrome, which can lead to visual impairment, are not necessarily stable and may degenerate as the dogs mature. Affected dogs are not considered suitable for either pets or breeding. These conditions include **excavation of the optic disc**, **detached retina** and **hyphema**. **Progressive retinal**

atrophy is a problem. Although neither the exact type nor the hereditary pattern have been determined, both the late onset variety and sight loss before a year of age have occurred. **Coloboma, distichiasis** and **corneal dystrophy** have also been seen in Collies.[9] Other eye problems are **heterochromia iridis (walleye)**[10] and **choroidal hypoplasia. Hip dysplasia** is relatively rare in the Collie; however, screening of breeding stock is recommended as a preventive measure.

The Collie is susceptible to all the **dermatoses**[11] which affect the modern dog. A proper diet and regular grooming will, to a large extent, prevent skin problems. Regular grooming of the long, dense coat will ensure early detection and treatment of any underlying condition which could otherwise become extensive. Many veterinary dermatologists feel that Collies are very susceptible to **demodicosis, hydradivitis** and **nasal pyoderma. Discoid lupus erythematosus (DLE)** is often confused with nasal solar dermatosis. They occur most commonly in Collies, Australian Shepherds, Shetland Sheepdogs and German Shepherd Dogs.[12,13] **Nasal Solar Dermatitis** and **DLE** are the more frequent causes of restricted nasal depigmentation.

Dermatomyositis has been reported. **Bullous pemphigoid** and **Vitiligo** have also been seen in Collies.[13]

Factor VIII deficiency (hemophilia A) has been described in Collies by Roswell, et al, in 1960. Its mode of inheritance is sex-linked recessive.[14] **Patent ductus arteriosus** was described by Mulvihill in 1971.[15,16,17,18] Young reports **deafness** of Collies in his 1955 article on inherited defects of dogs.[19] Saunders and Magrane reported **optic nerve hypoplasia** in 1952 and 1953.[20,21] **Inguinal and midline hernias**[22] were reported by Fox in 1963.

Epilepsy was reported as a congenital defect in Collies by Urbich in 1974.[23]

Cerebellar degeneration has been reported in the breed.[24]

BEHAVIOR

The Collie is sensitive, anxious to please, high-strung and grows deeply attached to the family. He is intelligent and easily trained and an effective watch-dog. He mistrusts strangers.

OLD AGE

The life span of a collie is about 8 to 12 years with the average about 10 years. Generally the Collie ages well, with different lines showing different tendencies. The most common failing of old dogs is arthritis, which may be minimized by drug therapy.

References

1. Brignac, Michele M. "Congenital and Breed Associated Skin Diseases in the Dog and the

Cat," *KalKan Forum*; December, 1989.

2. Mitchell, A.L. "Dominant Dilution and Other Color Factors in Collie Dogs," *J. Her.;* 1935: 26:424-430.

3. Priester, W.A. "Congenital Ocular Defects in Cattle, Horses, Cats, Dogs," *JAVMA* 155:1504-1511.

4. Donovan, R.H., et al: "Anomaly of the Collie Eye," *JAVMA;* 1969: 155:872-875.

5. Roberts, S.R. "The Collie Eye Anomaly," *JAVMA*; 1969: 155:859-865.

6. Wyman, E. and Donovan, E.F "Eye Anomaly of the Collie," *JAVMA;* 1969: 155:866-70.

7. Yakely, et al, "Genetic Transmission of an Ocular Fundus Anomaly in Collies," *JAVMA;* 1968: 152:457-461.

8. Yakely, W.L. "Collie Eye Anomaly: Decreased Prevalence Through Selective Breeding," *JAVMA;* 1972: 161:1103-1107.

9. Magrane, W.C. *Canine Ophthalmology.* (Lea & Febiger, Philadelphia, PA.,1977) 305.

10. Kirk, R.W. and Bistner, S.J. *Handbook of Veterinary Procedures and Emergency Treatment: Hereditary Defects of Dogs.* 1975: Table 124: 661.

11. Muller, G.H. and Kirk, R.W. *Small Animal Dermatology.* (W.B. Saunders, Philadelphia, PA; 1969).

12. Griffin, C., Kwochka, K., and MacDonald, J. *Current Veterinary Dermatology, the Art and Science of Therapy*, Mosby Yearbook, St. Louis, MO. 1993: 225.

13. Griffin, C., Kwochka, K., and MacDonald, J. *Current Veterinary Dermatology, the Art and Science of Therapy*, Mosby Yearbook, St. Louis, MO. 1993: 226, 231,310.

14. Sherwood, L., et al, "Canine Hemophilia Due to Antihemophilic Factor Deficiency: A Case Report," Mich.State U. Vet. 1966: 26:52.

15. Mulvihill, J.J. and Priester, W.A. "Congenital Heart Disease in Dogs: Epidemiologic Similarities to Man," *Teratology;* 1973: 7: 73-78.

16. Patterson, D.F. "Epidemiologic and Genetic Studies of Congenital Heart Disease in the Dog," *Circ. Res.;* 1968: 23: 171-202.

17. Patterson, D.F. "Canine Congenital Heart Disease: Epidemiological Hypotheses," *J. Sm. Anim. Prac.*; 1973: 12: 73-78.

18. Young, G.B. "Inherited Defects of Dogs," *Vet. Rec.;* 1955: 67: 15-19.

19. Young, G.B. "Inherited Defects of Dogs." *Vet. Rec.*; 1955: 67: 15-19.

20. Gelatt, K.N. and Leipold, H.W. "Bilateral Optic Nerve Hypoplasia in Two Dogs," *Canad. Vet. Journal;* 1971:12:91-96.

21. Saunder, L.Z. "Congenital Optic Nerve Hypoplasia in Collie Dogs," *Cornell Vet.*; 1952: 42:67-80.

22. Phillips, J.M. and Felton, T.M. "Hereditary Umbilical Hernia in Dogs," *J. Hered.*; 1939: 30:433-435.

23. Urbich, R. "Untersuchunger zur Amtiolog: Klink der zerebralen Anfullsleiden beim Schottischen Schaferhund (Collie)," *Vet. Med. Griesen*; 1974: 1133-1137.

24. Ettinger, S.J. *Textbook of Veterinary Internal Medicine: Diseases of the Dog and Cat.* W.B. Saunders Co. Philadelphia, PA 1989: 597-598.

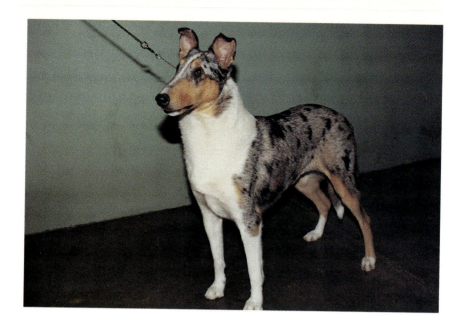

COLLIES (SMOOTH)

Smooth coated Collies can be found in a breeding of two roughs. In general the smooths tend to be a bit more aggressive. There is a noticeable increase of stamina and vitality in the smooths, perhpas explained by a concentration on a different gene pool.

Without the insulation of the heavy coat, the smooth variety is more at the mercy of extreme weather.

There are no physical aspects at variance with those of the rough variety, although some breeders report **bloat** more common in the smooth than in the rough Collie. Perhaps the lack of a long hair coat allows bloat to be diagnosed in an earlier stage.

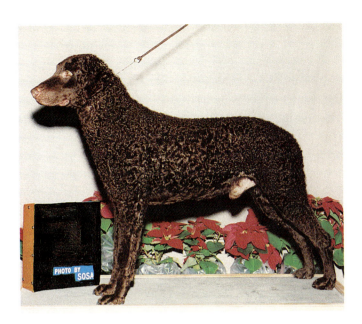

CURLY COATED RETRIEVER

ORIGIN AND HISTORY

The Curly Coated Retriever is popularly believed to be descended from the 16th century English Water Spaniel and from the retrieving setter. Some maintain that the Irish Water Spaniel was its ancestor. Since both liver and black are recognized colors for the Curly, it is very likely that the cross did occur. Whichever spaniel was its progenitor, it is supposed that the St. John's Newfoundland was added to the mixture about 1835. It is thought by some that in 1880 the Curly was again crossed with the Poodle (one-time retriever of France), with the object of giving his coat a tight curl.

DESCRIPTION

The only recognized colors are liver and black. A white spot on the chest is undesirable, although a few white hairs would be allowed in an otherwise good dog. Curlys are noted for having an even temperament and can be protective without being aggressive. Front dewclaws are usually removed, but removal is not a requirement for shows. If back dewclaws occur, they should be removed.

THE SHOW RING

Dogs should weigh between 75 and 85 pounds and stand 26 to 28 inches. Bitches should weigh from 65 to 75 pounds and should be 22 to 26 inches high.

The tight, curly coat should begin at the middle or rear of the ear line and extend all the way to the tip of the tail. Saddle backs are dogs with smooth to wavy hair over the back. They are acceptable in Australia, but not in the United States for show purposes.

There are no disqualifications in the show ring for this breed.

BREEDING AND WHELPING

Litters average seven in number, although a range of one to 15 puppies has been reported. Normal puppies weigh between 8 and 14 ounces.

RECOGNIZED PROBLEMS

Many breeders have noted a bilateral **alopecia** on the caudal aspect of the rear legs which appears at about 4 months of age and usually returns to normal at about 2 years. No explanation is offered. Generalized hair loss is common during lactation.

Members of the Medical Problems Research Committee[1] of the parent club report the following as occurring in the breed:

1. **Cushing's Syndrome**
2. **Pseudo-Cushing's Syndrome**
3. **Low thyroid**
4. **Inability to metabolize calcium**
5. **Juvenile osteoparesis**
6. **Bilateral alopecia, not thyroid related and not responsive to therapy**.

The Committee feels that surgery should not be considered for puppies exhibiting **entropion**, as this problem may be resolved as the dog matures. They also caution that the **thyroid** rating of the Curly Coated Retriever is at the lowest of the normal range, and that **pyometra** occurs more often than in dogs of other breeds.

BEHAVIOR

The Curly Coat is affectionate, loyal and easy to train.

OLD AGE

The average life span is from 8 to 12 years.

Reference
1. Caldwell, Marillyn, 1116 N. 38th, Lincoln, NE 68503.

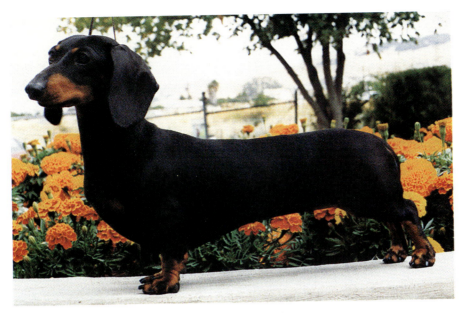

Smooth Dachshund

DACHSHUND

ORIGIN AND HISTORY

Taking its name from the German meaning "badger dog," the Dachshund breed of today traces its history to a specialized hunting dog of Middle Europe.[1] The earliest depictions of this "Teckel" or "tracking dog" in Germany are late 16th-century woodcuts of a "low, crooked-legged specie," as described in hunting literature.[2] They were especially effective in burrowing for badgers, but they also were used against wild boars, foxes and deer.

During the 17th century, the name Dachshund was firmly established.[3] By 1848, before recorded registrations, specialized breeding had begun which led to the three varieties of coats in Dachshunds: smooth-haired, long-haired and wire-haired. The smooth was first produced as a result of selective breeding of the smooth, long-haired hunting dog with Miniature French Pointers and Pinschers.[2] Breeders retained the long-haired Dachshund by breeding the smooth Dachshund with the Spaniel. The last coat developed was the wire-haired. The first individuals were recorded in the 1890s as a result of interbreeding with Pinschers, Schnauzers, Scotch Terriers and English Dandie Dinmonts.[2]

The first Dachshunds Club (for smooths only) was established in England in 1888. The Standard had been fixed earlier (1879) in Germany. From this period until the 1940s, the "modern type" smooth breed from German imports made up a high proportion of registered dogs in both Great Britain and the United States.[4] The AKC first registered smooths in 1885. Long-haired Dachshunds and wire-haired Dachshunds were not recognized in the United States until 1931.

201

The hunting ancestry of the Dachshund has not been forgotten, although few individuals are now imported for hunting in the United States. Dachshunds are still bred for hunting abilities (the AKC holds field trials) and separate stud books are kept for hunters in Germany.

DESCRIPTION

Dachshunds are playful, individualistic dogs that can be self-willed.[1] They are bred to maintain strength and stamina. The smooths and wire-hairs are more energetic, while the long-haired Dachshunds tend to be more dignified. The Dachshund of today comes in two sizes, three coats and several colors.

THE SHOW RING

Miniature Dachshunds are under 11 pounds in weight after 1 year of age, while the Standards are generally 16 to 32 pounds. There is no weight disqualification. It is essential the Dachshund be agile, trim and athletic.

Colors include red, brindle, black, chocolate, gray and fawn, and can have tan markings in specified areas. The Dachshund can also be dappled, which is a clear brownish or grayish or white ground with dark, irregular patches. Wall eyes are acceptable in dapples. Each of the coat textures comes in all colors.

The streamlined proportions of hunting skill are retained and exaggerated in the modern breed. In proportions, the height at the shoulder should be half the length of the body from breastbone to tail. The girth of the chest should be twice the height.[2] The forequarters should be muscular with straight, vertical forelegs at the deepest point of the chest. In the hindquarters, the hip is level to the shoulder with muscular hind legs, round buttocks, and arched, well-padded feet.[3] The tail is evenly tapered and well covered with hair.

The head and neck are prominent, with a long, tapered head and long, very muscular neck. The eyes are medium sized and almond-shaped, the darker the better, set off by a strong bridge bone. The ears are long and rounded, never narrow or folded.[3]

The bite is a strong scissors or level. Any deviation, undershot or overshot, is a fault.

The common faults are loose shoulders, bowed legs, long or twisted feet, poor angulation of front or hindquarters, goggle eyes and dewlaps. A small or narrow chest is also a fault as well as any weak pigmentation or albino characteristics (light eyes, pink or clear noses).[2]

Each coat variety has its own coat standards. For the smooth (either solid color or two-colored), the coat should be short, thick and shiny. There should not be too much tan and no white in the coat. Faults include bald patches, thin coat, leathery ears or a brush tail.[3]

The long-haired Dachshund coat should be soft and silky, with especially long hair under the neck and behind the legs. It should not have leather ears (little or no hair) or too much long hair on the feet. Too profuse a coat which masks type, equally long hair over the whole body, a curly coat or a pronounced parting on the back are all faults. [1,3] The wire-haired Dachshund has a double coat — a hard, thick outercoat and a dense undercoat. It should have a bearded chin. A flag tail is a fault.

Knuckling over of front legs is a disqualification in all three coat varieties.

RECOGNIZED PROBLEMS

Skull measurements were taken on 66 dogs of seven breeds using mostly data from breeders' studbooks. Litter size averaged 4.37±1.79 in the Dachshund, 3.51±1.48 in the Miniature dachshund.[5] **Ectasia syndrome (chorioretinal dysplasia)** is one of several eye disorders common in the Dachshund breed. Indications are excavation of the optic disc and retinal detachment. **Ectasia of the sclera, (staphyloma)**, is also possible. This condition is a weakening of the wall indicated by thin, blue or bulging sclera.[6]

Heterochromia iridis ("walleye") occurs in Dachshunds as an incomplete dominant trait. The two irises may develop as two different colors, or only part of one iris may differ. There is no indicated loss of vision.[8]

Microphthalmia is a condition in which the eyeball is diminished in all directions.[8] Though not rare in any breed, it occurs frequently in the Dachshund. Depending on the individual, the eyes may be functional, but may develop **congenital cataract** or **detached retina**.[8]

Entropion, glaucoma and progressive retinal atrophy has been reported in Longhaired Mini-Dachshunds.[8,9] **Districhiasis** and **persistent pupilary membrane** are found in the Dachshund.[10] **Keratoconjunctivitis sicca** is seen in this breed commonly, as are **dermoid cysts** and **atypical pannus**.

Uveodermatologic syndrome has been reported in the Dachshund.[7] They are at increased risk for **generalized demodectic mange** and **pemphigus foliaceous**.[7]

Intervertebral disc disease is a particularly dangerous and, unfortunately, common crippler of Dachshunds. The breed is predisposed because of its conformation; several studies confirm the high incidence of disc disease in chondrodystrophoid (short-legged) breeds at an early age (3 to 6 years) rather than as a geriatric condition.[11] The accompanying dehydration and calcification make the structure lose its shock-absorbing ability and tend to cause vertebral protrusion or extrusion. The results are upper motor neuron lesion, pain and bilaterally symmetrical pelvic paresis. Dachshunds are affected in the thoracolumbar region. **Achondroplasia** is a congenital defect found in some Dachshunds. The **abnormal ossification of the long bones** is inherited as an autosomal dominant trait.

Another bone disorder common to Dachshunds is **osteopetrosis**, a condition similar to the "swimmer pups" that develop in Bassets, English Bulldogs and Scotch Terriers.[5] The cause is unknown. As early as 2 weeks of age, puppies may be weak and unable to stand, although they nurse and grow normally. Since the trunk is not supported in a standing position, the limbs tend to spread laterally. A rough surface for daily exercise can improve mild cases.

Panniculitis is a multifactorial inflammatory condition of the subcutaneous fat. Thirteen out of 22 cases seen were Dachshunds.[12]

Two problems Dachshunds may exhibit are **cystinuria (excessive cystine in the urine)** and **renal hypoplasia** resulting in **polydipsia** and **polyuria**. Cystinuria is a sex-linked recessive trait (occurs in males). Similar to renal failure, renal hypoplasia calls for a special diet.[13]

They are also known to have calcium oxalate and struvate stones.[14,15] In a study of 839 **uroliths** submitted by veterinarians for analysis, 562 (67%) were composed of at least 70% magnesium ammonium phosphate, and 57 (6.8%) at least 70% calcium oxalate. Most were found in the bladder. Uroliths occurred more frequently in females than in males, but there was little difference in prevalence between dogs aged 1 to 12 years. The uroliths were found in 60 known breeds of dog, including the Dachshund.[16]

Although the mode of inheritance is not determined, Dachshunds tend to develop **diabetes mellitus**. This chronic metabolic disease is the result of decreased secretion of insulin from the pancreas, indicated in dogs by a renal threshold of 175 to 220 mg. insulin per 100 ml.[5] Early signs of the disorder are polyuria and polydipsia, progressing to weight loss and ketosis.

Breeding studies have shown a genetic basis for **idiopathic epilepsy**.[17]

Two defects whose mode of inheritance has not been determined are **deafness** and **clefts of the lip and palate**. The long-haired Dachshund is particularly liable to have problems with undershot or overshot jaws because of abnormal relative growth. A German study has described **sensory neuropathy** in Longhaired Dachshunds, with information on symptoms, diagnosis, prognosis and treatment.[18] Affected puppies have decreased superficial and deep sensation over the entire body, urinary incontinence and proprioceptive deficits in the pelvic limbs. Patellar reflexes are normal but flexor muscles are absent due to the lack of pain sensation. There is no paresis or muscle atrophy present. Dachshunds often develop **pattern baldness**. It is an inherited alopecia that begins before the dog is 1 year old. Males have **bilateral alopecia** of ear pinnae and females have **alopecia** of the ventral body. There is no known treatment.

Dachshunds as a breed have an increased incidence of **hyperadrenocorticism** and **hypothyroidism**.[19,20] Dachshunds are also known to have **alopecia**[21] associated with the gene for dilution. It has been reported that Dachshunds are predisposed to **cutaneous mast cell tumors**[22] and **ununited anconeal process**. There is a higher incidence of **cryptorchidism** reported in Miniature Dachshunds.[23]

BEHAVIOR

Dachshunds are gentle, tranquil, tenacious and cheerful. They can also be cunning and stubborn. They will try to train their owners rather than be trained. They are intelligent and make excellent companion dogs.

References

1. Johnson, N.H. *The Complete Puppy and Dog Book.* (Atheneum, New York, NY.,1973); 12, 27, 278-279.
2. Jones, A.F. and Hamilton, F., Eds., *The World Encyclopedia of Dogs.* (Galahad Books, New York, NY, 1971) 336, 337, 358.
3. American Kennel Club, *The Complete Dog Book.* 18th ed. (Howell Book House, New York, NY, 1992) 169-175.
4. American Kennel Club, *The Complete Dog Book.* 18th ed. (Howell Book House, New York, NY,1992) 169-175.
5. Hahn, S. "Variation of Skull Traits and Reproduction in Breeds of Small Dogs," Thesis, Tierarztliche Hochschule Hannover, Ger. Fed. Rep. 1988: 130; 11 ref.
6. Magrane, W.G. *Canine Ophthalmology.* (Lea & Febiger, Philadelphia, PA. 1975).
7. Griffin, C., Kwochka, K., McDonald, J. *Current Veterinary Dermatoloty, the Art and Science of Therapy.* Mosby Yearbook. St. Louis, MO. 1993.
8. Barnett, K.C. "Inherited Eye Disease in the Dog and Cat," *J. Sm. Anim. Prac.* 1988: 29:7, 462-475; 33 ref.
9. Rubin, L.F. *Inherited Eye Diseases in Purebred Dogs.* Williams and Williams, 1989: 101.
10. Christmas, R. DVM, *D.C.A. Newsletter*, Sept. 1992: p 20-21.
11. *Current Veterinary Therapy-VI.* R.W. Kirk, Ed. (W.B. Saunders Co., Philadelphia, PA, 1977); 841-848, 905-906, 1001-1009, 1137-1141, 1178.
12. *Small Animal Dermatology.* (Maller, Keith & Scott; 831 4th Ed.)
13. Hoskins, H.P., Eds., *Canine Medicine.* (Vet. Publ. Inc., Santa Barbara. CA.,1977); 82, 93, 398-399, 531, 583, 593.
14. *American Kennel Club Gazette.* September, 1992: 76.
15. Hesse, A. and Bruhl, M. "Urolithiasis in Dogs, Epidemiological Data and Analysis of Urinary Calculi," *Kleintierpraxis*; 1990: 35:10, 505-512; 18 ref.
16. Osborne, C.A., Clinton, C.W., Bamman, L.K., Moran, H.C., Coston, B.A.R., and Frost, A.P. "Prevalence of Canine Uroliths: Minnesota Urolith Center," *Vet Clinics of N. Amer., Sm. Anim. Practice;* 1986: 16:1, 27-44; 6 ref.
17. Graves, T.K. "Seizures in Dogs," *The American Kennel Club Gazette*; March, 1992.
18. Bichsel, P. "Neuromuscular Diseases of Young Dogs," Jahresversammlung. Schweizerische Vereinigung fur Kleintiermedizin. 2.-4. Juni 1988. Bazel 1988, 43-50. Zool Bern, Switzerland; c/o H.Heinimann, Schweis. Serum und Impfinstitut, Postfach 2707.
19. Brignac, Michele M. "Congenital and Breed Associated Skin Diseases in the Dog and Cat," *KalKan Forum;* December, 1989.

20. Larsson, M. "The Breed, Sex and Age Distribution of Dogs with Primary Hypothyroidism," *Svensk-Veterinartidning.* 1986: 38:15, 181-183; 3 ref.
21. *American Kennel Club Gazette*; 109, September, 1992.
22. Veterinary News. *The American Kennel Club Gazette;* April, 1990: 44.
23. Bell, Jerold S. DVM; "Sex Related Genetic Disorders: Did Mama Cause Them?" *American Kennel Club Gazette*, Feb. 1994; 76.

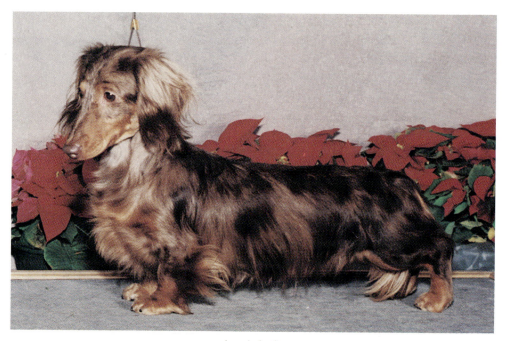

Longhaired

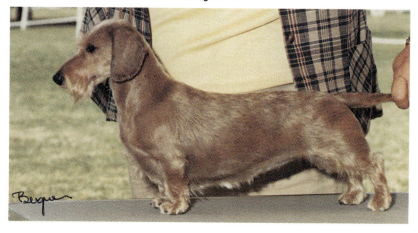

Miniature Wirehaired

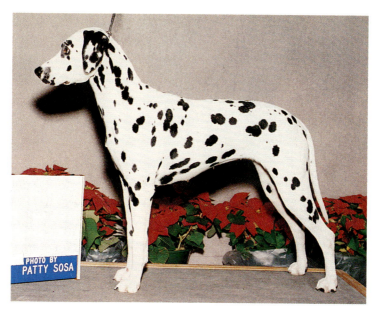

PHOTO BY
PATTY SOSA

DALMATIAN

ORIGIN AND HISTORY

According to Frankling,[1] evidence is lacking that the Dalmatian actually originated in Dalmatia even though dogs with spotting patterns similar to the present-day Dalmatian were portrayed in paintings from Eastern Mediterranean countries as early as the 14th century.

The breed, as we now know it, came from hunting dogs in England during the 19th century. There, Dalmatians were trained to travel with and guard their owners' horses and carriages. Primarily a running dog, the Dalmatian still retains many characteristics in common with English Pointers.

DESCRIPTION

Some breeders are successful in breeding Dalmatians who are friendly to anyone whom their masters make welcome. However, the basic nature seems to be that of a watch dog that distrusts all strangers. In a dog whose ancestors were used for guarding, suspicion would be characteristic.

Dalmatians are a popular choice of obedience exhibitors, as the breed is highly trainable and one which seems to enjoy obedience exercises.

THE SHOW RING

According to the American Standard of the breed, the desired height of dogs and bitches is between 19 and 23 inches at the withers, **a height over 24 inches being a disqualification.** A height of 23 to 24 inches for dogs and 22 to 23 inches for bitches is stated as the ideal in the

British Standard. Thus, descendants of Dalmatians imported from Great Britain tend to be oversize.

Dalmatian puppies should be born with white hair and small pigmented spots in the skin. **Those born with large pigmented patches in the coat, as is typical of an English Pointer, would be subject to disqualification.** At about 2 weeks the white hairs within the margins of the small pigmented spots are replaced with pigmented hairs. The pigment in the spots should be eumelanin, either black or brown (liver) in color. **Animals having spots of both brown and black color or pigment of any other type, such as phaeomelanian (lemon), would be subject to disqualification in the conformation ring.** At maturity the spots should be distinct (having no white hairs intermixed at the margins) and should vary in size from that of a dime to a half-dollar. Incomplete pigmentation of the eye rims or nose is considered a major fault. The coat should be short, dense and glossy. **Undershot or overshot bites are disqualifications.** A scissors bite is ideal. **Trichiasis, entropion** and **ectropion** are major faults. According to the Standard of the breed, the dewclaws may be removed.

BREEDING AND WHELPING

Litter-size is large in Dalmatians; eight to 10 is usual but 12 to 15 is not uncommon. Most of the puppies weigh between 11 and 15 ounces at birth.

RECOGNIZED PROBLEMS

Incompletely pigmented eye rims and **noses, patches, blue eyes** and **deafness**[2] can each occur in Dalmatian puppies. There is probably a genetic basis for each characteristic as the frequency of each trait differs somewhat in different bloodlines of the breed. The relative, as well as actual, size of the pigmented areas in the skin and in the iris of the eye tend to increase with age as a result of pigment cell migration.[3] It is difficult even for the experienced breeder to predict whether or not a partially pigmented nose, eye rim or iris will become completely pigmented by the time the animal reaches maturity. Patches will become larger and thus more objectionable with age. Unpigmented iris (blue eyes) is considered a fault in Great Britain but not in the United States regardless of whether it occurs unilaterally or bilaterally. Microscopic studies of deaf Dalmatian puppies that underwent euthanasia at different ages indicate that deafness is a degenerative process.[4,5] Puppies that could hear to some degree at 6 weeks of age have been known to become deaf by 3 months.

Two recent studies reported results of an investigation that included almost 2,000 Dals. By surveying these dogs with brainstem auditory emission response (BAER) tests, Dr. Terrell Holliday, et al, and Dr. George M. Strain, et al, concluded that the incidence of hearing disorders is currently close to 30%.[6]

Following is an abstract from a study done by Dr. George Strain, et al. "To screen for congenital deafness, brainstem auditory-evoked response (BAER) testing was performed on 1031 Dalmatians from three geographically separated areas. Phenotypic marker assessment was done to determine markers possibly associated with deafness. Markers included sex, hair coat color, pigmentation of different areas of skin (eye rims, nose and ears), presence of a patch, spot size and marking (density of spotting), sire and dam BAER status and presence of iris and retinal tapetal pigmentation. Combined data from all test sites showed 8.1% bilateral deafness (N==83 dogs) and 21.6% unilateral deafness (N==223), or an overall 29.7% incidence of hearing disorders. Significant (P<0.05) associations with deafness for the data from all the test sites combined were seen for patch, sire and dam BAER, iris pigment and retinal pigment. However, results differed for several of the significant phenotypic markers when analyses were done on the data from the individual test sites; changes from significant to not significant were found. This suggested the existence of multiple populations of deafness patterns, and reinforced the precautionary conclusion that associations of phenotypic markers with deafness are not necessarily functionally significant.[7]"

In a recent study of 839 **uroliths** submitted by veterinarians for analysis, 562 (67%) were composed of magnesium ammonium phosphate, and 57 (6.8%) at least 70% calcium oxalate. Most were found in the bladder. Uroliths occurred more frequently in females than in males, but there was little difference in prevalence between dogs aged 1 to 12 years. The uroliths were found in 60 known breeds of dog including Dalmatians.[8]

Urinary calculi of the urate type, **bacteriuria,** and a characteristic **dermatitis** which includes discoloration of the skin and white hair are common ailments of the Dalmatian that are considered a possible syndrome.[9,10] The basic cause is inability to metabolize uric acid to allantoin. This metabolic defect, resulting in a high level of uric acid excretion in the urine, is unique to the Dalmatian breed of dogs. It has been shown that by reciprocal transplants of livers between Dalmatians and mongrel dogs that the liver is the primary defective organ, the amount of uric acid excreted in the urine being determined by the donor liver.[11]

The dermatitis is characterized by hive-like eruptions of the skin which persist much longer than true hives. These eruptions first cause the overlying hairs to spread and stand erect. The damage is sufficiently severe to produce hair loss in the affected areas which leads to a "moth-eaten" appearance of the haircoat. While this pattern is most likely to appear over the back, it may affect all skin surfaces. The discoloration is very similar to the color produced by chronic licking. However, licking is not the cause in this syndrome because the discoloration appears in areas inaccessible to the tongue. Affected individuals are often restless to irritable, and males tend to lick at the penile sheath with unusual intensity. Individuals so affected usually react positively when tested for **inhalation allergy**, although the significance of this to the syndrome manifested is not clear. The authors have observed complete remission of the dermatitis by feeding the meat-free diet recommended for reduction of uric acid excretion in chronic stone formers.[12] Any concurrent urinary tract infection should be treated. The dermatitis is apparently due to an interaction between the elevated uric acid levels typical of Dalmatians, the tendency to **inhalation allergy**[13] and (in some cases) the urinary-tract infection. Presumably, the dermatitis could be relieved by hyposensitization but the simpler dietary management is preferable.

Additional treatment with allopurinol has been recommended in severe cases of **urolithiasis/dermatitis syndrome**.[6,5] This breed is at increased risk for generalized **demodicosis**.[14]

Tubular transport dysfunction has been discussed in a Cornell report on canine hereditary nephropathies.[15]

In a recent study, compared with mixed-breed dogs there were eight breeds at higher risk of developing **glaucoma**, one of which was the Dalmatian.[16]

Globoid cell leukodystrophy has been reported in Dalmatians.

Muscular Dystrophy, a rare x-linked recessive disease that is fatal, has been identified in Dalmations.[17]

BEHAVIOR

As a companion dog the Dalmatian is patient, gentle and obedient. They are distant with strangers and are excellent guard dogs. The "Dal" needs human company, without which it becomes melancholy.

OLD AGE

Life expectancy is from 10 to 12 years for a Dalmatian. Continued migration of pigment cells into the skin results in the development of "tick" spots in the white background of the coats of some individuals in old age.

References
1. Frankling, E. *The Dalmatian*. 4th ed, (Howell Book House, New York, N.Y., 1974).
2. Gewirtz, E.W. "Researching Dalmatian Deafness," *The American Kennel Club Gazette;* January, 1991.
3. Schaible, R.H. and Brumbaugh, J.A. "Electron Microscopy of Pigment Cells in Variegated and Nonvariegated Piebald-Spotted Dogs," *Pigment Cell;* 1976: 3:191-200.
4. Johnsson, L.G., et al, "Vascular Anatomy and Pathology of the Cochlea in Dalmatian Dogs," In *Vascular Disorders and Hearing Defects*; A.J.D. de Lorenzo, Ed. (Univ. Park

Press, Baltimore, Md, 1973) 249-293.

5. Mair, I.W.S. "Hereditary Deafness in the Dalmatian Dog," *Arch. Oto-Rhino-Laryng.;* 1976: 212:1-4.

6. *Journal of Veterinary Internal Medicine*; Volume 6, Number 3, May/June, 1992

7. Strain, George M., et al, "Brainstem Auditory-Evoked Potential Assessment of Congenital Deafness in Dalmatians: Associations with Phenotypic Markers," *Jour. of Vet. Int. Med.*; 1992: 6:175-182.

8. Osborne, C.A., Clinton, C.W., Bamman, L.K., Moran, H.C., Coston, B.R., and Frost, A.P. "Prevalence of Canine Uroliths: Minnesota Urolith Center," *Vet. Clinics of N. Amer, Sm. Anim. Prac.;* 1986: 16:1, 27-44; 6 ref.

9. Lowrey, et al: "Allopurinol in the Treatment of an Intractable Metabolically-Derived Dermatosis in a Dalmatian Dog," *VM/SAC*; 1973: 68: 755-762.

10. Hesse, A. and Bruhl, M. "Urolithiasis in Dogs, Epidemiological Data and Analysis of Urinary Calculi," *Kleintierpraxis*; 1990: 35:10, 505-512; 18 ref.

11. Kuster, G., et al, "Uric Acid Metabolism in Dalmatians and Other Dogs," *Arch. Intern. Med.;* 1972: 129: 492-496.

12. Osbaldiston, C.W. and Lowrey, J.C. "Allopurinol in the Prevention of Hyperuricemia in Dalmatian Dogs," *VM/SAC;* 1971: 66: 711-715.

13. Ackerman, Lowell, DVM, "Allergic Skin Diseases," *American Kennel Club Gazette;* September, 1990.

14. Griffin, C., Kwochka, K., McDonald, J.: *Current Veterinary Dermatology, the Science and Art of Therapy.* Mosby Yearbook, St. Louis, MO. 1993: 74.

15. Picut, C.A. and Lewis, R.M. "Comparative Pathology of Canine Hereditary Nephropathies: An Interpretive Review," *Vet. Res. Comm.*; 1087, 11:6, 561-581; 91 ref.

16. Slater, M.R. and Erb, H.N. "Effects of Risk Factors and Prophylactic Treatment on Primary Glaucoma in the Dog," *JAVMA;* 1986: 188:9, 1028-1030; 7 ref.

17. Bell, Jerold S. DVM; "Sex Related Genetic Disorders: Did Mama Cause Them?" *American Kennel Club Gazette.* Feb. 1994; 75.

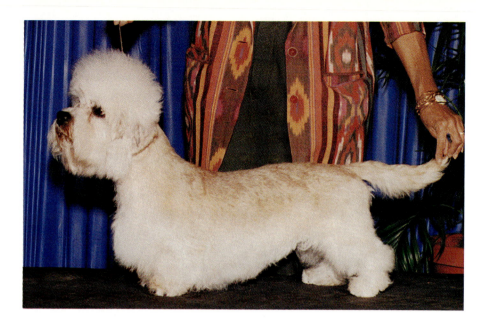

DANDIE DINMONT TERRIER

ORIGIN AND HISTORY

Dandie Dinmont Terriers originated in the border country between England and Scotland, where they hunted badgers, foxes, rats and weasels.

DESCRIPTION

"Dandies" are playful, affectionate and even-tempered. They are calmer than many other terrier breeds, and gentle with children. Dandies attach themselves to one master more than do dogs of most breeds. Although tolerant of others, they make excellent watch dogs. Dandies do not demand constant attention and are content to lie quietly in a favorite chair or corner.

THE SHOW RING

In 1876, the Dandie Dinmont Terrier Club of England specified 14 to 24 pounds in their Standard as the desirable weight range for Dandies, with 18 pounds the preferred weight and 24 pounds the upper limit. Although that weight range still applies, a dog weighing more than 24 pounds is not disqualified. However, a Dandie weighing more than 20 pounds would have difficulty going to the ground. This terrier has pendulous ears and a coat consisting of soft, silky hair on the head, and crisp, rough hair on the body. Dandies are of two colors, pepper or mustard. The pepper type ranges from bluish-black to silvery grey. The mustard type varies from a reddish brown to a pale fawn. **The breed Standard for Dandie Dinmonts lists no automatic disqualifications**, but it does list some faults. Because the Dandie needs a strong grip to hold its prey, correct bite is important to the breed. The teeth must meet, and the muzzle must not be too short. The ratio of muzzle to dome should be 3:5.

Undesirable markings are also faulted. For example, a mustard dog sometimes has an overabundance of pepper hairs and grey undercoat in the saddle region of the back. This marking, known as saddleback, is faulted. Front and back dewclaws should be removed. Ears should not be cropped, nor tails docked.

DENTITION

Full dentition is usual in Dandie Dinmonts, but the breed has its share of undershot and overshot bites. Occasionally, canine teeth or incisors will be missing in some individuals. Selective breeding to achieve shorter muzzles often results in a lack of molars and premolars.

RECOGNIZED PROBLEMS

Like most long-bodied dogs, Dandies are susceptible to **intervertebral disc syndrome** because of the conformation, length and flexibility of their spines. A disc can be ruptured by involuntary movements, or by pressure on the spine when the body is at an unfavorable angle. Sometimes a disc protrudes into the spinal cord, producing pressure and severe pain. Results may range from transient signs of pain to severe hemorrhage and death. Mildly affected dogs may show only slight discomfort at the site of the displaced disc, slight stiffness, slightly abnormal gait, reluctance to move and an apprehensive temperament. For seriously affected individuals, moving is acutely painful. Complete paralysis of the hind legs and tail may occur, together with fecal and urinary retention. A period of spinal shock may last two to three days. This syndrome usually occurs in dogs that are 6 to 8 years old.

Hip dysplasia and **medial subluxation of the patella** are related conditions sometimes reported in the Dandie Dinmont. It is thought that in dwarf dogs, hip dysplasia results from improper development of the acetabulum secondary to a poor fitting of the femoral head in the acetabulum. As the affected femur and its head twist, the hip socket develops into a large, shallow opening, creating an unstable joint. In affected dogs, the femur tends to be excessively bowed. The stifle tilts outward and frequently the patella subluxates medially. As the patella slips in and out, the dog walks normally for a while and then suddenly favors a hind leg. The affected leg has a pigeon-toed appearance. Persistent luxations cause continuous lameness or abnormal or hopping gaits.

Although the Dandie Dinmont's achondroplastic features are desirable, breeders must avoid breeding in the exaggerated forms that can affect movement of the legs. The breeder's goal must be dogs with stable joints, sound movement and stride and legs that look straight from both the front and back.

Luxation and subluxation of the shoulder and elbow joints occur in Dandie Dinmonts and are difficult to treat. Often surgical intervention is required to stabilize the joint.

Because the long bones of the Dandie Dinmont are rather short, **traumatic fractures** usually occur at the ends rather than the midshafts of the humerus and femur. Usually fractures of the humerus occur just above the elbow. Fractures of the femur occur either just above the stifle or just below the hip. Repairing fractures of a Dandie's long bones is difficult. Their shape does not lend itself to stabilization with a plaster cast. Neither pinning nor plating the chondrodystrophoid long bone is easy. **Dislocation** secondary to trauma is reported. The hip, elbow and hock are most commonly affected. These dislocations usually can be reduced by manipulation followed by bracing or support. Occasionally open reduction is necessary.

In stifle and shoulder joints, **torn ligaments**, rather than dislocation, are more likely to occur secondary to trauma. **Rupture of the anterior cruciate ligament** is most common. To prevent instability of the joint, surgical repair is often necessary.

Dandies are subject to **ear infections** because of their flop ears. Also, hair in the ear tends to trap dirt and foster infection. Ear infections can also be secondary to infestation by the ear mite Otodectes. Clinical signs of infestation are shaking or scratching of the head, holding an ear to one side and rubbing an ear along the ground.

Dandies are one of a specified group of breeds with a higher risk for canine **lymphoma**.[1,2,3]

Cushing's disease has been identified in The Dandie Dinmont Terrier.[4]

BEHAVIOR

The Dandie is an excellent companion dog. He is pleasant and playful, adaptable and extremely loyal. He is an excellent watch dog with a big bark for his size.

OLD AGE

The average life span of the Dandie Dinmont is approximately 10 to 12 years, although some live 15 years.

References
1. Madewell, Bruce R., VMD, MS, "Canine Lymphoma," *Vet Clinics of North America: Sm. Anim. Prac.*; Vol.15, #4, July: 1985.
2. McCaw, Dudley, DVM, "Canine Lymphosarcoma," AAHA's 56th Annual Meeting Proceedings, 1989.
3. Rosenthal, Robert C., DVM, MS, PhD, "The Treatment of Multicentric Canine Lymphoma," *Vet. Clinics of N. America: Sm. Anim. Prac.*; July, 1990: Vol. 20, #4.
4. Wilford, Christine, DVM; "Veterinary News" *AKC Gazette*, April 1994: 34.

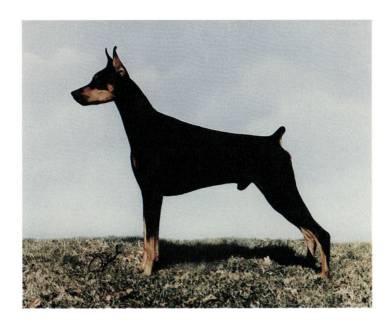

DOBERMAN PINSCHER

ORIGIN AND HISTORY

The Doberman Pinscher is a relatively new breed, developed in the 1870s by Herr Louis Doberman of Germany. By using crosses of the smooth-haired German Pinscher, Rottweiler, and certain shepherd strains, a rough form of the desired breed was produced by 1890. The Doberman Pinscher Club of America was formed in 1921, and the breed quickly gained approval of the American public.

DESCRIPTION

The Doberman is not recommended for anyone who is not a true dog lover, nor for someone only concerned with protection, nor as an outdoor dog. This breed demands training with affection. The Doberman needs close contact with human beings that can be filled by living as a house dog and member of the family. Although many people believe that Dobermans are "one man" dogs, they are actually friendly with all members of the family as well as with friendly visitors. They are, of course, one of the best home-protective breeds.

The Doberman is highly intelligent as well as beautiful. Unfortunately, the dog is often found in unsuitable homes where it is denied the affection it needs, either through indifference or ignorance of its needs.

Dobermans come in four colors — black, red, blue and fawn, all with rust markings. They have short coats that make them ideal for the house. They require only regular brushing to remove any excess shedding. The blues and fawns do have coat problems. It is dishonest for breeders to sell these colors as being "rare and valuable" when they know there is a chance the puppy in question may have a coat problem. Blues and fawns can in some cases be almost bald by the time they are 6 years old. They are often sold for more money to unsuspecting novices when in truth they should be sold for less than the other colors. Also, the owners should be informed about the extra care that blues and fawns require to keep their coats.

THE SHOW RING

The Standard calls for a breed of medium size with the ideal for dogs of 27 1/2 inches at the withers; for bitches, the ideal is 25 1/2 inches. **The only disqualifications are overshot more than 3/16 of an inch, undershot more than 1/8 of an inch, dogs not of an allowed color and four or more missing teeth. The Standard calls for a judge to dismiss from the ring any shy or vicious Doberman.**

BREEDING AND WHELPING

Owners should be discouraged from breeding their bitches unless they have a quality dog. Even then, they must realize that it takes a great deal of time, effort and money to raise a litter properly. Dobermans are, as a rule, easy whelpers. The puppies should weigh about 1 pound at birth and gain weight rapidly. The average size litter is about eight, but 12 is not uncommon. The smaller litters seem to give the most problems whelping. Dobermans grow fast; they must get a good diet during this period in order to develop properly.

GROWTH

Tails should be docked and dewclaws removed when the puppy is 3 days old. Since Dobermans have rather short tails, docking is often a problem. The tail should be cut at half an inch from the anus, then the skin pulled back and more bone removed. This procedure will usually leave the tail the right length for that dog.

Ears are best cropped at 6 to 7 weeks. In a litter in good condition, the puppies should weigh 10 to 12 pounds at 6 weeks. There are many methods for taping the ears after surgery, but the cut edge should never be covered with tape. It is far better for the cut edge to remain exposed to the air. Either apply 1 1/2 inch tape to each side of the ear with two layers of tape, and use a brace between the ears to hold them in a natural upright position, or use foam rubber between the puppy's ears. Stitches should be left in for only one week.

Show puppies should be chosen at 8 to 9 weeks of age since this age gives a good indication of what they will be like when mature. The puppy should be compact, have a good top line, tight feet and good depth of brisket. Head shape can change a great deal after this age, but eye shape and ear placement usually do not change. Of course, the care the puppy receives during the peak growth period is very important, and many a good puppy has been ruined for show by lack of proper feeding and care.

RECOGNIZED PROBLEMS

Cervical vertebral instability (CVI), often referred to as **wobbler syndrome**, is a serious problem in Dobermans. It often does not show up until the dog is well past his or her prime and after it has already been used in a breeding program. The signs range from minimal rear leg incoordination to complete paralysis. The cause is unknown. Clinical studies indicate that both genetics and diet may be involved. One study indicated that excess intake of protein, calcium and phosphorous accelerates growth and can lead to changes similar to wobbler syndrome. Instability usually involves the last three cervical vertebrae. All animals used in a breeding program should be x-rayed, no matter how sound they appear to the eye.

Deafness has been reported in the Doberman Pinscher.[1]

Craniomandibular osteopathy is a disease characterized by bilateral irregular osseous proliferation of the mandible, tympanic bulbar and occasionally of other bones of the head. This disease has been reported in Dobermans.[2]

Polyostotic fibrous dysplasia (a cortical defect characterized by osteophytes and cyst formation in distal metaphysis of the ulna and radius) has been reported in the breed.[3,4,5] **Bundle of His degeneration** has been implicated as a cause of sudden death in Dobermans.[6,7]

Congenital renal dysplasia[8] has been reported in Dobermans. This is a similar condition to that found in Norwegian Elkhounds, Lhasa Apsos, Shih Tzus, and Cocker Spaniels. **Glomerulopathy** in Dobes is discussed in a Cornell study of hereditary canine nephropathies.[9]

Alopecia,[10,11] a condition characterized by dry, lusterless hair coat, scaliness and papules is most commonly found in blue Dobermans and was formerly called blue Doberman syndrome. The condition also occurs in some red Dobermans, blue Dachshunds and blue Whippets. Most dogs with this syndrome have normal coats at birth and while young. Soon "moth-eaten" alopecia and scaly skin appear. In some, but not all, there is papule formation. The papules are cystic hair follicles, devoid of hair, which develop into pustules and after several years, almost all hair of the trunk and body are lost. The head, legs and tail are least affected.

The disease is incurable, although the skin can be helped with treatment. Frequent submerged baths and dressings will hydrate the skin. Anti-seborrheic shampoo will help remove scales. Alpha-Keri spray applied daily will make the coat look shinier and helps lubricate the dry, brittle hairs. If thyroid tests reveal a low or low — normal level, thyroid supplementation is justified and seems helpful in some cases.

Vitiligo is more commonly observed in Rottweilers and Dobermans. **Vitiligo** is a genodermatosis affecting the production of melanin in the skin and hair.[12]

Follicular dysplasia has been reported in adult black and red Dobes.[13]

Dobermans may be at higher risk for **pemphigus foliaceous** and **bullous pemphigoid**.[12] This breed has an unusually high incidence of **demodicosis**.

Von Willebrand's disease (VWD) (pseudohemophilia[14]) is characterized by prolonged bleeding time, low Factor VIII, reduced platelet adhesiveness, and abnormal prothrombin consumption time. Patients may exhibit **recurrent melena, prolonged estrual bleeding, excessive bleeding after trauma and subcutaneous hematoma.**

Other signs include **hematuria**, serosanguineous otitis externa; **protracted bloody diarrhea** irritated by stress, parasites or infections. Dogs with this disease may appear to have **eosinophilic gastroenteritis**, since both states are marked by eosinophilia, shifting leg lameness and similar radiographic changes.

Because **VWD** is usually less severe than hemophilia A, affected animals frequently survive to reproduce. It is becoming more important that animals used for breeding be tested for this condition. VWD in the Doberman is caused by a defective dominant gene with incomplete penetrance.[15] Cryoprecipitates given twice daily for one or two days are the treatment of choice.[9]

Dobes are one of the breeds at greatest risk for developing **osteosarcomas**.[16]

In a study at the U. of Pa. Veterinary Hospital, Dobes were consistently shown to be at increased risk of canine parvovirus enteritis. It is concluded that there are significant breed differences in susceptibility to CPV enteritis, but the pathogenesis for this has not been determined.[17] Personal communication and experience lead us to believe this increased susceptibility is due to the high incidence of Von Willebrand's disease in the Doberman.

Flank sucking occurs almost exclusively in Dobermans.[18] The animal may rest for hours with the head directed toward the flank and the jaws opened and resting on the skin in the flank region. The skin in the flank does not appear to be excessively irritated, although it is frequently covered with saliva. The habit is often reported to occur at puberty and to be lost in adulthood. There is no known therapeutic approach to the syndrome.

Narcolepsy is a problem in Dobermans. A recent study by the Stanford Sleep Research Center has proven that the disease is hereditary. This disease is similar in dogs and cats.

Dancing Doberman disease presents with an adult Doberman holding up one pelvic limb while standing; no underlying bone or joint disease can be detected. The clinical signs can remain the same for years, with only one limb affected. Other dogs may progress to the other limb, so while standing the animal alternately flexes and extends each pelvic limb in a dancing motion, then sits down. Over several months to years the gastrocnemius, semitendimosus, and semimembranosus muscles atrophy and mild pelvic limb weakness and conscious proprioceptive deficits develop. A simultaneous degeneration and regeneration process of the distal nerves is suspected. The genetic basis of this disorder is not known, but it appears to be a breed predisposition.[19]

Immune complex disorders (ICD) is a hereditary problem in Doberman Pinschers. Signs include pyoderma, generalized demodectic mange, generalized erythema, pruritus and alopecia.[20] The adrenal cortex is probably involved in the hereditary transfer of ICD.

Dobermans also are subject to **Chronic Active Hepatitis**. They also have an increased breed incidence of **hypothyroidism** and may have a familial hypothyroidism. It has been suggested that the breed is predisposed to **acral lick dermatitis (acral lick granuloma) because they are an active breed with superior intelligence and are easily bored by inactivity.**[21]

Dilated cardiomyopathy has been reported in the breed.[22,23]

OFA has reported **elbow dysplasia** in the Doberman Pinschers.[24]

Microphthalmia and **persistent hyperplastic primary vitreous** have been reported in Dobermans.[25]

Atherosclerosis was diagnosed PM in 21 dogs between 1970 and 1983. Nine dogs had died and 12 were destroyed because of complications associated with the disease. The mean age was 8.5± 0.5 years; 18 dogs were male. Three breeds had a higher prevalence of the disease than other breeds, including Dobes. Common clinical signs were lethargy, anorexia, weakness, dyspnoea, collapse and vomiting.

Hypercholesterolemia, lipidaemia and hypothyroidism were common in affected dogs tested, and protein electrophoresis revealed high values for alpha 2 and beta fractions in all dogs tested. ECG indicated conduction abnormalities and myocardial infarction in three of seven dogs. Affected arteries (including coronary, myocardial, renal, carotid, thyroidal, intestinal, pancreatic, splenic, gastric, prostatic, cerebral and mesenteric) were yellow-white, thick and nodular and had narrow lumens.

Myocardial fibrosis and infarction also were observed in the myocardium. Histologically, affected arterial walls contained foamy cells or vacuoles, cystic spaces, mineralized material, debris with or without eroded intima and degenerated muscle cells.[26]

BEHAVIOR

Data were obtained on 245 cases of **aggressive behavior** in dogs of 55 breeds. Aggression involved barking, growling and biting. Dominance aggression was found in the Doberman.[27]

The Doberman is a born guard dog. He is intelligent, quick and strong. With proper training he can also be a stable, devoted companion dog. The male is more impetuous and less sensitive than the female. Training is most important for Dobermans who are to be family companion dogs.

PUPPY	2 WKS.	3 WKS.	4 WKS.	5 WKS.	6 WKS.	7 WKS.	SEX
			GROWTH CHART				
A	2 lb 8	4 lb 2	6 lb 8	8 lb	10 lb	13 lb 1	MALE
B	2 lb 11	4 lb 5	6 lb 12	8 lb 8	11lb 8	14 lb 1	MALE
C	2 lb 14	4 lb 1	6 lb 8	8 lb 8	12 lb 4	13 lb 8	MALE
D	2 lb 12	4 lb	6 lb 4	7 lb 12	10 lb 4	13 lb	MALE
E	2 lb 4	3 lb 7	5 lb	6 lb 12	9 lb	11lb 8	BITCH
F	2 lb 8	3 lb 12	5 lb 8	7 lb 4	9 lb 7	12 lb 5	BITCH
G	2 lb 9	3 lb 13	5 lb 8	6 lb 12	8 lb 8	11 lb 8	BITCH
H	2 lb 4	3 lb 6	5 lb 5	7 lb	9 lb 4	11lb 8	BITCH
I	2 lb 8	3 lb 12	5 lb 8	7 lb 4	9 lb 11	12 lb 4	BITCH
J	2 lb 10	4 lb	5 lb 12	7 lb	9 lb 9	12 lb 5	BITCH

These are fairly representative weights for a litter of ten. Puppies from smaller litters may be larger. The subject puppies received bottle feeding to supplement the mother's milk.

References

1. Strain, G.M. "Deafness in Dogs and Cats," *Proc. 10th ACVIM Forum*; 1992.
2. Watson et al, "Craniomandibular Osteopathy in Doberman Pinschers," *J. Sm. Anim. Prac.;* 1975: 16:11-19.
3. Canig, C.B. and Seawright, A.A. "A Familial Canine Polyostotic Dysplasia and Subperiosteal Cortical Defects," *J. Sm. Anim. Prac.;* 1969: 10:397-405.
4. Kirk, R.W. and Bistner, S.I. *Handbook of Veterinary Procedures and Emergency Treatment: Hereditary Defects in Dogs*. Table 124, 1975: 661.
5. Canig, C.B. and Seawright, A.A. "A Familial Canine Polyostotic Fibrous Dysplasia with Cortical Defects," *J. Sm. Anim. Prac.*; 1965: 10.
6. James, T.N. and Drake, E.H. "Sudden Death in Doberman Pinschers," *Henry Ford Hosp. Bull.*; 1965: 13:183-190.
7. James, T.N. and Drake, E.H. "Sudden Death in Doberman Pinschers," *Annual of Int. Med.;* 1969: 68:821-829.
8. Erickson, et al: "Congenital Defects of Dogs, Part II," *Can. Prac.*; 1977: 4,(5):51-61.
9. Picut, C.A. and Lewis, R.M. "Comparative Pathology of Canine Hereditary Nephropathies: An Interpretive Review," *Vet. Res. Comm.;* 1987: 11:6, 561-581; 91 ref.

10. Muller, G.H. and Kirk, R.W. *Sm. Anim. Dermatology.* 2nd ed. (W.B. Saunders, Philadelphia, PA., 1976).

11. Miller, W.H., Jr., "Color Dilution Alopecia in Doberman Pinschers with Blue or Fawn Coat Colors," *Veterinary Dermatology.* 1990: 1:113-122.

12. Griffin, C., Kwochka, K., McDonald, J. *Current Veterinary Dermatology, the Science and Art of Therapy.* Mosby Yearbook, St. Louis, MO. 1993: 142, 171, 226, 231.

13. Miller, W.M., Jr., "Follicular Dysplasia in Adult Black and Red Doberman Pinschers," *Veterinary Dermatology.* 1990: 1: 181-187.

14. Dodds, J.W. "Inherited Hemorrhagic Defects," *Current Veterinary Therapy VI.* (W.B. Saunders, Philadelphia, PA.,1977). 444-445.

15. Bell, J.S. "Identifying and Controlling Defective Genes," *American Kennel Gazette*; July, 1993: 85.

16. *JAVMA*; Vol. 196, No. 9, May 1, 1990.

17. Glickman, L.T., Domanski, L.M., Patronek, G.J., and Visintainer, F. "Breed-Related Risk Factors for Canine Parvovirus Enteritis," *JAVMA;* 1985: 187:6, 589-594; 22 ref.

18. Hart, B.L. "Canine Behavior," *Can. Prac.*; 1977: 4 (6):14.

19. Ettinger, S.J. *Textbook of Veterinary Internal Medicine: Diseases of the Dog and Cat.* W.B. Saunders Co., Philadelphia, PA. 1989: 725.

20. Plechner, A.J. and Shannon, M.S., VM/SAC, references: Muller & Kirk, *Small Animal Dermatology*; (W.B. Saunders, Philadelphia, PA 1976).

21. Brignac, Michele M. "Congenital and Breed Associated Skin Diseases in the Dog and Cat," *KalKan Forum*; December, 1989.

22. "Cardiomyopathy in Doberman Pinschers," *American Kennel Club Gazette*; June, 1989.

23. Ettinger, S.J. *Textbook of Veterinary Internal Medicine: Diseases of the Dog and Cat.* W.B. Saunders Co., Philadelphia, PA. 1989: 1104.

24. Bodner, Elizabeth, DVM, "Genetic Status Symbols," *The American Kennel Club*; Sept. 1992.

25. Barnett, K.C. "Inherited Eye Disease in the Dog and Cat," *J. Sm. Anim. Prac.*; 1988: 29:7, 462-475; 33 ref.

26. Liu, S.K., Tilley, L.P., Tappe, J.P., and Fox, P.R. "Clinical and Pathologic Findings in Dogs with Atherosclerosis: 21 cases," *JAVMA;* 1986: 189:2, 227-232; 33 ref.

27. Borchelt, P.L. "Aggressive Behavior of Dogs Kept as Companion Animals," *Applied Animal Ethology;* 1983: 10, 45-61; 24 ref.

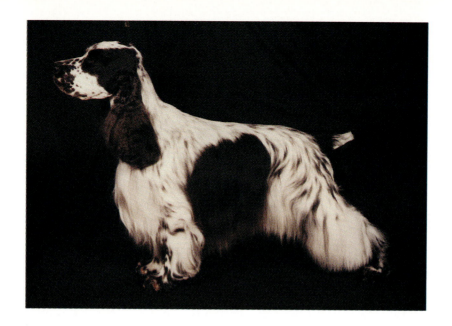

ENGLISH COCKER SPANIEL

ORIGIN AND HISTORY

Descending from Water and Toy Spaniels, the smallest of the upland bird hunters acquired the name "cocker" because of their skill in routing woodcocks from dense cover. A spaniel resembling the modern English Cocker appears in a 17th-century Van Dyck portrait. Taller and stronger than its American cousin, the English Cocker also differs by having a much longer muzzle.

In England, the Cocker (English Cocker) flourished and became the top breed for many years, but in the United States it is still a semi-rare breed placing about 70th in the AKC's list of dogs registered annually.

DESCRIPTION

By temperament, the English Cocker is equable and loving, happy with his work. In fact, the word "merry" has become synonymous with the English Cocker, and veterinarians find it a placid and easy dog to treat. English Cockers are either solid color — black, red, golden and very occasionally black and tan — or partis. The latter run the gamut: dark and light blue roans, black and white and black/white ticked, liver roan, liver and white, orange roan, orange and white; the tricolors consist of blue/roan and tan, black/white and tan, liver/roan and tan, and liver/white and tan. Disqualifications in the show ring consist of white hair on the solids other than in the chest area. Nostrils should be black, but brown is permitted in the lighter colors.

Black markings such as ears, mask and patches are easily discernible at birth. Dark blues can be picked out by the black pads of the feet. The differences between lighter blues and black/whites cannot be accurately predicted until the puppy is several weeks old. In fact, as ticking appears as the puppy grows, the demarcation line between a black/white ticked dog and a light blue roan is sometimes hard to distinguish. The blue roans range from very light to almost black. Orange is a recessive color and must be carried by both dam and sire to appear. At birth the orange puppies' color often appears white.

THE SHOW RING

The Standard calls for a dog not more than 17 inches at the shoulder and from 28 to 34 pounds. The bitch should not exceed 16 inches and should weigh from 26 to 32 pounds. Because this is a very active hunting dog, it should be compact, sturdy, with good bone and muscle and should have the depth of chest and spring of rib to enable it to work long hours in the field. It also needs strong, well-angulated hindquarters for good driving power. Its head, with fine chiselling and equal proportions, is its most distinctive feature.

There are no breed disqualifications.

Major faults comprise anything that detracts from the breed's purpose — to be a good hunting dog and companion. Faults include narrow chests with corresponding slab sides; "snipy" foreface with undershot or overshot jaw; excessively heavy or curly woolly coat; loose haws; poor hindquarters; bad temperament. Tails should be docked and dewclaws removed around the fourth day. The tail should be cut at the point where it starts to taper, at about the fourth or fifth vertebra or approximately 1/3 the length.

BREEDING AND WHELPING

Ovulation occurs from the 9th to the 14th day of estrus. The gestation period averages 61 days and the average number of pups is five, although it can range from one to eleven.

With normal health and good nutrition, an English Cocker bitch is easy to breed and will have no problems during gestation or whelping. The bitch should be exercised daily, for she will remain active right up to whelping time. Weight at birth ranges from 2 to 4 ounces. Occasionally there is a swimmer in a litter. A flattened chest prevents the puppy from using its front legs normally. It is not noticeable until about 2 weeks of age when the pup's eyes open and it starts walking. This "swimmer" condition can last from several days to several weeks but usually corrects itself. Some English breeders use a knitted harness to correct the condition.

GROWTH

An English Cocker puppy's rate of growth is rapid from birth to 6 months. Then it tapers off to a slow maturing with a deepening and widening of brisket, more layback of shoulders, an increase of height at the withers and a widening and deepening of muzzle and skull. The slow maturing English Cocker puppy should be given a lot of exercise, especially hill climbing, to build bone and muscle.

DENTITION

In smaller dogs and bitches, mouths should be watched at teething time to see that new teeth are not misplaced by retained baby teeth.

RECOGNIZED PROBLEMS

There are few health problems that seem to have a breed incidence. One condition is the progressive loss of vision in some individuals after middle age, **(progressive retinal atrophy)**.[1,2,3] Some have a **retinal degeneration** and others may develop **cataracts**. **Glaucoma** has been found in the breed.[4] Second, there is an incidence of **cryptorchidism** in the breed. These conditions are probably hereditary in nature, but it has not been proven.

Familial 78XX male **pseudohermaphroditism** has been reported in the breed.[5] **Hermaphroditism** in one case affected two littermates and one subsequent sibling.

The English Cocker is prone to **ear problems** if the hair is not removed from inside the ear. **Hemophilia A,**[6] **juvenile amaurotic idiocy**[6] and **neuronal ceroid lipofuscinosis**[6] have also been reported in the English Cocker.

The **"short toe anomaly"** occurs occasionally in the English Cocker.[7]

In a Swedish study the high incidence of **chronic liver disease** and **liver cirrhosis** in certain breeds, among them English Cockers, seem to indicate that hereditary factors may be of importance in the development of these conditions.[8]

In studies by Strain, English Cockers were listed fourth in incidence of **deafness**. Of 144 studied, 13.9% were unilaterally or bilaterally deaf.[9]

Dilated cardiomyopathy has been described in the breed.[10]

BEHAVIOR

The English Cocker is a gentle, playful companion dog. He is submissive and interested in his owner's life. He is independent and intelligent and does not care for young children.

OLD AGE

Unfortunately, the one problem that confronts the English Cocker breeder is that the older dog — 8 years and older — too often has eye problems, mostly in the form of **cataracts**[11] and consequently is often blind by 10 years of age.

The English Cocker's life span is from 10 to 14 years.

References

1. Barnett, K.C. "Abnormalities and Defects in Pedigree Dogs, IV, Progressive Retinal Atrophy," *J. Sm. Anim. Prac.*; 1963: 4:465-467.
2. Barnett, K.C. "Genetic Anomalies of the Posterior Segment of the Canine Eye," *J. Sm. Anim. Prac.;* 10:451-455.
3. Barnett, K.C. "Canine Retinopathies, III — The Other Breeds," *J. Sm. Anim. Prac.;* 6:185-196.
4. Bedford, P.G.C. "The Etiology of Primary Glaucoma in the Dog," *J. Sm. Anim. Prac.* 16:217-239.
5. Hare, W.D.C., et al, "Familial 78XX Male Pseudohermaphroditism in Three Dogs," *J. Reprod. Fert.;* 36:207-210.
6. Kirk, R.W. and Bistner, S.I. *Handbook of Veterinary Procedures and Emergency Treatment.* 3rd ed. (W. B. Saunders, Philadelphia, Pa., 1981) 822.
7. English Cocker Spaniel column, *American Kennel Club Gazette;* July, 1990.
8. Anderson, M. and Sevelius, E. "Breed, Sex and Age Distribution of Dogs with Chronic Liver Disease: A Demographic Study," *J. Sm. Anim. Prac.*; 1991: 32:1, 1-5; 20 ref.
9. Strain, George M., et al, "Deafness in Dogs and Cats," *Proc. 10th ACVIM Forum*; 1992.
10. Ettinger, S.J. *Textbook of Veterinary Internal Medicine: Diseases of the Cat and Dog.* W.B. Saunders Co. Philadelphia, PA. 1989: 1104.
11. Barnett, K.C. "The Diagnosis and Differential Diagnosis of Cataract in the Dog," *J.. Sm. Anim. Prac.*; 1985: 26:6, 305-316; 20 ref.

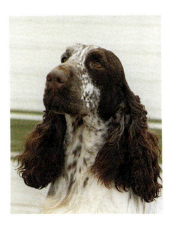

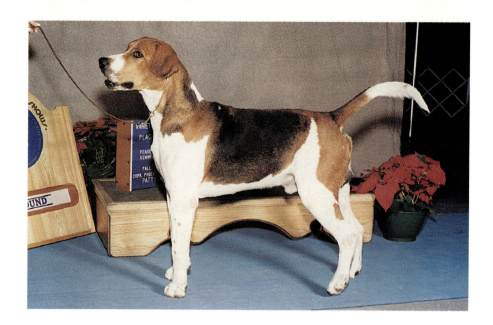

ENGLISH FOXHOUND

DESCRIPTION

The appearance of the English Foxhound is far stouter than his American cousin.

THE SHOW RING

Either pig-mouth (overshot) or undershot mouths are a disqualification.

RECOGNIZED PROBLEMS

Researchers have not differentiated between American and English Foxhounds, so problems named in the American Foxhound chapter would apply to the English Foxhound.

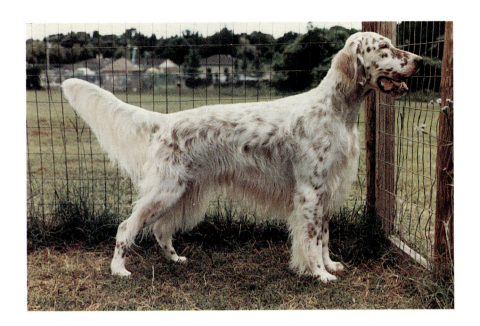

ENGLISH SETTER

ORIGIN AND HISTORY

The English Setter was bred for centuries to hunt with and for man. The breed was first perfected in consistent quality by two English breeders, Mr. Laverack and Mr. Llewellin, in the 1800s.

The term "Llewellin Setter" is used often, sometimes to refer to a strain bred primarily for hunting ability; however, no Llewellin Setters exist today. Stock from that kennel has long since been diluted by crosses with other strains.

DESCRIPTION

Dogs of this breed are sensitive and cooperative, with an intense desire to please. They possess keen scenting ability and will relinquish their natural instinct to capture and kill their own prey in an effort to gain approval from their companion, man.

A sharp temperament is almost unknown. A vicious English Setter should be considered sick or under extreme stress or pain. These dogs excel as family pets and thrive as household members.

THE SHOW RING

English Setters are a medium-large breed, dogs about 25 inches at the shoulders and bitches about 24 inches. They have soft, silky coats and long feathers on the chest, ears, legs and tail. Their coats are white with orange, black, liver or lemon flecks. They are referred to as orange beltons, blue beltons, etc., and as tricolors (black or liver with tan points). Large patches of color on the body are undesirable. A finely chiseled, long and lean head, and gentle, dark, expressive eyes are characteristic of the breed. Full dentition is usual, but undershot bites do occur in the breed. Overshot bites of as much as 2.5 cm will correct as late as 14 months.

Removal of dewclaws is recommended but not required.

There are no disqualifications for showing this breed in conformation.

BREEDING AND WHELPING

Season and length of gestation in English Setters follows a normal pattern, but time of ovulation is irregular. Some bitches conceive when bred on the eighth day; others conceive when bred as late as the 24th day. If conception does not result from a mating, a much earlier or later breeding date should be considered.

Onset of puberty in the dog is as variable as ovulation in the bitch. Although some dogs have successfully served at stud when they were only 6 1/2 months old, others are still sexually immature at 20 months of age.

English Setters are subject to **eclampsia**. To overcome **uterine inertia**, many bitches require a calcium injection at whelping.

Bitches in some bloodlines produce excess milk and require milk removal by hand even with large litters. These bitches must be treated with moist, hot compresses to prevent caking. The average litter size is six to 10, although litters as large as 15 are not rare.

Puppies are born white, or white with black ears and with pink noses, eyerims and footpads. Rarely an orange marking will be present at birth. Pigmentation begins to appear a few days after birth and ticking (body spotting) is evident in the third week. Breeders consider the 21st day the day to observe coat color, admire pigmentation and to test for deafness.

RECOGNIZED PROBLEMS

Congenital deafness is encountered in English Setters. Strain has reported that in his study approximately 18% of the English Setters tested were either bilaterally or unilaterally deaf.[1]

Disturbance of bone growth rarely occurs, but it has been seen, as has **hypoglycemia.**

Neuronal ceroid lipofuscinosis (juvenile amaurotic familial idiocy[2,3] or **AFI or Battens Disease)** occurs because of inborn errors in metabolism that create a basic metabolic defect. A **lipidosis** is defined as a genetically determined disorder primarily affecting lipid metabolism and manifested by abnormal concentrations or certain lipids or lipoproteins in tissue or extracellular fluid. The condition is heritable as a recessive trait. Clinical manifestation of this syndrome does not usually occur until the dog is at least 1 year old. The first signs, usually reduced vision and increasing dullness, are noticed when the dog is between 15 and 18 months old. The dog becomes less vital and loses contact with its surroundings. The gait becomes stiffer and signs of ataxia appear. Food intake is usually normal. At about 18 months of age, affected dogs may show spasms of the muscles, especially the masseter muscles. The dogs seem cramped in the jaw and begin to click their teeth with subsequent development of seizures and tonic-clonic convulsions. Death often occurs during an acute attack of cramp. Very few affected dogs survive to the age of 2 years.

Necropsy reveals enlargement of lymph nodes and possibly a brain cortex that is slightly yellower than normal. The normal brain of an English Setter weighs about 90 gm; in dogs suffering from AFI, the brain weight may be reduced to as little as 60 gm.[1]

Progressive retinal atrophy affects many breeds of dogs, but occurs primarily in hunting breeds such as the English Setter.[4]

Hemophilia A has been reported as a sex-linked, recessively inherited condition.[5] Although reported, this condition is extremely rare.

English Setters are predisposed to **tonsillitis**. The breed, with its profuse feathering and its sometimes long, excessive estrus flow, seems particularly inclined to **bacterial infection of the vagina**.

A hereditary trait thought to be recessive that is found in English Setters is **craniomandibular osteoarthropathy**. This excessive ossification of the lower jaw and back of the skull causes added weight and is visible in x-rays.

The whiter English Setters with less heavily pigmented skin are prone to **dermatitis**. They are one of the breeds predisposed to **atopy**.[6] **Staphylococcus pyoderma** and **demodectic mange** are also commonly seen in the breed. Some individuals of this breed show an allergic reaction to newsprint, so the common use of newspapers in the whelping box or as bedding is discouraged. Insecticide dips have stimulated acute moist dermatitis in these dogs.

English Setters tend to be **long sleepers**. Acetylpromazine, demerol and phthalofyne anthelmintics should be used with caution. **Anaphylactic reaction** to routine immunization is seen in this breed.

English Setters should be kenneled in runs more than 5 feet wide because they can injure their tails when they stand and wag them in one that is too narrow. Once a tail is "bloodied," the condition is increasingly difficult to overcome.

BEHAVIOR

An English Setter can be a dog for all seasons in that many are family pets, hunters and also compete in the show ring. They are the softest in temperament of the three setters, and require patience, patience and more patience when training in obedience work. They are not dumb; they simply avoid doing anything which might be wrong and displease.

OLD AGE

The life expectancy of English Setters is about 14 years. A large percentage die of **lymphosarcoma** and **carcinomas of the oral and nasal cavities**.

References
1. Strain, George M., "Deafness in Dogs and Cats," *Proc. 10th ACVIM Forum*; 1992.
2. Koppand, N. "Neuronal Ceroid-Lipofuscinosis in English Setters," *J. Sm. Anim. Prac.*; 1970: 10: 639-644.
3. Kirk, R.W. and Bistner, S.I. *Handbook of Veterinary Procedures and Emergency Treatment: Hereditary Defects of Dogs*. Table 124. 1975: 661.
4. Magrane, W.G. *Canine Ophthalmology*. 3rd ed. (Lea & Febiger, Philadelphia, PA.,1977); 305.
5. Sherwood, L., et al, "Canine Hemophilia Due to Antihemophilic Factor Deficiency: A Case Report," Michigan State University; Vet.1966: 26: 52.
6. Griffin, C., Kwochka, K., McDonald, J. *Current Veterinary Dermatology, the Science and Art of Therapy*. Mosby Yearbook, St. Louis, MO. 1993: 101.

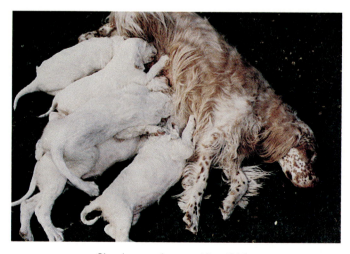

Showing puppies are white at birth.

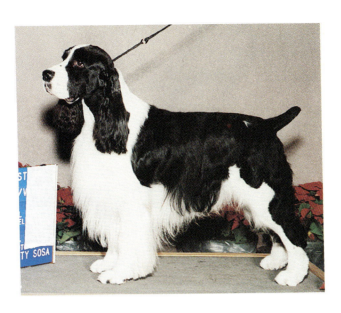

ENGLISH SPRINGER SPANIEL

ORIGIN AND HISTORY

Their zest for pursuing game to its source gives the English Springer Spaniel its name. Thought to be the pheasant dog depicted in paintings dating from 1637, the breed knows no peer as a "hunter of feathers."

DESCRIPTION

The Springer is felt to be the most robust of the spaniels, and is probably the forebear of most spaniel breeds.

The English Springer is ideal for hunters who hunt alone. It is quick to learn, obedient, easy to train and eager to please. It enjoys the company of a family and is patient and affectionate with children. Somewhat reserved with strangers, the English Springer makes an excellent watchdog. This is an ideal breed for people interested in obedience training and competition.

THE SHOW RING

The ideal shoulder height for dogs is 20 inches; for bitches 19 inches. The English Springer is a square dog. In judging the English Springer Spaniel, the overall picture is a primary consideration. The English Springer Spaniel is first and foremost a sporting dog of the spaniel family and he must look and behave and move in character.

There are no disqualifications for this breed.

BREEDING AND WHELPING

Springer Spaniels are a hardy breed, rarely having problems during gestation and whelping. The bitches tend to gain too much weight during pregnancy. The average number of whelps per litter is seven or eight, and the weights can range from 9 to 14 ounces with an average of 11 ounces.

GROWTH

Nose pigment is incomplete at birth and patches of solid color on the body will be smaller than they will be in the adult. Nose pigment can fill in as late as 12 months. Tails and dewclaws should be removed, with care taken not to cut the tails too short. Leave 1/3 of the tail. Obesity is a common problem between 3 and 6 months of age. The average bitch will reach adult height and weight at 18 months, while the dogs will take 24 to 30 months to reach full maturity. Undershot bites are common in the breed. Many dogs do not develop the condition until 9 to 12 months of age.

RECOGNIZED PROBLEMS

A prevalent health problem in this breed is **chronic ear infections.** A proper ear cleaning routine, followed regularly, will help prevent most ear problems.

Retinal dysplasia[1] has been described as hereditary to this breed,[2] as has **progressive retinal atrophy.**[3] Another eye problem in Springer Spaniels is **central progressive atrophy**.[4,5,6,7,8] This hereditary trait is suggested to be dominant with incomplete penetrance. Usually affecting dogs 3 to 5 years of age, this condition is evident in mottling and increased reflectivity of the centralis, loss of central vision and apparent best vision in dim light.

Other eye problems include **ectropion, entropion, glaucoma** and **distichiasis**.[9]

Congenital seborrhea has been reported by Austin.[10]

Dr. Urs Giger, Associate Professor of Medicine and Medical Genetics at the School of Veterinary Medicine, University of Pennsylvania, has described **PFK (phosphofructokinase)** in English Springer Spaniels. PFK, a major regulatory enzyme in all cells of the body, catalyzes the metabolism of sugar and is pivotal in the production of energy to maintain normal cell function. Dogs with this enzyme deficiency have diseased red blood cells and muscle cells.

The first molecular genetic screening test for a common inherited disease in companion animals has been developed in Dr. Giger's laboratory. The test identifies carriers and affected dogs with PFK. PFK deficiency can present as a mild to life-threatening episodic illness. A hallmark sign of this disease is intermittent dark urine, with the color of the urine ranging from orange to dark coffee-brown, which commonly develops after strenuous exercise, prolonged barking and excessive panting. These conditions accelerate the destruction of red blood cells in affected dogs, resulting in dark brown urine, and in severe forms, pale gums (anemia) or jaundice with fever and poor appetite. Clinical manifestations usually resolve within hours to days. Affected dogs have a relatively normal life expectancy; however, situations that can precipitate such crises should be avoided.[11]

Some English Springer Spaniels also suffer from a blood deficiency known as **Factor XI or PTA (plasma thromboplastin antecedent)**.[12] The mode of inheritance is autosomal, incompletely dominant. **Seizures** have been reported[13] and are known to be a sex-related genetic disorder.[14] **Hip dysplasia** is a common problem in this breed. **Elbow dysplasia** has been reported by the OFA.[15] **Ehlers-Danlos syndrome (cutaneous asthenia)** is a condition in hyperextensibility and fragility of skin.[16,17,18] Severe lacerations are sometimes the result of minimal trauma in Springer Spaniels affected by Ehlers-Danlos syndrome. The mode of inheritance is dominant.

Lichenoid-psoriasiform dermatosis has been reported in the English Springer Spaniel.[19]

Myasthenia gravis has been seen in English Springers.[20,21] There is now a screening test available to diagnose **fucosidosis** in English Springer Spaniels.[22]

BEHAVIOR

Data were obtained on 245 cases of **aggressive behavior** in dogs of 55 breeds. Aggression involved barking, growling and biting. Dominance aggression was found in the English Springer.[23] The **"Rage Syndrome"** has been observed in the English Springer Spaniel.

Most English Springers are easily trainable, eager to please and obedient. They make excellent family dogs and are good with children. Springers make good watch dogs as they are somewhat reserved with strangers.

OLD AGE

Springers live to be quite old, 15-year-old Springers are quite common. They retain health and vigor into later years, if given proper care. Obesity is usually a problem in the older animals, so their diets should be adjusted accordingly.

References
1. Barnett, K.C. "Inherited Eye Disease in the Dog and Cat," *J. Sm. Anim. Prac.*; 1988: 29:7, 462-475; 33 ref.
2. Kirk, R.W. and Bistner, S.I. *Handbook of Veterinary Procedures and Emergency Treatment.* (W.B. Saunders, Philadelphia, PA, 1981) 822.
3. Rubin, L.F., DVM, *Inherited Eye Diseases in Purebred Dogs.*
4. Erickson, F., et al, "Congenital Defects in Dogs: A Special Reference for Practitioners," Ralston Purina Co. (reprint from Canine Practice), *Vet. Publ. Co.*; 1977.
5. Barnett, K.C. "Abnormalities and Defects in Pedigree Dogs, IV, Progressive Retinal Atro-

phy," *J. Sm. Anim. Prac.*; 1963: 4:465-467.

6. Barnett, K.C. "Canine Retinopathies, III, The Other Breeds," *J. Sm. Anim. Prac.*; 1956: 6:185-196.

7. Barnett, K.C. "Genetic Anomalies of the Posterior Segment of the Canine Eye," *J. Sm Anim. Prac.*; 1969: 10:541-455.

8. Barnett, K.C. "Primary Retinal Dystrophies in the Dog," *JAVMA;* 1969: 154:804-808.

9. Magrane, W.G. *Canine Ophthalmology.* 3rd ed. (Lea & Febiger, Philadelphia, PA., 1971).

10. Austin, V, "Congenital Seborrhea of the Springer Spaniel," *Mod. Vet. Prac.;* April, 1973: 53-55.

11. Giger, Urs "PFK Deficiency," *The Canine Chronicle*; November, 1993: 39.

12. Kirk, R.W. *Current Veterinary Therapy,VI.* (W.B. Saunders, Philadelphia, PA, 1971).

13. Bell, Jerold S. DVM "Sex Related Genetic Disorders: Did Mama Cause Them?" *American Kennel Club Gazette*, Feb. 1994; 76.

14. English Springer Spaniel column, *The American Kennel Club Gazette*; March, 1990.

15. Bodner, Elizabeth, DVM, "Genetic Status Symbols," *The American Kennel Club Gazette*; Sept. 1992.

16. Hegreberg, G.A., et al, "A Connective Tissue Disease of Dogs and Mink Resembling Ehlers-Danlos Syndrome of Man, II, Mode of Inheritance," *J. Hered.*; 1969: 60:249-254.

17. Hegreberg, G.A., et al: "Connective Tissue Disease of Dogs and Mink Resembling Ehlers-Danlos Syndrome, III, Histopathological Changes of the Skin," *Arch. Path.;* 1970: 90: 159-166.

18. Hegreberg, G.A., et al, "A Heritable Connective Tissue Disease of Dogs and Mink Resembling Ehlers-Danlos Syndrome in Man, I, Skin Tensile Strength Properties," *J. Invest. Derm.* 54:377-380.

19. Griffin, C., Kwochka, K., McDonald, J.: Current Veterinary Dermatology, the Science and Art of Therapy. Mosby Yearbook, St. Louis, MO 1989: 171.

20. *Cornell University Animal Health Newsletter.* Feb.,1991: Vol. 8 # 12.

21. Kern, Maryanne, DVM, "Diseases of the Esophagus," *The American Kennel Club Gazette*; January, 1993.

22. Bell, Jerold S. "Identifying and Controlling Defective Genes," *American Kennel Gazette*; July, 1993: 85.

23. Borchelt, P.L. "Aggressive Behavior of Dogs Kept as Companion Animals: Classification and Influence of Sex, Reproductive Status and Breed," *Applied Animal Ethology*; 1983: 10:1, 45-61; 24 ref.

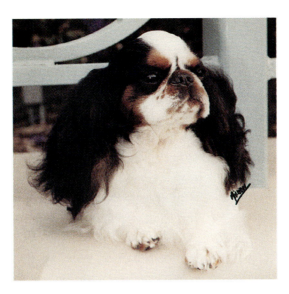

ENGLISH TOY SPANIEL

ORIGIN AND HISTORY

The origins of the English Toy Spaniel are lost in obscurity. The first written reference in England, the home of this breed, is about 1570.

These Spaniels were always court dogs and royal favorites during the reign of Charles I and II, and ladies' pets through the reign of the Edwardians (1910), but gradually lost ground to the Chinese Pekingese.

This breed almost disappeared during World War II when so many dogs were euthanized for fear of raids as well as for feeding problems. After the war, a few enthusiasts began working to reestablish the breed.

Now it is again popular in England, and it is hoped it will also become popular in the United States.

DESCRIPTION

The English Toy Spaniel is a gentle dog, a good mixer with other dogs.

They are generally devoted to one person and like to choose their masters. If brought up with children, they make excellent companions.

THE SHOW RING

Weight varies from 8 to 14 pounds. There are four colors. The Blenheim is a white dog with well scattered chestnut patches, red ears and markings around the eyes. The Prince Charles is a tricolored white dog with well scattered black patches, and with chestnut markings above the eyes, lining the ears, under the tail and inside the legs. The King Charles is a black dog with chestnut markings as in the Prince Charles. The Ruby is a rich mahogany red dog.

235

The coat is silky and straight with long fringes to ears, chest, body, legs and tail.

Special characteristics include the massive head with the skull well domed and full over the eyes. The nose is black, very short and upturned. The stop should be deep and well defined.

The breed has a definite undershot bite but the lips should meet to give a good finish. The eyes are very large and dark, deep set and wide apart.

This Spaniel has two distinct types of feet: the round, cat-like foot and the foot with the center pad and nails fused as one. The latter is an inheritance from a small water dog, the Pyrame. This foot is normal for the breed. The nails must be kept quite short.

Serious faults include a **hanging tongue** and a **luxating patella**.

The nose should always be black. The Black and Tan and the Ruby should not have any white markings.

Dewclaws are usually removed, if they occur. The tail should be docked at 3 to 5 days of age, leaving about 1 1/2 inches. This should give an adult a 3-inch tail.

There are no breed disqualifications.

BREEDING AND WHELPING

The estrous cycle generally begins at about 12 to 14 months of age, and the seasons are the normal 6 to 8 months. The male generally reaches maturity at about 12 months, but has been reported as occasionally taking longer.

Delivery is usually easy, but some bitches have problems in extremely cold or hot and humid climates.

Litters average from two to five puppies. The breed produces large whelps for the breed size, averaging from 3 to 7 ounces. The pink noses become black. The gene for dilution is carried by some, and occasional dilute blues and livers have been born.

The most commonly reported birth defects are **cleft palates**.

RECOGNIZED PROBLEMS

The domed shape of the English Toy Spaniel's head and the occasional large puppy may make **cesarian section** necessary as often as 50% of the time depending on the strain. Breeders report **incomplete fontanel** closure. Fontanels have been known to close as late as 1 year. Dental hygiene is of the utmost importance as English Toy Spaniels often have premature tooth loss. A grossly long **lazy tongue** that never fully retracts will dry out and become leather-like. Partial amputation may be necessary.

The **Luxating patella** is the breed's most important problem; it has been reported for more than 100 years. Considerable improvement in the problem has been achieved in the past

30 years through careful breeding. **Congenital femoral shift** predisposes the dog to dislocations in 95% of the cases in luxation of the patella. Careful examination and diagnosis is most important before attempting surgical repair. The problem may never be eliminated, as this predisposition seems to be a weakness of many toy breeds.

Breeders report a possible **bone growth disturbance** seen between 6-12 months of age. This is temporary and best treated by allowing free exercise once luxation of the patella has been ruled out.

Umbilical hernias are fairly common. This defect should be selectively bred out of the breed, since surgical repair produces a cosmetic solution.

Diabetes mellitus has been reported in the breed. It usually affects the middle-aged to older bitches. Symptoms are increased thirst and increased urination. Occasionally star-shaped **cataracts** form which are diagnostic of the problem. Early diagnosis and treatment can prolong useful life of these individuals by 2 to 3 years.

Juvenile cataracts have been seen.

Fused toes with odd toenails, sometimes between the toes, occur in this breed.

Breeders report the occurrence of **congestive heart defects**, including **patent ductus arteriosus (PDA)**.

Epilepsy has been diagnosed in the breed.

Anesthesia can be a problem with English Toy Spaniels due to the unique conformation of the muzzle.

BEHAVIOR

The English Toy Spaniel is strictly a companion dog. This dog is timid with people it doesn't know but is very sociable with its friends and family.

OLD AGE

The life span of the English Toy Spaniel is from 8 to 14 years, and some individuals live to 16 years of age.

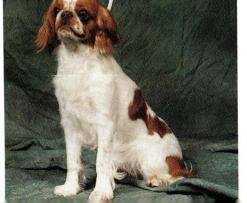

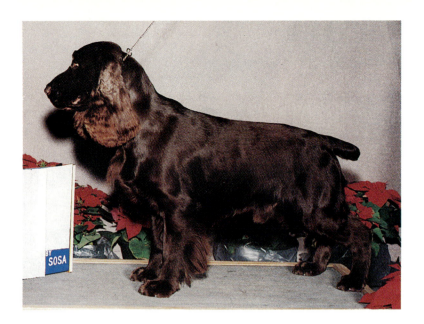

FIELD SPANIEL

ORIGIN AND HISTORY

The Field Spaniel is maybe the rarest dog recognized by the American and British Kennel Clubs. There are approximately 400 in the United States and a similar number in England.

At one time the breed was nearly extinct. After 1929 there were none in the United States and during World War II the number in England was reduced to six. Through concerted British efforts, and through inter-breeding with Springer Spaniels, the breed was preserved and reintroduced into the United States in 1967. At that time C. Tuttle of Virginia and Richard Squier of Ohio imported three dogs and established the breed in the United States. At present there are only a few active breeders in the United States, but the Field Spaniel Society of America was formed in 1980.

DESCRIPTION

They are staunch, strong hunting companions and able retrievers. The breed is characterized as a gay sporting spaniel with a strong, reaching field gait.

238

THE SHOW RING

The male Field Spaniel should be about 18 inches at the shoulder; bitches should be about 17 inches. They should weigh from 35 to 50 pounds.

Most Field Spaniels are liver-colored, although some are black, liver-roan, blue-roan or liver and tan.

BREEDING AND WHELPING

Because of interbreeding with Springer Spaniels, a liver and white or liver-roan puppy occasionally results from breeding two liver Field Spaniels. Because of the limited gene pool, an occasional defective puppy is born and should be euthanized.

Pure liver puppies have resulted from mating sibling liver-colored Field Spaniels with white chests. One solid liver spaniel has sired seven champions to date, all solid liver.

Because the Field Spaniel is such a rare breed, few veterinarians will see Field Spaniel puppies in their practice.

Tails should be docked and dewclaws removed at 3 to 5 days of age. One-third of the tail should be left after docking.

RECOGNIZED PROBLEMS

Some female Field Spaniels have developed a **hypothyroid** condition, usually after breeding.

An unusual **sensitivity to anesthetics** along with slow recovery is seen in some Field Spaniels.

Hip dysplasia has been reported in the breed.

Breeders report a recurring problem with **pyometra**.

BEHAVIOR

Owners of Field Spaniels feel that this dog has the best temperament of all the spaniels. He is intelligent, stable and calm.

OLD AGE

Most Field Spaniels live to be 12 to 14 years of age.

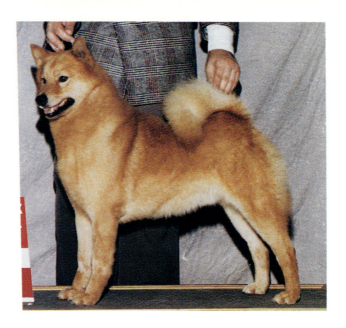

FINNISH SPITZ

ORIGIN AND HISTORY

After a long period of decline, the Finnish Spitz was rescued from deterioration during the late nineteenth century. In 1892 Finland's Kennel Club established a Standard for the present day Finnish Spitz. It was many years before the dog became well-known outside its own country. In 1927, Sir Edward Chichester imported a pair of Finnish Spitzes into England, and the breed was recognized by the British Kennel Club in 1935. One of the pioneer British breeders, Lady Kitson, called the dog a "Finkie" — a nickname still popular with many of the breed's fanciers. The Finnish Spitz was approved for competition in the Non-Sporting Group in 1988.

DESCRIPTION

The *Suomenpystykorva*, known in English as the Finnish Spitz, is found virtually everywhere in its native land. In the city it is a companion; in the country it is still a working dog. The Finnish Spitz has a friendly disposition, loves children and is an excellent watch dog.

THE SHOW RING

The dog is considerably larger than the bitch. Height at the withers in dogs: 17 1/2 to 20 inches; in bitches: 15 1/2 to 18 inches. The Finnish Spitz is a square dog, its substance and bone in proportion to size.

RECOGNIZED PROBLEMS

The Finnish Spitz may be at higher risk for **pemphigus foliaceous**.[1]

Cleft palates are seen in some strains as is **ectasia**.

Only 3% of the radiographs submitted to the OFA are not certified free of **hip dysplasia**. **Patellar luxation** is occasionally seen but concerned breeders here and in Finland are reducing the incidence.

Adult onset **seizures** or **epilepsy** are reported. A one year old dog, on necropsy showed a possible **copper storage** problem but further research has not confirmed that diagnosis.

Breeders warn that low doses of medication are needed due to muscle to fat ratio in this breed.

BEHAVIOR

The Finnish Spitz is a good companion dog. He is friendly, faithful and loyal to his family. He is playful, particularly with children. He is an alert watchdog. He can be a barker, because that is how he hunts in his native land.

OLD AGE

The average life span of the Finnish Spitz is 13 to 14 years of age.

References
1. Griffin, C., Kwochka, K., McDonald, J. *Current Veterinary Dermatology, the Science and Art of Therapy*. Mosby Yearbook, St. Louis, MO. 1993: 142.

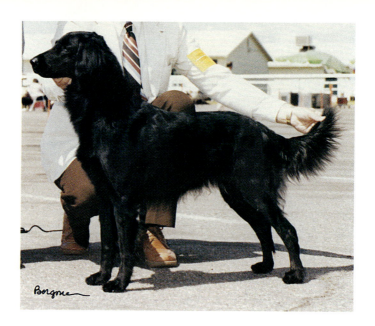

FLAT COATED RETRIEVER

ORIGIN AND HISTORY

The Flat Coated Retriever is thought to be the product of a cross between a Labrador Retriever and a Newfoundland. This breed was developed between 1859 and 1873 from integrated stock in England, principally by E. Shirley. H. R. Cooke owned large numbers of dogs, which kept the breed healthy although there were relatively few owners.

Since 1900 the Flat Coated Retriever has been greatly outnumbered by Labradors and Goldens. Fortunately, the number of dogs has increased since World War II, when the breed's existence was seriously threatened.

DESCRIPTION

Partly because of its relative obscurity in the past few decades, the Flat Coated Retriever has retained good hunting qualities. It can retrieve well both in heavy cover and from water.

THE SHOW RING

The dog should be from 23 to 24 1/2 inches at the shoulder; the bitch should be from 22 to 23 1/2 inches at the shoulder. Animals should be in lean, hard condition, free of excess

242

weight. The eyes are dark brown and obliquely set rather than straightforward. The set of the small ears is also important. They should be set quite close to the side of the head.

The forequarters should be those of the deep-chested retriever, with a rather long neck, deep, broad chest and only a gradual spring in the ribs. The back is short and square.

The legs and feet of the Flat Coated Retriever are important features in judging. Forelegs are straight, feet are round and strong, though rather small. A Flat Coated Retriever is disqualified for show if it is yellow, cream or any color other than black or liver.

RECOGNIZED PROBLEMS

Flat Coated Retrievers have a low incidence of **hip dysplasia** but **luxating patellas** are a common problem.

Only two cases of **Progressive Retinal Atrophy** have been reported in the breed, however **glaucoma** (see Bassets) is more common.

Epilepsy and **diabetes insipidus** are documented in this breed. **Thyroid imbalance** and **megaesophagus** are occasionally see.

Of current concern to breeders is the early death of Flat Coated Retrievers diagnosed as having **histiosarcoma**.

BEHAVIOR

The Flat-Coat is affectionate, patient and companionable with family and friends. He is an active and outgoing dog.

OLD AGE

Most Flat Coated Retrievers live from 10 to 14 years of age.

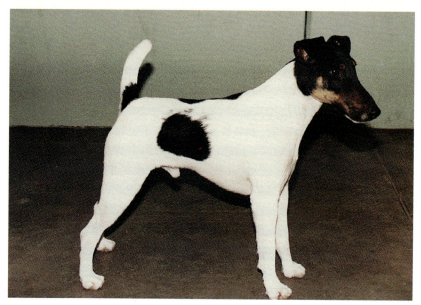
Smooth Fox Terrier

FOX TERRIER — WIREHAIR AND SMOOTH

ORIGIN AND HISTORY

The Fox Terrier is widely known throughout the English speaking world. There are two strains — the Wirehair and the Smooth. The Smooth was the first bred of the two, developed from the smooth-coated Black and Tan Bull Terrier, Greyhound and Beagle. The Wire is a descendant of the Welsh Black and Tan.

To develop a white coat and straight head for the Wire, a number of cross-breedings of the Smooth and Wire were done.

This practice was discontinued several decades ago, so that breeders could maintain the Fox Terrier Standard as established in England in 1876.[1] The American Fox Terrier Club was established in 1885.

DESCRIPTION

Originally a hunting dog, the Fox Terrier is now chiefly a companion animal.

It can adapt to city or country life.

As long as its human family is near, it is happy. The Fox Terrier is devoted, loyal and an excellent watch dog.

THE SHOW RING

The Breed Standards for the Smooth and Wirehair Terriers were separated in February of 1991. The Wire's coat should be hard and stiff, never woolly or silky, and only moderately

244

long. The Smooth's coat is flat, dense and quite short.

The head shape of the Fox Terrier is very important. The skull is flat and narrow, with very little stop. Ears are v-shaped and small. Tulip, prick or rose-shaped ears are faulted in both varieties. Although the jaws should be strong and muscular, they should not be like those of the greyhound or English Terrier. The muzzle is long and sloping to a black nose.

Facial distinctions are the deep-set dark eyes.

Carriage is also important in judging. The straight forelegs should be carried straight ahead in movement. Long, muscular thighs are characteristic of champion Fox Terriers. The correct proportions call for a dog that is not too leggy, one that measures about 15 1/2 inches in height and about 12 inches down the back.

The dominant color is white, with only three colors faulted if found as secondary colors: brindle, red and liver.

Disqualifications are the same for both the Smooth and the Wire. They include a white, cherry or spotted nose, ears in a prick, tulip or rose shape and the mouth much undershot or overshot.

BREEDING AND WHELPING

Fox Terriers have very few problems with breeding or whelping. Wire puppies at birth are black and white or all white. As they get older, although white remains white, the black turns to tan on the face, as does some of the black on shoulders, hips and tails. Noses at birth can be black, black and pink or pink. They gradually turn black by the age of 8 weeks.

As early as 3 months of age, the Wire puppy should be exposed to grooming and brushing, combing and gradual stripping.

GROWTH

Tails should be docked and dewclaws removed at the same time. The best time for removal on the healthy puppy is from the third to the fifth day after birth. Tail docking in Wires is most important, as too short a tail can ruin the appearance of an otherwise beautiful dog. The general rule is to remove a scant 1/3, but it is best to have the puppy held with the head up and a mark placed on the tail, level with the head.

Tails vary in length, and each individual puppy should be given special consideration. A chunky tail may have only the tip removed. The overall balance of the dog is of utmost importance. If any doubt, a tail too long can be remedied, but one too short ruins the dog for show.

RECOGNIZED PROBLEMS

Deafness[2] and **goiter** are two problems found in some Fox Terriers.[3,4]

Some of the eye defects of this breed are **lens luxation,**[5,6] **distichiasis** and **cataract.**[7] Lens luxation often produces **secondary glaucoma. Recessive ataxia** is a hereditary defect of the breed, due to **bilateral demyelination of the spinal cord.**[8,9] Onset is usually between 2 and 4 months of age. Initial progress is rapid, with paralysis resulting in most cases.

Dislocation of the shoulder[10,11] is also a problem in Fox Terriers. **Legg-Perthes** disease is another skeletal problem. Radiographs will often reveal aseptic necrosis of the femoral head and neck. **Oligodontia** (fewer teeth than normal) has been reported in some dogs. **Pulmonic stenosis** has been reported in Fox Terriers.[12,13,14] The cause of the narrow artery at its origin has not been determined.

Myasthenia gravis has been reported in Smooth Fox Terriers.[15,16]

Atopic dermatitis is a possible hereditary immunologic disorder reported in this breed.

Persistent aortic arch and **esophageal achalasia** have been encountered.

Fox Terriers are predisposed to **cutaneous mast cell tumors.**[17]

Eye injuries are common in Fox Terriers of all ages, probably because of the great physical activity of the breed. Older dogs often develop **cataracts. Hip dysplasia** is seldom found in the breed. Fox Terriers are one of several breeds reported to be at a higher risk of developing **colonic disease.**[18] **Ectopic ureter** was diagnosed in 228 dogs. The female to male ratio was 217:11. Six breeds, among them Fox Terriers, were identified with greater frequency of diagnosis than expected. The strength of association in certain purebred dogs suggests a familial relationship.[19]

The Wirehair Fox Terrier is a breed in which **idiopathic epilepsy** has been detected.[20]

BEHAVIOR

The Fox Terrier is adaptable and will be happy either in the city or in the country as long as its "people" are near. It is a lively, active, devoted companion and an excellent watch dog.

OLD AGE

The life span of the Fox Terrier averages about 10 to 13 years. As the dog grows older, its temperament remains generally the same, its activity decreases and it sleeps more. Deafness, blindness and loss of smell frequently develop. Stiffness of joints becomes apparent, and warts are found, making grooming difficult. In old males, atrophy and tumors of the testicles commonly occur, as does prostatic hypertrophy.

References
1. American Kennel Club, *Complete Dog Book.* (Howell Book House. New York, N.Y. 1992); 355-362.
2. Strain, George M. "Deafness in Dogs and Cats," *Proc. 10th ACVIM Forum;* May,1992.

3. Young, G.B. "Inherited Defects in Dogs," *Vet. Rec.;* 1955: 67:15-19.

4. Kirk, R.W. and Bistner, S.I. *Handbook of Veterinary Procedures and Emergency Treatment: Hereditary Defects of Dogs.* Table 124:1975: 661.

5. Formston, C. "Observations on Subluxation and Luxation of the Crystalline Lens in the Dog," *J. Comp. Path.*; 1945: 55:168-184.

6. Lawson, D.D. "Luxation of the Crystalline Lens in the Dog," *J. Sm. Anim. Prac.*; 1969: 10:461-463.

7. Dodds, W.J. "Inherited Hemorrhagic Defects," *Current Vet. Therapy VI.* R.W. Kirk, Ed. (W.B. Saunders, Philadelphia, PA., 1977) 438-445.

8. Bjork, G., et al, "Hereditary Ataxia in Smooth-Haired Fox Terriers," *Vet. Rec.*; 1957: 69:871-876.

9. Bjork, G., et al, "Hereditary Ataxia in Fox Terriers," *Acta. Neuro. Suppl.*; 1962: 1:45-48.

10. Campbell, J.R. "Shoulder Lameness in the Dog," *J. Sm. Anim. Prac.*; 1968: 9:189-198.

11. Vaughan, L.C. "Congenital Dislocation of the Shoulder Joint in the Dog," *J. Sm. Anim. Prac.*; 1969: 10:1-3.

12. Mulvihill, J.J. and Priester, W.A. "Congenital Heart Disease in Dogs: Epidemiologic Similarities to Man," *Teratology;* 1973: 7:73-78.

13. Patterson, D.F. "Epidemiologic and Genetic Studies of Congenital Heart Disease in the Dog," *Circ. Res.;* 1968: 23:171-202.

14. Patterson, D.F. "Canine Congenital Heart Disease: Epidemiological Hypotheses," *J. Sm. Anim. Prac.*; 1971: 12:91-96.

15. Cornell Univ. Animal Health Newsletter. February, 1991: Vol.8 #12.

16. Kern, Maryanne, DVM, "Diseases of the Esophagus," *The American Kennel Club Gazette;* January, 1993.

17. Veterinary News, *"The American Kennel Club Gazette*"; April, 1990: 44.

18. Houston, D.M. "An Integrated Study of Colonic Disease in the Dog," Dissertation-Abstract-International.-B,-Sciences and Engineering; 1989: 50:4, 1278-1279.

19. Hayes, H.M., Jr., "Breed Associations of Canine Ectopic Ureters: A Study of 217 Female Cases," *J. Sm. Anim. Prac.;* 1984: 25:8, 501-504; 12 ref.

20. Bell, Jerold S. DVM "Sex Related Genetic Disorders: DId Mama Cause Them?" *American Kennel Club Gazette*, Feb. 1994; 76.

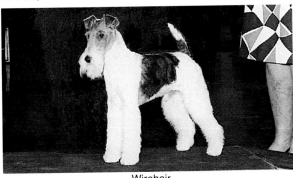

Wirehair

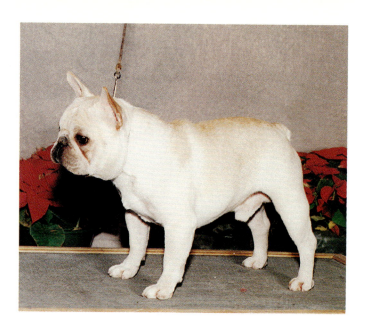

FRENCH BULLDOG

ORIGIN AND HISTORY

The French Bulldog was created when the French began crossing the Miniature English Bulldog with several French breeds. Although the breed had long been a household pet, it was not standardized until it reached the United States.

DESCRIPTION

French Bulldogs are courageous little dogs and loving pets. They can be stubborn but are usually tractable. The breed is not vicious or mean. Because they are house dogs, French Bulldogs do not adapt well to kennels.

THE SHOW RING

Recognized colors in the breed are brindle, white, cream, fawn and brindle with white (pied).

The French Bulldog is the only canine breed with bat ears. Tails should not be docked, nor ears trimmed. Any dewclaws on the hind legs should be removed. Free or normal dentition is usual.

Disqualifications, according to the breed Standard, are: coats of white with black,

black with white, black and tan, liver, mouse or solid black (black means black without any trace of brindle); nose other than black, except light nose with white, cream or fawn coat; any alteration other than removal of dewclaws; weight more than 28 pounds; ears not characteristically bat-shaped.

BREEDING AND WHELPING

The length of gestation is 63 days. During pregnancy, bitches are affectionate and seek human companionship. The need for **cesarean section** is common in this breed, because the puppies have large heads.

Eclampsia is uncommon in French Bulldogs. The average size of a litter is four or five puppies. The puppies vary in size at birth, averaging 6 to 8 ounces. French Bulldog puppies at birth characteristically look like full-grown specimens of the breed, complete with the pushed-in face. The most common defects at birth are **cleft palates** and **cleft lip**. Sometimes a single puppy has both. Some are born with an **elongated soft palate,** which makes breathing and swallowing difficult. The rate of growth for dogs is shown in Table 1. Bitches are born with the same weight as dogs, but grow more slowly. At maturity, bitches weigh 22 to 26 pounds.

RECOGNIZED PROBLEMS

Hip dysplasia is not a serious problem in French Bulldogs. The breed is particularly susceptible to **tonsillitis** and **upper respiratory problems**, as are most brachiocephalic breeds.[1] Also, they have many cases of **allergic dermatitis**.

The occurrence of **congenital alopecia** in a litter of four female French bulldogs is described in an English study. With the exception of the haircoat the affected bitch was clinically normal. The distribution of the sparse hair (head, tip of tail and paws) mimicked that seen in the Chinese Crested dog. Histopathological examinations of skin biopsies revealed features frequently observed in congenital alopecia — a reduction in number of hair follicles, hypoplasia or absence of epidermal appendages and pronounced follicular hyperkeratosis. Abnormalities of collagen and elastic fibers were not detected.[2]

A recent publication reports the laboratory diagnosis of **Hemophilia A and B**[3,4] in a single family of French Bulldogs. Indistinguishable clinically, the deficiencies are diagnosed by special laboratory procedures. **Hemivertebra** is listed as occurring in the breed.[5,6,7,8] Other problems reported in French Bulldogs are **brachyury (short tail)** and **short skull**.[9]

BEHAVIOR

The "Frenchie" is a very adaptable and satisfactory companion. He is very responsive to affection. He will romp with the children or lie quietly with the older folks. He is also a ruthless mouse hunter.

OLD AGE

A large percentage of this breed die of **carcinoma**. Dogs are prone to carcinoma of the genital-urinary tract, and bitches are prone to carcinoma of the breast.

Table 1 — Growth Rate of Male French Bulldogs	
Age	**Weight**
Birth	6 oz.
4 weeks	3 lb 8 oz.
3 months	16 lb.
6 months	22 lb.
9 months	25 lb.
12 months	26 lb.
18 months	27 lb.

References
1. French Bulldog column, *American Kennel Club Gazette*; June 1990.
2. Marks, A., Van den Broek, A.H.M., and Else, R.W. "Congenital Hypotrichosis in a French Bulldog," *J. Sm. Anim. Prac.;* 1992: 33:9, 450-452; 11 ref.
3. Splappendel, R.J. "Hemophilia A and Hemophilia B in a Family of French Bulldogs," *Lydschr, Diergenesk 100;* 1975: 1075-1088.
4. Ettinger, S.J.: Textbook of Veterinary Internal Medicine, Diseases of the Dog and Cat. W.B. Saunders Co., Philadelphia, PA 1989: p 2259.
5. *Canine Practice*; August, 1977: 59.
6. Done, S.H., et al, "Hemivertebra in the Dog: Clinical and Pathological Observations," *Vet. Rec.;* 1975: 96:313-317.
7. Drew, R.A. "Possible Association Between Vertebral Development and Neonatal Mortality in Bulldogs," *Vet. Rec.;* 1974: 94: 480-481.
8. Pearson, H. and Gibbs, C. "Abnormal Vertebral Development in Bulldogs," *Vet. Rec.;* 1974: 95:27-28.
9. Kirk, R.W. and Bistner, S.I. *Handbook of Veterinary Procedures and Emergency Treatment: Hereditary Defects of Dogs.* 1975: Table 124, 661.

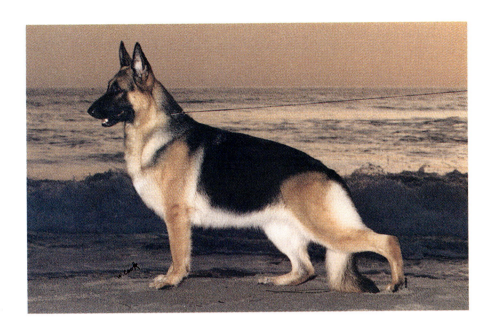

GERMAN SHEPHERD

ORIGIN AND HISTORY

Today's German Shepherd is a highly refined composite of herding types of previous centuries. At the end of the 19th century, a few German breeders sought to preserve the splendid working qualities of their Shepherd dogs. Cavalry Captain Max Von Stephanitz crusaded in 1889 to standardize the breed and succeeded in forming the largest breed club in the world.

The German Shepherd has a proud tradition of service to man as a companion, pet and working dog.

DESCRIPTION

The German Shepherd is a loyal and obedient dog, possessing sound character and temperament. The breed's intelligence and ability to learn are remarkable. Throughout the years, people have come to misinterpret the German Shepherd's temperament, associating the breed with "police dogs" and treating them accordingly. A German Shepherd that has been trained for protection purposes should be handled only by a professional handler. As pets, German Shepherds adapt well to human beings and can provide excellent companionship. They are sensitive and instinctively know when to guard lives or property.

The Standard's ideal of the German Shepherd is: "Stamped with a look of quality and nobility, difficult to define but unmistakable when present. The breed has a distinct personality, marked by self-confidence, a certain aloofness which does not lend itself to indiscriminate friendships. The dog is poised but eager and alert, both willing and able to serve in its capacity as watch dog, companion, guardian, guide dog, herding dog, tracking dog and in the armed forces. The ideal Shepherd is a working animal with an incorruptible character."

THE SHOW RING

The adult Shepherd's body proportions are a 10 to 8 1/2 ratio of body length to height. The proper length to height ratio is created by angulation and breadth of fore and rear quarters rather than by a long back. A Shepherd should have a short, strong back without dip and roach. The loin should be short and fairly broad. The dog should have good substance of bone and body, a gently sloping croup and a saber-like tail, hanging at least to the hock joint. Seen in profile, the Shepherd should give the impression that a drop of water placed between his ears would run off to the end of his tail.

A Shepherd's gait should be smooth and outreaching with no wasted motion. Seen front and rear at a trot, there should be no looseness in elbow and hock, no crossing over or toeing out.

At full trot a Shepherd should single track, with his feet coming in to the center line of his body, which is the center of gravity. Faults of gait seen front, side or rear are listed by the Standard as very serious. In size, a dog should stand 24 to 26 inches at the withers and a bitch, 22 to 24 inches. Slight variations are permissible. The Standard grades faults as serious, very serious, and disqualifying.

Disqualifying faults are: cropped or hanging ears; cropped tail; undershot bite; white dogs; dogs with noses not predominantly black; and any attempt to bite the judge.

Serious faults are long coats, overshot bites, missing teeth (except first pre-molars), blue, liver or pale, washed-out colors and tails too short or with clumpy ends.

BREEDING AND WHELPING

A Shepherd puppy is usually one of a litter of eight to 10 and weighs from 12 ounces to 1 pound at birth. As a puppy the German Shepherd is cub-like and clumsy with big bones and a clumsy head, particularly the male. The pastern joints and paws are big and the ears are soft. Even at birth, some qualities which will be present at maturity can be identified. Fore and rear skeletal assemblies should form right angles. The shoulder blade should be well-laid-back, the upper arm set at a 90-degree angle to it and about equal in length. The lower arm or leg bone should be 90 degrees to the upper arm and the pastern should have a slight spring — about 25

252

degrees. The rear assembly should match this with the upper thigh bone parallel to the shoulder blade, the stifle bone parallel to the upper arm. Shepherds may or may not be born with dewclaws on the hind legs. If present, the dewclaws are usually removed.

GROWTH

Through puppyhood and youth Shepherds grow rapidly in bony frame and attain full body height and length before they fill out in weight. Ears become erect at a variety of times — as early as 3 months, but may be as late as 7 to 8 months. They may come up crooked or separately. The ears may go back down as second teeth come in, but this is nothing to be concerned about. If the ears are large and thin and hang like a hound's ears, they will remain soft.

Some Shepherds reach full maturity at 16 months. Usually, however, the dogs reach full maturity at 3 years and the bitches at 2 years.

RECOGNIZED PROBLEMS

Skeletal disorders are prevalent in this breed and **hip dysplasia** is one of the most frequently encountered. A Norway study of 5519 radiographs of Shepherds revealed 22% as dysplastic.[1] Over 14,000 radiographs of the spine of ten breeds were examined for abnormal vertebrae in the lumbosacral region, which were manifested by different types of fusing. There was some link between these abnormalities and hip dysplasia. Such abnormalities were seen in 11% of 5682 German Shepherds.[2]

Elbow dysplasia occurs in the German Shepherd. The term elbow dysplasia has been applied to disorder of the elbow joint that led to acute pain, dysfunction, and/or chronic progressive degenerative joint disease. Ununited anconeal process caused some elbow dysplasia and osteochondrosis of the medial condyle of the distal humerus was also involved. Most recently, the importance of fragmentation of the medial coronoid process has been elucidated.

Recent work on developmental anomalies of the elbow have determined that all three developmental lesions of the elbow are themselves secondary to anatomic abnormalities of the developing elbow joint.

The unifying theory of elbow dysplasia states that all three lesions result from faulty development of the trochlear notch of the ulna. This creates an incongruity between articular surfaces of the proximal ulna and the distal humerus. The incongruity results in too much contact in the area of the anconeal and medial coronoid process, and too little contact between the center of the trochlear notch and the humeral trochlea.

Panosteitis is a disorder of endosteal ossification in the shafts of the long bones.

Panosteitis often occurs in dogs with **Von Willebrand's disease**, a blood coagulation defect caused by deficiency of functional Factor VIII and abnormalities in platelet aggregation. The abnormal Factor VIII and platelet aggregation persist throughout life although clinical signs tend to disappear with age.[32]

The **intractable diarrheas** of Shepherds deserve special mention, for the owners should invest in gastrointestinal diagnostic services rather than in medicine. Many possibilities exist as to the cause of **malabsorption syndrome** — an illness resulting from disease of the absorbing cells lining the intestine. **Eosinophilic gastroenteritis**, causing a chronic small bowel diarrhea associated with fluctuating high eosinophil counts is frequently encountered. These are two of the more common causes of chronic diarrhea seen in the German Shepherd. Ettinger suggests treatment of 2.5 mg. prednisone per kg, reduced to 0.5 mg/kg daily.

Progressive Posterior Paresis occurs in middle-aged and older dogs with some predilection for males. There is a gradual onset with increasing weakness and ataxia of the rear legs. Neurological examinations reveal the following signs: asymmetric strength in the rear limbs, crossed extensor reflexes, exaggerated knee and ankle jerk reflex, intact flexor and abnormal proprioceptive reflex. Dropped tail, absence of pain and presence of sensation and varying degrees of muscle atrophy occur. Differential diagnosis must be made with care and it should be noted that most of the other problems involve the loss of sensation where this syndrome does not. Little data have been compiled to explain the hereditary basis for this syndrome but there is a distinct predilection for the breed. Most therapies are to little avail. A German study describes **axonopathy** in German Shepherd Dogs and has information on symptoms, diagnosis, prognosis and treatment.[3]

A description is given of the clinical, neurological and radiological symptoms in 57 dogs with the **cauda equina syndrome;** 45% of the dogs were German Shepherds.[4] Most of the animals became diseased at an early age (av. = 6.3 yrs.) and showed partly progressive, partly fluctuating movement disturbances in the hind legs, tail paresis, pain in the lumbar-sacral region and trouble with micturition.

Studies by Strain et al have reported **congenital deafness** in German Shepherds.[5]

Fifty percent of the reported cases of **Calcinosis circumscripta of the tongue** occur in the German Shepherd. (Muller, Scott, Kirk; 7th ed.)

Pituitary dwarfism, an inherited trait in German Shepherds, causes hypofunction of the pituitary gland. These puppies don't grow and have hormone abnormalities.

Skin problems seen are **bilateral symmetrical alopecia, hyperpigmentation**, and retention of puppy coat.[6,7]

Pancreatic insufficiency (EPI) in German Shepherds is thought to be controlled by polygenic inheritance.[8]

Nodular dermatofibrosis with renal cystadenocarcinoma is a syndrome in the German Shepherd dog characterized by multiple cutaneous nodules and bilateral multifocal renal cystadenocarcinomas. It was first reported in Switzerland in 1983. Since then there have been additional reports. This syndrome occurs most frequently in middle-age dogs of either sex. An increased frequency of **uterine leiomyomas** has been reported in affected females. Pedigree analysis suggests that the syndrome is inherited in an autosomal dominant fashion. Dogs initially are presented with cutaneous nodules of the extremities. Nodules arising on the feet may ulcerate and cause lameness. As the disease progresses, nodules increase in size and number and may occur elsewhere on the body, especially on the head. Nodules range in size from a few millimeters to several centimeters in diameter. Some are haired, while others have a glabrous or slightly pitted surface. Skin pigmentation is variable. Histologically these nodules consist of hyperplastic dermal collagen. Similar skin lesions have been termed "collagenous nevi."

Renal abnormalities usually are not recognized until late in the course of disease and often are documented only at necropsy. Both kidneys usually are affected. Kidney enlargement is due to the presence of numerous renal cortical cysts of varying size. The content of these cysts has been described as varying from a clear or yellow fluid to a brown, red, or gray soft mass. Cysts are believed to originate from renal rubules which become occluded by papillary projections of initially hyperplastic, and later neoplastic, tubular epithelium. The syndrome progresses slowly, and the dogs usually succumb either to renal failure or to results of metastasis of the carcinoma. One case involving renal cystadenoma (instead of cystadenocarcinoma) has been reported. The author (and others) have seen this syndrome in mixed-breed dogs, including one which had no German Shepherd dog in its ancestry.

Diseases of the urinary tract reported in the German Shepherd are **prostatic diseases, cystinuria**,[9,10] and **silica uroliths**. German Shepherd Dogs are one of the breeds reported to have **hypoplasia of the penis** and **congenital phimosis**.[11]

German Shepherds may be predisposed to acute **moist dermatitis (hot spots)** due to their thick hair coat.[12] German Shepherds are susceptible to **inhalant** and **food allergies**.[13] German Shepherds are also predisposed to **yeast dermatitis** caused by **Malassezia**.[14] They are also one of the breeds at increased risk for **generalized demodectic mange**.[15]

Cutaneous (discoid) lupus erythematosus occurs most frequently in Collies, German Shepherd Dogs, Siberian Huskies and Shetland Sheepdogs. **Cutaneous lupus erythematosus** is considered to be a mild form of **systemic lupus erythematosus**. Antinuclear antibody test are usually negative. The most common sign (90%) is a **nasal dermatitis**

characterized by varying degrees of **depigmentation, erythema, ulceration** and **erosions**. A possible female predilection has been reported.[33] Other skin diseases occasionally reported in German Shepherds are **uveodermatologic syndrome, Vitiligo** and **canine nasal dermatitis**.[16]

German Shepherds are one of several breeds reported to have significantly higher disposition for **malignant neoplasms**.[17] Of 13,974 dogs presented at a clinic in Germany from 1977 to 1985, 699 (5%) had neoplasms. The commonest site was the mammary gland (31%), and the breeds most involved were Poodle (17%) and German Shepherd (16%).[18]

Diseases of the eye reported in the German Shepherd Dog are **eversion of the nictitating membrane**,[19,20] **ectasia**,[15] **bilateral cataract**,[21,22] and **pannus**.[14]

Hemopoietic system disorders reported in the German Shepherd Dog are **hemophilia A**[16,23] and **Von Willebrand's Disease**.[24]

Disorders of the cardiovascular system include **Subaortic stenosis**,[16,25,26,27,28] and **persistent right aortic arch**[23,24,25].

Cleft lip and **palate**[29] and **conjunctival dermoid cysts** are also reported.

The German Shepherd is a breed in which **idiopathic epilepsy** has been reported.[30]

BEHAVIOR

The most frequent problems seen in German Shepherds concern their **personality** and **temperament**. The inheritance of behavior and temperament is complex, for the characteristics of a breed comprise a combination of several independently inherited traits which are modified by genetic factors. The German Shepherd is an excellent working dog, but some may be unpredictable, aggressive or extremely shy and difficult to socialize.

This inherited abnormality becomes more prevalent as the breed becomes more popular and is bred to satisfy public demand.

The reputation of the breed was damaged by inept handling and indiscriminate breeding. In many incidences involving aggressiveness, it is the master's fault for not knowing how to train the dog or how to control it. If properly trained when young, the German Shepherd can be trained to do almost anything, and will be loyal, faithful and obedient when mature.

Data were obtained on 245 cases of aggressive behavior in dogs of 55 breeds. Incidence of protective aggression and fear-elicited aggression was found in the German Shepherd.[31]

OLD AGE

German Shepherds live an average of 12 years.

References

1. Lingaas, P. and Heim, P. "A Genetic Investigation of the Incidence of Hip Dysplasia in Norwegian Dog Breeds," *Norsk-Veterinaertidsskrift*; 1987: 99:9, 617-623; 22 ref.

2. Winkler, W. "Transitional Lumbosacral Vertebrae in the Dog," Dissertation, Fachbereich Veterinarmedizin der Freien Universitat Berlin. 1985: 143; 50 ref.

3. Bichsel, P. "Neuromuscular Diseases in Young Dogs," *Jahresversammlung. Schweizerische Vereinigung fur Kleintiermedizin*. 2.-4. Juni, 1988. Bazel. 1988, 43-50. Zool Bern, Switzerland; c/o H. Heinimann, Schweis. Serum und Impfinstitut, Postfach 2707.

4. Jaggy, A., Lang, J., and Schawalder, P. "Cauda Equina Syndrome in the Dog," *Schweizer-Archiv-fur-Tierheilkunde*; 1987: 129:4, 171-192; 15 ref.

5. Strain, George M. "Deafness in Dogs and Cats," *Proc. 10th ACVIM Forum*; May, 1992.

6. Andresen, E., et al, "Pituitary Dwarfism in German Shepherd Dogs: Genetic Investigations," *Nord. Vet.*; 1974: 26: 692-701.

7. Trueblood, M.H. Washington State Univ. College of Veterinary Medicine Newsletter, 1976.

8. Bell, Jerold S. "Identifying and Controlling Defective Genes," *American Kennel Gazette*; July, 1992: 84.

9. Kirk, R.W.; Bistner, Sl. Handbook of Veterinary Procedures and Emergency Treatment: Hereditary Defects of Dogs. Table 124, 1975; 661.

10. Patterson, D.F. and Medway, W. "Hereditary Diseases of the Dog," *JAVMA*; 1966: 149:1741-1754.

11. Ettinger, S.J. *Textbook of Veterinary Internal Medicine*. W.B. Saunders Co. Philadelphia, PA 1989: 1883-1884.

12. Brignac, Michele M. "Congenital and Breed Associated Skin Diseases of the Dog and Cat," *KalKan Forum*; December, 1989.

13. Ackerman, Lowell, DVM, "Allergic Skin Diseases," *American Kennel Club Gazette*; September, 1990.

14. Griffin, C., Kowchka, K., McDonald, J. *Current Veterinary Dermatology, the Science and Art of Therapy*. Mosby Yearbook, St. Louis, MO. 1993: 45.

15. Griffin, C., Kowchka, K., McDonald, J. *Current Veterinary Dermatology, the Science and Art of Therapy*. Mosby Yearbook, St. Louis, MO. 1993: 74.

16. Griffin, C., Kowchka, K., McDonald, J. *Current Veterinary Dermatology, the Science and Art of Therapy*. Mosby Yearbook, St. Louis, MO. 1993: 218, 231, 310.

17. Kusch, S. "Incidence of Malignant Neoplasia in Dogs Based on PM Statistics of the Institute of Animal Pathology, Munich, 1970-1984," Inaugural Dissertation, Tierarztliche Fakultat, Ludwig Maximilians Universitat, Munchen, German Federal Republic. 1985: 22; of ref.

18. Fabricius, E.M., Schneeweiss, U., Schroder, E., Dietz, O., Wildner, G.P., Schmidt, W., Baumann, G., Benedix, A., Weisbrich, C., and Stuhrberg, U. "Serological Diagnosis of Neoplasms in Dogs With a Clostridium Butyricum Spore Preparation," *Monatshefte fur Vet.*;1986: 41:7, 220-224; 40 ref.

19. Magrane, W.G. *Canine Ophthalmology*; 3rd ed. (Lea & Febiger, Philadelphia, PA., 1977) 305.

20. Priester, W.A. "Congenital Ocular Defects in Cattle, Horses, Cats, and Dogs," *JAVMA;* 1971: 160:1504-1511.

21. Kirk, R.W.; Bistner, SI. Handbook of Veterinary Procedures and Emergency Treatment: Hereditary Defects of Dogs. Table 124, 1975; p 661.

22. von Hipple, E. "Embryolgische Utersuchungen uber Vererhung Angeborener Katarakte uber Schichlstar des Hundes Sowie uber eine Bessondere Form von Kapselkatarakt," *Graefes Arch. Opth.*; 1930: 124:300-324.

23. Cotter, S.M., et al, "Enostosis of Young Dogs," *JAVMA* ; 1958: 153:401-410.

24. Dodds, W.J. "Canine von Willebrand's Disease," *J. of Lab. and Clin. Med.*; 1970: 76:713-721.

25. Mulvihill, J.J. and Priester, W.A. "The Frequency of Congenital Heart Disease (CHP) in Dogs," *Teratology;* 1971: 4:236-237.

26. Mulvihill, J.J. and Priester, W.A. "Congenital Heart Disease in Dogs: Epidemiologic Similarities to Man," *Teratology;* 1973: 7:73-78.

27. Patterson, D.F. "Epidemiologic and Genetic Studies of Congenital Heart Disease in the Dog," *Circ. Research* 23:171-202;1968

28. Patterson, D.F. "Canine Congenital Heart Disease: Epidemiological Hypotheses," *J. Sm. Anim. Prac.;* 1971: 12:263-287.

29. Jurkiewiez, M.J. and Bryant, D.L. "Cleft Lip and Palate in Dogs: A Progress Report," *Cleft Palate J.;* 1968: 5:30-36.

30. Bell, Jerold S. DVM "Sex Related Genetic Disorders: Did Mama Cause Them?" *The American Kennel Club Gazette*, Feb. 1994; 76.

31. Borchelt, P.L. "Aggressive Behavior of Dogs Kept as Companion Animals: Classification and Influence of Sex, Reproductive Status and Breed," *Applied Animal Ethology;* 1983: 10:1, 45-61; 24 ref.

32. Ettinger, S.J. *Textbook of Veterinary Internal Medicine.* W.B. Saunders Co. Philadelphia, PA 1989: 2360.

33. Ettinger, S.J. *Textbook of Veterinary Internal Medicine.* W.B. Saunders Co. Philadelphia, PA 1989: 2312.

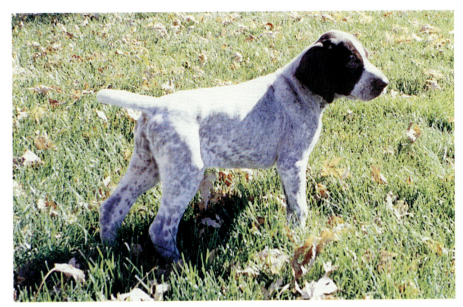
Puppy

GERMAN SHORTHAIRED POINTER

ORIGIN AND HISTORY

The ancestors of the German Shorthaired Pointer are the old Spanish Pointer, English Foxhound and German tracking hounds. It was popular in Germany as an all-purpose hunting dog, and imports began to appear in the United States in the 1920s. The principal goals of obedience and good temperament are still evident in these dogs.

The German Shorthaired Pointer was first admitted to the AKC stud book in 1930.[1] Field trials have been important throughout the breed's history, and the prime consideration in their judging is the animal's ability to perform as a gun dog.[2,3]

DESCRIPTION

German Shorthaired Pointer puppies are born pure white with liver patches, or solid liver with or without white markings on chest and/or toes. Ticking begins to appear in the pure white by 10 days to 2 weeks, and permanent coloration is established in 6 to 8 weeks.

THE SHOW RING

The only allowable colors in purebred German Shorthairs are liver (dark brown) and white in any combination, or solid liver. Tails must be docked, usually on the fourth day after whelping. Slightly more than half of the tail should be removed. A too-short tail spoils the overall balance of the dog. Dewclaws are prone to injury in this field breed and the leg looks cleaner without them. Dewclaws on the hind legs must be removed.

The height of dogs, measured at the withers, should be 23 to 25 inches. The height of bitches measured at the withers should be 21 to 23 inches. Deviation of more than one inch above or below the described heights are to be severely penalized. Dogs should weigh between 55 and 70 pounds, while bitches should weigh between 45 and 60 pounds.

Major faults in the breed are mainly physical or mental problems which interfere with the dog's chief purpose in life — that of a hard working field dog. Barrel chest, steep shoulders, straight stifles, out-at-elbows, pinched elbows, cowhocks and fiddle fronts all prevent the dog from covering the fields and heavy brush easily and effortlessly and are considered major faults.

Disqualifications for this breed are: china or wall eyes, flesh colored nose, extreme overshot or undershot, and a dog with any area of black, red, orange, lemon or tan, or a solid white dog.

BREEDING AND WHELPING

German Shorthair Pointers do not present unusual problems during pregnancy. A diet high in meat protein and mineral supplement, plus regular exercise helps maintain top condition. Most bitches in this breed whelp without complication and seem to have a high degree of maternal instinct. They do not seem to have postpartum problems, although **eclampsia** can occur, especially with large litters.

Mastitis sometimes occurs in heavy milkers. The average litter is eight or nine, but may range from six to fourteen.

Many German Shorthair bitches have false pregnancies, whether bred or bred without conceiving. This condition corrects itself in time and no medication is necessary.

GROWTH

A German Shorthair puppy of substantial bone and standard size (21 or 23 inches in the mature bitch and 23 to 25 inches in the mature dog) will weigh around 18 to 20 pounds by 8 weeks (less for a bitch), 25 to 30 pounds by 12 weeks, 35 to 40 pounds at 4 months. Weight may slow down in proportion to height from this point on to full height development (10 months or so). Physical maturity continues to develop until 2 ½ to 3 years.

Illness or injury during the fast growth period may slow down or stop all growth and development. Once the condition has been remedied, growth will usually catch up.

DENTITION

Mild overshots usually correct themselves by physical maturity, but undershots never do. Missing teeth do not seem to be a problem. The loss of baby teeth and the appearance of permanent teeth occur smoothly and there is seldom a problem of retention of baby teeth.

RECOGNIZED PROBLEMS

The adult German Shorthair Pointer should have a calm, stable temperament, one that is easy to work with and easy to live with. A nervous, high-strung dog is not desirable. **Hip dysplasia**[4] and **entropion** are faults which occur in the breed. Stubborn **ear problems** have been noted occasionally as in other hanging-ear type dogs. "**Hot spots,**" or **weeping eczema** may occur in the summer. In some strains, **bloat** is proving to be a problem.

A non-painful, pitting edema known as **lymphedema**[5] is a severe problem in German Shorthaired Pointers. Two blood disorders of the breed are **Von Willebrand's disease** and **thrombocytopathy (a platelet disorder).**[6]

This pointer has the following eye problems: **pannus**[7] and **eversion of the nictitating membrane.**[8] **Subaortic stenosis,**[9,10,11,12] **amaurotic idiocy,**[1] **fibrosarcoma**[13] and **melanoma**[13] are also reported.

Familial **hypothyroidism** is suspected in German Shorthaired Pointers.[14]

Breeders report **pseudohermaphroditism** is found in some bloodlines.[15]

BEHAVIOR

The German Shorthair Pointer is one of the best all-round hunters. He is also an excellent family pet. He is energetic, amiable and fits well into family life. Like all hunting dogs he acts foolish if confined too long without adequate exercise.

OLD AGE

German Shorthairs, barring accidents or unusual illness, tend to be long lived. It is not unusual to find 13- and 14-year-old dogs in good health. Kidney failure, heart attacks and strokes usually end the lives of very old dogs. Severe arthritis and rheumatism make euthanasia necessary for some aged dogs.

References

1. American Kennel Club, *The Complete Dog Book*. (Howell Book House, New York, N.Y. 1992); 45-49.
2. von Dewitz, Seiger, *The Complete German Shorthaired Pointer.*
3. Maxwell, C.B. *The German Shorthaired Pointer.*
4. Kirk, R.W. and Bistner, S.I. *Handbook of Veterinary Procedures and Emergency Treat-*

ment: Hereditary Defects of Dogs; Table 124, 1975: 661.

5. Saunders, D. "Congenital Hereditary Lymphedema," *Southwest Vet* ; 1971: 24:139-140.
6. Kirk, R.W. *Current Veterinary Therapy, VI.*; (W.B.Saunders, Philadelphia, PA. 1975).
7. Magrane, W.G. *Canine Ophthalmology;* 3rd ed. (Lea & Febiger, Philadelphia, PA 1977); 305.
8. Martin, C.L. and Leach, R. "Everted Membrane Nictitans in German Shorthaired Pointers," *JAVMA*; 1970: 157:1229-1232.
9. Mulvihill, J.J. and Priester, W.A. "The Frequency of Congenital Heart Defects in Dogs," *Teratology;* 1971: 4:236-237.
10. Mulvihill, J.J. and Priester, W.A. "Congenital Heart Disease in Dogs: Epidemiologic Similarities in Man," *Teratology*; 7: 73-78.
11. Patterson, D.F. "Epidemiologic and Genetic Studies of Congenital Heart Disease in the Dog," *Circ. Res.;* 1968: 23: 171-202.
12. Patterson, D.F. "Canine Congenital Heart Disease: Epidemiological Hypotheses," *J. Sm. Anim. Prac.*; 1971: 12: 263-287.
13. Kirk, R.W. and Bistner, S.I. *Handbook of Veterinary Procedures and Emergency Treatment: Hereditary Defects in Dogs.* 1981: Table 119: 823.
14. Brignac, M. "Congenital and Breed Associated Skin Diseases in the Dog and Cat," *KalKan Forum;* December, 1989.
15. Bell, Jerold S. DVM "Sex Related Genetic Disorders: Did Mama Cuase Them?" *American Kennel Club Gazette*, Feb. 1994; 76-77.

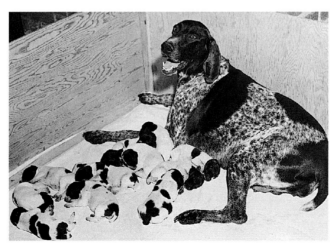

Bitch with litter of 12

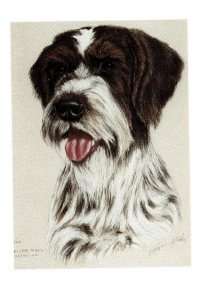 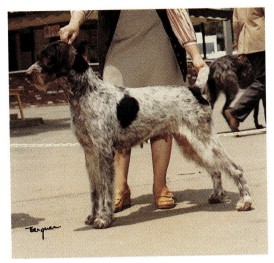

GERMAN WIREHAIRED POINTER

ORIGIN AND HISTORY

The German Wirehaired Pointer is one of the all-purpose hunting dogs developed in Germany after 1850. It combines the pointing and tracking ability of the Pointer with the retrieving enthusiasm of the retrievers. The Wirehaired Pointer Club of Germany first accepted a variety of interbred retrieving pointers, but later accepted only the German Wirehair, Pudelpointer, Griffon and Stichelhaar.

The breed was first recognized in Germany in 1870. In the United States, German Wirehairs were imported in the 1920s and admitted by the American Kennel Club in 1959.[1]

DESCRIPTION

The German Wirehaired Pointer was bred for ruggedness, ability to track all types of game and retrieving in all terrains. For these purposes, the breed's coat is the most important feature; the all-weather, water repellent harsh coat has a dense undercoat, with an insulating and water repellent overcoat. Long tufts on the brow bone, neck, and back sides of limbs are protective in undergrowth.

The German Wirehaired Pointer has several characteristics of pointer appearance, including sturdiness and a lively, intelligent personality. A rugged, hard-going dog, it is not the ideal house pet, but is a good companion in an outdoor environment.

THE SHOW RING

The head should be slightly long and broad, with a medium stop. The teeth should occlude in a true scissors bite. The nose is dark brown with wide nostrils.

Slightly longer than tall (by ratio of 10 to 9), the German Wirehaired Pointer has a straight, short back. It has the broad hips and deep chest of the retrievers in its heritage. Weight varies with the hunting purpose, but the dogs should be no taller than 26 inches, the bitches no shorter than 22 inches. Color should be liver and white, liver and roan, liver with white ticking or solid liver. Faults include a feather tail, flat feet, smooth coat, long or woolly coat, black in the coat and a spotted or flesh-colored nose.[1]

There are no breed disqualifications.

BREEDING AND WHELPING

German Wirehaired Pointers frequently whelp large litters, 12 to 14, and raise them all. Birth weight of the whelps ranges from 9 to 15 ounces. Dewclaws should be removed and tails docked at 3 to 5 days of age. Leave slightly less than 1/2 of the tail (approximately two-fifths).

RECOGNIZED PROBLEMS

A review of literature and personal experience of veterinarians interviewed revealed few hereditary or congenital problems. **Sebaceous cysts** and **malocclusion** are seen in a high percentage. A German study reports there was significant decrease of litter size as ages of sire and dam increased.[2]

BEHAVIOR

The German Wirehair is steady and lively. He is very affectionate with his master and is jealous of other dogs.

References

1. American Kennel Club, *The Complete Dog Book*; (Howell Book House. New York, N.Y., 1992) 50-53.
2. M. Kock, "Statistical and Inheritance Studies on the Breeding Situation, Defects and Behavioural Characters in the German Long-Haired Pointer," Thesis, Tierarztliche Hochschule Hannover, German Federal Republic. 1984: 151; 8 ref.

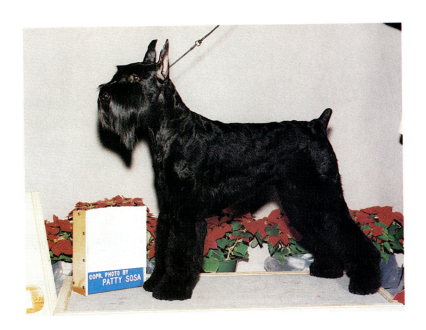

COPR. PHOTO BY
PATTY SOSA

GIANT SCHNAUZER

ORIGIN AND HISTORY

Cattle drovers in Germany admired the Standard Schnauzer, but, desiring a larger dog to serve their purpose, they carefully developed the Giant Schnauzer. With the advent of automation, Giant Schnauzers declined in popularity until the early 1900s, when their keen intelligence made them an obvious choice for police work.

DESCRIPTION

Giant Schnauzers are good companions and family protectors. They are reliable with children and are usually not one-person dogs. A shy or mean Giant Schnauzer is abnormal and undesirable. Unstable or excessively aggressive dogs may reflect an owner's mishandling rather than an inherent defect.

Giant Schnauzers do not develop well if raised in a kennel. They thrive on human contact and need proper outlets for their above-average intelligence, initiative, energy level and stubbornness.

Most Giant Schnauzers are black. (For color information on salt and pepper, consult the chapter on Standard Schnauzer.) Puppies are black at birth. A small white spot on the chest is permitted, providing that it is no larger than dime size at 6 weeks.

265

THE SHOW RING

The average weight for a bitch is 75 pounds and for a dog, 95 pounds. The height averages 23 1/2 to 27 1/2 inches. The Giant Schnauzer's bone structure is somewhat heavier than the Doberman's, but not as heavy as the Rottweiler's. **Disqualifications are: over or undershot bites and markings other than specified in the Standard.**

BREEDING AND WHELPING

Giant Schnauzers weigh from 6 ounces to more than 1 pound at birth. Large litters can be expected, with an average of seven to nine puppies.

Giant Schnauzers do not reach full maturity until 2 years of age. Rapid growth begins at 12 weeks. Often a Giant Schnauzer's adult weight can be estimated by doubling its weight at 17 weeks.

GROWTH

Tails should be docked and dewclaws removed at 2 to 4 days. Tails must be cut at either the second or third vertebra. To prevent a squared appearance they should be sutured. The tail should measure 2 to 3 inches at maturity. Removal of front dewclaws is optional; rear dewclaws, which seldom occur, must be removed. Ear cropping is optional. Ears should be cropped between 6 weeks and 3 months of age. Most Giant Schnauzers that are shown have cropped ears. Since breeders have not paid attention to the nice, natural, high-set terrier type ear, which drops neatly forward, most Giants with uncropped ears have large, heavy, hound ears. These ears do little to enhance the bold, alert, spirited appearance typical of the breed. Styles of cropped ears vary from a short, stubby, Bouvier des Flandres-like cut to a long Great Dane cut. An ear shaped similar to a Doberman's ear is preferable.

DENTITION

Full dentition is usual. Overshot bites are seen more than undershot bites. Both are disqualifications under the breed Standard.

RECOGNIZED PROBLEMS

The Giant Schnauzer is prone to the same problems experienced by the other large breeds. Veterinarians who have treated Giant Schnauzers have reported isolated cases of **urinary-tract infections**, **hemorrhagic gastroenteritis**, **osteochondritis dissecans** and skin problems such as **seborrhea** and **dermatitis**. Treatment of long-bone injuries, particularly in puppies, is reportedly lengthy and difficult.

Hip dysplasia is a problem. The official breed club is stressing a program of radiographing dogs for **hip dysplasia** and breeding only those that are declared free of the condition by OFA or radiologists at accredited veterinary colleges.

Inherited selective intestinal **malabsorption of cobalamin (Cb1)** was observed in a family of Giant Schnauzers. Family studies and breeding experiments demonstrated simple autosomal recessive inheritance of this disease.[1]

In a Swedish study Giant Schnauzers were reported to have a higher-than-average incidence of **primary hypothyroidism.**[2]

Three black Giant Schnauzers, mother, daughter and son, developed single or multiple primary **squamous cell carcinomas** of the nail bed between the ages of nine and twelve years. Radiographic evidence of osteolysis of the third phalanx, especially in a middle-aged to older large-breed, black dog would warrant the amputation and histopathological examination of the digit because of the likelihood of squamous cell carcinomas.[3,4]

BEHAVIOR

The Giant Schnauzer is trainable, steady, calm and patient with children. He is an excellent companion but is not suited for apartment life. He needs space.

OLD AGE

The normal life span of the Giant Schnauzer is 10 to 12 years. A frequent cause of death is the automobile. Giant Schnauzers seem indifferent to cars and traffic, and an all-black dog is nearly invisible to drivers after dark.

References
1. Fyfe, J.C., Giger, U., Hall, C.A., Jeryk, P.F., Klumpp, S.A., Levine, J.S., and Patterson, D.F. "Inherited Selective Intestinal Cobalamin Malabsorption and Cobalamin Deficiency in Dogs," *Pediatric Research*; 1991: 29:1, 24-31; 37 ref.
2. Larsson, M. "The Breed, Sex and Age Distribution of Dogs with Primary Hypothyroidism," *Svensk-Veterinartidning*; 1986: 38:15, 181-183; 3 ref.
3. Paradis, M., Scott, D.W., and Breton, L. "Squamous Cell Carcinoma of the Nail Bed in Three Related Giant Schnauzers," *Vet. Record*; 1989: 125:12, 322-324; 20 ref.
4. Lettow, E., Middel-Erdmann, I., and Keil, S. "Diseases of the Distal Phalanx in the Dog," *Kleintierpraxis*; 1988: 33:9, 345-346; 8 ref.

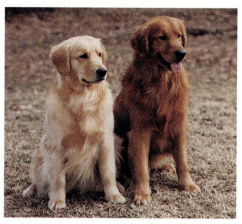

GOLDEN RETRIEVER

ORIGIN AND HISTORY

Golden Retrievers first came into prominence in England during the early part of the 19th century. To obtain the type desired, breeders crossed setters, water spaniels and other sporting breeds with light-built Newfoundlands, the St. John's Newfoundland. These dogs were noted for their endurance, excellence in swimming and skill in retrieving.

DESCRIPTION

Breeders sought to produce a strong dog of moderate size. They also produced one which has proved to be remarkably gentle and one which mixes well with the other dogs. They are ideally suited for obedience work and for use as guide dogs.

THE SHOW RING

In size the dogs should be 23 to 24 inches at the withers and the bitches should be 21 1/2 to 22 1/2 inches. The length from the breastbone to the point of the buttocks should be slightly greater than the height. Weight for the dogs is 65 to 75 pounds and for bitches, 55 to 65 pounds.

The coat should be dense and water-repellent with good undercoat. The color should be lustrous golden, of various shades. White hairs (other than a few on the chest) are not desirable.

Disqualifications in the show ring include deviations in height of more than an inch and undershot or overshot bite.

Front dewclaws are removed. Rear dewclaws are not usually found, but should be removed if they occur.

BREEDING AND WHELPING

The first estrus can be expected between 9 and 11 months. The most common gestation time is 60 to 61 days. This is a breed where free whelping is the rule. Average litter size is six to eight whelps and birth weight varies greatly between family lines.

In newborns, **cleft palates** and **hernias** are not common. Occasional **swimmer puppies** are born.

Although most puppies thrive on an adequate diet of quality materials, some puppies in this breed require a calcium supplement.

RECOGNIZED PROBLEMS

Hip dysplasia is commonly found in the breed, as is **elbow dysplasia.** In a Norwegian study of 2809 radiographed Goldens 29% were affected by hip dysplasia.[1] Isolated cases of **pseudodwarfism** have been reported. **Central progressive retinal atrophy** is a problem in Golden Retrievers.[2] **Von Willebrand's disease** is reported by Dodds.[3] **Entropion** is reported by Magrane.[4]

Cataract is a familial problem in Golden Retrievers.[5] In many instances the cataract is not complete, but appears as a triangular subcapsular opacity at the posterior pole of the lens. The lesion is therefore not readily apparent to the owner. Test breedings seem to indicate that cataract in Golden Retrievers is a dominant trait. If this hypothesis is valid, those dogs with triangular cataracts would be heterozygotes while those with complete cataracts would be homozygotes. These cataracts may not become visible to the owner or even under veterinary examination for a year or more. Two thousand two hundred and fifty-one Goldens were examined for certification under the BVA/Kennel Club eye examination scheme. Cataracts were diagnosed in 7.4% of the Goldens.[6]

Golden Retrievers are commonly seen for **acute moist dermatitis (hotspots)**. This is a surface bacterial infection caused by self induced trauma as the animal rubs or scratches to alleviate an itch. **Otitis externa, allergenic skin disease**, external parasites or matted, dirty-hair coat can cause the initial scratching. Dense, heavy undercoats predispose this breed and care should be taken to keep dead hair removed from the dense coat by regular, vigorous brushing. Treatment is to clip the hair and clean the area with an antiseptic. Cortisone is often given orally or by injection. Oral antibiotics, and topical cortisone/antibiotic creams and ointments may also be helpful.[7] Goldens may be predisposed to food allergy.[8]

Goldens are susceptible to **inhalant allergies**[9] and at higher risk of developing food allergies.[10] **Uveodermatologic syndrome** has been reported in the breed.[16] **Subvalvular aortic stenosis (SAS)** is a heritable heart defect that affects several breeds and is common in Golden Retrievers.[11]

Golden Retrievers have an increased breed incidence of **hypothyroidism**.[5]

Golden Retrievers commonly develop **acral lick dermatitis (acral lick granulomas)**.[5]

269

Cerebellar hypoplasia has been reported by Knecht, et al (1979).[12] Cerebellar hypoplasia is most commonly observed in cats as a result of a prenatal infection. Although reported in the dog, a specific etiology has not been established. Heredity has been suggested in progressive ataxia in smooth-hair terriers and in cerebellar abiotrophy in Kerry Blue Terriers. In the latter, the clinical signs were progressive; two of the animals reported by Knecht showed nonprogressive signs and one affected dog became clinically normal with age.

Some microscopic features were found in all dogs necropsied. Marked gliosis and demyelination of the cerebellum were not observed. Focal diminution of the granular cells was occasionally seen. Degenerative changes of the Purkinje cells were not present and the deep cerebellar and olivary nuclei were normal.

The occurrence in six out of 14 dogs born to clinically normal parents indicates an autosomal recessive mode of transmission. In recessive transmission, consanguinity of the parents is expected when a litter from normal parents contains approximately one affected progeny in four animals. Examination of the five-generation pedigree of one affected dog revealed no ancestor common to both paternal and maternal lineage. Thus, if the transmission of cerebellar hypoplasia is recessive, it occurs in more than one bloodline and may even be widespread in the breed.[6] The Golden Retriever is one of a group of breeds at greatest risk of developing **osteosarcomas.**[13]

A study was made of 335 dogs (Labs, Rottweilers, Retrievers) with **elbow osteochondrosis** that had been seen at the Royal Veterinary College from 1977 to 1987. Males were affected more often than females. The condition was bilateral in 50% of the cases and the peak age for onset of lameness was 4 - 6 months. In Rottweilers the lesions found at exploratory arthrotomy were predominantly abnormalities of the coronoid process, while in Retrievers and Labs lesions most commonly affected the medial humeral condyle or the coronoid process.[14] A Swedish study reports the incidence of **osteochondrosis** significantly higher than average in several large breeds, including Goldens.[15] Inherited forms of **muscular dystrophy** linked to the "x" chromosome are being studied and have been identified in the Golden Retriever.[16]

Congenital **phimosis** is reported in Golden Retrievers.[17]

The Golden Retriever is a breed in which **idiopathic epilepsy** has been detected.[18]

Diaphragmatic hernia is inherited as an autosomal recessive defect of the left dorsal caudal diaphragmatic crop. Puppies die shortly after birth of respiratory distress.[19]

BEHAVIOR

The Golden is patient and gentle with children. He is obedient, trainable and intelligent.

He is an ideal family companion.

OLD AGE

In old age, the Golden Retriever often develops cysts and/or warts. The life expectancy is from 10 to 13 years.

References

1. Ingaas, F. and Heim, P. "A Genetic Investigation of the Incidence of Hip Dysplasia in Norwegian Dog Breeds," *Norsk-veterinaertidsskrift*; 1987: 99:9, 617-623; 22 ref.
2. Rubin, L.F. "Cataract in Golden Retriever," *JAVMA* ; 1974: 156:458-475.
3. Dodds, W.J. "Blood Coagulation, Hemostasis, and Thrombosis," In *Handbook of Laboratory Animal Science II*; E.C. Milby and N.H. Altman, Eds. (CRC Press, Cleveland,O: 1974).
4. Magrane, W.G. *Canine Ophthalmology*. 3rd ed. (Lea & Febiger, Philadelphia, PA.:1977); 305.
5. Gelatt, K.N. "Cataracts in the Golden Retriever Dog," *VM/SAC*; 1972: 67:1113-1115.
6. Curtis, R. and K.C. Barnett, "A Survey of Cataracts in Golden and Labrador Retrievers," 1989: 30:5, 277-286; 14 ref.
7. Brignac, Michele M. "Congenital and Breed Associated Skin Diseases in the Dog and Cat," *KalKan Forum;* December, 1989, 9-16.
8. Werner, A. "Aspects of Food and Food Supplements in Skin Disease," *Pedigree's Breeder Forum*; 1993: Vol. 2, #1.
9. Ackerman, Lowell, DVM, "Allergic Skin Diseases," *American Kennel Club Gazette*; September, 1990.
10. Griffin, C.; Kwochka, K., McDonald, J. *Current Veterinary Dermatology, the Science and Art of Therapy*. Mosby Yearbook, St. Louis, MO 1993: 123, 28.
11. Golden Retriever column, *American Kennel Club Gazette*; September,1990.
12. Knecht, C.D., et al, "Cerebellar Hypoplasia in Chow Chows," *JAVMA;* 15(1):51-53; 1979.
13. *JAVMA*; May 1, 1990: Vol. 196, #9.
14. Guthrie, S. "Use of a Radiographic Scoring Technique for the Assessment of Dogs With Elbow Osteochondrosis," *J. Sm. Anim. Prac.*; 1989: 30:11, 639-644; 5 ref.
15. Bergsten, G. and Nordin, M. "Osteochondrosis as a Cause of Claims in a Population of Insured Dogs," *Svensk-Veterinartidning*; 1986: 38:15, 97-100.
16. Veterinary News, *The American Kennel Club Gazette*; October, 1991.
17. Ettinger, S.J. *Textbook of Veterinary Internal Medicine*. W.B. Saunders Co., Philadelphia, PA 1989: p 1884.
18. Jerold, S. DVM: "Sex Related Genetic Disorders: Did Mama Cause Them?" *American Kennel Club Gazette*, Feb. 1994; 76.
19. King, L.G. DVM: "Respiratory Congenital Disorders."Western Veterinary Conf. Feb. 1994.

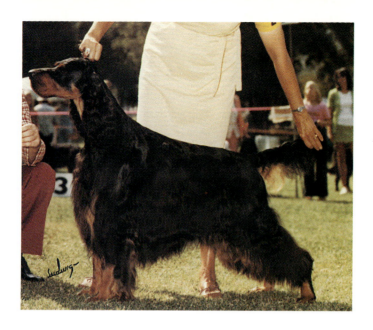

GORDON SETTERS

ORIGIN AND HISTORY

The black and tan setter was known as far back as two centuries ago. However, it became popular as a distinct breed in Scotland beginning in the late 1700s, when the Duke of Gordon established a kennel. It was from this strain that the first pair, "Rake and Rachel," were brought to America in 1842 by George W. Blunt. "Rachel" was later owned by Daniel Webster. From this pair, along with other importations, an American strain of gun dog was developed. The popularity of the breed reached a height at the turn of the century when the Gordon was in demand, not only as a gentleman's shooting dog, but as the commercial hunter's favorite.

DESCRIPTION

The official breed Standard states, "A good-sized, sturdily-built dog, well muscled, with plenty of bone and substance, but active, up-standing and stylish, appearing capable of doing a full day's work in the field. Strong, rather short back, well sprung ribs and short tail; fairly heavy head, finely chiseled; intelligent, noble and dignified expression, showing no signs of shyness; clear colors and straight or slightly waved coat. A dog that suggests strength and stamina rather than extreme speed."

While most breeders prefer a hunting dog with show potential or a show type with

272

hunting ability, there is a definite tendency for the hunter or field trainer to want a small or medium size dog and the show handler seems to seek to impress the judges with a larger dog. The Gordon is an affectionate, intelligent dog and responds well to obedience training. His desire to please makes him a biddable hunting companion as well as an ideal house pet. He is considered to be excellent with children.

As with all hunting breeds, the Gordon Setter should not be allowed to run loose without supervision. The scent of game, or even the sight of the neighbor's cat, may cause him to start a chase that could end in tragedy.

The Gordon in the field is a close working dog, although he can be encouraged to range further ahead of the hunter as is desired in field trial competition. He quarters his ground thoroughly and seeks out likely cover. If the bird is there, he will locate it but will need some training to be "steady to wing."

THE SHOW RING

In size, dogs run from 24 to 27 inches at the shoulder and 55 to 80 pounds in weight. Bitches are generally smaller, measuring 23 to 26 inches at the shoulder and 45 to 70 pounds in weight.

The color is black with tan markings. The tan should be a rich chestnut or mahogany. The locations of the tan color are specific in the standard.[1]

Predominantly tan, red or buff dogs which do not have the typical pattern of markings of a Gordon Setter have a disqualifying fault.

BREEDING AND WHELPING

While the mating cycle may be variable, bitches are usually ready to breed between the 10th and 14th day of their season. Some breeders report their bitches conceive as early as the 8th day and as late as the eighteenth. The gestation period can be 58 to 65 days but is usually 61 days.

The Gordon Setter litter averages eight to 12 whelps weighing 10 to 12 ounces each. Birth defects are not common. The Gordon bitch is an easy whelper and is usually able to nurse even a large litter without help.

Breeders have reported puppies born with deformities of the last two or three vertebrae of the tail.

The tan color on a puppy is obvious at birth and should deepen in color by 8 weeks. While it is not usual, a puppy can be born solid red. Some breeders destroy red puppies. While red puppies are ineligible for showing, they can now be registered with the AKC. They should not be used for breeding as the breed Standard calls for a "black and tan."

273

GROWTH

Kennels report an extreme range in the caloric requirements of Gordon Setters.

Gordon Setters are relatively slow to mature. Breeders expect the dog to be at its physical peak as late as 6 to 8 years of age.

RECOGNIZED PROBLEMS

The following have been reported in Gordon Setters:

1. **Hip dysplasia**
2. **Thyroid imbalance**[2]
3. Generalized **progressive retinal atrophy**[3,4]

Cerebellar cortical abiotrophy[5,6,7] has been described in Gordons from 6 to 24 months of age. Although a few cases of **ataxia** have been severe, no dog has become unable to stand. A prancing gait and poor coordination in a Gordon Setter 6 months of age or older could indicate this disorder. Going up or down stairs, the afflicted dog displays consistent overshooting of the feet.

Dogs do not recover from gait disorder, and are eventually euthanized. Necropsies have revealed diffuse degeneration of neurons in the cerebellar cortex. Evidence suggests an autosomal recessive mode of genetic transmission of this disease. The trait is not sex-linked; both sexes are affected. The important thing for owners of Gordon Setters to remember is that both parents of the affected dogs carry this trait; they are obligate heterozygotes. Therefore, two of the grandparents must also carry the trait. In addition, approximately 50% of the dog's littermates are carriers of the trait, but these can be identified only by breeding studies. Breeders can trace family lines to establish which puppies are carriers.

Hypothyroidism has been reported in Gordons.[8]

The Gordon Setter is a breed in which **idiopathic epilepsy** has been detected.[9]

BEHAVIOR

The Gordon is very adaptable to guarding and family life. He is sincere, helpful and polite. He is very affectionate with his family but can be reserved with strangers.

OLD AGE

The average life span of the Gordon is 12 years.

References

1. American Kennel Club, *The Complete Dog Book*. 18th ed. (Howell Book House Inc., New York, N.Y., 1992) 79-83.

2. Scott, C.W. and Paradis, M. "A Survey of Canine and Feline Skin Disorders Seen in a University Practice," Small Animal Clinic, University of Montreal, Saint-Hyacinth, Quebec, 1987-1988: *Can. Vet. Jour.* 1990: 31:12, 835-839; 50 ref.

3. Hodgman, S.F.J., et al, "Progressive Retinal Atrophy in Dogs I: The Disease in Irish Setters (Red)," *Vet. Rec*; 1949: 61:185-190.

4. Magnusson, H. "About Retinitis Pigmentosa and Consanguinity in Dogs," *Arch. Vergh. Ophthal.*; 1911: 2:147-163.

5. De LaHunta, A., et al, "Hereditary Cerebellar Cortical Abiotrophy in the Gordon Setter," *JAVMA;* Sept., 1980: 177:538-541.

6. Gorham, M.E. "Brittany Spaniels and Gordon Setters Plagued by Hereditary Muscle Disease," *DVM;* March, 1982: 13(3):52-54.

7. Ettinger, S.J. *Textbook of Veterinary Medicine, Diseases of the Dog and Cat.* W.B. Saunders, Co. Philadelphia, PA. 1989: 597-598.

8. Scott, C.W. and Paradis, M. "A Survey of Canine and Feline Skin Disorders Seen in a University Practice," Small Animal Clinic, University of Montreal, Saint-Hyacinth, Quebec, 1987-1988: *Can. Vet. Jour.;* 1990: 31:12, 839-835; 50 ref.

9. Bell, Jerold S. DVM "Sex Related Genetic Disorders: Did Mama Cause Them?" *American Kennel Club Gazette*, Feb. 1994; 76.

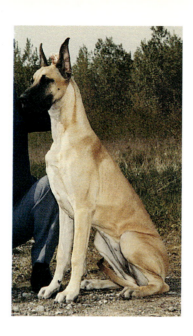

GREAT DANE

ORIGIN AND HISTORY

Magnificent size and supple grace characterize the "Apollo" of dogs—the Great Dane. The dog of today was originally bred in Germany to run down and fight the wild boar. Sixteenth-century etchings depict Great Danes hunting with great agility. In the 18th century one observer reported "No equipage can have arrived at the acme of grandeur until a couple of harlequin Danes precede the pomp."

Today's gentle Dane remains an alert guard dog that conducts itself with tact even in small apartments.

DESCRIPTION

Stable, sweet temperament with proper training is most important in the Great Dane. Unusual temperament is caused by environment and training, physical conditions, and inheritance. Any unpredictable vicious tendencies in a Great Dane are unforgivable, and the owner should not hesitate to have the dog euthanized.

Fawn and brindle puppies look very dark at birth—almost black—but gradually change to the normal expected color within 3 to 5 weeks. The pink feet and nails turn black within the first week. Blue puppies are also darker at birth and the skin often looks blue when wet. Black puppies are born black. Excessive white on any puppy (other than Harlequin) is most objection-able. (See Great Dane disqualifications).[1] Harlequin puppies are white with irregular torn black patches. On Harlequins, the pink skin, feet and especially the nose turn black more slowly. The tiny black spots on the nose gradually enlarge and spread together at a time rate according to the number and size of spots. Harlequin color is very unpredictable and each individual varies. The color sometimes changes during the first year by developing more spots, ticking or by the patches growing larger and running together. Mismarks (colors other than described in the Great Dane Standard) such as merles, solid white or predominantly white puppies are euthanized by many breeders, as they often carry lethal genes, deafness and many unforeseen problems that may develop.

Rear dewclaws are most unusual but should be removed if present. Front dewclaw removal is optional. Do not dock tails—a crook in the tail is rare, but if present at birth, can sometimes be corrected by squeezing the tail and rolling it between the fingers until it is straight, then splinting with stiff tape.

Ear cropping is optional but desired by owners. Ears are cropped medium-long (4 to 5 inches from top of skull to top point of ear). This may look long but the head will grow into the size. The best time to crop is at 25 pounds, or 12 weeks, as size varies in litters. Cropping does **NOT** make ears stand. The postoperative care plus consistent taping (with or without frames) to support the ear is the answer to standing ears.

THE SHOW RING

Great Danes' height must be at least 28 inches for bitches and 30 inches for dogs. Average age of maturity is 2 1/2 to 3 1/2 years. Usually the slower maturing Danes live longer. Average approximate weights for dogs are: small, 115 pounds; medium, 130 pounds; and large, 150 pounds. Weights for bitches are: small, 110 pounds; medium, 120 pounds; large, 130 pounds. There is no maximum limit on height or weight.

DISQUALIFICATION FAULTS

Disqualification faults include Danes under minimum height; any color other than those described under "Color, Markings, and Patterns"; docked tails and split noses.

BREEDING AND WHELPING

The normal Great Dane requires no special care during gestation other than good-quality food and exercise. Litter size averages eight to 10, with older bitches whelping slightly fewer in number. All bitches need close watching the first three days after whelping, as puppies are often suffocated by the bitch unknowingly lying on them. Birth weight ranges from 3/4 to 1

1/2 pounds. Large litters often need some supplemental feeding, using regular baby-size nipples and bottles. A standard commercial formula is the safest and best to use. Feed at 6- to 12-hour intervals, depending on need, leaving the puppies with the mother between times for cleaning, warmth and the natural need to nurse. Puppies will suck each other if unable to get to their mother.

Weaning begins at 21 days or sooner if possible as Great Dane puppies usually have teeth by 3 weeks of age. Puppies should be weaned by 4 to 5 weeks.

GROWTH

The most rapid and stressful growing time is from 4 to 10 months. During this period the tendency to over-vitaminize is most common. This often causes stress and improper nutritional balance that can lead to faulty assimilation and utilization of the food. A natural, well balanced, wholesome diet is the safest and best way to feed, although a high protein stress type of diet is sometimes necessary. Common stress signs caused by improper diet are **splay feet**, **broken down or enlarged pasterns and hocks**, **dull dead coat**, **drooping ears**, **arching the back**, **pot bellies** and **excessive soft stools**. Nutritional problems are best checked by doing a hair analysis and/or a blood calcium phosphorous ratio.

DENTITION

Permanent teething starts at about 4 months. A scissors bite is correct. Any variance such as wry or missing teeth, overshot and undershot bites should be watched for. On a young developing mouth, a tight or even bite may go undershot (a serious fault). Often, the slightly overshot bite is more apt to develop into the correct scissors bite. Teething may have an effect on ear training because of the extra calcium drain on the animal's system.

RECOGNIZED PROBLEMS

Bloat (gastric torsion or dilatation) can appear at almost any age except early puppyhood.[2] Usual symptoms are rapid distention of the stomach area, dry or foamy retching, a pained fixed look with the head and neck extended forward. Immediate emergency help is necessary to relieve the pressure by tubing or surgery. Early diagnosis and treatment is most critical to ensure the best chance of survival.

BREED	# CASES	# CONTROL	RISK RANK
Great Dane	299	37	1
St. Bernard	81	19	2
Weimaraner	49	13	3
Irish Setter	180	65	4
Gordon Setter	24	10	5
Standard Poodle	57	33	6
Basset Hound	39	34	7
Doberman Pinscher	139	130	8
Old English Sheepdog	27	29	9
German Shorthaired Pointer	25	28	10
Newfoundland	13	15	11
Airedale Terrier	12	15	12
German Shepherd	202	246	13
Alaskan Malamute	23	29	14
Chesapeake Bay Retriever	10	14	15
Boxer	28	39	16
Collie	39	71	17
Labrador Retriever	72	182	18
English Springer Spaniel	18	45	19
Samoyed	13	42	20
Dachshund	26	81	21
Golden Retriever	37	158	22
Cocker Spaniel	14	115	23

Bloat risk ranking for 24 pure breeds, compared with risk for all dogs combined.
(Taken from *Bloat Notes* School of Veterinary Medicine, Purdue University)

Bone problems are common during the first year of growth. Nutrition, trauma and heredity are the three most probable causes. **Elbow dysplasia** has been reported in the breed.[3] **Osteosarcoma** is a well known problem among all large purebred dogs. By the time of diagnosis, the condition is usually inoperable. Growing young Danes are very prone to **tonsillitis**.

Many Great Danes have a low tolerance to tranquilizers. **Demodectic mange** most often occurs during the stress period of teething (4 to 6 months) or during the first year. **Acne** has been recognized in Great Danes.[4]

Many Great Danes do not tolerate milk. Continuous soft stools are a symptom of this intolerance. They can tolerate raw suet or fat but cooked grease or fat may cause diarrhea. Great Danes **DO NOT DO WELL** if raised in a small kennel or cement facility.

Calcium Phosphate Deposition disease causes progressive incoordination and paralysis in Great Dane puppies one to two months old. **Periarticular calcium phosphate mineralization** and **bone deformities** occur. The bones are short, have a thin cortex and increased medullary trabeculae. The caudal cervical vertebrae canal becomes narrowed due to dorsal displacement of C7. This causes spinal cord compression and the clinical signs. It seems to be a familial disease. Serum calcium and phosphate are normal but blood Ph is lower in affected dogs. The mineralization of soft tissue and bone deformities are considered a primary change rather than secondary to any other underlying disease process. There is no known treatment.[5] **Hypertrophic osteodystrophy** has been described in the breed. It often occurs in well nourished puppies 4 to 7 months of age. Affected dogs run an elevated temperature of 103 to 107½, their legs are swollen and they walk with great pain.

Great Danes may have **Wobbler syndrome**, a compression of the spinal cord caused by **caudal cervical vertebrae malformation** and **malarticulation**.[1] The problem seems to be associated with young growing dogs. The principal clinical sign most often noticed by the owner is the ataxia of the pelvic limbs. Evidence suggests a role of nutrition as well as genetics in the development of this syndrome.[6]

Common eye problems of Great Danes include **eversion and inversion of membrane nictitans**[7] and **heterochromia iridis (Walleye)**.[8] **Microphthalmia** has also been reported.[9,10] Deafness is seen in this breed.[11]

BEHAVIOR

Great Danes are steady, patient and affectionate. Good with children in the family, they can be reserved with strangers.

OLD AGE

The average age of the Great Dane is a short 5 to 8 years. Older Danes hold their weight on little food and are generally easy keepers. Often small black growths (like moles) appear anywhere on the body and are best left alone unless they are growing rapidly or draining. Some degree of arthritis is most common in older Danes. A thick 2 to 4 inch soft, warm draft-free bed is needed for comfort as well as for avoiding callouses that can become sore or develop into a lick granuloma or related problems. The most common causes of death are trauma, kidney failure, bloat and assorted forms of spinal degeneration.

References
1. American Kennel Club, *Complete Dog Book*. (Howell Book House, New York, NY. 18th ed.1992) 262-266.

2. Trotter, E.J., et al, "Caudal Cervical Vertebrae Malformation-Malarticulation in Great Danes and Doberman Pinschers," *JAVMA;* 1976: 168(10): 917-930.

3. "Veterinary News," *American Kennel Club Gazette;* June, 1990.

4. Griffin, C., Kwochka, K., McDonald, J. *Current Veterinary Dermatology, the Science and Art of Therapy.* Mosby Yearbook, St. Louis, MO. 1993: 171, 266.

5. Ettinger, S.J.: Textbook of Veterinary Medicine. W.B. Saunders, Co., Philadelphia, PA 1989: 640.

6. Conrad, C. Radiology Section. Purdue University, W. Lafayette, IN., Personal Communication. 1975.

7. Magrane, W.G. *Canine Ophthalmology.* (Lea & Febiger, Philadelphia, PA.,1968) 232.

8. Kirk, R.W. *Current Veterinary Therapy VI.* (W.B. Saunders, Philadelphia, PA. 1977) 73.

9. *Canine Practice.* 4(4): 60 August, 1977.

10. Mitchell, A.L. "Dominant Dilution and Other Color Factors in Collie Dogs," *J. Hered.;* 1935: 26: 424-430.

11. Strain, George M. "Deafness in Dogs and Cats," *Proc. 10th Forum;* May, 1992.

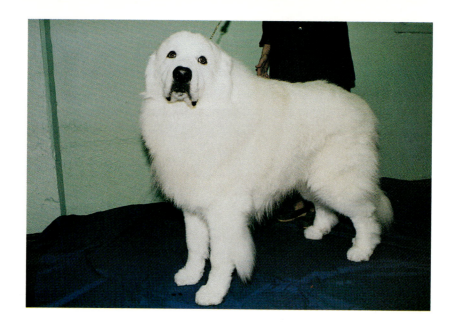

GREAT PYRENEES

ORIGIN AND HISTORY

The Great Pyrenees was developed long ago in the rugged mountains between Spain and France. In this isolated region, the dogs guarded the shepherd's flock and house. They developed a gentle temperament and a fierce loyalty to man. The breed has no extant ancestor.

DESCRIPTION

Pyrenees are instinctive, benevolent guardians. Because they are somewhat introverted, calm and contemplative, they are ideal family dogs. They adapt to most climates. Puppies should be acquired when they are 7 to 12 weeks old and should be socialized while young to prevent shyness or aggressive behavior. Males may become over-assertive at around 10 months of age and should be firmly corrected.

The eyes of the Pyrenees are rich, dark brown. Frequently, the embryonic vein that feeds the retinal nerve *in utero* does not resorb. It resembles a frayed circle of string suspended in the cornea. The breed's normal temperature, 100.8 degrees F, is unusually low. These dogs also have small, deep veins, slow pulse and low metabolism. Extreme caution should be used when anesthetics are administered. A shepherd's crook at the tip of the tail is characteristic.

THE SHOW RING

The adult coat is profuse and white or principally white with gray or badger markings. Eye rims, nose, and lips are black. The skin is pink with random black patches. A 27-inch dog weighs about 100 pounds; a 25-inch bitch weighs about 85 pounds.

Serious faults are incorrect bite (which should be level or scissors), unsound bone structure, missing pigmentation, missing dewclaws, light eyes, loose eyelids, droopy jowl and shyness or aggressiveness. Aggressiveness is usually the result of abuse or improper training.[1]

Pyrenees have several distinctive characteristics. They have single dewclaws on their front legs and double dewclaws on their rear legs. **The dewclaws must not be removed.** Briards and Pyrenees are the only two breeds recognized by the AKC **whose standards cite the lack of double back dewclaws as a fault.**

There are no breed ring disqualifications in this breed.

BREEDING AND WHELPING

Bitches frequently have their estrus at 1 year. Thereafter estrus occurs at six-month intervals. Ovulation is erratic, and conception may occur from the 5th to the 23rd day. Gestation averages 61 days. **Eclampsia** is rare. Bitches are usually easy whelpers, so if labor lasts more than three hours without the birth of a puppy, a **cesarean section** should be considered. Puppies are whelped at approximately half-hour intervals. Litters average six to seven puppies. The bitch and litter should be watched closely for at least five days after whelping, because bitches roll on the puppies and smother them. Puppies weigh about 1 pound at birth and are white, sometimes with black spots that gradually fade to gray or badger.

GROWTH

Pigment should be complete within 5 weeks. Growth is rapid. Puppies should be weaned when they are 3 weeks old. They require a diet high in calcium and protein, because by 4 months old they may be gaining as much as 3/4 pound a day. The breed is mature at 18 months to 2 years. Once mature, they require less food than most large breeds, because of their low metabolism.

RECOGNIZED PROBLEMS

Pyrenees are subject to certain congenital conditions: **inverted eyelids, hip dysplasia, slipped patella, achondroplasia, blue eyes (smoky yellow at maturity), swimmer puppies, over or undershot bite** and **missing dewclaws.**

Other defects, such as **missing eyeball, deafness, congenital hernia, monorchidism,** cryptorchidism, cleft palate, brittle bone syndrome, defective heart and missing thoracic wall, are rare. Pyrenees recover easily from common infections, such as kennel cough and gastrointestinal infections. Pyrenees sometimes develop cataracts when they are 2 to 3 years old. However, blindness is not common, even in dogs as old as 15 years.

Factor XI deficiency, PTA (Plasma Thromboplastin Antecedent) has been described in Great Pyrenees.[2]

BEHAVIOR

The Great Pyrenees' sweet expression makes him look slow and lethargic, but he is alert and intelligent. He adapts well to family life if he has room to exercise. He is gentle and patient.

OLD AGE

The breed is hardy and lives 12 to 15 years. Some Pyrenees have lived to 18 years. The older dog may be arthritic and appreciates a warm, soft bed. The most common problem in older males are kidney and bladder problems. Metritis is seen frequently in unspayed, nonproducing bitches. Lymphosarcoma, bone cancer and spondylitis have been seen in older dogs.

References
1. The American Kennel Club, *The Complete Dog Book*. (Howell Book House. New York, N.Y. 1992) 267-271.
2. Ettinger, S.J.: Textbook of Veterinary Internal Medicine, Diseases of the Dog and Cat, A.B. Saunders, Co., Philadelphia, PA 1989: 2259.

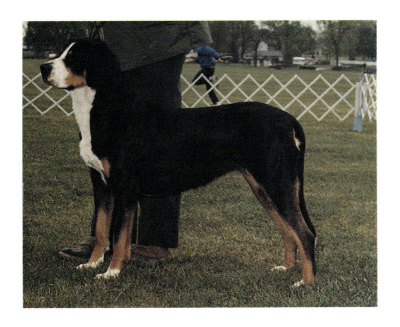

GREATER SWISS MOUNTAIN DOG

ORIGIN AND HISTORY

The Greater Swiss Mountain dog, a larger relative of the Bernese, had a fixed breed type by 1905. The four types of Swiss Mountain Dog are believed to be descended from the Tibetan Mastiff. The breed was well-known in the middle ages, when it accompanied its Swiss masters into battle as a bodyguard and attack dog.[1]

DESCRIPTION

This breed's specific work is as a herd dog and a stable dog, but he has been used very successfully as a guard dog and to pull a cart. He is good-tempered, patient and easily trainable, making him an excellent companion dog. Greater Swiss Mountain Dogs are good with children and have excellent memories. It is said they can recognize each member of their herd.

THE SHOW RING

Greater Swiss Mountain Dogs are 25 1/2 to 28 1/2 inches high for males and 23 1/2 to 27 inches high for bitches and weigh around 130 pounds. The dog should have a strong scissors bite, heavy thighs and short, round feet. Eye color varies from hazel to chestnut and its ears are triangular and pendent. The tail is carried down. The coat is soft and silky; wavy but not curled. He is jet black with brown-red on the cheeks, legs, the brisket and over the eyes. White markings on the head or brisket are essential. White paws and tip of tail are preferable.

Faults: eyes too light, ears or tail badly carried, faded or impure colors, white neck ring, absence of white markings.[2]

There are no disqualifying faults for this breed.

BREEDING AND WHELPING

Estrus in the Greater Swiss Mountain Dog bitch is usually first seen between 8 and 10 months of age. They are meticulous about cleaning themselves, so the owner must be observant.

Gestation is very normal, and whelping presents no unusual problems. The average litter is eight, weighing from 3/4 to 1 pound.

Rear dewclaws are removed, and removal of front dew claws is optional. Breeders suggest this be done on the second day as these are large boned whelps that grow at an amazing rate. At eight weeks a puppy can be expected to weigh from 16 to 22 pounds.

RECOGNIZED PROBLEMS

Many of these dogs are imports and some have not fared well on dog foods containing soybean meal. They are a particularly hardy breed and very rarely ill. Undershot mouths are seen in the breed.

An estimated 60 to 70% of Greater Swiss Mountain Dogs experience **panosteitis.** These dogs gain as much as 1 pound a day and growth related problems appear. **Hip dysplasia** is seen less often than might be expected considering the size of the dogs.

Von Willebrand's disease has been documented in Greater Swiss Mountain Dogs.

Puppies in the breed that are diagnosed as having **megaesophagus** become asymptomatic as they mature.

Seemingly excessive numbers of eyelashes are normal in this breed and create no problem.

BEHAVIOR

These dogs do not take well to a change of ownership after 18 months of age. Health problems may develop, or they may become too aggressive to manage. The Greater Swiss Mountain Dog needs lots of space. They may not adapt to confined city living.[2] They are easily trained, good with children, even-tempered and patient. They can be trusted to live congenially with other dogs.

OLD AGE

Greater Swiss Mountain Dogs live to be 11 to 13 years of age.

References
1. Illustrated Book of Dogs, *Reader's Digest*, 1989.
2. *Guide to Dogs*, (Simon and Schuster, 1980).

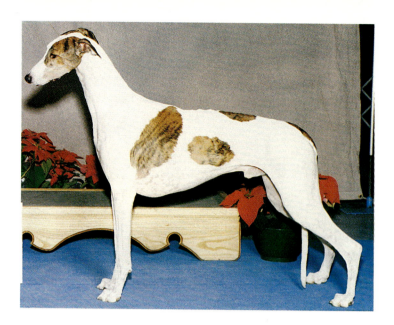

GREYHOUND

ORIGIN AND HISTORY

The Greyhound is a very old breed. Its many purposes—courser, racer, pet and investment—have been known for centuries.

There are many records of the Greyhound or "Gazehound" (running on sight of its quarry)[1] in ancient times. For example, in the Tomb of Amten in about 2500 B.C., in the Book of Solomon, in Ovid's writing, even earlier in wall paintings on the Nile the Greyhound is mentioned.

The breed was taken by merchants in caravans throughout Iraq, Persia and Russia. In Britain, Saxon chiefs owned Greyhounds. In 1016, the Laws of Canute established the limits to which common persons could use Greyhounds in hunting.[2] Later, Britain declared that only royal-blooded men and noblemen could own Greyhounds.[1]

Greyhounds were brought to North America in the 1500s by the Spanish explorers for hunting purposes. They have been popular with professional soldiers for centuries; General George Custer kept racing Greyhounds.[3]

The Greyhound is now rarely used for hunting but still runs in the sport of coursing (hare hunting) and mechanical racing (pursuing mechanical hares in structural tracks). The earliest organized coursing was in England in the first Waterloo Cup Event in 1836.[4] In the United States Greyhound racing is a high-draw sport that is still growing in popularity.

The Greyhound was first specified in Islington in 1859.[1] Its popularity has continued in England, particularly in Cornwall. The breed was listed in American Kennel Club history, too, with its first registration in the second stud book.[3]

DESCRIPTION

The Greyhound is built for running and in its most perfect form presents a picture of elegance, strength and harmony. As versatile as its qualities are, its various ways of performance are all related to the functional qualities of its build: leanness, depth of chest, strong muscular development, elongated head, long neck and long body. In a Greyhound of fine quality, the coat should be fine and smooth. The feet should be hard and close, well knuckled up, more hare than cat feet.

The Greyhound is intelligent and loyal. Their sensitiveness is paired with sweetness and unaggressiveness. These qualities are even present among racers. Their quality as a companion dog is unsurpassed.

THE SHOW RING

The height of the mature dog is 27 to 30 inches. The AKC weight for dogs is 65 to 70 pounds and for bitches 60 to 65 pounds.

Puppies are born in all colors; solid, brindle and parti-color. Color is immaterial according to the Standard of the American Kennel Club. Some of the colors seen at birth will change after a few weeks—a silvery gray will change into fawn, a chocolate brown into red.

Greyhounds bred for show are registered with the American Kennel Club. The Greyhound Club of America, a member of the AKC, has set up the Standard which specifies the qualities necessary for perfection. The conscientious breeder breeds selectively, having in mind not only the perfection of appearance but equally the avoidance of any genetic imperfections or defects.

There are no disqualifying faults in the breed ring.

BREEDING AND WHELPING

Beginning of estrus is at about 11 months of age, but a belated start is not abnormal. First estrus may be as late as 2 1/2 years of age, as it was with one of the most famous Greyhound bitches in the United States. The estrus cycle of the Greyhound is 8 months or greater.

Some males are **"lazy breeders"** and an artificial insemination may be required.[5]

Typically no special problems during the gestation nor at the time of delivery occur. Litter size may be as many as 10 to 15 puppies. The delivery is often a lengthy process, since a period of inertia may set in after the majority of puppies are born. Experience has shown that home environment is usually preferable to hospitalization because the bitch is quite dependent upon individual attention and reassurance.

Puppies are born with proportionately long tails. Extra care should be taken during delivery not to damage the tail or aggravate a congenitally deformed tail. Young animals may trip on their long tails. Breeders should be especially alert to abrasions on the tail since young Greyhounds will "race" about spontaneously.

Birth weights of puppies vary. Dogs may weigh between 1 1/4 and 1 1/2 pounds while bitches usually weigh somewhat less.

A Greyhound has reached its height at about 9 months of age, but full physical maturity requires 2 to 3 years.

RECOGNIZED PROBLEMS

Greyhounds have a hereditary problem with **hemophilia A (Factor VIII deficiency)**. The condition is passed to offspring as a sex-linked recessive trait. Excessive bleeding usually begins after weaning. Bleeding occurs most often in limbs and joints, where lameness may result. Diagnosis may be problematic, especially in young animal's fractures. Prolonged bleeding is important because the Greyhound's swiftness and impulsive racing make them prone to injuries. Vitamin K should be kept available if hemophilia is suspected.

Von Willebrand's disease has been reported in the breed.[6]

Tail irritations and **broken tails** are also a problem in adult life.

Esophageal achalasia is common in Greyhounds. This condition, also called **cardiospasm**, is characterized by dysfunction of the esophageal wall and failure of the terminal sphincter to close in the esophagus. The mode of inheritance of this neuromuscular imbalance has not been determined.

The Greyhound is predisposed to **dystocia**. In addition to inertia in the dam, fetal anatomical peculiarities are a contributing factor. The incidence of fetal death is relatively high.

In the past, Greyhounds were risky candidates for anesthesia, probably due to the small amount of fatty tissue they possess which might interfere with proper elimination of the drugs used. Improvement of techniques and experience have greatly diminished this risk.

A **short spine** is an autosomal recessive trait inherited in some Greyhounds. They also have predisposition to **luxation of the lens**.

Bloat has been reported as a problem occurring in the breed.

Greyhounds are remarkably free of **hip dysplasia**.

RACING GREYHOUNDS

Greyhounds or mixed Greyhounds used in hunting in the prairies of the West are called staghounds. These dogs hunt on sight and are automatically released from vehicles when game is sighted.

Racing Greyhounds are registered with national racing associations, such as the National Greyhound Association in the United States. As well as the conventional identification by color and sex, racing Greyhounds are registered by characteristic colors of each toenail. Registration is required soon after birth, within 60 days. Ear tattoos are given each dog—the litter number is recorded on the left ear, the month and year of birth and puppy number are recorded in the right ear.

RACING RELATED INJURIES

Racing Greyhounds are run often (every 3 to 4 days) and injuries are common. Blood and urine samples are taken regularly. Most injuries are the result of the stress of racing: **Luxation, fractures and impacts on the foot pads are common.**

Dropped muscle is traumatic rupture of the muscle sheath or the tendon attachment, either in the front or hind legs. The result is bulging of the muscle and later a visible cavity. Incidence is most common in the gracilis; another location is the long head of the triceps at the proximal origin of the scapula. **Stopper injury**, an injury to the accessory carpal bone, is a fracture often caused by racing. It is a common source of lameness. The fourth metacarpal is also often fractured, a condition called **quarter bone injury**. An external splint is usually sufficient if the joints are not involved.

A **jack** is a traumatic injury with swelling and hematoma or sertoma of the medial surface of the hock. The term comes from the dog's racing form, in which a jackknife shape is seen. The injury is caused when the thoracic limb clashes with the medial surface of the pelvic limb.

Unlike some other breeds for which research on injuries is fairly recent, the Greyhound has been studied exhaustively because of his role in racing. Therefore, descriptions of injury frequency, severity, etc. are quite specific. Prole (1976) found that the left front foot and leg were more often injured (when all injuries were counted), than the right front leg, right rear leg and left rear leg, respectively.

The majority of injuries to toes occurred to toes three and four, the longer digits. The web between toes is often split, occurring on both front and rear toes. A condition known as **"track leg"** occurs when the left tibia strikes the lateral epicondyle of the lower end of the left humerus. Swelling and bruising result, but the injury is not necessarily severe enough to remove the animal from his regular race schedule. Lameness of racing Greyhounds is directly proportional to the race season itself, i.e., a wet season keeps the speeds low, with fewer injuries. A dry season allows faster times and a higher incidence of lameness. Luxations occur in the third and central tarsal bones. They can be confirmed by X-rays. **Bowing of the hock** is an injury to the plantar ligament.

Severely injured digits (fractures and luxations) indicate a need for amputation. Amputation causes relative disability depending on which digit is involved. Removing digits I and IV causes some disability, but amputating digits II or III is so disabling that the dog probably could not race again. **Acute arthritis** in the leg joints is another problem of racing Greyhounds, including the carpus, tarsus, elbow and stifle. The patient is acutely ill, febrile, anorectic and loses weight. One treatment is penicillin streptomycin and betamethazone.

An **azoturia-like disease** often occurs in Greyhounds. Symptoms including stiffness, anorexia and reluctance to move, usually beginning the day after overexercise. Later, the dog develops severe cramping and rigidity. Treatment includes large amounts of fluids, steroids and rest. Phlebotomy may be used if 48 hours of continuous fluids fail to lower the PCV levels.

Racing Greyhounds have a skin condition called **"Alabama rot."** Researchers at the Kansas State School of Veterinary Medicine are close to a breakthrough for a control or a cure. The syndrome is characterized by skin lesions and kidney failure. The disease is believed to be related to a human kidney disease that occurs in adolescence and is probably the result of bacteria-produced toxin. It occurs in small, local outbreaks and doesn't seem to spread between kennels and dogs and it does not have to be fatal. The Kansas State research team believes that they will either develop a vaccine or be able to recommend specific changes in environment to prevent "Alabama rot."

UNUSUAL CHARACTERISTICS OF RACING GREYHOUNDS

The Greyhound can be characterized as having a naturally occurring, significantly higher mean arterial pressure and cardiac output with a lower total peripheral resistance compared to the mongrel. Cardiac output is significantly reduced in the Greyhound in response to pentobarbital, and is associated with a much greater reduction in stroke volume for the Greyhound than for the mongrel.

Angiostrongylus vasorum, a helminth of the pulmonary artery and the right ventricle, has been reported in Ireland and England in Greyhounds. Slugs and snails are the intermediate hosts. Symptoms are large subcutaneous swellings in dependent areas such as the submandibular space, thorax, and legs. There is a distinct murmur on the right side. There is lameness only if the legs are affected. The first stage of larvae is found in the feces; the larvae and ova are also found in the tracheal mucus. Treatment is with Levamisole (10 mg/kg per day for three days).

BEHAVIOR

The Greyhound, if properly exercised, can be a quiet and agreeable house pet. He is loyal, vain, proud, intelligent and reserved with friends and strangers.

References

1. A.F. Jones and F. Hamilton, Eds., *The World Encyclopedia of Dogs.* (Galahad Books, New York, N.Y.,1971) 357,361,363,416,620..
2. N.H. Johnson, *The Complete Puppy and Dog Book.* (Athenaeum, New York, NY, 1973) 29-30.
3. The American Kennel Club, *The Complete Dog Book.* (Howell Book House, New York, NY.,1992) 182-185.
4. The American Kennel Club, *The Complete Dog Book.* (Doubleday and Co.,Inc..,Garden City, N.Y.1968) 51, 78, 168-170, 372.
5. Chris Walkowicz, "The Mechanics of Breeding," *American Kennel Club Gazette;* June, 1990: 68.
6. J.D. Littlewood, M.E. Herrtage, N.T. Gorman and N.J. McGlennon, "Von Willebrand's Disease in Dogs in the United Kingdom," *Vet. Record;* 1987: 121:20, 463-468; 28 ref.

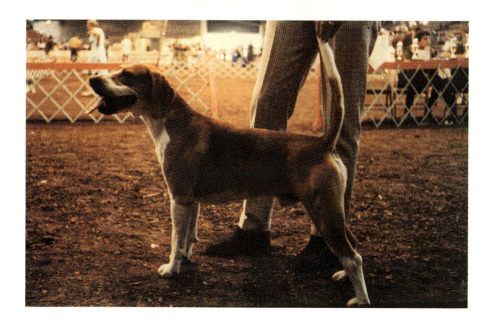

HARRIER

ORIGIN AND HISTORY

The Harrier is believed to have originated in England from Southern Hound and Greyhound crosses. The first pack of Harriers in England was the Penistone, established by Sir Elias de Midhope in 1260. Hunting the hare has always had great popularity throughout the British Isles, and in some ways enjoyed greater favor than fox hunting. One great cause of its popularity was that a pack of Harriers could be followed on foot. Despite all stories of the ancient origin of Harriers, it is the general belief that the dog of today is merely a smaller edition of the Foxhound, and that he has been bred down from the larger hound by selective breeding.

DESCRIPTION

Harriers have an even temperament and make very good family pets since they require minimal grooming and medical care.

THE SHOW RING

Harriers are one of the few breeds whose Standard calls for them to toe in. They should be 19 to 21 inches at the shoulder. Proportion is slightly off square.

There are no disqualifying faults.

BREEDING AND WHELPING

The average litter seems to be seven or eight, and puppies should weigh 8 to 10 ounces.

RECOGNIZED PROBLEMS

Harriers are extremely healthy dogs with no major hereditary defects. **Malocclusion** can be a problem.

BEHAVIOR

The Harrier is a robust, healthy dog but is first and foremost a hunting dog. He is not really suitable as a house dog. He is a pack animal and prefers to live with the pack.

OLD AGE

Most Harriers live to be 12 to 15 years old.

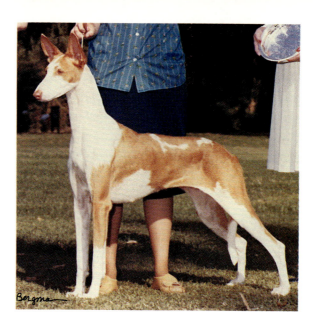

IBIZAN HOUND

ORIGIN AND HISTORY

The Ibizan Hound is one of the oldest of purebred dogs, having originated in ancient Egypt. Around the 8th Century B.C., the Phoenicians carried the breed to the Balearic Islands off the coast of Spain, where the people of Ibiza have retained them essentially as working hunters, keeping only the ones who could feed their families.

DESCRIPTION

According to the revised Standard of the Ibizan Hound Club of the U.S. (not the current AKC Standard), "...as a gazehound, the Ibizan is unequaled and has the ability to hunt by day or by night, singly, in pairs, or in packs. He is called the "Three-Way Hunter," incorporating highly developed sight, scent, and hearing abilities. Particular to the breed are large, erect ears that are highly mobile...; oblique, amber eyes, alert to every movement; and a prominent, flesh-colored nose. The Ibizan is an agile, ... intelligent and docile dog; a tall, graceful dog, fine, but never giving the appearance of lacking strength...In top show or hunting condition, the last few ribs and points of the hip bones will be in evidence."

The Ibizan Hound is a natural breed. No cropping or cutting of ears or tail is allowed. Removal of dewclaws is optional. Most breeders remove dewclaws when puppies are 2 days old. Ears stand at any age between 4 weeks and 6 months. Taping of ears is not encouraged as it hides genetically weak ears. If taping is used, it should be noted in records.

The dog should be shown in its natural state, with no trimming of the feathering on back of thighs or on the tail. Exhibitors are encouraged not to remove whiskers.

Ibizans are highly trainable and excel in obedience. They generally do not range as far from owners as some other sighthounds. They have incredible endurance and can retain a fast trot for hours. Ibizans love coursing and are great distance runners, doing best on 800-yard courses or longer. The distinctive gait is a floating, suspended, single-tracking trot, just skimming the ground. The speed is comparable to that of the Afghan or Saluki. In jumping, great heights can be reached from a standstill.

Ibizans do not do well in kennels. Many will pace up and down and not retain weight if kept away from human company. They make excellent house dogs, staying clean and shedding little. They are very affectionate and like to rub against their owners. In playing with other dogs, they may growl and click their teeth. This should not be mistaken for aggressiveness. In spite of being enthusiastic hunters, these dogs do not bother small animals around the home.

THE SHOW RING

Dogs range from 23 1/2 to 27 1/2 inches in height, weighing about 50 pounds. Bitches range from 22 ½ to 26 inches and weigh about 42 to 49 pounds.

Ibizans have two types of coat, smooth and wire. The wire coat will be from 1 to 3 inches long with a possible moustache. Both types of coat often appear in a single litter. The wire coat is sometimes not apparent until about a year; and conversely, some seemingly wire coats in young puppies turn out to be smooth. Colors are combinations of red and white, or solid red (from light yellowish-red called "lion" to deep red) or white. **Any color other than red or white is a disqualification.** A lozenge marking (or "Ax Mark") on the forehead, is desirable, but its absence is not to be considered a fault. The standard calls for a flesh-color nose.

Breeders consider the following as faults: Extreme shyness or viciousness; bent or broken ears; front feet in a definite East-West attitude; undershot or overshot bite; structure that is heavy or massive; structure which is fragile, lacking in strength; feet which are broken, splayed or paper in appearance; bulging muscles, thereby losing elegance in appearance; coarse or heavy head; wide hips; and bulging veins.

BREEDING AND WHELPING

Ibizans are still very close to the wild canines because many bitches have only one estrus every 10 months to a year. Many bitches do not have their first estrus until almost 2 years of age. Some bitches now come in at the age of 8 months and have two seasons annually.

Bitches are easy whelpers and good mothers, even at times regurgitating their own food for the puppies.

Litters average from 6 to twelve. At birth, puppies generally weigh slightly under 1 pound and are very sturdy. The red ones are usually born rather pale and darken with age. Puppies can be started at 3 weeks on puppy chow made into a gruel, and then weaned at 5 weeks.

GROWTH

These dogs grow very fast, although they are not truly mature until 3 years of age. They need a well balanced diet of puppy chow with lots of powdered milk for the first year. Great care must be taken not to oversupplement. It is normal for a healthy Ibizan Hound to eat considerable amounts of grass without upsetting its digestion.

RECOGNIZED PROBLEMS

Some dogs are born with **missing teeth**; this deficiency should be considered in any breeding program, even though it is not mentioned in the Standard. The breed tends to have rather extreme **false pregnancies**, and it is advisable to spay nonbreeding stock.

At this time there are few hereditary problems in the breed, except an occasional **unilateral cryptorchid**.

Bloat has been reported in the breed.[1]

Hereditary seizures have been reported that seem to concentrate in specific lines.[2] **Axonal dystrophy**, a disease affecting the muscles and nerves is rarely seen, but the genetic potential involves almost every Ibizan Hound.[2] Dr. Bell of Cornell reports that axonal dystrophy is thought to be inherited as an incomplete dominant. The condition manifests itself with tiny fibrous cysts throughout the central nervous system. The symptoms copy those of the "Wobbler" syndrome. Affected dogs will stagger and then progress to convulsions. It is usually fatal by fourth year.

Ibizans are listed as one of the breeds with **congenital deafness**.[3]

Ibizan Hound breeders are in the enviable position of having an unspoiled natural breed, many dogs being only third-generation American. This is the time to prevent the many hereditary defects that plague other purebred dogs from becoming entrenched in the breed. It is recommended that all breeding stock be x-rayed for hip dysplasia and eyes examined for hereditary eye defects. No dog or bitch should be bred before it is 2 years old because problems common to other breeds are not apparent until then.

Some Ibizans are predisposed to **skin problems**, so puppy acne and staph must be guarded against. Ibizans should be kept very clean, although cleanliness is not usually a problem.

Some individuals suffer from **hives** on occasion; this can be controlled with antihistamines or steroids. Some are allergic to tick and flea collars, and also great care must be taken with dips and sprays because Ibizans wash themselves like cats. As in all sighthounds, anesthesia is to be administered with caution.

BEHAVIOR

The Ibizan is also known as the Spanish Greyhound. It is not as quiet and reserved as a greyhound. Hunting packs can only have one male in them as two males in a pack will fight. They are more aggressive than greyhounds. They need space and adapt well to country living.

OLD AGE

Mature dogs often become quite lazy and will lounge about all day unless encouraged to exercise. All Ibizans would benefit greatly from at least two 20-minute walks a day, at a brisk trot, along with an occasional run in a safe area or on a lunge line. Actually, the breed can take all the exercise offered. Ibizans are always playful and age well if given proper care. Life span should be from 12 to 14 years.

References
1. *American Kennel Club Gazette*, Ibizan column, 132; November, 1990.
2. Puskas, L. "Ibizan Hounds Column," *American Kennel Club Gazette*; September, 1993.
3. Strain, George M. "Deafness in Dogs and Cats," *Proc. 10th ACVIM Forum*; May, 1992.

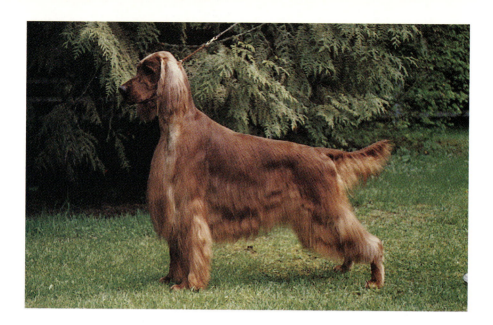

IRISH SETTER

DESCRIPTION

Characteristically, the breed is large, mahogany red, and devil-may-care. Irish Setters require play, exercise, affection and above all, patience and understanding. They can be snobs or clowns, but are always loyal to their owners. These dogs may be supersensitive or hardheaded, though they rarely lack intelligence. Often they like to play dumb, and no dog is more adept at acting than the Irish Setter.

THE SHOW RING

The ideal Irish Setter dog is 27 inches at the withers and weighs about 70 pounds; the ideal bitch is 25 inches tall and weighs 60 pounds. The correct specimen always exhibits balance, whether standing or in motion.

There are no disqualifying breed faults.

BREEDING AND WHELPING

Irish Setter bitches can have very erratic estrous cycles. Some bitches regularly come into estrus at six-month intervals, but others go as long as two or three years between periods. First estrus may not occur in some individuals until they are 3 years old.

False pregnancies, often severe, are common after a fertile season. Not every season is fertile. A bitch should never be spayed solely because of the natural occurrence of false pregnancy. Whelping bitches should be watched carefully and attended constantly. **Uterine inertia** is common. **Cesarean section** is often required when a bitch whelps part of the litter and then quits. **Dystocia** is occasionally caused by malpresentation of a fetus, generally in one of three positions: 1) the back presented against the birth canal with the head in one horn and the buttocks in the other; 2) the head turned back over a shoulder; or 3) one front leg forward and the other turned backward.

Irish Setter bitches frequently develop **eclampsia**. They may also become hyperactive after whelping. During the first three days after whelping, they should be watched closely because they may carelessly step on their puppies or constantly move them around. Usually the dam eventually calms down and becomes a good mother.

Mastitis is seldom a problem.

Irish Setters are notoriously prolific, although in some bloodlines, small litters of three to five puppies are usual. The average size of a litter is eight to 10, but often 14 or more are seen. Frequently, in large litters, the first and/or last puppy is born dead. The usual birth weight of Irish Setter puppies is 16 ounces.. However, weights may range from 6 to 26 ounces. Weight at birth is not an indicator of adult size. Color at birth varies from almost black-mahogany to light fawn. Adult color cannot be determined until the puppies start to lose their baby fuzz and develop a dark streak down their backs and tails. The fringes of the ear tips often indicate adult color.

White markings can be found on most puppies; some strains have more white than others, and a few have none. White markings should never be considered a fault in puppies, because most of the white disappears as the animals mature. White spots on the back or side can also disappear with adulthood. Occasionally, black markings occur. These, too, usually vanish with the puppy coat. Pure black puppies are rare.

Dewclaws may or may not be removed.

Field-stock Irish Setters are generally smaller than other strains, both at birth and as adults. Their estrous cycles are more regular, but breeding difficulties occur as often as in large strains of the breed. The growth rate of the smaller dogs is slower and bone development is not as rapid, but these smaller dogs usually mature faster. Puppies of the nonfield strain grow as rapidly as Great Dane puppies, reaching maturity after only 30 to 36 months.

DENTITION

Baby **canine teeth** must often be pulled. Underbites and overbites are common. The underbite often is not apparent until a puppy is 9 months old. At this time the head stops growing but the lower jaw continues to grow. For this reason a slight overbite is preferred in puppies.

RECOGNIZED PROBLEMS

Congenital malformations seen occasionally in Irish Setters include **stub tails**, **club feet** and, very rarely, **cleft palates**, **harelip** and part of the internal organs outside the head or body. **Malformed vertebrae** are extremely common, resulting in a smaller or larger "kink," usually at the tip of the tail. Unless this kink constitutes a severe deformity, it should be ignored and the puppy allowed to live.

Irish Setter puppies are not for the faint of heart, for they demand a great deal from their owners. They are unusually accident prone. If the owner of an Irish Setter can endure the first year and one-half of the dog's life, he might make it the rest of the way. **Broken bones** are common.

Disturbances of growth are being seen with increasing frequency, most commonly **hypertrophic osteodystrophy**, **osteochondritis dissecans**, **panosteitis**, **rickets** and an array of problems that may be related to over-nutrition.

Because Irish Setters are not mentally, physically or emotionally mature until they are 3 years old, they should not be pushed too hard until they reach that age.

The incidence of **hip dysplasia** in the breed is estimated at 35 percent and appears to be decreasing.

Uveodermatological syndrome has been reported in the Irish Setter, among other breeds.[1,2]

Generalized **progressive retinal atrophy**[3,4] occurs in Irish Setters in all sections of the country. A candidate gene, the hereditary material suspected of being responsible for PRA in the Irish Setter, has been identified.[5] **Cataracts** are common, mostly in older dogs. The incidence of **juvenile cataracts** is increasing, however, together with other eye diseases that are often mistaken for progressive retinal atrophy.

Hemophilia A (due to Factor VIII deficiency) in the Irish Setter was originally reported in 1946 and has been reported twice since.[7,8,9]

Granulocytopathy is a disease caused by neutrophil dysfunction in Irish Setters. Clinically there is increased susceptibility to infection. In puppies studied clinically and with neutrophil function tests there was fever, gingivitis, destruction of bone and bone proliferation in the mandibles. radius and ulna. Leukocytosis and impaired phagocytosis are characteristic of the disease, which is caused by an autosomal recessive gene. Prognosis is poor, and treatment with antibiotics and cortico-steroids gives only temporary relief.[10]

Congenital carpal subluxation is considered a sex-linked recessive trait. Carpal subluxation was first seen in a colony of Irish Setters with Hemophilia A.

Surveys conducted in 1968[11] indicated a breed predisposition to **persistent right aor-**

tic arch,[12,13,14,15] and **primary megaesophagus**.[16]

Generalized **myopathy**[17] and **quadriplegia with amblyopia**[18] are other problems some breeders have encountered.

The Irish Setter is one of the breeds at greatest risk of developing **osteosarcomas**.[19] Irish Setters are susceptible to **inhalant allergies**.[20]

Penicillin reactions are frequent. Overreaction to anesthetics can occur but incidence is not high. **Otitis externa** is a severe problem. **Inter-digital cysts**, **mammary tumors**, **salivary gland disorders**, **entropion**,[5] **ectropion**, **plugged tear ducts**, **infected anal glands**, **enlarged prostate**, **vaginitis**, **metritis, pyometra** and **melanomas** are encountered frequently in the adult Irish Setter. Irish Setters have an increased breed incidence of **hypothyroidism**.[21]

Wheat-sensitive enteropathy was explored in a litter bred from two Irish Setters with a naturally occurring enteropathy. Jejunal biopsies from all eight progeny exhibited morphological changes comparable to those in the parents, while biochemical abnormalities appeared to be related to age. In biopsies obtained from the first group of four dogs at eight months, the activities of alkaline phosphatase and leucyl-2-naphthyl-amidase were almost undetectable while disaccharidases were unaltered.

In contrast, analytical subcellular fractionation of biopsies obtained from the second group of four dogs at 9 months showed that specific activities now reflected a major deficiency of brush border alkaline phosphatase, and normal brush border leucyl-2-naphthylamidase accompanied by elevated soluble activity. Further studies are indicated to determine whether these findings represent an age-related abnormality affecting specific microvillus membrane proteins.[22]

Other bowel disorders and **intussusception** occur because Setters frequently ingest foreign materials.

The adult dog should be kenneled in an area at least 6 feet wide and 20 feet long. Pea rock is recommended as a ground surface in the run, because it passes safely through the digestive tract.

Trimethoprim-Sulphonamide hypersensitivity has been reported in the Irish Setter as well as in other large breeds of dogs. The cases reported showed clinical signs of polyarthritis, joint pain and pyrexia. Cases reported were in Weimeraners, Irish Setters, Golden Retrievers, Labrador Retrievers, Flat Coat Retrievers, Dobermans and one Cocker Spaniel.[23]

The Irish Setter is a breed in which **idiopathic epilepsy** has been detected.[24]

BEHAVIOR

The Irish Setter was bred for the country and some of them fare poorly as city dogs. A house-bound Irish Setter may be tagged as a crazy dog because the owners don't realize how much exercise this big red dog needs. If the Irishman is properly trained he is a joy to have as a companion. He is intelligent and independent and this combination can cause problems if he is not properly controlled.

OLD AGE

The 6- or 7-year-old Irish Setter is a joy to be around, for it rarely has health problems. Cardiac disease, nephritis or cancer of the lungs, prostate, lymphatic system and occasionally, the mouth or digestive system do occur.

Strokes are common in aged dogs. The likelihood of **bloat**, a threat from puppyhood, increases dramatically as the dog ages. Loss of sight and hearing also occurs, and incontinence may be a problem. Usually the problems of the aging Irish Setter are similar to those of old age in other breeds. A survey of 356 breeders conducted by the health committee of the Irish Setter Club of America found the average life span of Irish Setters to be 11.1 years.

With a minimum of specialized care, the Irish Setter can live a full life, once past the perils of puppyhood.

References

1. Romatowski, J. "A Uveodermatological Syndrome in the Akita Dog," *JAAHA;* 1985: 21:6, 777-780; 7 ref.
2. Griffin, C., Kowchka, K., McDonald, J.: Current Veterinary Dermatology, the Science and Art of Therapy. Mosby Yearbook, St. Louis, MO. 1993: 101, 218, 239, 266.
3. Hodgman, S.F.G., et al, "Progressive Retinal Atrophy in Dogs I: Disease in Irish Setters (Red)," *Vet. Rec.*; 1949: 6l:185-190.
4. Magnusson, H. "About Retinitis Pigmentosa and Consanguinity in Dogs," *Arch. Vergh. Ophthal.*; 1911: 2:147-163.
5. James A. Baker Institute for Animal Health. Personal Communication, *American Kennel Club Gazette*; September, 1993: 34.
6. Magrane, W.G. *Canine Ophthalmology*. 3rd ed. (Lea & Febiger, Philadelphia, Pa., 1977).
7. Kirk, R.W. and Bistner, S.I. *Handbook of Veterinary Procedures and Emergency Treatment: Hereditary Defects of Dogs.* Table 124, 1975: 661.
8. Brinkhous, K.M. and Graham, J.B. "Hemophilia in the Female Dog," *Science III*; 1948: 723-724.
9. Hutt, F.B., et al, "Sex-linked Hemophilia in Dogs," *J. Hered.;* 1948: 39:3-9.
10. Wigh, G.T. "Granulocytopathy in Irish Setters," *Svensk-Veterinartidning*; 1990: 42:5, 221-222. 2 ref.
11. Patterson, D.F., et al, "Hereditary Cardiovascular Malfunctions of the Dog: Birth Defects," Original article series V, XV, Card. Syst., National Foundation, 1972: 100-174.

12. Mulvihill, J.J. and Priester, W.A. "Congenital Heart Disease in Dogs, Epidemiological Similarities to Man," *Teratology;* 1973: 7: 73-78.

13. Patterson, D.F. "Epidemiologic and Genetic Studies of Congenital Heart Disease in the Dog," *Circ. Res.;* 1968: 23: 171-202.

14. Patterson, D.F. "Canine Congenital Heart Disease, Epidemiological Hypotheses," *J. Sm. Anim. Prac.*; 1971: 12: 263-287.

15. Naylor, R.J. "Persistent Aortic Arches," *JAVMA*; 1957: 130:283-284.

16. Kern, Maryanne, DVM, "Diseases of the Esophagus," *The American Kennel Club Gazette*; January, 1993.

17. Wentink, G.H., et al, "Myopathy with a Possible Recessive X-Linked Inheritance in a Litter of Irish Setters," *Vet. Path.;* 1972: 9: 328-349.

18. Palmer, A.C., et al, "Hereditary Quadriplegia and Amblyopia in the Irish Setter," *J. Sm. Anim. Prac.;* 1973: 14: 343-352.

19. *JAVMA*; May 1, 1990: Vol. 196, #9.

20. Ackerman, Lowell, DVM, "Allergic Skin Diseases," *American Kennel Club Gazette;* September, 1990.

21. Brignac, Michele M. "Congenital and Breed Associated Skin Diseases in the Dog and Cat," *KalKan Forum;* December 1989: 9-16.

22. Batt, R.M., Carter, M.W., and McLean, L. "Wheat-Sensitive Enteropathy in Irish Setter Dogs: Possible Age-Related Brush Border Abnormalities," *Research in Veterinary Science*; 1985: 39: 1, 80-83. 11 ref.

23. Gray, A. "Trimethoprim-Sulphonamide Hypersensitivity in Dogs," *Veterinary Record;* 1990: 127; 23, 579-580.

24. Bell, Jerold S. DVM: "Sex Related Genetic Disorders: Did Mama Cause Them?" *American Kennel Club Gazette*, Feb. 1994; 76.

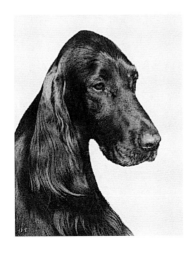

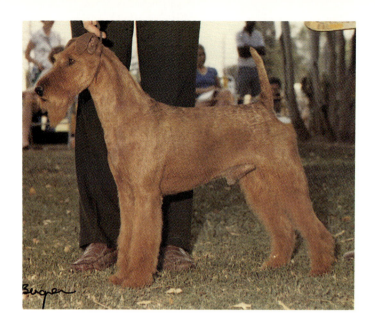

IRISH TERRIER

ORIGIN AND HISTORY

The Irish Terrier is one of the older terrier breeds. Its solid red coat and long, sleek body distinguish it from other terriers. The breed's high intelligence and even temperament have made it a favorite of both young and old.

DESCRIPTION

Irish Terriers are excellent family dogs. They are small enough to adapt to any environment, but large enough to be convincing watch dogs. They are lively and full of fun but are not "yappy" and remain calm indoors. They are extremely affectionate and gravitate to children. Male Irish Terriers are naturally aggressive to other males of any breed, so it is not advisable to keep two males as house pets.

THE SHOW RING

Irish Terriers must be a solid color, ranging from red wheaten to dark red. Occasionally a puppy is whelped with a pink nose or a white toenail, but these disappear in a few weeks. A small white patch on the chest is acceptable.

There are no disqualifying breed faults.

BREEDING AND WHELPING

The Irish Terrier bitch whelps easily and is usually an excellent mother. Size of the litter ranges from four to eight. Live litters of nine have been seen, all of which reached a healthy maturity. Irish Terrier puppies weigh approximately 8 ounces at birth.

GROWTH

Dewclaws should be removed and tails docked by the fourth day after birth. Tails should be docked carefully, because the appearance of many Irish Terriers has been spoiled by a too-short tail. A good general rule is to remove 1/4 of the tail. An imaginary line drawn from the top of the skull to the tip of the cut tail should be horizontal. It is better to leave the tail too long than too short, as it can always be shortened later.

Maintaining good ear carriage is probably the biggest problem in this breed. Novice owners of Irish Terrier puppies should be encouraged to keep their dogs' ears pasted to proper carriage. The tip of the ear should come to the outer corner of the eye. The problem ear should be pasted at the age of 3 months and should remain pasted until 1 year, or until the ear holds proper carriage without support. A good surgical glue should be used.

DENTITION

Bad bites are infrequent in this breed. A slight overbite will often correct itself by 7 or 8 months.

RECOGNIZED PROBLEMS

Irish Terriers are one of the 14 breeds having a predilection to **cystine stones**, occurring only in male dogs.[1,2]

Tubular transport dysfunction in Irish Terriers is discussed in a Cornell study of canine hereditary nephropathies.[3]

Inherited forms of **muscular dystrophy** linked to the "X" chromosome are being studied and have been identified in the Irish Terrier.[4]

A German study has described **hereditary myopathy** in Irish Terriers with information on symptoms, prognosis and treatment.[5]

Irish Terriers with heavier coats are subject to hot spots in warm weather. Daily combing and brushing will keep them clean and odor-free. Frequent bathing is not recommended. Shedding is minimal if the coat is cared for properly. Coats should be plucked to keep the harsh texture and good color, never clipped or scissored. Many people who are allergic to other dogs are not allergic to Irish Terriers.

BEHAVIOR

The Irish Terrier is a reckless and bold daredevil. He is apt to quarrel with other dogs, but is a gentle companion to his owners. He needs a lot of exercise if he is to be a satisfactory house dog.

OLD AGE

This adaptable breed has a life expectancy of 12 to 15 years. No ailments are unique to Irish Terriers in their old age.

References
1. Bovee, K.C. and Segal, S. "Canine Cystinuria and Cystine Calculi: The Newer Knowledge About Dogs," *Proceedings of the 21st Gaines Veterinary Symposium*; 1971.
2. Kirk, R.W. *Current Veterinary Therapy VII: Catalog of Genetic Disorders of Dogs.* (W.B. Saunders, Philadelphia, Pa., 1980) 96.
3. Picut, C.A. and Lewis, R.M. "Comparative pathology of Canine Hereditary Nephropathies: An Interpretive Review," *Vet. Res. Comm.*; 1987: 11:6, 561-581; 91 ref.
4. Veterinary News, *The American Kennel Club Gazette*; October, 1991.
5. Bichsel, P. "Neuromuscular Diseases of Young Dogs," Jahresversammlung. Schweizerische Vereinigung fur Kleintiermedizin. 2-4. Juni 1988: Bazel 1988, 43-50. Zool. Bern, Switzerland; c/o H.Heinimann, Schweis. Serum und Impfinstitut, Postfach 2707.

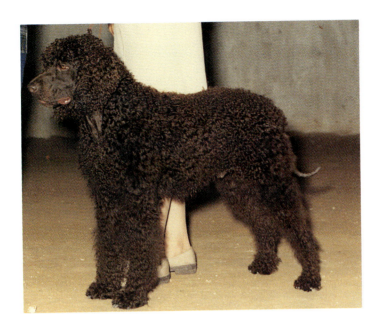

IRISH WATER SPANIEL

ORIGIN AND HISTORY

The Irish Water Spaniel originated in the Iberian peninsula. Early in the 19th century, Mr. Justin McCarthy began recording this breed's history.

DESCRIPTION

The Irish Water Spaniel is a powerful swimmer whose coat offers protection from the coldest water. Its coat and size tend to slow it in briar and thicket. Largest of the spaniels, the Irish Water Spaniel has a brown, harsh, curly coat, a topknot, and a tapered tail which has short and smooth hair with no feathering except for a 3-inch clump of curls at its root. The face has smooth, short hair with the topknot growing to a widow's peak and falling to or over the eyes. There is a short beard and sideburns. Some lines of the breed have a distinctive coat pattern. The longer, curly hairs of the coat end abruptly in a line that runs lengthwise down the middle of the hind leg. The front of the neck may have short, smooth, silky hair in a pattern similar to that of a shaved poodle.

THE SHOW RING

Dogs and bitches vary little in weight. The Standard prefers dogs standing 22 to 24 inches at the shoulder and weighing 55 to 65 pounds; bitches should be 21 to 23 inches measured at the highest point of the shoulder and weigh 45 to 58 pounds. Solid liver is the only color. White hair or markings are objectionable. You should keep in mind the importance of the various features, mentioned in the Breed standard, toward the basic original purpose of the breed. A stable temperament is essential in a hunting dog. **There are no disqualifying faults.**

BREEDING AND WHELPING

Few bitches need a **cesarean section**. The eyes of the Water Spaniel often appear light green in early puppyhood but darken to hazel as the puppies mature. White on the chest is undesirable. Many puppies are born with white on the chest or on a couple of toes. The white disappears in about 6 to 8 weeks and if the few remaining white hairs are pulled out, they do not reappear.

GROWTH

The longer hair of the topknot usually does not appear until the puppies are 4 to 5 months old. Few puppies have a heavy, mature topknot before 10 months.

The puppies retrieve early. Some retrieve soft toys at 6 weeks old. Some swim at approximately 8 weeks, but others take much longer to become accustomed to water.

RECOGNIZED PROBLEMS

The Irish Water Spaniel is one of the most trouble-free of all breeds. They have no eye problems. **Hip dysplasia** is seen occasionally. **Malocclusion** is seen, but healthy teeth are a strong point in the breed. Irish Water Spaniels can have a congenital **hypotrichosis** which is associated with abnormal teeth.[1]

BEHAVIOR

The Irish Water Spaniel is cheerful, obedient and intelligent. He is difficult to keep in the house because of his oily coat and his proclivity for rolling in the grass to keep his coat less greasy. He is an excellent water retriever.

OLD AGE

Life expectancy is the average for a breed of this size.

References
1. Brignac, Michele M. "Congenital and Breed Associated Skin Disease in the Dog and Cat," *KalKan Forum*; December, 1989: 9-16.

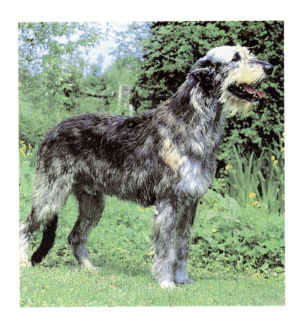

IRISH WOLFHOUND

ORIGIN AND HISTORY

The Irish Wolfhound is the tallest and rangiest of dogs. The breed is renowned for gentleness. Although Irish Wolfhounds were formerly used to hunt deer, wolf and boar, their activities in this field are now restricted by the reduction in the number of game, by game laws and by increasing opposition to the killing of wild animals.

DESCRIPTION

Irish Wolfhounds growl or bark in unusual situations and can thus deter burglars, but they are not aggressive guard dogs. They are very intelligent and do well in obedience work. Although they are sighthounds, a few have qualified in tracking.

THE SHOW RING

Disqualifications are not mentioned in the Irish Wolfhound Standard. Dogs more than 18 months old are penalized if they are less than 32 inches high or weigh less than 120 pounds. Bitches less than 30 inches high and weighing less than 105 pounds are also penalized. Faults listed in the Standard include too light or heavy a head, too highly arched frontal bone; large ears and those hanging flat to the face; short neck, full dewlap; too narrow or too broad a chest; sunken or hollow or quite-straight back; bent forelegs; overbent fetlocks; twisted feet, spreading toes; too curly a tail; weak hindquarters and a general want of muscle; too short in body; lips or nose that are liver colored or lacking pigmentation.

BREEDING AND WHELPING

Irish Wolfhound bitches generally show estrus for the first time at 14 to 18 months old and thereafter every 6 to 9 months. Some do not show estrus until 2 years old. The Irish Wolfhound Club of America (IWCA) Guidelines state that "A bitch should be bred only from the age of 2 to 7 years. She should not be bred if the result would be a litter more than once every 12 months."

In a study of one breeder's experience of 49 litters, 24 consisted of one puppy and 25 of multiple births of two to 12 puppies. The average number of puppies in multiple-birth litters was 6.6 puppies. The average of all litters was 3.9 puppies.

The average weight of newborn puppies is 1.5 pounds for dogs and 1.3 pounds for bitches. Puppies are usually dark at birth, and some have white markings. As they grow older, their color may become gray, brindle, wheaten, fawn, red, black or any variation. All are acceptable. Dewclaws should be removed at 3 days.

Irish Wolfhound puppies' food requirements do not differ from other breeds, except in quantity. The IWCA recommends that they be fed four or five times a day until they are a year old, then twice a day. For a puppy 3 months old, it advises 2 ½ to 3 pounds of meat and 4 to 6 cups of kibbled dog food or meal daily.

For a year-old pup, the IWCA recommendation is 2 pounds of meat a day, mixed with 5 to 6 cups of kibble. Less is recommended for older dogs. Some breeders recommend that, after weaning, a commercial dog food be fed, without any additives, three times a day. Although adult dogs may be fed only one large portion a day, three feedings a day serve as a precaution against bloat. Water should be available.

GROWTH

Since Irish Wolfhounds grow so rapidly, judicious exercise is of the utmost importance. Confinement in cages affects puppies physically, mentally and temperamentally. Free running is the best exercise for this breed. The IWCA recommends that puppies not be sold until they are 12 weeks old.

Irish Wolfhounds are close to their maximum height at 1 year, but do not fully mature until 3 or 4 years old.

RECOGNIZED PROBLEMS

Irish Wolfhounds are subject to **tail injury** and **elbow hygroma**. Care must be exercised that the hound is not praised or otherwise excited when his wagging tail could encounter a hard object. If the tip does not bleed, ordinary care plus bandaging may result in healing. If the dog pulls the bandage off, replace it with a bandage padded at the tip of the tail to the top. Apply the tape loosely and press it against the tail so circulation is not impeded. Replace the bandage every five days.

Medication may be a problem with Wolfhounds. Dosages of anesthesia and worm medicine should not be determined strictly according to weight. Due to the low percentage of body fat, this breed is very sensitive to barbiturate anesthetics. Anesthetics should be given slowly, just to effect rather than by body weight.

Rhinitis syndrome[1] appears often in Irish Wolfhounds puppies. It is evident as watery nasal discharge which may progress into a chronic condition. **Hip dysplasia** and **metabolic bone diseases** including **osteochondritis dessicans** occur in this, as in all giant breeds. OFA reports **elbow dysplasia** in Irish Wolfhounds.[2] Irish Wolfhound breeders have reported incidences of **heart disease, osteosarcoma, progressive retinal atrophy** and possibly **cataracts**.[3]

BEHAVIOR

His patient, thoughtful, intelligent character makes him an ideal companion dog, but he needs a large exercise area. He is good with children but reserved with strangers.

OLD AGE

The life span of Irish Wolfhounds, like that of all large dogs, is relatively short. In one study, average ages of death of 240 hounds which survived to 1 year were 5.0 years for dogs and 6.6 years for bitches.

The absence of sufficient data precludes writing authoritatively about causes of death in Irish Wolfhounds. Some of the main causes appear to be bloat, cancer and diseases of the heart and intestinal organs.

References

1. Wilkinson, G.T. "Some Observations on the Irish Wolfhound Rhinitis Syndrome," *J. Sm. Anim. Prac.*; 1969: 10: 5-8.
2. Bodner, Elizabeth, DVM, "Genetic Status Symbols," *The American Kennel Club Gazette*; Sept. 1992.
3. Irish Wolfhound Column. *The American Kennel Club Gazette*; June, 1993.

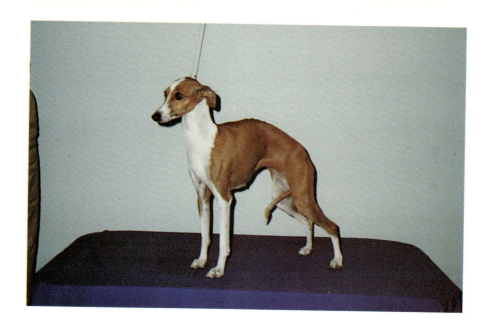

ITALIAN GREYHOUND

ORIGIN AND HISTORY

The elegant Italian Greyhound was adored by ladies 2000 years ago. The breed was undoubtedly bred by selection from the Greyhound. The dog was a favorite of Frederick the Great and entered English history in the 17th century.

DESCRIPTION

Italian Greyhounds are gentle, playful, loving companions. They generally prefer their own human family and are slow to befriend strangers. However, a person once accepted as a friend is seldom forgotten. Dogs that snap or bite should not be bred. Italian Greyhounds have for centuries been companions of both royalty and commoners. They are most content in constant contact with human beings, and they are excellent travelers.

THE SHOW RING

The average adult weight is 7 to 10 pounds, depending on bone size and structure; ideally 13 to 15 inches high at the withers.

Most colors and markings are acceptable, although **a dog with tan markings normally found on black and tan dogs of other breeds is disqualified, as is a dog with brindle**

314

markings. All shades of fawn, red, blue, black and piebald (predominantly white with patch markings of one other color) may be found in one litter. The coat of the Italian Greyhound is thin, smooth, fine and glossy.

BREEDING AND WHELPING

Bitches sometimes do not begin estrus until 18 months old; some do not begin until 2 years old. Once estrus begins, seasons adhere to the usual six-month pattern. Most bitches ovulate and conceive between the 9th and 14th day of estrus. The average litter is three to four pups; however, litters of six are not unusual. The Italian Greyhound bitch has few problems whelping, although a few experience uterine inertia. The puppies are surprisingly active at birth. Their average weight is 3 to 7 ounces. This weight usually doubles the first week of life. The puppies gain an average of 1 to 2 ounces a day, weighing about three pounds at 6 weeks. Dewclaws should be removed between 2 and 5 days old. They generally occur only on the forelegs.

Puppies should be checked for **cleft palate**. **Esophageal achalasia** and **persistent right aortic arch** may be found at 5 to 6 weeks.[1] The mode of inheritance of these conditions is thought to be autosomal recessive. The percentage of occurrence is small.

GROWTH

Full skeletal height is usually reached between 9 months and 1 year of age. Italian Greyhounds should measure 13 to 15 inches at the withers. The brisket continues to deepen until 18 months old. The skull and jaw also may continue to grow until the dog is 18 months old. Full maturity of the skeleton and musculature is reached between 18 months and 2 years.

The ear carriage from birth to 8 weeks is haphazard, generally flop or button. At 6 to 8 weeks old, the dog begins to hold the ears in the correct fold and, when alert, to carry them at right angles to the head. During teething the ears sometimes fly or stand erect. The ears should be correct when teething is finished. On the adult dog, an erect or button ear is a fault.

DENTITION

Milk teeth must sometimes be pulled to make room for the permanent canine teeth. Crooked incisors and canine teeth that protrude are becoming a problem in the breed. Badly under or overshot bites are faults in adult dogs. A scissors bite is preferred.

RECOGNIZED PROBLEMS

Male Italian Greyhounds are often 9 months to 1 year old before testicles are secured in the scrotum. However, this is not the norm. **Monorchidism** does occur but is not considered a major problem in the breed. Dilute color alopecia, once called **Blue Doberman syndrome** and sometimes called **color mutant alopecia** is found in the Italian Greyhound. It is characterized by partial alopecia, dry, lusterless skin, scaliness and papules. It can occur in any dog of dilute color. **Epilepsy** or epileptic-like convulsions are becoming a problem in the breed. The mode of inheritance has not been established. The **convulsions** occur between birth and 3 years of age and can be controlled with medication. Dogs that have had convulsions should not be bred.

Leg fractures during the dog's first two years of life can be a problem. Italian Greyhounds have little fear of jumping from any height and have been known to scale a wire fence like a monkey. Most fractures in the breed involve the distal radius and ulna. Setting fractures with a permanent pin or by plating have been the most successful methods. Because of the small diameter of the radius, obtaining the proper-size pin or plate is difficult. Getting the bones to mend correctly can be difficult.

Broken tails are not unusual because the tail is long and thin. These can be set with a spiral wrapping of Dericel cloth or paper tape. Wrap clockwise and counterclockwise, being careful not to wrap too tightly. A slight crook in a mended tail is not a fault. Ring tails and gay tails are faults. Some Italian Greyhounds have **receding gums,** with subsequent loss of the upper incisors by 5 years of age. Daily massage of the gums with peroxide solution and regular cleaning of teeth are recommended. Gas anesthesia is recommended for Italian Greyhounds, because they are sensitive to barbiturate anesthetics. Flea collars may cause an **allergic reaction** and should not be used on this breed.

BEHAVIOR

The "I.G." is mild and calm. He is an excellent companion in a serene household. He does not care for noise and activity. His trembling frequently signals emotion rather than fear or cold. A soothing pat from his owner, to whom he is strongly attached, assures him.

OLD AGE

Age does not change Italian Greyhounds' beautifully sculptured figures. Their eyes remain bright and they retain their spritely, fancy gait. The average life expectancy is approximately 15 years.

References
1. Erickson, F., et al "Congenital Defects in Dogs, A Special Reference for Practitioners," Ralston Purina Co. (reprint from *Canine Practice*, Vet. Prac. Publ. Co.) 1978.

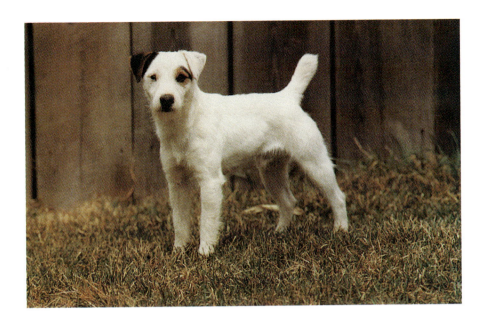

JACK RUSSELL TERRIER

ORIGIN AND HISTORY

This breed was developed in England in the last century by a clergyman, Reverend John Russell. It is not recognized by any all-breed canine organization, which is exactly what Jack Russell Terrier fanciers want.

The Jack Russell Terrier Club has developed a standard that keeps the breed pure and prohibits any further introduction of other breeds.

DESCRIPTION

The Jack Russell Terrier is similar to the Fox Terrier, with shorter legs, and is about 10 inches high. He has a narrow chest with legs set not too wide apart, giving an athletic appearance, ears folded down and carried wide, and dark, deep-set eyes. His coat may be smooth, broken or rough. He is predominantly white with tan, brown or black markings on his muzzle and body.

BREEDING AND WHELPING

The first estrus in the Jack Russell Terrier is often a "silent season" at 6 or 7 months. Most bitches then cycle on a 6-month schedule, although there are a few who have only one estrus a year. The gestation period is normal, 59 to 63 days, and a litter of 4 to 6 whelps is average. Some few are born with umbilical hernias.

Occasionally a brindle color puppy is born but these are not used in an ethical breeding program.

DENTITION

Missing pre-molars are a problem in some strains and over and undershot mouths are seen. Breeders report a few parrot mouths.

RECOGNIZED PROBLEMS

Hereditary **ataxia** has been reported in this breed.[1]

The breed is listed as one where deafness is found.[2] **Legg-Perthes** disease and **luxating patellas** are concerns of the National Breed Club.

BEHAVIOR

The Jack Russell Terrier is a "bounce-back" breed, a small breed that thinks big. He is obedient, courageous, devoted and has a merry disposition. They are active and require a secure environment as they consider anything with hair as fair game. It is said, "where the fox can go, so must the terrier."

References
1. Ettinger, S.J. *Textbook of Veterinary Internal Medicine: Diseases of the Dog and Cat.* (W.B. Saunders Co., Philadelphia, PA 1989) 660.
2. Strain, G.M. "Deafness in Dogs and Cats," *Proc. 10th ACVIM Forum; May, 1992.*

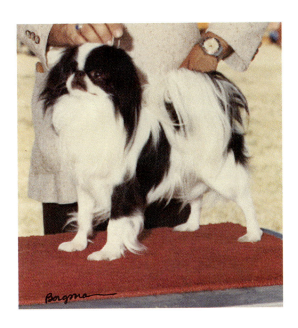

JAPANESE CHIN

ORIGIN AND HISTORY

The Japanese Spaniel, or Japanese Chin, originated in China centuries ago. It is reported that one of the Chinese emperors gave a pair to an emperor of Japan. They were owned only by the nobility and frequently were used as gifts of esteem to diplomats and foreigners who had rendered outstanding service to Japan. In August of 1977 the Japanese Spaniel became known officially by the American Kennel Club as the Japanese Chin.

DESCRIPTION

The Japanese Chin is a lively little dog with dainty appearance, smart, compact carriage and profuse coat. These dogs should be essentially stylish in movement, lifting the feet high when in action, carrying the tail (which is heavily feathered, proudly curved or plumed) over the back.[1]

THE SHOW RING

The majority of dogs are black and white, although there are whites with lemon and red markings, including all shades from pale lemon to deep red as well as brindle. The nose color must be black except in the red and white, where it can be self-colored. Eyes should be dark in

319

all colors. **In black and whites, a nose any color other than black is a disqualification.** Dewclaws may be removed, but removal is not required by the Standard.[2]

The smaller Japanese Chins are preferred if type and quality are maintained.

When divided by weight, classes should be under and over 7 pounds.

BREEDING AND WHELPING

Litters average three to five depending on the size of the bitch. Puppies should weigh 6 to 8 ounces at birth. **Cesarean section** is sometimes necessary in the smaller bitches and in those that have the preferred large head.

RECOGNIZED PROBLEMS

Monorchidism or **cryptorchidism** are common problems.

Achondroplasia is an incompletely dominant autosomal trait of this breed. It causes **shortened limbs**, **metaphyseal flaring**, **depressed nasal bridge** and **shortened maxilla**. Often **wedge or hemivertebrae** occur and **elbow luxations** and **medial patellar luxations** can occur secondary to joint laxity.[3]

BEHAVIOR

The Chin is the ideal companion dog. He is charming, graceful, intelligent, fun-loving and clean. He is devoted to his family and can be reserved with strangers.

OLD AGE

Most Japanese Chins live from 12 to 14 years of age.

Reference
1. *The Complete Dog Book*, The American Kennel Club. 18th edition, 1992.
2. *The Complete Dog Book,* The American Kennel Club. (Howell Book House, New York, NY., 18th ed. 1992); 443-445.
3. Ettinger, S.J. *Textbook of Veterinary Internal Medicine*. (W.B. Saunders Co. Philadelphia, PA, 1989); 2383.

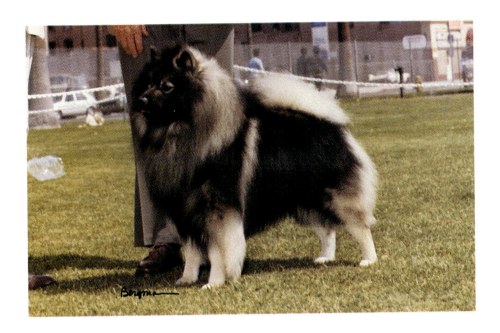

KEESHOND

ORIGIN AND HISTORY

The Keeshond (plural, Keeshonden), national dog of Holland, undoubtedly finds its origin in the Arctic or Subarctic sled dogs, yet as a "barge" dog has been called upon to serve as more of a companion-watch dog than a puller of sleds. Pictured in drawings over 200 years old, and in early paintings by Jan Steen, the dog has changed little through the years. Interest in the breed in the 1920s found scattered representation amazingly uniform and the dogs seen today are indistinguishable from early specimens.

DESCRIPTION

Keeshonden have sound, even temperaments and are very intelligent. They are exceptionally good with children and have lively, happy dispositions, but they can be stubborn at times. The breed is easily trained and does well in obedience. Keeshonden are clean and carry no doggy odor. They have acute hearing and are excellent watchdogs. The breed gives warning by barking, but is not aggressive. They are family dogs and should live in houses, never exclusively outside. If left on their own outside, Keeshonden sometimes bark excessively. Without human companionship they are miserable and bored.

Keeshonden reach full height by 9 to 10 months, but continue to mature until 2 or 3 years. At birth, puppies are predominantly black. Their coats are short and smooth. Puppies may have a little white on the feet and chest. The white on the feet usually disappears by 8 weeks. The white on the chest sometimes remains. Shoulder markings will be discernible at birth or within a couple of days.

Between birth and 8 months, several changes in coat color and texture occur. At 8 weeks, a puppy's coat is quite profuse, with a thick pale grey or cream undercoat and black-tipped outer hairs. Their legs have lightened to gray or cream. Any dark gray markings on the feet usually disappear within 5 months. Heavy black markings on the feet, however, usually do not completely disappear. Removal of dewclaws is recommended but not required.

THE SHOW RING

The ideal height, measured to the withers, is 18 inches for dogs and 17 inches for bitches. **There are no disqualifications for this breed.** Faults are: pronounced white markings, black stockings more than halfway down the foreleg (penciling excepted); and a white foot or feet. Very serious faults are entirely black or white or any solid color and any pronounced deviation from the color as described.

BREEDING AND WHELPING

Keeshond bitches normally begin estrus at 8 months to 1 year old, but occasionally a bitch does not begin until 18 months. An interval of 7 or 8 months between cycles is usual. Bitches are usually ready for breeding between the 11th and 15th days after first showing color, but bitches with prolonged estrous flow have conceived from breedings as late as the 18th day. They usually whelp between the 60th and 64th day, but litters have been whelped as late as the 70th day without problems. Keeshond bitches rarely require **cesarean section**.

Keeshond bitches carry their puppies without problems, provided they have adequate exercise and are not allowed to gain too much weight. Posterior presentations are common but rarely create problems. Keeshond bitches are good mothers and usually have adequate milk. The average size of a litter is five to seven puppies, although litters of 10 to 11 or two to three are not rare.

GROWTH

Well groomed, Keeshonden shed little hair. At 10 to 12 months, Keeshonden completely shed their undercoats. Daily grooming brushes out the undercoat.

Without daily grooming, the coat falls out in large tufts and the skin flakes. Often the owners assume that the loss of coat is due to a skin disorder. If hair becomes matted against the skin, the dog scratches severely and hot spots or a skin infection can result. Dogs usually shed

322

12 months after birth; bitches shed after each estrus. Bitches also shed extensively for 6 or 7 weeks after whelping. Keeshond puppies weigh 8 to 12 ounces at birth.

DENTITION

The Keeshond's teeth should meet in a scissors bite. Undershot and overshot mouths are rare, but dogs sometimes lack premolars.

RECOGNIZED PROBLEMS

The breed has **hip dysplasia**, but it has not been as serious a problem as it is in some of the large breeds. The OFA reported that hip dysplasia had a 48.7% decrease in Keeshonden from 1974 to 1984.[1] Dogs should be x-rayed before breeding. **Heart problems** are rare but not unknown. **Thyroid imbalance** is often responsible for a dull, dry, broken coat, with bare patches and dark skin around the shoulders and on the rump. **Growth-hormone-responsive dermatosis** and **castration-responsive dermatosis** have been described in the Keeshond.[2]

Recently, a study of congenital heart disease in the dog uncovered a syndrome consisting of **conus septal defects**,[3] including **tetralogy of Fallot** that occurred with unusually high frequency in the Keeshond. In the study 61 percent of a family of dogs had this defect.[4,5] Most breeders never encounter this syndrome.

Epilepsy is common in the breed,[6,7,8,9,10] usually appearing as a major problem at about 3 years of age. Some researchers report that an EEG may detect the condition at an earlier age; however, Margaret Wallace of the Department of Genetics, Cambridge University, reports that her work with 321 Keeshonden and 108 of their close ancestors did not support any diagnostic value from EEG readings. New findings indicate that such seizures are comparatively rare in the breed and they occur four times more often in dogs than in bitches. The dark pigment of **skin tumors** in Keeshonden may predispose the tumors to **melanoma** formation, as it does in many dark-pigmented animals. **Renal cortical hypoplasia** has been seen in Keeshonden. Signs: **polydipsia, polyuria, vomiting, convulsions, anemia** and **weakness**. First signs appeared at 10 to 13 weeks of age.[11] **Aberrant cilia** are found in this breed.

Keeshonden seem relatively free from problems encountered in many breeds, although growths and tumors in aging Keeshonden, **sebaceous cysts, rare umbilical hernias** and **birth defects** have been encountered. Fight wounds and injuries in kennel dogs, **congestive heart failure** in older dogs, generalized seasonal **allergic rashes** due to pollen, dust, fleas, **Addison's disease, hypothyroidism** and reproductive problems such as **postparturient metritis** and **pyometra** occur. Obesity is also a problem. Keeshonden tolerate all modern anesthetics and do not exhibit a high rate of adverse reactions to drugs. Keeshonden rarely have anal-sac problems.

BEHAVIOR

The "Kees" makes an excellent companion and watch dog. He is intelligent and easy to train. He is lovable, vivacious and always on the alert.

OLD AGE

The Keeshond matures slowly and stays active until 12 years old, if not allowed to become overweight. After 12 years, Keeshonden slow down and sleep more. Most live to 14 or 15 years. Older bitches can develop **mammary neoplasia** and pyometra, but if spayed at an early age, they have the same life expectancy as dogs. Bitches kept as pets should be spayed early in life.

References

1. Corley, E.A. and Hogan, P.M. "Trends in Hip Dysplasia Control: Analysis of Radiographs Submitted to the Orthopedic Foundation for Animals, 1974 to 1984," *JAVMA;* 1985: 187:8, 805-809; 8 ref.
2. Griffin, C., Kwochka, K., and McDonald, J. *Current Veterinary Dermatology: the Science and Art of Therapy*, Mosby Yearbook, St. Louis, MO.; 1993: 289, 299.
3. Kirk, R.W. and Bistner, S.I. *Handbook of Veterinary Procedures and Emergency Treatment: Hereditary Defects in Dogs.* 1981: Table 19, 824.
4. Patterson, et al, *Am. J. Cardiology* ; 1974: 34:187-205.
5. Mulvihill, J.J. and Priester, W.A. "Congenital Heart Disease in Dogs: Epidemiologic Similarities to Man," *Teratology;* 1973: 7:73-79.
6. Kirk, R.W. and Bistner, S.I. *Handbook of Veterinary Procedures and Emergency Treatment: Hereditary Defects of Dogs.* 1975: Table:24, 661.
7. Burns, M. and Frasier, M.N. *Genetics of the Dog*, Oliver and Body, London, England 1966.
8. Croft, P.G. and Stockman, M.J.R. "Inherited Defects in Dogs," *Vet. Rec*; 1963: 76:260-261.
9. Croft, P.G. "The Use of the Electro-Encephalogram in the Detection of Epilepsy as a Hereditary Condition in the Dog," *Vet. Rec.*; 1968: 82:712-713.
10. Wallace, M.E. "Keeshond: A Gentle Study of Epilepsy and EEG Readings," *J. Sm. Anim. Prac.*; 1975: 16:1-10.
11. Kloper, U., et al: "Renal Cortical Hypoplasia in a Keeshond Litter," *VM/SAC;* 1975: 1081-1083.

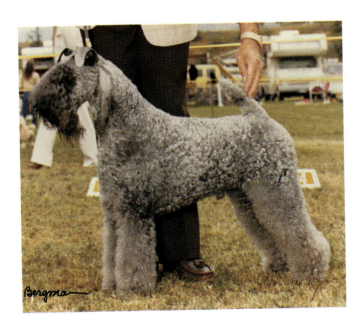

KERRY BLUE TERRIER

ORIGIN AND HISTORY

The Kerry Blue Terrier was developed in County Kerry, Ireland. It is probably a cross between a now-extinct herding dog and the Irish Wolfhound. It has been recognized as a pure-bred breed for over 100 years.

These dogs are large, robust trailers, and have been put to many uses, including retrieving, cattle herding, and in England, police work.

DESCRIPTION

The Kerry Blue does not like other dogs, but loves people.

They are very outgoing animals.

A veterinarian should never suggest a Kerry for anyone who plans to let his dog run loose. Most dogs are fighters, as well as some bitches. They will not get along with the neighboring dogs, which can be a problem.

The Kerry coat can begin to change color at any age. Those that start very early may turn too light a shade.

They may be any color of blue from light to dark; the very light ones are called silvers.

THE SHOW RING

There are two disqualifications in the breed: solid black and dewclaws on the hind legs.

There is no disqualification on height: the ideal, however, is between 18 and 19 1/2 inches for a dog, and 17 1/2 to 19 inches for a bitch.

BREEDING AND WHELPING

Kerry Blue Terrier puppies rarely have a full 63-day gestation, 60 to 61 days being their norm.

All puppies should be born black. They may have some white on chest, feet, and a few white hairs on the belly. If there is too much white on the chest, it may not grow out. If very small, it will disappear or at least will not show after the puppy changes color (black to blue). If a puppy is born brown with a pink nose, it should be euthanized because its coordination will be bad and its color very poor. This coloration should not be confused with a slight brown cast to its coat at birth.

Whelping problems are not common in the breed. Puppies will weigh 8 to 12 ounces at birth. Tails and dewclaws are removed at 3 days by most veterinarians if the puppies are strong. Years ago there were instances of dewclaws on all four feet, but this has not been seen recently. If one does occur it should be removed. Tails should be left fairly long so the puppy is in balance when mature. The tail should be even with the top of the head at maturity. If the tail is short and thick, more should remain than if it is long and skinny. Everyone has his own strong opinion on tail length.

A Publication of the Kerry Blue Club of America gives explicit instructions for setting Kerry ears (See page 330).

RECOGNIZED PROBLEMS

Hair follicle tumors are a problem in the breed.[1]

Spiculosis,[2] also called "Hard Hairs," "Rose Thorns," "Bristles," or "Spikes" is widespread in the breed, perhaps more prevalent in some lines than in others. The spicules are usually more numerous in dogs than in bitches, and they appear most numerous as the males reach sexual maturity, then begin to diminish. Those with somewhat coarser coats seem slightly more prone to having them than those whose coats are truly soft. The normal Kerry Blue hair coat is, as described in the standard, "soft, dense, and wavy." Thus, when brushing and combing it is easy to feel these stiff bristles. They are most frequently around the elbows and hocks; often in the feet between the toes; sometimes in the eyebrows, on the neck, sides, on the tail, etc. They are usually removable by hand...just pull out with fingers. But some are more deeply embedded, or the follicle "root" is rounded and more difficult to remove and hemostats are necessary...sometimes even needlenose pliers. If the spicule "root" remains undiscovered and grows, an incision and surgical removal become necessary.

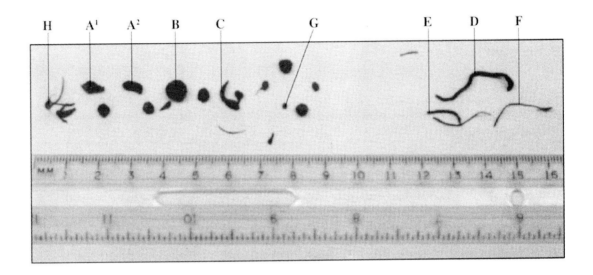

In the photo, the bristles marked H and the slim one below C and above D are the usual size and shape.

In the photo, A1 and A2 are pieces of the same long, thick spicule that was located near the tendon of the hock of a 12-month-old intact male. An incision had to be made to remove it, and there were some smaller soft pieces included. A couple of stitches were needed to close the incision.

In the photo, B, the largest round follicle "ball" had to be removed surgically from over the ribs of the same male dog. The external spike had been pulled off and broken, and this large ball was impossible to remove without opening the skin.

In the photo, C was located on the front of the foreleg and was removed intact with hemostats. The pointed end was external, and the rounded base was under the skin.

In the photo, D is an apparent cluster of hairs, solidified into one 2.3 cm rigid bristle that was deep inside the ear of a 3-year-old Kerry bitch. E shows two other bristles removed from the same ear, and F was in the other ear.

Ears are normally plucked so that wax and dirt don't build up, and this bitch had scrupulously clean ears; yet she whimpered when the side of her head was touched. She was tranquilized, and the otoscope revealed this unusually large spicule deep in the canal, which was

327

removed intact.

The male from which the large ball-ended spicules were extracted had an incredibly large number of them. He was anesthetized for dentistry and was carefully gone over by a surgical tech, who was able to find and remove 100+ spicules from every part of his body except for the underbelly and inner thighs. His owner had been treating him for a couple of months prior to this with a drawing salve called "Prid's Salve." She then stood the dog in a tub of warm water containing a heavy dilution of Epsom Salts. After he had soaked a while, she would use a small rubber brush and scrub up and down his legs to the elbows and above the stifle, and rub around the feet and toes. When she finished the tub would contain black "sand" made up of tiny round follicles and spicules of every length that she had rolled out with the brush. The smallest round follicle, G, is the size that she could brush out this way.

If the hairs don't readily penetrate the surface, if they just become ingrown, a patch of them can look like a fungal infection.[2]

The coordination of some Kerry Blues at 9 to 16 weeks old shows **cerebellar cortical and extrapyramidal nuclear abiotrophy**[3] with effects such as limb stiffness and head tremor. The earliest stiffness occurs in the pelvic limb, progressing to the thoracic limbs within two to four weeks. By eight to 10 weeks after onset of signs, side to side and to and fro oscillations make walking difficult. After 20 weeks the dogs are usually unable to stand.

There is no clinical evidence of cerebral cortical dysfunction. The affected dogs remain alert and respond to affection.

Kerry Blue Terriers suffer from several eye disorders, including the following: **narrow palpebral fissure**, **entropion**, **keratoconjunctivitis sicca**, and **distichiasis**. The breed is listed as being subjected to **ununited anconeal process**.[4]

Kerrys do have digestive-system problems. They cannot tolerate grease or changes in their diet without getting upset.

The health section of the Kerry Blue Terrier Club of America Handbook reports several other concerns of Kerry breeders: **cryptorchidism**, **pseudohermaphroditism**, **footpad keratoses**, **nasodigital keratoses**, **hypothyroidism**, **auto-immune diseases**, **Factor XI deficiency**, **hip dysplasia** and **subluxation of the patella**.[5]

BEHAVIOR

The "Kerry" is an affectionate and gentle companion. He is intelligent and exuberant. He is readily trainable but can be stubborn. He can be quarrelsome with other dogs.

OLD AGE

While Kerry Blue Terriers once lived to be 15 and 16 years, owners are now losing them at 12 years with a **malignancy**. Previously, they died of strokes or old-age problems.

Older Kerrys are more prone to **sebaceous cysts** than other breeds.

References

1. Kirk,R.W.;Bistner,S.I.: *Handbook of Veterinary Procedures and Emergency Treatment: Hereditary Defects of Dogs.* 1975; Table 124, p 661.
2. Martin,Thomas C., DVM. Personal Communication 1993.Adair Gardens Pet Hospital,1808 N. Belt West, Belleville, Il. 62223
3. Delahunta,A.;Averill, D.R., Jr.: "Hereditary Cerebellar Cortical and Extra-pyramidal Nuclear Abiotrophy in Kerry Blue Terriers." *JA* 1681: 1119-1123; 1976
4. Magrane, W.C.; *Canine Ophthalmology.* 3rd. Ed. Lea & Febiger, Philadelphia, PA 1977; 305
5. Collage, Scott, DVM. "The Kerry Blue Terrier and Health" *Kerry Blue Terrier Club Handbook.*

Setting Kerry Ears

Kerry ears vary in size, shape, thickness of leather and point where they are placed on the skull. No setting method suits every type of ear, but some generalizations can be stated to start the novice at ear pasting. Nine to 10 weeks of age is time enough to start. The ears will probably need pasting until 5 months of age and as long as up to 9 months in some cases.

Inner-ear cleanliness is a prerequisite to a symmetrically set final result. Start by trimming with a clipper, removing hair from the top of the ear flap and around the opening. Use a coarse clipper or scissors on underside of ear flap and top of skull so that 1/4 inch of hair is left for pasting. More rather than less is needed to get a good bond between ear and skull with liquid adhesive, which can be purchased at drug stores under the name of Due Liquid Adhesive, or at sewing counters under the name of Jiffy Sew. Pull hair from inside of ear. An artery clamp, or hemostat, is a good tool for hair pulling. Some hair may be removed from the upper part of the ear canal with it. It is best to tie the puppy to a grooming pole so that it cannot jump while being worked on in its ears. Four hands are better than two. Open the ear—holding it gently at D—and start cleaning the inner-ear bay, inserting a cotton swab forward and downward. Six-inch sticks with two long cotton ends are most satisfactory. If the stick comes loose from the cotton, the longer swab will be easier to remove from the inner ear. Well padded, homemade swabs are the best to use. A dry swab will clean the ear satisfactorily and will not sting. Alcohol, witch hazel, etc. are not needed—some may be left inside the ear. Slowly twist the dry swab and then withdraw it. Do this a few times and the excess hair and deposits will be removed. A veterinarian can supply an antibiotic ear drop that may be used after the cleaning. When clean, the ear is ready for pasting.

Place a box of tissue handy for wiping off the excess adhesive. Spread the adhesive on the underside of the ear flap from the tip C toward A and B, an inch in length on each side to form a V of adhesive. Place the ear on the skull as shown and press lightly. Hold the head to prevent the puppy from shaking the ear loose. Paste the material from the rear as well as from the front. (The last pasted ear can be picked up and reset if done immediately). When satisfied with the set, keep the puppy on the pole and distract it by brushing its coat. After five minutes the puppy may be put on the floor. It will shake its head and scratch at the ears. If not properly bonded, the set will not hold.

After three or more weeks, enough hair should have grown so that the ears may be cut loose. With very small strokes, snip at the hair with the tips of the scissors pressing towards the adhesive so as to leave the maximum amount of hair for the next pasting. Clean the ears as described. The ears may be reset immediately or allowed to hang free for a few hours.

At about 5 months of age, or when the permanent incisor teeth are in, leave the ears loose for a few days. The ears may seem uneven at first, but they usually even up by themselves. After 3 or 4 days, a determination can be made whether they are high enough, close enough to the head and carried with good expression. Some ears are properly set before the dog is 5 months old.

Should the ears, after being down between pastings, appear too high, let them hang free for a day or two. They will probably come down again. When they do, reset them as before. If one ear appears too far out, away from the head, reset that ear a bit further towards the middle of the head. Do not underestimate the importance of getting ears placed evenly at each setting. Time is required to obtain the best results.

When properly set, ears held forward in alert position will rest against the side of the cheeks. Line A-B will be a fold, not a roll. A roll may be used to set a very large ear in an attempt to minimize its size, but it is not correct. Read the Standard of Perfection for a description of proper ear carriage.

Never paste infected ears. Leave them loose until they are well. When the adhesive has stuck, let time unstick it. If a whole litter plays together, ears are torn loose. Try to repaste, skipping over the places where there is no hair. If not possible, or if the skin is bruised, wait a few days before repasting. If puppies take ear-tearing as a hobby, paste the ears and then place 1/2-inch adhesive tape from one cheek, over the flaps and down the other cheek, or all the way around the head, as an adjunct to, not a substitute for, pasting.

This procedure is not easy for the novice. If at all possible, experienced help should be sought.

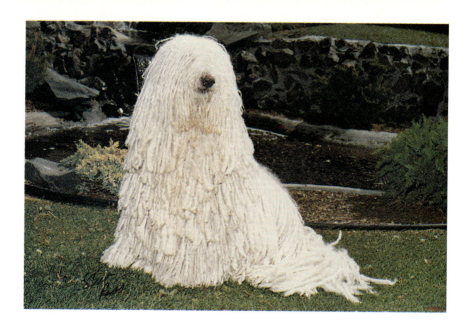

KOMONDOR

ORIGIN AND HISTORY

The Komondor (plural Komondorok) is the largest Hungarian livestock guard dog. The breed was used to guard the flocks while the smaller Puli did the herding. The mature coat falls into heavy protective cords which are practically impervious to predators and harsh weather conditions and give the dog a mop-like appearance. The dog is highly esteemed in Hungary today; the Standard for the breed is adapted from the one used there.

DESCRIPTION

The Komondor has impressive size and an imposing nature. The ideal temperament is that of a serious, conservative guard dog. This disposition must be understood if the dog is to be protective or friendly at the appropriate times. Most Komondorok have a stable temperament, although a few are unduly shy. As in all breeds, shy temperaments should not be perpetuated.

The dogs respond well to obedience training, which is strongly recommended. Handling amplifies the positive side of the dog's personality. At birth the breed is pure white, usually with pink pigmentation. Newborn coats are curly.

THE SHOW RING

A mature dog weighs over 100 pounds. Bitches are usually significantly smaller. Dogs are faulted if they are below 25 1/2 inches, and bitches should be over 23 1/2 inches.

Disqualifications are blue-white eyes; color other than white; bobtails; flesh-colored nose; short, smooth hair on head and legs; and failure of the coat to cord by two years of age.

BREEDING AND WHELPING

Bitches usually begin estrus at 12 months. Many cycle eight months or more apart. As in most large breeds, estrus is relatively long (a full three weeks), and ovulation often occurs late in the cycle. Ovulation at 14 to 16 days is common, but earlier and later dates of conception do occur.

Komondor puppies weigh 12 to 18 ounces at birth. The average size of a litter is seven or more puppies. Milk comes in late and many puppies are lost during the first week. It is advisable to be prepared with formula, bottles, feeding tubes and instructions.

Puppies are very sensitive to temperature changes. Surveillance is recommended.

GROWTH

Rate of growth is highly variable. Some puppies grow rapidly and stop early, others continue to grow until more than a year old. Usually the dogs are slow to mature, both physically and emotionally.

The nose begins to darken within days after birth, and the skin, especially on the ears, takes on a grayish cast. Pads darken to black, and pigment is usually complete in a few weeks. Occasionally a white spot on the nose develops later. The earlier a puppy's nose darkens, the better the pigment, and the less likely the nose is to fade at maturity. By 5 weeks a puppy's eyes should be brown. Blue eyes at this age are likely to be very light in the adult.

The corded coat, obvious at 1 year, is clearly corded by the age of two. The coat does not look mature until 3 years or older. At 5, the coat can reach the ground.

Some Komondorok are "unthrifty eaters," that is, they are picky eaters that do not gain weight. A low-residue diet may help unthrifty eaters; patience is required for the picky eaters. Prescribed steroids are the drugs of choice for appetite enhancement. With maturity, many dogs improve both in appetite and in weight maintenance.

DENTITION

Underbites and misaligned teeth in the lower jaw (especially the two front-central incisors) are common. Underbites become worse with maturity. Bites that are even at 5 months tend to become underbites later. Even scissors bites can become undershot as late as 9 months. Permanent teeth often come in before baby teeth are shed. Sometimes these baby teeth must be removed. Occasionally a dog lacks a tooth, usually a first premolar.

RECOGNIZED PROBLEMS

As in many working breeds, **hip dysplasia** is a problem. Although it cripples few dogs, x-rays show that some are unsuitable for breeding. Komondorok are rare, so most owners have their dogs x-rayed. As in all breeds, overwhelming preference for breeding is given to dogs with clear x-rays, in order to keep the incidence of hip dysplasia low.

Skin problems are common. **Staphylococcus infections** appear clinically as tiny, horseshoe-shaped lesions. **Pustular dermatitis** is fairly common in puppies just after weaning but is easily controlled. The breed is not immune to **allergic dermatitis** (hot spot) with the concomitant itch, but this responds to standard treatment. Bitches have a clear tendency to lose their coat from the middle forward, even without obvious skin problems.

The breed has more **cysts** than other breeds. These can be removed usually with an uneventful recovery.

BEHAVIOR

The Komondor is a gentle, loyal house pet. He is reserved with strangers. Grooming can be a problem unless his owner has some grooming expertise or uses a professional groomer. He needs space for the adequate exercise needed for a large dog.

OLD AGE

Life expectancy is 10 to 12 years.

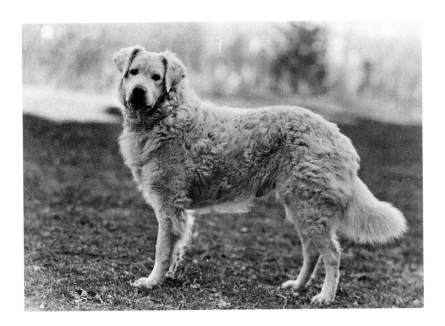

KUVASZ

ORIGIN AND HISTORY

Originating in Tibet, the Kuvasz (Hungarian plural: Kuvaszok) was developed to its present form in Hungary as a herding dog. Five to eight centuries ago they were the faithful companions of many European rulers. The Kuvasz is most similar to the Maremma Sheepdog and the Pyrenees Mountain Dog or Great Pyrenees, to which it is believed to be related.

The breed became renowned in Hungary during the latter half of the 15th century, when numerous private efforts were made to perpetuate the best specimens in order to use them to hunt large game animals.

King Matthias I of Hungary (1458-1490) had a profound effect on the development of the breed. As one of its foremost proponents he maintained extensive kennels and breeding colonies of the best specimens of that time and often gave puppies to visiting dignitaries. Kuvaszok were not acquired by the general population until later when the controls regarding their ownership were made less strict.[1]

DESCRIPTION

The breed as a whole exhibits a stable, kind temperament. Kuvaszok are intelligent and generally do not have nervous dispositions. The length of the coat of the Kuvasz makes this breed, in spite of its size, quite acceptable as a house dog.

The coat itself is short, straight and dense. The head, ears, feet, hindquarters and backs and sides of the forelimbs are usually coated with short hairs, while the neck and tail have longer hair.

THE SHOW RING

Dogs of this breed usually stand 28 to 30 inches at the shoulder. Bitches usually measure 26 to 28 inches. The weight of an adult dog may range from 100 to 115 pounds, while an adult bitch may weigh from 70 to 90 pounds. As befits a working dog, the Kuvasz should appear sturdy and give the impression of strength and agility.

The only acceptable coat color for this breed is pure white. A yellow saddle is seen in some specimens. This is a definite fault according to the Standard. Such individuals should not be bred.

The outer coat of an adult Kuvasz is rough in texture and wavy, with a fine-textured woolly undercoat. Faults of the breed include excessively domed skull, yellow eyes, pendulous eyelids and lips, ears close against head or thrown back, yellowish coat or yellow markings and light gray skin coloring.

Disqualifications include colors other than white, overshot or undershot bite, dogs smaller than 26 inches and bitches smaller than 24 inches.

Dewclaws on the forelegs should not be removed. Dewclaws on the hindlegs should be removed.[2]

BREEDING AND WHELPING

The Kuvasz does not exhibit any unusual characteristics concerning the age at which most bitches reach puberty. Normal estrous cycles are usually seen with this breed and dystocias are not common. Large litters are common with eight or more puppies being the rule rather than the exception.

RECOGNIZED PROBLEMS

There are few reported abnormalities involving the Kuvasz. As large dogs, though, they are susceptible to **hip dysplasia**. They are not generally plagued by extensive allergies or drug sensitivities, although **skin irritations** can develop as the result of tangled or matted coats.[3] The Kuvasz is one of the breeds affected with congenital **deafness**.[4]

BEHAVIOR

The Kuvasz is robust, gentle and intelligent. He is reserved, suspicious of strangers and not very affectionate.

OLD AGE
The average life span of the Kuvasz ranges from 6 to 9 years.

References
1. Lecaldano, P., Ed.: *The Encyclopedia of Dogs.* (The Crowell Co., New York, N.Y., 1970); 59-60.
2. Dangerfield, S. and Howell, E., Ed.: *The International Encyclopedia of Dogs.* (McGraw-Hill Book Co., Inc., New York, N.Y., 1971); 272.
3. Arnold, M., Personal Communication. Lincoln, Ne.
4. Strain, George M. "Deafness in Dogs and Cats," *Proc. 10th AVCIM Forum*; May, 1992.

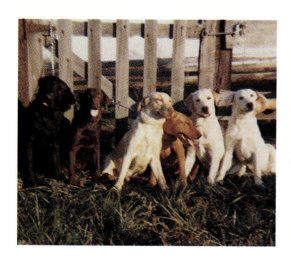 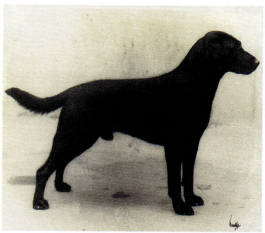

LABRADOR RETRIEVER

ORIGIN AND HISTORY

The Labrador Retriever has ancestors from Newfoundland rather than from Labrador.[1] The Labrador should geographically be called the St. John's Newfoundland, as it was in the early 1800s in England.[2] The excellent water dogs imported in the 19th century were bred with several other types of retrievers, always keeping two goals in mind—the water-repellent coat and the otter-like tail still evident on the modern Labradors.

The International Pointing Labrador Association has issued its first certification tests. The IPLA wants to establish the Labrador as a pointer.[3]

DESCRIPTION

General appearance of the Labrador Retriever should be that of a strongly built, short coupled, very active dog. He should be fairly wide over the loin and strong and muscular in the hindquarters.

The texture of the coat is important. It must be short and very dense. One test of the correct coat is that it feel hard to the touch. The undercoat beneath the water-repellent outer coat sheds yearly.

Color Anomalies: There is abundant evidence that other color genes are common in the breed.[2] The "tan point" gene is the one most observed, with tan markings such as those on the Doberman, or an otherwise black dog. "Brindle" is also seen in a variety of lines, with bicolored hair shafts. Since the Standard allows a small amount of white on the chest, it is

338

obvious that a gene for some kind of spotting is present, but subdued by the dominant gene for self-coloring. Occasionally, the recessive gene for "Irish" spotting combines, resulting in a white collar, chest, feet, head blaze and tip of tail such as are seen on many sheep-herding breeds. "Reverse" spotting has also been observed, both black spotting on yellows and yellow spotting on chocolates. These spots are usually small and occur in the expected places, such as point of chest or vent.

Several Labrador Retrievers have been reported that could be described as "Blue," as in the Doberman or Great Dane. These occurrences are so rare that the nature of the genes involved is indeterminate; however, a gene for "dilution" (such as in merle) could be a factor.

Although the existence of these other color genes has been documented, it must be remembered that any color anomaly in serious deviation from the accepted Standard should be destroyed or rendered sterile for the maintenance of desired breed characteristics.

THE SHOW RING

Dogs should be 65 to 80 pounds and 22 1/2 inches to 24 1/2 inches at the shoulder. Bitches should be 55 to 70 pounds and 21 1/2 inches to 23 1/2 inches at the shoulder.[1]

The colors are black, yellow or chocolate and are evaluated below:

Black

All black with a small white spot on chest permissible.

Yellow

Yellows may vary in color from fox red to light cream with variations in the shading of the coat on ears, the underparts of the dog, or on the back. A small white spot on the chest is permissible. Eye coloring should be the same as that of blacks with black or dark brown eye rims. The nose should also be black or dark brown, although fading to pink in winter is not serious.

Chocolate

Shades ranging from light sedge to chocolate. A small white spot on chest is permissible. Eyes are light brown or hazel. Nose and eye rim pigmentation is brown.

Any dewclaws on back legs should be removed. Dewclaws on the front legs are removed by most exhibitors of Labradors, but removal is not required.

Disqualifications in the breed standard are as follows:

⇑ **Any deviation in the height;**

⇑ **A thoroughly pink nose or one lacking in any pigment;**

⇑ **Eye rims without pigment;**

⇑ Docking or otherwise altering the length or natural carriage of the tail;

⇑ Any color or a combination of colors other than black, yellow or chocolate as described in the Standard.

BREEDING AND WHELPING

Average litter size is seven, with each whelp weighing approximately 12 ounces.

RECOGNIZED PROBLEMS

Receptor dystrophy has been reported in Labrador Retrievers according to a new study.[4] Dark adapted single flash and light adapted 30 Hz photopic flicker electroretinograms (ERGs) were recorded from a litter of seven Labrador Retrievers bred from parents affected with generalized progressive rod-cone dystrophy. After an initial increase of b-wave amplitudes from 5 weeks to 4 months similar to the controls, the b-wave amplitudes of the litter were significantly decreased at 7 months. At 21 months the b-wave amplitudes were very low, although some response to 30 Hz photopic flicker was still left. The ERG changes indicated a late onset of progressive rod-cone dystrophy which developed after maturation of the retina. The development of this photoreceptor dystrophy has not been previously described. Other eye problems such as **coloboma, dacryocystitis, distichiasis, persistent hyaloid artery** and **persistent pupillary membrane** have been diagnosed.

Labrador Retrievers have been reported to have **bilateral cataracts** as a dominant trait.[5,6] One thousand three hundred and ninety-nine Labs were examined for certification under the BVA/Kennel Club eye examination scheme. Cataracts were diagnosed in 6.6 percent of the Labs.[7] Other eye problems of the breed include **retinal dysplasia**[8] and **central progressive retinal atrophy**.[9,10,11,12,13] **Retinal dysplasia**[14,15] is a recessive hereditary trait that is evidenced by a progressively detached retina resulting in blindness. It is also associated with **dwarfism**[9,16,17] in the breed. **CPRA** is suggested to be a dominant with incomplete penetrance. Its signs are loss of central vision in dogs 3 to 5 years old. Affected animals have difficulty seeing stationary objects, with best vision in dim light. **Entropion** is another eye defect in some Labs.[18]

Postnatal cerebellar cortical degeneration is an inherited autosomal recessive disease in several breeds. Clinical and pathological descriptions of this disease have been reported in the Lab for the first time.[19]

Evidence for hereditary **copper toxicosis** is strong for Labrador Retrievers. Diagnosis is primarily by live biopsy samples. Penicillamine is the treatment drug of choice.[20]

Hemophilia A (Factor VIII deficiency) is a sex-linked recessive trait which results in prolonged bleeding, hemorrhagic episodes and prolonged PTT.[21,22]

Congenital Factor IX deficiency was diagnosed in a 15-week-old male Lab. Clinical signs included subcutaneous hematomas, profuse hemorrhage from a surgical wound and hemarthrosis. The signs abated when the dog was treated with fresh whole blood or plasmas. Specific clotting-factor assays confirmed the diagnosis in the patient and three male littermates and identified the carrier state in one female littermate.[23]

Another sex-linked recessive hereditary trait found is **cystinuria**.[11,12,24]

Bilateral carpal subluxation is an X-linked recessive trait in this breed.[25] The gene for the subluxation is allelic to the gene for hemophilia A.

Craniomandibular osteopathy is found in some Labradors.[11,26,27] The extensive ossification of the mandible and tympanic bulla causes discomfort and fever beginning at 4 to 7 months of age.

Hip dysplasia[28] is very common, but the incidence is improving. In Norway 22% of 2215 Labs radiographed between 1972-1984 were affected by hip dysplasia.[29] In addition, **ununited anconeal process** has been reported in the breed.

Skeletal muscles from six healthy dogs and three Labs with hereditary **muscular dystrophy** were examined morphologically and histochemically and were analyzed biochemically for sodium, potassium, calcium, magnesium, zinc, copper and chloride ions, total muscle water and total neutral lipid content. Flame atomic absorption spectrophotometer was used for elemental quantitation of hydrochloric and tissue extracts. Muscle samples from dystrophic dogs contained substantially increased concentrations of Na, Ca, Zn, Cu and Cl, and a considerable reduction in the content of K and Mg compared with samples from healthy dogs. Total muscle water and total fat content was higher in muscles from dystrophic dogs. Most muscle samples from dystrophic dogs had a type-2 fibre deficiency and an increase in number of fibers with internal nuclei.[30]

Three male littermates developed abnormal gait at 3 weeks of age followed by increasing muscle stiffness. The most remarkable clinical finding was a stimulus-responsive extensor rigidity. Five littermates (four male, one female) were normal. Myoclonus or seizures had occurred in other progeny of the grandsire. Post Mortem examination revealed only mild precordial oesophageal dilatation in two puppies. The condition is suggested to be similar to that of the spastic mouse, and deficiency of glycine function may be involved.[31]

Muscular dystrophy has also been reported in Labrador Retrievers in a German study.[35] A diagnosis of muscular dystrophy was made in a Lab puppy based on clinical signs of generalized muscle atrophy, depressed spinal reflexes and a "bunny-hopping" gait.[36]

A **muscle disorder** of Labrador Retrievers characterized by deficiency of type II muscle fibers was reported by Kramer et al.[37,38] Following is a summary of that report.

"A muscle disorder was detected in five Labrador Retrievers. The date of onset was less than 6 months. The clinical signs, which were exaggerated with exercise, cold or excitement, included abnormal head and neck posture, and a stiff, forced, hopping gait. A marked deficiency of skeletal muscle mass resulted in poor conformation. Both black and yellow Labrador Retrievers were affected, and pedigree studies indicated the disorder may have been inherited as an autosomal recessive trait. Some relief of the clinical signs was afforded by treatment with diazepam.

Marked creatinuria and low serum creatine phosphokinase activity were the only consistent abnormal laboratory findings. Histologic and cytochemical examinations of muscle biopsy specimens revealed a relative predominance of type I and a deficiency of type II skeletal muscle fibers. Electromyographic studies of the affected dogs indicated a myotonic defect."

Canine myopathies may be caused by inflammatory or degenerative diseases. **Labrador Retriever myopathy** is an inherited and degenerative disease. It can be transmitted by a simple autosomal recessive mode. Clinical signs are usually not apparent in the parents of affected dogs. By 3 months of age, the affected animal demonstrates an abnormal gait and limited exercise capability. Exercise causes weakness and collapse of the forelimbs. Cold weather may aggravate this disorder. Marked deficiency of skeletal muscle mass is evident by the time the dog reaches 6 months of age.

Apparently signs do not progress after 6 months of age. Some dogs have lived as long as 6 years without further development of signs. Routine laboratory profiles are typically within normal limits. Diagnosis can be based on history, clinical signs, EMG, nerve-conduction velocities and histologic and histochemical examinations of muscle biopsy material.[39]

A retrospective study was made of 135 dogs (Labs, Goldens and Rottweilers) with **elbow osteochondrosis** that had been seen at the Royal Veterinary College in 1977 to 1987. Males were affected more often than females. The condition was bilateral in 50% of the cases and the peak age for the onset of lameness was 4-6 months. In Rottweilers, the lesions found at exploratory arthrotomy were predominantly abnormalities of the coronoid process, while in Retrievers and Labradors lesions most commonly affected the medial humeral condyle or the coronoid process.[32] A Swedish study reports that the incidence of **osteochondrosis** was significantly higher than average in several large breeds, including Labradors.[33] The occurrence of osteochondrosis in a breeding colony of Labs during an 11-year period was investigated. The incidence in progeny varied between different sires and dams and was associated with the severity of radiographic evidence of elbow arthritis in sires and dams, with dams contributing significantly more than sires, suggesting a "maternal" effect.[34]

Labrador Retrievers are among the top breeds in the incidence of **shoulder dysplasia, elbow dysplasia, hypertrophic osteodystrophy, hypoglycemia, hypothyroidism,**[40] **missing** teeth, diabetes and **melanoma**. **Prolapsed rectum** and **prolapsed uterus** have also been reported by many breeders and veterinarians. **Congenital phimosis** is seen in this breed.[41] Labrador Retrievers are reportedly predisposed to **cutaneous mast cell tumors.**[42]

An associated **ocular and skeletal dysplasia** in Labrador Retrievers is caused by one abnormal gene which has recessive effects on the skeleton and incomplete dominant effects of the eye. The forelimbs of normal and affected pups were radiographed between birth and 156 days of age and the length of the radius and ulna measured. There was a significant difference in the mean length of these bones in normal and affected pups at birth and this difference was maintained over the period of observation. Similar differences were observed in purebred Labs and in Labrador Retriever-Beagle crosses. It is concluded that the length of the radius and ulna could be used to identify pups affected by this syndrome if test matings with affected animals were done to identify carrier animals. Abnormal shape of the radius and ulna, which is seen in animals affected with this syndrome, should be used to augment the accuracy of identification of puppies affected by this syndrome.[43]

Canine congenital hypotrichosis is seen in black Labrador Retrievers and is associated with abnormal teeth. Affected areas have fewer numbers of hair follicles and sebaceous glands.[44]

There appears to be an increased incidence of **primary megaesophagus** in this breed.[45]

In a Swedish study it was found that a high incidence of chronic **liver disease** and **liver cirrhosis** indicated that hereditary factors may be of importance in the development of these diseases.[46]

Leukotrichia was reported in one litter of Labrador Retriever puppies.[47]

Vitamin A responsive dermatosis has been found in Labrador Retrievers.[48] They are also at increased risk for **food allergy.** This allergy manifests itself so similarly to sarcoptic mange that it is often mistaken for scabies.[49]

Atherosclerosis was diagnosed postmortem in 21 dogs between 1970 and 1983. Nine dogs had died and 12 were destroyed because of complications associated with the disease. The mean age was 8.5±0.5 years; 18 dogs were male. Three breeds, including Labs, had a higher prevalence of the disease than other breeds. Common clinical signs were lethargy, anorexia, weakness, dyspnoea, collapse and vomiting. Hypercholesterolemia, lipidemia and hypothyroidism were common in affected dogs tested, and protein electrophoresis revealed high values for alpha 2 and beta fractions in all dogs tested. ECG indicated conduction abnormalities and myocardial infarction in three of seven dogs. Affected arteries (including coronary, myocardial, renal, carotid, thyroidal, intestinal, pancreatic, splenic, gastric, prostatic, cerebral and mesenteric) were yellow-white, thick and nodular, and had narrow lumens. Myocardial fibrosis and infarction also were observed in the myocardium. Histologically, affected arterial walls contained foamy cells or vacuoles, cystic spaces, mineralized material, debris with or without intima and degenerated muscle cells.[50]

Idiopathic epilepsy has been detected in the breed.[51]

Super ventricular tachycardia with atypical atriventricular accessory pathways is reported in the breed.

BEHAVIOR

The Lab is an excellent companion dog. He is intelligent, readily trainable and patient and gentle. He is being used as a "sniffer" dog by drug enforcement agents and as a "hearing" dog by the deaf.

OLD AGE

Labradors have an average life span of 10 to 12 years.

References

1. *The Complete Dog Book*, The American Kennel Club, (Howell Book House, New York, N.Y., 1992); 72-74.
2. Jones, A.F. and Hamilton, F., Eds.: *The World Encyclopedia of Dogs*. Galahad Books, New York, N.Y., 1971); 238-243.
3. Mueller, L. "Hunting Dogs: Certified Pointing Labs," *Outdoor Life*; April, 1990: pp 25-27.
4. Kommonen, B. and Karhunen, U., and "A Late [Onset of] Receptor Dystrophy in the Labrador Retriever," *Vision-Research*; 1990: 30: 2, 207-213; 30 ref.
5. Barnett, K.C. "Types of Cataract in the Dog," *JAAHA;* 1972: 8: 2-9.
6. Bjerkas, E. "Hereditary Cataract of Dogs in Norway," *Norsk-Veterinaeartidsskrift;*1991: 103:1, 5-14; 21 ref.
7. Curtis, R. and Barnett, K.C. "A Survey of Cataracts in Golden and Labrador Retrievers," *J. Sm. Anim. Prac.*; 1989: 30:5, 277-286; 14 ref.
8. Barnett, K.C., et al: "Hereditary Retinal Dysplasia in the Labrador Retriever in England and Sweden," *J. Sm. Anim. Prac.;* 1970: 10:755-759.
9. Barnett, K.C. "Abnormalities and Defects in Pedigree Dogs, IV: Progressive Retinal Atrophy," *J. Sm. Anim. Prac.*; 1963: 4:465-467.
10. Barnett, K.C. "Canine Retinopathies, III: The Other Breeds," *J. Sm. Anim. Prac.*; 1965: 6:185-196.
11. Barnett, K.C. "Genetic Anomalies of the Posterior Segment of the Canine Eye," *J. Sm. Anim. Prac.;* 1969: 10:451-455.
12. Barnett, K.C. "Primary Retinal Dystrophies in Dogs," *JAVMA;* 1969: 154:804-808.
13. Garmer, L. "Progressive Retinal Atrofi (PRA) hos Labrador Retriever," *Svensk-Veterinartidning*; 1986: 38:15, 120-123;3 ref.
14. Carring, et al: "Retinal Dysplasia Associated with Skeletal Abnormalities in Labrador

Retrievers," *JAVMA;* 170(1): 49-56.

15. Wikstrom, B. "Retinal Dysplasia," *Svensk-Veterinartidning;* 1986: 38:15, 129-130; 10 ref.

16. Farnum, C.E., Jones, K., Riis, R., and Wilsman, N.J. "Ocular-Chondrodysplasia in Labrador Retriever Dogs: A Morphometric and Electron Microscopical Analysis," *Anatomical Record;* 1992: 232:4, 32A; American Assoc. of Anatomists 150th Annual Meeting, March 11-14, 1992, New York, NY.

17. Carrig, C.B., Sponenberg, D.P., Schmidt, G.M., and Tvedten, H.W. "Inheritance of Associated Ocular and Skeletal Dysplasia in Labrador Retrievers," *JAVMA;* 1988: 193:10, 1269-1272; 6 ref.

18. Magrane, W.G. *Canine Ophthamology.* 3rd Ed. (Lea & Febiger, Philadelphia, Pa., 1977); 305.

19. Perille, A.L., Baer, K., Joseph, R.J., Carrillo, J.M., and Averill, D.R. "Postnatal Cerebellar Cortical Degeneration in Labrador Retriever Puppies," *Canadian Vet. Journal;* 1991: 32:10, 619-621; 11 ref.

20. Thornburg, L.P., Polley, D., and Dimmitt, R. "The Diagnosis and Treatment of Copper Toxicosis in Dogs," *Canine Practice;* 1984:11;5,36-39; 13 ref.

21. Kirk, R.W. and Bistner, S.I. *Handbook of Veterinary Procedures and Emergency Treatment: Hereditary Defects in Dog*s. 1975: Table 124, 661.

22. Archer, R.K. and Bowden, R.S.T. "A Case of True Hemophilia in a Labrador Dog," *Vet. Res.;* 1959: 71:560-561.

23. Verlander, J.W., Gormon, N.T., and Dodds, W.J. "Factor IX Deficiency (Hemophilia B) in a Litter of Labrador Retrievers," *JAVMA;* 1984: 185:1, 83-84; 4 ref.

24. Patterson, D.F. and Medway, W. "Hereditary Diseases of the Dog," *JAVMA;* 1966: 149:1741-1754.

25. Pick, J.R., et al: "Subluxation of the Carpus in Dogs: An X-Chromosomal Defect Closely Linked with the Locus of Hemophilia A," *Lab. Inv.;* 1967: 17:243-248.

26. Riser, W.H. and Fankhouser, R. "Osteopetrosis in the Dog: A Report of Three Cases," *J. Am. Vet. Rad. Soc.;* 1970: 11:29-34.

27. Erickson, R., et al: "Congenital Defects in Dogs: A Special Reference for Practitioners," Ralston Purina Co. (reprint from *Canine Practice*) Veterinary Prac. Publ. Co.; 1978.

28. Willis, M.B. "Hip Scoring Scheme Update," *Vet. Record;* 1987: 121:7, 140-141.

29. Lingaas, F. and Heim, P. "A Genetic Investigation of the Incidence of Hip Dysplasia in Norwegian Dog Breeds," *Norsk-Veterinaeretidsskrift;* 1987: 99:9, 617-627; 22 ref.

30. Mehta, J.R., Braund, K.G., McKerrell, R.E., and Toivio-Kinnucan, M. "Analysis of Muscle Elements, Water, and Total Lipids from Healthy Dogs and Labrador Retrievers with Hereditary Muscular Dystrophy," *Am. Jour. of Vet. Research;* 1989: 50:5, 640-644; 42 ref.

31. Fox, J.G., Averill, D.R., Hallettt, M., and Schunk, K. "Familial Reflex Myoclonus in Labrador Retrievers," *Am. J. of Vet. Research;* 1984: 45:11, 2367-2370; 8 ref.

32. Gutherie, S. "Use of a Radiographic Scoring Technique for the Assessment of Dogs With Elbow Osteochondrosis," *J. Sm. Anim. Prac.;* 1989: 30:11, 639-644; 5 ref.

33. Bergsten, G. and Nordin, M. "Osteochondrosis as a Cause of Claims in a Population of Insured Dogs," *Svensk-Veterinartidning*; 1986: 38:15, 97-100.

34. Studdert, V.P., Lavelle, R.B., Beilharz, R.G., and Mason, T.A. "Clinical Features and Heritability of Osteochondrosis of the Elbow in Labrador Retrievers," *J. of Sm. Anim. Prac.*; 1991: 32;11, 557-563; 36 ref.

35. Bichsel, P. "Neuromuscular Diseases of Young Dogs," *Jahresversammlung. Schweizerische Vereinigung fur Kleintiermedizin.* 2-4, Juni 1988.Bazel.1988, 43-50. Zool Bern, Switzerland; c/o H.Heinimann, Schweis. Serum und Impfinstitut,Postfach 2707.

36. Braund, K.G. "Challenging Cases in Internal Medicine: What's Your Diagnosis," *Vet-Med.*; 1988: 83:12, 1202-1212. 4 ref.

37. Kramer, et al: "A Muscle Disorder of Labrador Retrievers Characterized by Deficiency of Type II Muscle Fibers," *JAVMA*; 1976: 169:817-820.

38. McKerrell, R.,Anderson, J.R., Herrtage, M.E., Littlewood, J.D., and Palmer, A.C. "Generalized Muscle Weakness in the Labrador Retriever," *Vet. Record*; 1984: 115:11, 276; 4 ref.

39. Hoskins, J.D., DVM, PhD: Root, C.R., DVM, M.S., "Myopathy in a Labrador Retriever," *Vet. Med/Sm. Anim. Clin.*; September, 1983: 1387-1390. 8 ref.

40. Huntington,Ann L., DVM, "Hypothyroidism," *The American Kennel Club Gazette*; January, 1991: 104.

41. Ettinger, S.J. *Textbook of Veterinary Internal Medicine.* (W.B. Saunders Co., Philadelphia, PA 1989); 1884.

42. Veterinary News. *The American Kennel Club Gazette*; April, 1990: 44.

43. Carrig, C.B., Schmidt, G.M., and Tvedten, H.W. "Ocular and Skeletal Dysplasia in Labrador Retrievers," *Veterinary-Radiology*; 1990: 31:3, 165-168; 3 ref.

44. Brignac, Michele M. "Congenital and Breed Associated Skin Diseases in the Dog and Cat," published in *KalKan Forum* (December 1989)

45. Kern, Maryanne, DVM, "Diseases of the Esophagus," *The American Kennel Club Gazette*; January, 1993.

46. Andersson, M. and Sevelius, E. "Breed, Sex and Age Distribution in Dogs With Chronic Liver Disease: A Demographic Study," *J Sm. Anim. Prac.*; 1991: 32: 1, 1-5; 20 ref.

47. White, S.D. and Batch, S. "Leukotrichia in a Litter of Labrador Retrievers," *JAAHA*; 1990: 26:3, 319-321; 14 ref.

48. Ettinger, S.J. *Textbook of Veterinary Internal Medicine.* (W.B. Saunders Co., Philadelphia, PA 1989); 1884.

49. Griffin, C., Kwochka, K. and McDonald, J. *Current Veterinary Dermatology, the Science and Art of Therapy*, Mosby Yearbook, St. Louis, Mo. 1993: 123, 171.

50. Liu, S.K., Tilley, L.P., Tappe, L.P., and Fox, P.R. "Clinical and Pathological Findings in Dogs with Atherosclerosis: 21 cases," (1970-1983) *JAVMA*; 1988: 189:2, 227-232; 33 ref.

51. Bell, Jerold S. DVM "Sex Related Genetic Disorders: Did Mama Cause Them?" *American Kennel Club Gazette*, Feb. 1994; p 76.

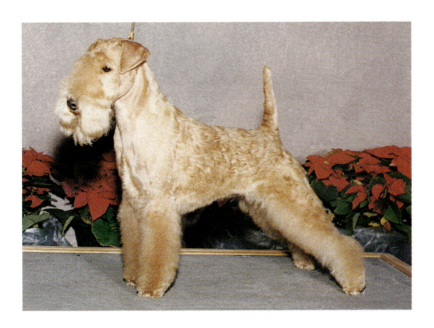

LAKELAND TERRIER

ORIGIN AND HISTORY

The Lakeland Terrier was originally known as the Patterdale Terrier. Originating in England's Lake District, it was bred by farmers to hunt fox and otter.

In 1871, a Lakeland Terrier is said to have crawled 25 feet under rock in pursuit of an otter. To free the entombed dog required three days of blasting.

DESCRIPTION

Lakeland Terriers are calmer and less excitable than the other long-legged terriers of the British Isles. Some are hyperactive, however, when not in familiar surroundings.

If a dog has behavior problems, obedience training and restructuring of the environment are advised. Its heritage of hunting quarry often larger than itself has made the Lakeland relatively insensitive to pain when excited; thus physical punishment is seldom very effective.

Lakelands make excellent playmates for children because they seldom resent rough treatment.

This breed is affectionate and sensitive to their owner's wishes.

THE SHOW RING

The ideal height for these dogs is 14 1/2 inches from withers to ground, with 1/2 inch deviation in either direction permissible. The weight of the well-balanced male in hard show condition is 17 pounds. The dog is squarely built and the bitch may be slightly longer. Balance and proportion are of primary importance.

The "Lakie" comes in a variety of colors: blue, black, liver, red and wheaten. The saddle may be blue, black, liver or varying shades of grizzle.

Disqualifications are: overshot or undershot bites.

BREEDING AND WHELPING

Lakeland Terrier bitches exhibit normal estrus. Highest rates of conception can be obtained by breeding every other day for standing heat. The interval between seasons varies. Intervals of 12 to 15 months are not uncommon.

Onset of the first estrus as late as 20 to 24 months of age should not be considered abnormal.

The average litter is three or four puppies. Provided the bitch is not allowed to gain too much weight, whelping is usually easy. There is no evidence of predilection for breeding problems or problems in rearing puppies.

Lakeland Terrier puppies vary in weight according to the size of the bitch and the number of whelps. By 3 months of age, size at maturity can be predicted. Dogs should weigh 7 to 8 pounds at 3 months, and bitches should weigh 6 to 7 1/2 pounds.

GROWTH

The whelps are almost solid black at birth. If a puppy has tan points, the mature color will be black and tan, black or red grizzle and tan, or blue and tan. Red puppies are born self-colored. Liver and tan dogs are rare. In saddled specimens, the color begins to "break" at 2 to 8 weeks.

Generally, the earlier the black color begins to recede, the more restricted the saddle will be. The color may continue to grizzle until the 2nd or 3rd year. White markings on the throat, feet, belly and back of the neck may occur and are sometimes extensive. Elongated markings on the midline tend to disappear, as do markings on the toes.

Dewclaws should be removed, and tails should be docked so that they will be level with the top of the skull when the dog matures. However, there is no formula for docking that is agreed upon by everyone.

Some puppies born with short tails will need only about 1/2 inch removed.

RECOGNIZED PROBLEMS

Cryptorchidism is prevalent in the breed, and there is a high incidence of **undershot**

bites.

The breed is listed as having some incidence of **ununited anconeal process**,[1] **lens luxation** and **distichiasis**.[2]

Due to the small genetic base of the Lakeland Terrier, breeders are concerned by the appearance of **Legg-Perthes disease**[3] and **Von Willebrand's disease**.[4] Both are insidious and can be misdiagnosed.

BEHAVIOR

The Lakey is a lively, friendly companion dog. His acute hearing makes him an excellent watch dog.

OLD AGE

The Lakeland Terrier remains vigorous into old age, living for 15 years or longer.

References
1. Foley, C.W., et al, *Abnormalities of Companion Animals*. 1975: 104.
2. Quinn, A.J. Personal Communication.
3. Lee, R. and Fry, P.D. "Some Observations on the Occurrence of ECP in the Dog," *J. Sm. Anim. Prac.* 10: 309-317; 1696.
4. Dodds, W. Jean, Personal Communication.

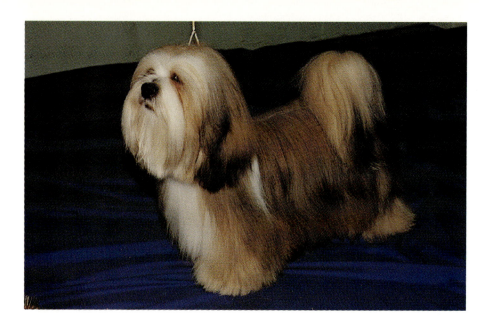

LHASA APSO

ORIGIN AND HISTORY

The Lhasa Apso originated in Tibet, in the holy city of Lhasa. Even though the breed is small, it was originally used as a guard dog.

DESCRIPTION

The personality of the Lhasa Apso is aloof and they tend to be wary of strangers. The Lhasa Apso is a good warning dog with a gentle and even temperament.

This medium-sized dog requires only moderate exercise. Because of the quantity of coat it carries, the Lhasa Apso should be provided with a well-drained exercise yard of either stone or concrete.

Color inheritance is quite mixed, even though the first animals brought to the United States were base colors of black, white and cream.

THE SHOW RING

Lhasas are usually 10 to 11 inches high at the shoulder, and longer than tall. All colors are equally acceptable. **There are no breed disqualifications.**

BREEDING AND WHELPING

As the Lhasa Apso is a brachycephalic breed, the bitch requires special prenatal care.

While the bitch is usually a free whelper, the delivery should be attended. The undershot bite does not permit the bitch to sever the cord easily. Lhasa Apsos suffer from hereditary **umbilical hernias** (gnawing the cord frequently results in a more severe hernia). **Inguinal hernias**[1] are also a problem.

Delivery problems may occur because of the large, blunt, round shape of the head of the fetus. Other problems may be associated with the bitch's being overweight from improper diet and weak-muscled from inadequate exercise.

To reduce maternal **dystocia**, the bitch should be fed a high-protein diet, which prevents overeating, in an attempt to intake adequate protein. She should be exercised daily to develop stamina and musculature. Litter size is between three and five whelps, with as many as 10 being recorded in a single litter.

Lhasa Apso puppies average between 5 and 7 ounces at birth. Formerly puppies were born with a kink at the tip of the tail. This trait has almost disappeared from today's breeding programs. It is recommended that dewclaws be removed on the third or fourth day to facilitate grooming the long leg hair on the adult dog.

GROWTH

Growth is steady, with the dog reaching his mature weight at 12 to 15 months. Bitches will weigh between 15 and 18 pounds, and dogs between 17 and 20 pounds. Average weights seem to be increasing in the breed as a whole and some dogs may reach 25 pounds.

The puppy coat is replaced with the mature coat by about 8 months.

The adult coat is a double one with a soft undercoat and a stiffer outer coat. Regular grooming is important to prevent matting. Bitches frequently lose their undercoat after weaning a litter or going through false pregnancy. During the summer months, **pyoderma** or **hot spots** may develop.

DENTITION

The shortened muzzle of the Lhasa Apso results in an undershot jaw similar to many small dogs of oriental origin. Bites should be even or undershot; scissors and overshot bites are undesirable.

Teeth are frequently misaligned and there may be one or two missing incisors.

RECOGNIZED PROBLEMS

The major congenital defects of the breed are umbilical and **inguinal hernias,**[1] **patellar luxations** and **medial entropion**. **Distichiasis, aberrant cilia** and **progressive retinal atrophy** are other eye problems.[2] A puppy should be carefully examined for these conditions.

Renal cortical hypoplasia[3,4] is a serious cause of uremia in the breed. Symptoms begin at about one year of age. There is increasing evidence of renal failure in some lines because of a lack of the antidiuretic hormone (ADH). This is more commonly called the **water drinking syndrome**. An incidence of 40% has been observed in one strain.

The Lhasa Apso is one of the breeds reported to have a significantly higher risk for **uroliths** than most other breeds.[5] Breeders are expressing growing concern over evidence of **hip dysplasia.** OFA certification is desirable. The short nose of the breed often predisposes a rolling of the skin at the medial canthus of the eye. **Corneal ulcers** and **corneal pigmentation** commonly occur in individuals having hairs of the nasal fold rub on the eye. Lhasas are one of a group of breeds that are highly susceptible to **inhalant allergies.**[6] **Lissencephaly,**[7] a congenital absence of cerebrocortical convolutions, was discovered in two Lhasa Apso dogs by clinical and pathological evaluation. Neurologic abnormalities included behavioral, visual and convulsive disorders. The neurologic abnormalities were mild or delayed in onset after birth, indicating the canine is less dependent on the cerebral cortex for sensorimotor function than is man. **Congenital hypotrichosis** occurs in Lhasa Apsos and is associated with abnormal teeth.[8]

BEHAVIOR

The Lhasa is a robust, easily trained companion dog. He is not a good companion for lively children. He does not like changes in routine or being left alone. He has acute hearing and makes a good watch dog.

OLD AGE

Decreasing interest in physical activity results in a weight gain. Because of the short muzzle, respiratory difficulties are sometimes experienced by the older dog. Lhasa Apsos with abnormally long backs often have disc protrusions in later years.

References
1. Hayes, H.M. "Congenital Umbilical and Inguinal Hernias in Cattle, Horses, Swine, Dogs, and Cats: Risk by Breed Among Hospital to Patients," *Am. J. Vet. Res.;* 1974: 35:839-842.
2. Magrane, W.G. *Canine Ophthalmology*, 3rd ed. (Lea & Febiger, Philadelphia, PA.,1977).
3. Kaufman, C.F., et al: "Renal Cortical Hypoplasia with Secondary Hyperparathyroidism in the Dog," *JAVMA*; 1969: 155:1679-1685.
4. Picut, C.A. and Lewis, R.M. "Comparative Pathology of Canine Hereditary Nephropathies: An Interpretive Review," *Vet. Res. Comm.;* 1987: 11:6, 561-581; 91 ref.
5. Bovee, K.C. and McGuire, T. "Qualitative and Quantitative Analysis of Uroliths in Dogs: Definitive Determination of Chemical Type," *JAVMA;* 1984: 185: 9,983-987; 18 ref.

6. Ackerman, Lowell, DVM, "Allergic Skin Diseases," *American Kennel Club Gazette;* September, 1990.

7. Greene, C.E., et al: "Lissencephaly in Two Lhasa Apso Dogs," *JAVMA;* 1976: 169:405-409.

8. Brignac, Michele M. "Congenital and Breed Associated Skin Disorders in the Dog and Cat," *KalKan Forum*; Dec, 1989: 9-16.

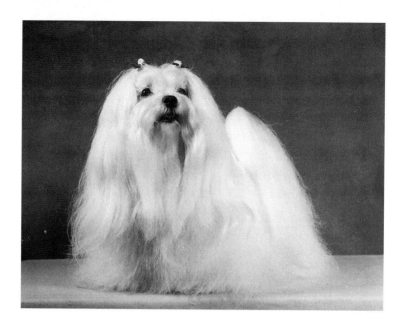

MALTESE

ORIGIN AND HISTORY

Originally from the ancient island of Malta, this tiny breed was a favorite of the Greeks, Phoenicians and Egyptians. They have been pets of the wealthy for centuries. They are Spaniel dogs, not Terriers, and are usually spirited and healthy.

DESCRIPTION

The adult Maltese tends to be extremely active, but his size precludes the necessity of large exercise areas. The average mature dog weighs 5 pounds. The breed is outgoing, inquisitive, friendly and often called the "dog of a million kisses."

THE SHOW RING

Weight should be under 7 pounds, with from 4 to 6 pounds preferred. Overall quality is to be favored over size.

The coat is long, flat and silky. Any suggestion of kinkiness, curliness or woolly texture is undesirable. The proper Maltese is pure white. Lemon on the ears is permissible but not desirable. **There are no breed disqualifications.**

BREEDING AND WHELPING

Maltese frequently have difficulty with delivery, especially in the first whelp with a small litter. Because of this tendency, breeding stock should be selected from lines having large litters (at least four or more), and bitches should be bred to small males. A prenatal examination on the 28th day to determine litter size and pelvic size can be used to forewarn the breeder of possible difficulties. While most Maltese are free whelpers, they occasionally need help in delivery of large puppies. A **cesarean section** may be required in small bitches. Litters average three to four puppies depending upon the size of the dam. **Eclampsia** is an occasional problem in the breed.

Maltese that will attain the mature weight of 5 pounds will weigh between 3 and 5 cunces at birth.

The black pigmentation of the nose and eye rims begins shortly after birth and is usually complete by the third week. In some lines, eye rims do not color completely and nose pigmentation fades as the dog ages.

Mating is usually successful on the 11th or 13th day, but individual bitches may vary.

It is recommended that dewclaws be removed on the third or fourth day to facilitate grooming the long leg hair of the adult dog.

GROWTH

The puppy coat is shed and replaced by the mature coat when the dog is about 8 months old. This change causes considerable matting. Bitches frequently lose their coats after weaning puppies or going through a false pregnancy. The adult coat grows continuously but more slowly in the older dog. The hair is delicate and easily broken and damaged. In the past, certain lines had a tendency to produce lemon-colored spots, usually on the ear. Selective breeding has minimized the problem. Show dogs sometimes have their hair wrapped and are crated on white paper to protect the coat from breaking and becoming discolored.

Growth is rapid, with the dog reaching full size between 8 and10 months. Weight of the adult dog may vary from 3 to 7 pounds. Dogs usually weigh more than bitches from the same litter. Stud dogs mature slowly, and many small males do not have sufficient stamina for natural breeding. Mating must often be assisted.

DENTITION

While full dentition is normal, incisors may be missing if the dog is extremely small or if the muzzle is narrow. Misaligned teeth are also a problem with the narrow muzzle. Temporary teeth which fail to come out naturally by 6 months of age must be removed. Overshot, under-shot or wry mouths have been reported but are not common.

Dental disease is common and should be prevented by good oral hygiene, especially removal of tartar every 6 to 12 months. Whenever gum redness (**gingivitis**) is noted, mouth-wash and cleaning of the teeth on a daily basis are necessary. Halitosis is an early indication of dental disease.

RECOGNIZED PROBLEMS

The hereditary defects most common in this breed are **poor pigmentation, malocclusion (undershot)** and **misalignment** produced by retention of temporary teeth. **Hydrocephalus, open fontanel, hypoglycemia** (due to glycogen storage disease) and **patellar luxation** are all common, as is **cryptorchidism. Patellar luxation** should be corrected early, before osteoarthritis changes can occur. Correction of the direction of stress on the patella usually corrects the condition.

Both **deafness** and **blindness** occur in the breed. The size and weight of the mature dog eliminate some of the problems of the larger breeds. **Hip dysplasia** is all but nonexistent, as are problems of the spine.

Tear stain on the face is common and is produced by inadequate drainage and frequently requires surgical correction. **Aberrant cilia (trichiasis)** are a frequent cause of drainage or excessive tearing.

Maltese, in a study of **hypertrophic pyloric gastropathy,** were one of two breeds most commonly affected.[1]

White-shaker dog syndrome (generalized tremor) which affects pure-bred Maltese in particular, can be called a disease for which there is a cure but no known cause. The condition exists primarily in young Maltese dogs and appears to be associated with certain neurological abnormalities, but the exact abnormality that triggers off the tremors cannot yet be identified. The syndrome does respond to corticosteroid treatment.[2]

BEHAVIOR

The Maltese is one of the hardiest of small dogs and makes a good companion for a family with children. He is playful and intelligent.

OLD AGE

The older dog has a decreased desire for activity. He is relatively free from physical ailments, with the exception of tooth problems and arthritis from patellar luxation. The teeth usually are very small and have thin enamel and short roots. If teeth begin to decay, they should be removed to prevent the possibility of infection. Many older dogs are completely toothless but healthy otherwise. The breed lives an average of 12 to 14 years.

Reference
1. Bellenger, C.R., Maddison, J.E., MacPherson, G.A. and Ilkiw, J.E. "Chronic Hypertrophic Pyloric Gastropathy in 14 Dogs," *Australian Vet. Jour.*; 1990: 67:9, 317-320; 19 ref.
2. "White-shaker Dog Syndrome" *Animal Health Newsletter*, Dec. 1993; Vol. II, #10; 2.

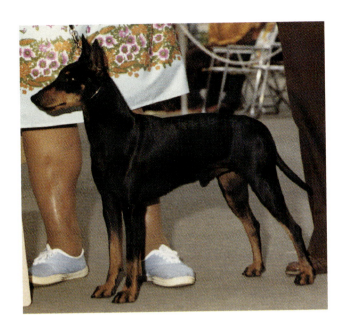

MANCHESTER TERRIER

ORIGIN AND HISTORY

The Manchester Terrier was developed when a rat-killing terrier was crossed with a Whippet to produce a dog that was good in coursing and ratting. The resulting Manchester is the only terrier to have a roached back.

DESCRIPTION

Manchester Terriers are of two varieties, Toy and Standard. Toys are up to 12 pounds; Standards are 12 to 22 pounds. For AKC registration, the two sizes are not differentiated. Serious breeders try to keep the two varieties separated, but most will cross them when seeking certain traits. The Manchester Terrier is a very active, aggressive dog throughout its life. It is usually affectionate to all humans, both adults and children, and it likes to be petted and loved. However, there is little generosity in its soul for other dogs, and this attribute can result in serious harm or death when it confronts a large and aggressive adversary.

THE SHOW RING

The breed standard for the Toy Manchester is the same as that for the Standard Manchester except for size and ears. Toys should not exceed 12 pounds and Standards should not exceed 22 pounds. Standard variety ears may be cropped, Toy ears may not be cropped.

Breed disqualifications are any color other than black and tan; white in any part of the coat, a patch or stripe measuring as much as 1/2 inch in its longest dimension; weight (Standard Variety) — over 22 pounds; ears (Toy Variety) — cropped or cut ears.

BREEDING AND WHELPING

The newborn of both varieties are remarkably uniform. At birth, the Standards and Toys will be about the same size, 5 to 6 ounces. Natural whelping is the rule, and unless a very small Toy bitch is bred, the dam will do everything for herself and the pups. With young mothers, darkened quarters for whelping will reduce excitability. The whelping area should be quite warm (around 80^0 F).

The newborn show little or no tan markings and appear nearly all black. The tan develops in its proper areas over the first 3 to 4 weeks. The thumb prints and pencil markings are somewhat slower to develop. Mismarkings such as a white spot on the chest, toes or tail usually are evident at birth or a few days after.

GROWTH

At about 3 to 5 days all dewclaws should be removed. Tails are left natural as specified by the Standard.

The ears of the Toy Manchester must not be elevated by surgery. Different dogs will raise their ears at different ages, from 3 weeks to 5 or 6 months. If a puppy goes to 6 months with soft, floppy ears, taping could be necessary. The usual mistakes made with Toy Manchesters are taping at too early an age and not taping continuously for a long enough period. Once taping is elected, it may be necessary to continue for 3 to 4 months. Taping should be done with 1/2 inch tape, starting at the base of the ears on the outside, laminating the tape, strip after strip, up to the tip. Each application should be overlapped about 1/2 the width of the tape. Another strip should be wrapped around the entire ear about 1/4 of its length from the base to pull the ear into a curve that would half encircle the average index finger. Another piece of tape is wrapped at the same level from one ear to the other to pull the ears toward each other.

The ears of the Standard Manchester in the United States are customarily cropped to a point. The cropping determines 50% and the aftercare 50% of the end result. The details of this procedure are involved, but three points should be emphasized. The ear should be a long crop when compared to the crop of a Miniature Schnauzer. The ears should be brought in tight to the skull at the base so there is no unsightly wing angling out at the side; pressure or hemostatic agents, like oxycel, are preferable to sutures to control hemorrhage from the two arteries involved. Serious hemorrhage rarely results from this surgery; sutures can leave unsightly scars on an otherwise attractive dog.

DENTITION

Dentition usually progresses uneventfully. A slight defect in the temporary teeth may correct in the permanent teeth. Occasionally, first pre-molars in the upper jaw are missing. Smaller dogs have a problem with temporary teeth remaining after permanent teeth appear. Extraction is indicated in this case.

RECOGNIZED PROBLEMS

Congenital defects are rather rare in pups from well-bred and good-conditioned parents. **Cleft palates** and **umbilical hernias**[1] have been reported in this breed, but they are rare. **Secondary glaucoma (luxating lens)** has been a problem in the breed.[2]

Manchesters are prone to upsets in growth and development, or even worse, to severe **reactions and anaphylactic shock following immunization.** Many breeders feel the distemper and hepatitis vaccines should be given at reduced dosage, although repeated doses may be necessary.

Hip dysplasia is practically unknown to the breed.

This breed is prone to **skin irritations,** and **low-grade skin infections** are often incorrectly labeled demodectic mange. A commercial dog bath containing lanolin is good for the skin and may bring back natural hair growth. An antibiotic topical ointment may be helpful.

Grand mal epilepsy may be encountered at any age. This is not a breed characteristic, but exists in certain families. The conscientious breeder will take steps to eliminate this trait, and will not sell or give away any afflicted dogs. Older dogs (7 to 8 or over) sometimes show minor attacks which are probably due to cerebral ischemia. Once the condition has set in, medication is useful in preventing attacks.

Cutaneous asthenia (Ehlers-Danlos syndrome)[3] has been reported in the breed. Clinical signs include fragility of the skin and peripheral blood vessels, hyperextensibility and laxity of the skin. Lacerations are easily produced. The skin of these animals has wide, pliable scars. Subcutaneous hematomas may develop at the site of injury. The skin has a moist, blanched appearance and is velvety in texture.

Cutaneous asthenia in dogs is genetically transmitted. It is a collagen abnormality inherited as an autosomal dominant trait with complete penetrance. Affected animals should be removed from the breeding program.

BEHAVIOR

The Manchester is lively and intelligent and makes a good companion dog.

OLD AGE

With reasonable care, Manchesters may easily reach 15 to 16 years of age, outliving some of the larger breeds. The old dog may lose its teeth or develop **cataracts** or **arthritis**.

References
1. Hayes "Congenital Umbilical and Inguinal Hernias in Cattle, Horses, Swine, Dogs and Cats: Risk by Breed and Sex Among Hospital Patients," *Am. J. Vet. Res.*; 1974: 35:839-842.
2. Magrane, W.G. *Canine Ophthalmology*. 3rd Ed. (Lea & Febiger, Philadelphia, PA., 1977).
3. Foley, C.W., et al: "Abnormalities of Companion Animals," Iowa State University Press, Ames, Ia., 1979: 135.

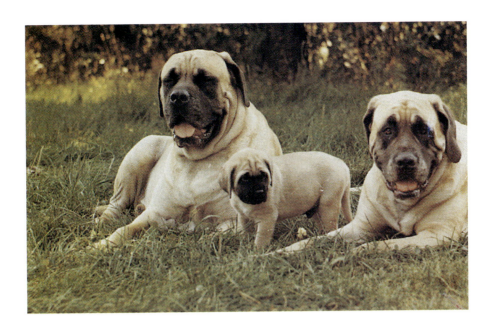

MASTIFF

ORIGIN AND HISTORY

Mastiff refers to a group of large, square-muzzled dogs that have been used for fighting, hunting and guarding since the days of the Roman Empire. In England during the Middle Ages, it was required that one Mastiff be kept for every two peasants, so the breed developed as a family dog. With this background, Mastiffs became companions that are aggressive with other dogs but loyal, faithful friends to man.

DESCRIPTION

Because many people confuse the Mastiff with the Bullmastiff, it is always best to refer to the breed by its full name.

Mastiffs are extremely sensitive, devoted and eager to please those they love. They need human companionship and constant reassurance, as they seem to lack self-confidence.

Dogs of Mastiff breeding are lethargic and usually do not roam. They are content to sit in the house all day, if their family is there, and go outdoors only when necessary. Because they are very serious about guarding their people, they make excellent watch dogs.

Mastiffs characteristically are rather aloof, not readily befriending strangers. The breed has serious faults of temperament. They are often extremely shy and since this trait is heritable,

361

shy individuals should not be used for breeding.

The Mastiff breed has three coat colors, silver fawn, which shades from almost creamy white to a dark-gray mousy color; apricot, which shades from stag red to pale tan; and brindle, which has dark stripes on a fawn background. If a brindle has one apricot parent, its ground color is reddish. Brindle-to-brindle matings have produced all three colors in the resulting litter. A black mask and ears and very dark eyes are required. Adult coat color is difficult to predict at birth. A Mastiff's jaw should be firm and pronounced. A scissors bite is preferred, but an underbite is permissible if the incisors do not show when the mouth is closed.

The Breed Standard includes no disqualifications. Undesirable features are white markings of any kind, lack of dark mask and ears, light eyes, dogs less than 30 inches tall, and bitches less than 27 1/2 inches.

BREEDING AND WHELPING

Mastiffs mature slowly and should not be used for breeding until they are 2 years old. Bitches do not usually come into first estrus before they are 11 or 12 months old. Ovulation is irregular, with conception possible any time from the 7th to the 21st day. Gestation ranges from 60 to 67 days. Five puppies are an average litter, although litters of up to 14 have been reported. Many bitches experience **uterine inertia** after whelping one or two puppies, probably resulting from the breed's characteristic lethargy. Thus, supervised exercise is essential for maintaining proper muscle tone. At birth, the puppies are generally uniform in size, weighing 1 to 1 1/2 pounds. Their eyes open at about 2 weeks. At this time the puppies should begin receiving supplemental food. The most satisfactory additive is raw beef, ground twice and with most of the fat removed. This supplement should be fed once a day, starting with one teaspoonful daily, gradually feeding more as the puppies demand it.

GROWTH

The desired growth rate is shown in Table 1. Continuing muscle development adds more weight after the dogs reach 12 months of age. The dogs usually weigh 195 pounds at 2 years of age, and the bitches 150 pounds.

RECOGNIZED PROBLEMS

Obesity is the curse of the Mastiff breed. Feeding these dogs too much or giving them too many vitamins or minerals is detrimental. However, many owners continue to overfeed their dogs in the mistaken belief that the heavy feeding increases the dog's size. OFA has reported **elbow dysplasia** in this breed.[1] Mastiffs have **ectropion** and **persistent pupillary membranes**.[2] **Vaginal hyperplasia** is a problem in the breed. **Bloat** is a hazard at any age.

BEHAVIOR

The Mastiff makes an excellent watchdog. He is good with children and eager for affection, but he needs firm handling while being trained, as do most large dogs.

OLD AGE

Arthritis, **nephritis** and **heart problems** are the infirmities that commonly affect aging Mastiffs. The average lifespan is 9 to10 years.

TABLE 1 GROWTH RATE OF MASTIFFS		
AGE	WEIGHT (LB)	
(Mos)	Males	Females
1	15	13
2	36	28
3	60	42
4	81	55
5	108	77
6	128	89
7	138	100
8	158	110
9	166	114
10	171	122
11	177	130
12	185	140

References
1. Bodner, Elizabeth A., DVM, "Genetic Status Symbols," *The American Kennel Club Gazette*; September, 1992.
2. Foley, C.W., et al: *Abnormalities of Companion Animals*. Iowa State University Press. Ames, Iowa, 1979: 35.

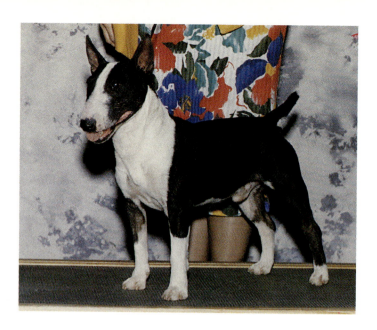

MINIATURE BULL TERRIER

ORIGIN AND HISTORY

The Miniature Bull Terrier was developed directly from the Bull Terrier breed, with some individuals reportedly weighing as little as 10 pounds.[1]

This strong little breed was first given separate breed status by the Kennel Club of Britain in 1939. The breed was recognized by The AKC in 1991.

DESCRIPTION

The Miniature Bull Terrier is a very active breed and makes a good, playful companion. As with the Standard breed, the bull-baiting ancestry shows itself in courage, strength and athletic ability.

Because of their great energy, Miniature Bull Terriers must be carefully trained. Some sources suggest bitches as a gentler animal for some homes.[2] This breed is not suitable for urban living, where exercise is limited.

THE SHOW RING

The Standard dictates size by height rather than weight.[3] The adult dog must not be over 14 inches at the shoulder.

364

The thin coat and tight skin of the breed are the same as in the Standard breed. Also, the big-boned chunkiness is retained in the Miniature.

RECOGNIZED PROBLEMS

No congenital defects have been documented in this breed. Some breeders have reported isolated cases of epilepsy. The problems encountered in Bull Terriers might be expected to appear, but have not been verified at the time of this publication.

BEHAVIOR

If trained with firmness the Miniature Bull Terrier makes a great companion for a lively, active child. He is suspicious of strangers and does not get along with other dogs.

References
1. Jones, A.F. and Hamilton, F., Eds., *The World Encyclopedia of Dogs*. (Galahad Books,New York, N.Y.,1971); 428.
2. Johnson, N.H. *The Complete Puppy and Dog Book*. (Atheneum, New York, N.Y., 1973); 63-64, 128.
3. *The Complete Dog Book*, The American Kennel Club, 18th ed., (Howell Book House. 1992); 382-384.

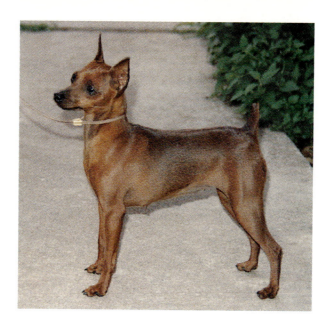

MINIATURE PINSCHER

ORIGIN AND HISTORY

The Miniature Pinscher was first developed around 1895 when the Pinscher Klub was formed in Germany.[1] Importations of the breed to the United States began after World War 1, with the Miniature Pinscher Club being formed in 1929.

DESCRIPTION

The Miniature Pinscher is a keen watch dog, often as aggressive as a large dog. Its high degree of activity and intelligence make it an excellent show dog, and it is often used in stage shows.[1] Miniature Pinschers make excellent house dogs, but they require discipline. Training should start at about 3 to 6 months with daily, short work sessions (about 10 to 15 minutes each). Miniature Pinschers respond to affection and make good obedience dogs. They tend to become attached to one master, exclusive of others, so an effort should be made to expose the dog to several people and regular human handling.

THE SHOW RING

In general, the appearance is that of a compact, short-coupled, smooth-coated toy breed. Serious faults include vicious or shy behavior, poor action, over-developed muscles or curly, uneven or dull coat.

It has a narrow head with a flat forehead and strong muzzle. Eyes should be slightly oval and very dark. Except on chocolates, the nose must be black.

The breed has catlike feet, well arched with blunt nails. Its tail should be held erect, docked 1/2 (two vertebrae remaining).[1] There are three accepted colors: solid red or stag-red, black with tan markings and chocolate with rust or tan markings.

Breed disqualifications include: under 10 inches or over 12 1/2 inches in height; any color other than listed; thumb mark (patches of black hair surrounded by rust on the front of the foreleg between the foot and the wrist; on chocolates, the patch is chocolate hair); and white on any part of dog which exceeds 1/2 inch in its longest dimension.

BREEDING AND WHELPING

One of the problems in breeding is finding an animal of correct size with good conformation. An ideal breeding pair would be a good bitch of 11 3/4 inches and a dog of no more than 11 to 11 1/2 inches. Successive generations bred from standard-size animals seem to produce dogs lacking in substance, so it is suggested that a dog of greater size and substance be used every two or three generations.

Larger Minpins (as breeders refer to them) often appear coarse, with Manchester-type heads, while the very small specimens have the "apple head" of the Chihuahua and are not as sound in leg as desired.

The Miniature Pinscher is an unusually hardy toy breed, and it has very little trouble during gestation and parturition. The bitch should be dewormed before breeding, exercised and kept within proper weight limits.

The bitch should be in a whelping pen 2 to 3 weeks prior to whelping. It is critical to prevent chilling since this is often the cause of infant mortality. Heating at least a section of the pen with a heating pad or a similar appliance is helpful. The pen should also be in an area free of draft and heavy traffic.

Cleft palates are common in this breed, so each newborn should be examined. Also, large litters often force some puppies to be pushed away at feeding time, so supplemental hand feeding may be necessary.

GROWTH

Newborns should be examined for excessive white spots and the black and rust puppies for thumb marks. The adult color of a dog is often hard to judge in the puppies. Often a light red will darken to a nice clear red, and true mahogany reds may appear almost black at birth.

Tails should be docked at 2 or 3 days. On the puppy, the tail should just cover the anal triangle. Dewclaws should be removed at this time.

Supplemental feeding is recommended for all puppies by the time they reach 3 to 4 weeks of age. A multivitamin supplement is also recommended.

At about 12 weeks the ears should be trimmed. The puppy should be dewormed and in good general health before trimming. The ear length is measured by folding the ear across to the ipsilateral medial canthus of the eye and marking at this point on both sides. This gives a realistic length for the ear. Clamp across the ear, beginning at the most distal portion where it is marked for length, and ending at the lateral end of a small linear ridge that is found inside, almost at the bottom. Take a sharp razor blade and cut along the hemostat. After this, take a curved hemostat to give a slight curve in the distal half of the ear with a fine tip. Clamp the ear after deciding exactly how much of a curve is wanted, and then again cut with a sharp razor blade. Following this, the lower portion of the bell of the ear is cut across right next to the head, giving a sharp impression without any flaring at the bell of the ear. Suture with several single sutures rather than a running suture, and cover the cut surfaces with an antiseptic ointment. Subsequently, take a large piece of styrofoam and sculpture a "dunce cap" for the puppy. With liquid adhesive, stand the ear and stick it to the lateral surface of the cap. Reinforce this with regular adhesive tape, leaving the cut edges open enough to remove stitches at about seven days. Daily application of ointment prevents puckering and reduces scarring. In 2 to 3 weeks, remove the cap and see if the ear stands. If not, pull the ears across the skull, folding them over each other to pull out any puckering, leaving for 2 or 3 days. Take them down and roll in a typical manner for Boxers and Dobermans.

RECOGNIZED PROBLEMS

Inguinal hernias are fairly frequent in the breed.

Aseptic femoral head necrosis (Legg-Perthes disease) is found in Miniature Pinschers, evidenced by limping at about 6 or 7 months of age. Whether or not this is a hereditary condition has not been determined. Temporary immobilization or surgery, depending on the severity of the condition, may be necessary.

Hip dysplasia is relatively rare in the Miniature Pinscher. **Skin diseases** of various types are common.

Progressive retinal atrophy[2] **(PRA)** has been recognized in Miniature Pinschers. With PRA, night vision gradually deteriorates while day vision remains normal. In the next stage, the dog becomes completely night blind and day vision deteriorates.

Deafness has been reported, but only infrequently.

Lack of pigment in the nose, nails, etc., and large white spots on the chest are common. Selective breeding can greatly decrease the incidence of this defect. Breeding black to black too frequently increases the incidence of "thumb marks," a characteristic which disqualifies the animal for show.

The gene for dilution is carried by some MinPins and an occasional blue will be born. As in other breeds, skin diseases are associated with these "dilutes."

Shoulder dislocation has been described in this breed.[3]

BEHAVIOR

Minpins are lively and active and make excellent watch dogs. They are easily trained and make excellent companions. The Miniature Pinscher is a barker and does feel the cold.

OLD AGE

Miniature Pinschers usually live to about 12 years.

Reference

1. *The Complete Dog Book,* The American Kennel Club. (Howell Book House. New York, NY. 1992); 450-452.
2. Foley, C.W., et al *Abnormalities of Companion Animals,* Iowa State University Press, Ames, Ia., 1979: 78-79.
3. Campbell, J.R. "Shoulder Lameness in the Dog," *J. Sm. Anim. Prac.*; 1968: 9:189-198.

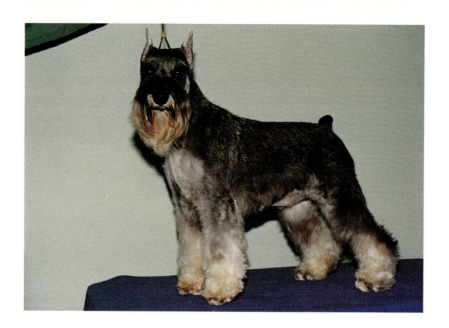

MINIATURE SCHNAUZER

ORIGIN AND HISTORY

Of German origin, Miniature Schnauzers have been bred in the United States since 1925. Useful as ratters, Miniature Schnauzers can guard houses and give alarms as well as larger dogs can. Their basic good health, good temperament, nonshedding and attractive appearance make them admirably suited as pets.

DESCRIPTION

The Miniature Schnauzer is a sturdy, robust dog standing from 12 to 14 inches at the shoulder. Ideally, it is as long as it is tall, giving a blocky, square appearance. In this breed, development of personality and temperament demand close association with human beings. Kennel isolation is particularly detrimental to mental well being. These dogs are "people lovers" and make ideal companions for a family.

THE SHOW RING

Color ranges through all shades of gray intermingled with black, giving a "salt and pepper" appearance. Permitted colors also include solid black or black and silver. In these latter two, there must be no off-colored hair in the body coat. To condition the Schnauzer coat

370

for the show ring, it is necessary to "pluck" or strip the body and head coat approximately 10 weeks before the show. The show coat will usually last only about 8 to 10 weeks before the process must be repeated. Breeders like to produce heavy-boned dogs with good spring of rib and profuse furnishings. The eye should be small and dark, giving an alert expression.

Breed disqualifications are: dogs or bitches under 12 inches or over 14 inches; color solid white or white striping, patching or spotting on the colored areas of the dog, except for the small white spot permitted on the chest of the black. The body coat color in salt and pepper and black and silver dogs fades out to light grey or silver white under the throat and across the chest. Between them there exists a natural body coat color. Any irregular or connecting blaze or white mark in this section is considered a white patch on the body, which is also a disqualification.

BREEDING AND WHELPING

Ovulation varies from as early as 7 days to as late as 16 days, with an average time being 10 days from onset of estrus. The gestation period can vary from 56 to 65 days. The top producing bitch in the breed routinely presented her well-developed puppies between the 56th and 58th day of pregnancy. Experience has been that Miniature Schnauzers on the whole are lazy whelpers, and about 15% have to be aided by a **cesarean section**. Schnauzer bitches are not as adept at removing the fetal membranes as the other breeds, and they should be given close attention during whelping. The average litter is between three and five puppies, but as many as 10 in a litter have been seen. Normal birth weights range from 4 to 9 ounces. The puppy should make daily gains of about one ounce, and it should double its birth weight by the end of the first week. Dewclaws and tails can be docked as soon as the puppy is making good progress. Usually this is done about the third or fourth day after birth.

GROWTH

Development of the puppy varies somewhat with the various strains, but as a general rule, the puppy should measure approximately 8 inches at 8 weeks, 10 inches at 12 weeks, 11 inches at 16 weeks and 12 inches at 5 months. These measurements should be average for the ideally sized 13 1/2-inch Schnauzer.

Tail length of the show dog is important. When docking, the tail is held in an upright position, and cut at about the demarcation of white and gray hair on the ventral surface of the tail. This may vary from dog to dog. A guide is to bring the tail down over the rectum and clip to a point where it just covers the rectum. In cutting the tail, care should be taken to leave more skin anteriorly than posteriorly so that the skin when sutured will cover the end of the tail, thus preventing a scarred end. This also aids in holding the tail erect. A properly cut adult tail will develop to about two inches above the back line, carried erect.

Ear cropping is usually done between 9 and 11 weeks. An otherwise fine show dog can be ruined by improperly cropped ears. Various techniques have been developed. Excellent results can be obtained by the "free-hand" method:

1. After obtaining surgical depth of anesthesia, ears are clipped with surgical blade #40, washed with alcohol and wiped with a gauze pad.

2. Next, a sharp indelible pencil is used with a ruler to make a mark on the anterior medial edge of each ear 1 3/4 inches up from the skull (varies by 1/8 inch either way depending upon the size of the dog).

3. A free-hand line is now drawn from the mark made on the ears down to the base of the auricular cartilage. To do this expertly requires a good knowledge of what a proper Schnauzer ear should look like.

4. Using a 3-inch cartilage scissor (slightly curved), make the cut downward from the original free-hand line. This should be done in one cut without stopping. Lay excised portion of the ear on top of the other ear to verify line accuracy. Be particularly careful to have as little bell as possible left in the ear. At the same time, do not take down to the point where the ear will not stand.

5. Next, a V-shaped portion of the basal auricular cartilage (tragus) is removed at the base of the incision on both ears. This cut results in a smooth appearance between the skull and the ear and, when done properly, gives the illusion of a narrower head and higher ear set.

6. 3-0 monofilament nylon with a swagged-on 3/8 inch cutting needle is used as a continuous suture, starting at the base of the V and continuing dorsally, ending 1/4 inch below the tip of the ear. The suture is knotted at both ends. Suturing through the cartilage offers no problem, but catching just the dorsal and ventral skin is preferable. If hemorrhage is a problem, the three small auricular vessels can be grasped with a small mosquito forceps and twisted, or they can be ligated with 5-0 cat. As a rule, hemorrhage is not significant. The main mistake with ear cropping the Schnauzer is too much bell or too wide an ear.

DENTITION

Undershot or **overshot** mouths are faults. Attention should be given to the mouth of the puppy during loss of deciduous teeth. The bite may be saved by extracting deciduous teeth that are interfering with proper development of the adult canines and incisors. Missing teeth are rarely a problem of this breed.

RECOGNIZED PROBLEMS

Abnormalities at birth are relatively rare. The breed does seem prone to urinary tract problems such as **nephritis, cystitis** and the formation of **uroliths.**[1] There are strong indications that genetic predisposition is a factor in producing some of these conditions. Care should be used in selecting breeding stock that is suspect of kidney disease. A study of pedigrees has indicated a genetic basis for **juvenile renal disease.**[2] Breeding studies in a strain of Miniature Schnauzer dogs with **persistent Mullerian duct syndrome (PMDS)** indicated that this syndrome is inherited as an autosomal recessive trait.[3]

A recent study at the University of Minnesota reports that Miniature Schnauzers are more than 11 times more likely than all other breeds to develop **calcium oxalate bladder stones (uroliths).**[4] Of 839 **uroliths** submitted by veterinarians for analysis, 562 (67%) were composed of at least 70% magnesium ammonium phosphate, and 57 (6.8%) at least 70% calcium oxalate. Most were found in the bladder. Uroliths occurred more frequently in females than in males, but there was little difference in prevalence between dogs aged 1 to 12 years. The uroliths were found in 60 known breeds of dog, but were most prevalent in Miniature Schnauzers (22.3%).[5,6]

A second rather common, but much less severe, problem is the **follicular dermatitis**[7] **(Schnauzer comedo syndrome)** that occurs along the dorsal midline from the neck to the tail. This seems to particularly plague Schnauzers that have been clipped. Etiology of this condition is not clear, but is probably genetic due to its exclusive occurrence in Miniature Schnauzers. Some feel it is a sensitivity reaction to clipping. Treatment consists of medicated baths with a benzoyl peroxide shampoo followed by 3 weeks of systemic antibiotics. If no response is seen, then isotretinoin (Accutane) at 1 to 2 mg/kg q 24 hour p.o. has been quite effective. After lesions resolve, most dogs can be maintained without signs of toxicity on alternate-day therapy.

Miniature Schnauzers are one of the breeds that may be predisposed to **food allergy**[8] and to **inhalant allergies.**[9] Some have reproductive problems with **pseudo-hermaphroditism, cryptorchidism** and **Sertoli cell neoplasia.**[10] Another reported problem is **sinoatrial syncope**, with accompanying fainting and nausea.[11]

Muscular dystrophy is a rare x-linked recessive disease that has been identified in the breed.[12]

A serious problem of the breed is **esophageal achalasia.**[13] It is suspected to have familial ties and is sometimes successfully treated by stomach tubes and special feeding. **Primary megaesophagus** has been determined to be an hereditary disease in Miniature Schnauzers.[14] **Pulmonic stenosis** is found in Miniature Schnauzers.[15]

In a clinical study the results indicate that the **hyperlipidemia** of Miniature Schnauzers is due to a familial disorder resulting in delayed clearance of triglyceride-rich lipoproteins from the circulation.[16] Miniature Schnauzers have been identified as the breed most likely to have **high cholesterol and triglycerides**. Medication and dietary modifications should be used to lower the risk of **diabetes** and/or acute **pancreatitis**, common life-threatening sequelae to these diseases in dogs.[17] Clinical experience dictates a high index of suspicion for acute pancreatitis when any older Miniature Schnauzer is vomiting and has an elevated temperature.[18] **Seizures** have been reported to be associated with elevated triglycerides and a diagnosis of **idiopathic hyperlipoproteinemia.**[19,20]

Some Miniature Schnauzers carry a recessive gene for a hereditary congenital juvenile **cataract**.[21] When affected, this particular type of cataract is always found bilaterally and in eyes that are smaller than normal and usually slightly elliptical in shape. Breed clubs, including the American Schnauzer Club, are actively attempting to eliminate the condition. They recommend slit-lamp examination of all litters to determine if any puppies are affected. Test breed the parents and eliminate sires and bitches carrying the gene.

Progressive Retinal Atrophy has been reported in the breed.[22] **Microphthalmia** has also been reported in Miniature Schnauzers.[23] **Legg-Perthes** disease[25] occurs in the breed. This aseptic necrosis of the femoral head results from the lack of blood supply. Certain families show a high incidence of the disease. A specific genetic factor has not been proved. The use of such animals for breeding is not suggested.

Von Willebrand's Disease (VWD)[6] has been described in Miniature Schnauzers. Affected dogs exhibit mild to severe bleeding diathesis (tendency to leak blood from vessels), recurrent shifting lameness with radiographic changes similar to eosinophilia panosteitis hematuria, recurrent stress-induced diarrhea, melena (dark stools), chronic serosanguineous otitis externa, prolonged estrual and postpartum bleeding and subcutaneous hematomas.

Atherosclerosis[24] was diagnosed Postmortem in 21 dogs between 1970 and 1983. Nine dogs had died and 12 were destroyed because of complications associated with the disease. The mean age was 8.5± 0.5 years; 18 dogs were male. Schnauzers were one of three breeds that had a higher prevalence of the disease than other breeds. Common clinical signs were lethargy, anorexia, weakness, dyspnoea, collapse and vomiting. Hypercholesterolemia, lipidemia and hypothyroidism were common in affected dogs tested, and protein electrophoresis revealed high values for alpha 2 and beta fractions in all dogs tested. ECG indicated conduction abnormalities and myocardial infarction in three of seven dogs. Affected arteries (including coronary, myocardial, renal, carotid, thyroidal, intestinal, pancreatic, splenic, gastric, prostatic and mesenteric) were yellow-white, thick and nodular and had narrow lumens. Myocardial fibrosis and infarction also were observed in the myocardium. Histologically affected arterial walls contained foamy cells or vacules, cystic spaces, mineralized material, debris with or without eroded intima, and degenerated muscle cells.[25]

A study reports an increased incidence of **spinaliomas** in Schnauzers.[26]

BEHAVIOR

The Miniature Schnauzer is a lively and energetic companion. He is lovable and easily trained. He needs frequent grooming and is a barker.

OLD AGE

The Miniature Schnauzer makes an ideal pet, even into its later years. It should remain active for 12 to 13 years.

References

1. Bovee, K.C. and McGuire, T. "Qualitative and Quantitative Analysis of Uroliths in Dogs:Definitive Determination of Chemical Type," *JAVMA*; 1984: 185: 9, 983-987; 18 ref.

2. Morton, L.D., Sanecki, R.K., Gordon, D.E., Sopiarz, R.L., Bell, J.S., and Sakas, P.S. "Juvenile Renal Disease in Miniature Schnauzer Dogs," *Vet. Path.*; 1990: 27:6, 455-458; 13 ref.

3. Meyers-Wallen, V.N., Donahoe, P.K., Ueno, S., Manganaro, T.F., and Patterson, D.F. "Mullerian Inhibiting Substance is Present in Testes of Dogs With Persistent Mullerian Duct Syndrome," *Biology of Reproduction*; 1989: 41:5, 881-889; 47 ref.

4. Hesse, A. and Bruhl, M. "Urolithiasis in Dogs: Epidemiological Data and Analysis of Urinary Calculi," *Kleintierpraxis*; 1990: 35:10, 505-512; 18 ref.

5. Osborne, C.A., Clinton, C.W., Bamman, L.K., Moran, H.C., Coston, B.R., and Frost, A.P. "Prevalence of Canine Uroliths: Minnesota Urolith Center," *Vet. Clinics of N. Amer, Sm. Anim. Prac.*; 1986: 16:1, 27-44; 6 ref.

6. Bovee, K.C. and McGuire, T. "Qualitative and Quantitative Analysis of Uroliths in Dogs: Definitive Determination of Chemical Type," *JAVMA;* 1984: 185:9, 983-987; 18 ref.

7. Mueller, G.H. and Kirk, R.W. "Small Animal Dermatology: Breed Predilection of Skin Disease," (W. B. Saunders, Philadelphia, PA 1976); 137.

8. Werner, A. "Aspects of Food and Food Supplements in Skin Disease," *Pedigree Breeder Forum*; 1993: Vol.2, #1.

9. Ackerman, Lowell, DVM, "Allergic Skin Diseases," *American Kennel Club Gazette*; September, 1990.

10. Brown, T.T., et al: "Male Hermaphroditism, Cryptorchidism, and Sertoli Cell Neoplasia in Three Miniature Schnauzers," *JAVMA;* 1976: 169 (8):821-825.

11. Hamlin, R.I., et al: "Sinoatrial Syncope in Miniature Schnauzers," *JAVMA;* 1972: 161 (9):1022-1028.

12. Bell, Jerold S. DVM "Sex Related Genetic Diseases: Did Mama Cause Them?" *American Kennel Club Gazette*, Feb. 1994; 75

13. Clifford, D.H., et al: "Management of Esophageal Achalasia in Miniature Schnauzers," *JAVMA;* 1972: 161 (9):1012-1020.

14. Kern, Maryanne, DVM, "Diseases of the Esophagus," *The American Kennel Club Gazette*; January, 1993.

15. Patterson, D.F. "Epidemiology and Genetic Studies of Congenital Heart Diseases in the Dog," *Cir. Research;* 1968: 23: 171-202.

16. Whitney, M.S. "Identification and Characterization of a Familial Hyperlipoproteinemia in Miniature Schnauzer Dogs," 1987: 48: 1, 65.

17. Veterinary News, *The American Kennel Club Gazette*; October, 1991.

18. Griffin, C., Kowchka, K., and McDonald, J. *Current Veterinary Dermatology, the Science and Art of Therapy. Mosby Yearbook*; St. Louis, MO. 1993: 186.

19. Bodkin, K. "Seizures Associated With Hyperlipoproteinemia in a Miniature Schnauzer," *Canine Practice*; 1992: 17:1,11-15;6 ref.

20. Richaardson, M. "Idiopathic Hyperlipoproteinemia in a Miniature Schnauzer," *Companion Animal Practice*; 1989: 19:4-5, 33-37; 3 ref.

21. Rubin, L.F., et al: "Hereditary Cataracts in Miniature Schnauzers," *JAVMA;* 1969: 154 (11): 1456-1458.

22. Parshall, C.J., Wyman, M., Nitroy, S., Acland, G., and Aguirre, G. "Photoreceptor Dysplasia: An Inherited Progressive Retinal Atrophy of Miniature Schnauzer Dogs," *Progress in Vet and Comp. Ophthalmology*; 1991: 1:3, 187-203; 21 ref.

23. Barnett, K.C. "Inherited Eye Disease in the Dog and Cat," *J. of Sm. Anim. Prac.*; 1988: 29:7, 462-475; 33 ref.

24. Foley, C.W., et al: "Abnormalities of Companion Animals," Iowa State University Press, Ames, Ia., 1979: 43.

25. Liu, S.K., Tilley, L.P., Tappe, J.P., and Fox, P.R. "Clinical and Pathologic Findings in Dogs with Atherosclerosis: 21 cases," *JAVMA*; 1986: 189:1, 227-232; 33 ref.

26. Halouzka, R. and Nechvatal, M. "Unusual Incidence of Spinaliomas in Schnauzers," *Veterinarni Medicina*; 1990: 35: 1, 49-56; 6 ref.

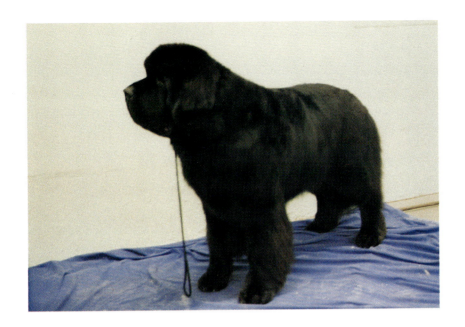

NEWFOUNDLAND

ORIGIN AND HISTORY

Developed on the island of Newfoundland, the Newfoundland is believed to be a descendant of native Indian and wild dogs. These dogs were then interbred with dogs brought to the island by Viking settlers. Newfoundlands became well-known in the 18th century, when they were carried on most ships as lifeguards.

DESCRIPTION

The Newfoundland is a large, powerful dog, ranging from 100 to 180 pounds. They have a thick double coat; a soft and dense undercoat and a longer water-resistant outercoat. They are generally black, but black and white (Landseer) and bronze and gray do occur. The breed is gentle and demonstrates extreme loyalty. They instinctively protect their masters without being overly aggressive. They are constantly on watch around children, trying to keep them from harm.

THE SHOW RING

Average height for adult dogs is 28 inches, for adult bitches, 26 inches. Approximate weight of adult dogs ranges from 130 to 150 pounds, adult bitches from 100 to 120 pounds.

Any sign of vicious behavior is a serious fault. Excessive shyness is also a fault as are yellow eyes, over or undershot bite, narrow skull and "snipy" or pointed muzzle. **Any colors or combination of colors not specifically described in the Standard will disqualify the dog from the show ring.**

BREEDING AND WHELPING

A bitch may show she is pregnant about 35 days after breeding. If she has a small litter, she may not show until late in the gestation period. With a large litter the whelping time may be as long as 24 hours and this may cause problems with the last puppies. These puppies may be born in a weakened condition (even stillborn) or the bitch may retain one or more placentas. Some bitches are not careful with their puppies. They can crush or smother them with their bodies. The average litter contains eight puppies, ranging in size from 3/4 to 2 pounds. The average size for a puppy is 1 1/2 pounds. Puppies should be checked for deformities. If rear dewclaws are present they should be removed. Growth rates vary but an average has been established. (Chart)

DENTITION

The Newfoundland should have a level or scissors bite. Teeth are generally small. **Undershot** bites and crooked teeth are common.

RECOGNIZED PROBLEMS

Acute gastric dilatation (bloat) and **gastric torsion** are problems due to the deep chest and general conformation of the breed. Vigorous exercise immediately after eating could be a contributing factor and should be avoided.

Another source of trouble is the Newfoundland's heavy, water-resistant coat. Cooling is of prime importance in hot climates. This breed should be observed closely when there is a danger of **heat stroke**. Their black color absorbs the heat and contributes to the problem.

Elbow dysplasia has been described in the breed.[1] The heavy coat is also a factor in the development of **acute focal moist dermatitis (hot spots)**. These should be cleansed and treated as soon as detected to avoid spreading. Among 30 Newfoundland dogs in which Type 1 **allergic dermatitis** was diagnosed, **hypothyroidism** was found in 14. The association of the two conditions was partly confirmed by the success of combined prednisone and triiodothyronine treatment. Most cases were young, possibly showing a hereditary disposition.[2]

In a study of the records of 4,489 dysplastic dogs, prevalence was highest in Newfoundlands (29.4%). Prevalence of dysplasia was similar in males and females, indicating no sex predilection for hip dysplasia.[3] Of 584 Newfoundlands x-rayed in Norway between 1972 and 1984, 38% were dysplastic.[4]

Ectopic ureter was diagnosed in 228 dogs. The female to male ratio was 217:11. Six breeds were diagnosed with greater frequency of diagnosis than expected, including Newfoundlands.[5]

Newfoundlands have been reported to be at significantly higher risk of having **pemphigus foliaceous**.[6] (see Akita) **Subaortic stenosis** and **eversion of the nictitating membrane** have been reported in Newfoundlands. Many of the everyday problems seen with Newfoundlands are manmade. In order to be healthy individuals, these dogs need daily attention, especially grooming and exercising. Removal of hair mats and foreign particles is very important. Prospective owners should be aware of the need for a large physical facility for handling this breed.

A WORD OF CAUTION: when administering a tranquilizer or anesthetic to a Newfoundland, be very careful of dosage. Some Newfoundlands require much smaller dosages than the recommended amounts. Large amounts can be fatal.

BEHAVIOR

The Newfoundland is a gentle, lovable pet that gets along with everyone. He loves children and other animals. He is a good guard dog. His devotion to his master is so unswerving that he hates to be separated, and a change of owners is very difficult.

AVERAGE GROWTH RATE	
Age	**Weight (Pounds)**
Birth	1 1/4
1 wk	2
2 wks	3
4 wks	10
8 wks	15
3 mo	40-50
6 mo	75-80
9 mo	100

OLD AGE

Average life span of the Newfoundland is 8 to 10 years. Older dogs seem to enjoy the water and continued activity.

References

1. "Veterinary News," *American Kennel Club Gazette*; June, 1990.
2. Kristensen, F. "Concurrent Hypothyroidism and Allergic Dermatitis, Type 1, in Dogs," *Dansk Veterinaertidsskrift*; 1989: 72:16, 939-941;5 ref.
3. Keller, G.G. and Corley, E.A. "Canine Hip Dysplasia: Investigating the Sex Predilection and the Frequency of Unilateral CHD," *Vet. Med.*; 1989: 84:12, 1162, 1164-1166; 13 ref.
4. Lingaas, F. and Heim, P. "A Genetic Investigation of the Incidence of Hip Dysplasia in Norwegian Dog Breeds," *Norsk-Veterinaertidsskrift*; 1987: 99:9, 617-623; 22 ref.
5. Hayes, J.M., Jr., "Breed Associations of Canine Ectopic Ureters: A Study of 217 female Cases," *J. Sm. Anim.Prac.*; 1984: 25:8, 501-504; 12 ref.
6. Ihrke, P.J., Stannard, A.A., Ardans, A.A., and Griffin, C.E. "Pemphigus Foliaceous in Dogs: A Review of 37 Cases," *JAVMA*; 1985: 186:1, 59-66; 58 ref.

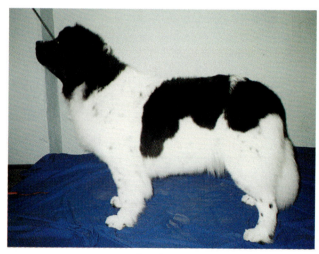

Landseer

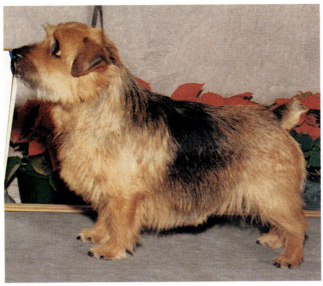
Norfolk Terrier

NORFOLK AND NORWICH TERRIER

ORIGIN AND HISTORY

Norwich Terriers were introduced in England in 1880 and soon became the pets of students at Cambridge University. After World War I, several were brought to America and bred by the Cheshire Hunt in Philadelphia. They make excellent ratters, rabbit dogs and ideal house dogs as their hard, close coat does not collect dirt. The Norwich Terrier, first recognized by the American Kennel Club in 1936, is now a well-established breed. In England and America the breed is divided by ear carriage into two breeds: The Norwich (Prick Ear) and the Norfolk (Drop Ear).

DESCRIPTION

Small, low, rugged terriers with stamina and spirit, they may be red, black and tan or grizzle in color. Their legs are short and powerful with sound bone. Their harsh, wiry coats need regular grooming, and when completely blown may be stripped with a small stripping comb, but never clipped or shaped. Both varieties go to ground and are good ratters.

These breeds, unspoiled and vigorous, good tempered and gregarious, have proved adaptable under a wide variety of conditions. Tails should be medium docked and dewclaws removed at 3 to 5 days. The tail, according to the story, should be long enough for a man to grasp and pull the dog out of a hole. This translates to removal of slightly more than half the tail.

THE SHOW RING

The Norwich Terrier has sensitive prick ears and a slightly foxy expression. The ideal height should not exceed 10 inches at the withers and the ideal weight is approximately 12 pounds. The Norwich is an approximately square dog. The Norfolk Terrier has expressive dropped ears. The height at the withers is 9 to 10 inches and the weight should be 11 to 12 pounds for a male. Bitches tend to be smaller than dogs. Length of back from point of withers to base of tail should be slightly longer than the height at the withers. Eyes should be bright and dark, not light or protruding. Their jaws, clean and strong, should have the ideal scissors bite. A mouth badly over or undershot is penalized in either variety.[1,2]

There are no breed disqualifications.

BREEDING AND WHELPING

Because of their short legs and conformation, some individuals may require help in mating. Again, because of size, assistance may be required during whelping. An occasional stillborn puppy occurs, but the cause is unknown.

Bitches are usually bred at their second or third seasons. Time of ovulation and breeding seems to be between the 9th and 13th day, depending upon the individual. The normal litter is three to four. At birth the average weight is 5 ounces. At 2 months they should weigh 3 pounds; at 3 months, 5 pounds; and at 6 months, 10 pounds.

RECOGNIZED PROBLEMS

Norwich and Norfolk Terriers are extremely healthy breeds. Some individuals are prone to **skin problems** in hot weather, the so-called **"summer eczema."** This is usually a flea bite allergy or allergic reaction to some antigen (foreign protein) in their environment. The incidence parallels other breeds. Insecticide dips stimulate acute moist dermatitis in some dogs.

BEHAVIOR

Active keen dogs, these Terriers are excellent family pets. Besides hunting, their greatest joy in life is to please their family.[3] They are good watch dogs and require little grooming.

OLD AGE

Life span is 13 to 14 years, and death can be due to any of many old-age problems, with no single cause.

References

1. *Complete Dog Book*, The American Kennel Club (Howell Book House, New York, NY. 1992); 389-394.
2. Larrabee and Read, (Eds.);*Norwich Terriers U.S.A.*, 1936-1966
3. Fournier, B,S, *How to Raise and Train a Norwich Terrier.*

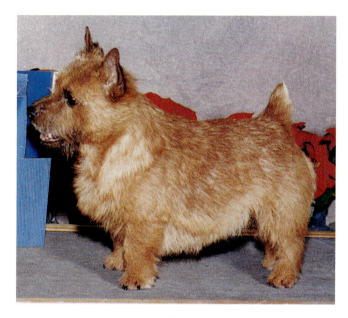

Norwich Terrier

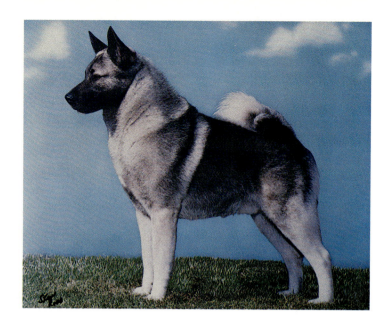

NORWEGIAN ELKHOUND

ORIGIN AND HISTORY

Skeletal remains notably similar to today's Norwegian Elkhound have been dated as early as the Stone Age by archaeologists. Scandinavians refer to the Elkhound throughout their history. The first record of the Norwegian Elkhound in the United States is in a 1913 AKC Stud Book. This great northern hunting dog was placed in the hound group in the United States because of a mistranslation of its name, *Elg hund*, which literally means "moose dog."[1]

DESCRIPTION

Norwegian Elkhounds are friendly, bold and energetic. They are effective guardians, with great dignity, poise and independence. They are independent scent hunters and were bred to have the stamina and agility to survive for days in harsh terrain and weather.

THE SHOW RING

Elkhounds are medium-sized dogs. They are balanced within their square profiles. They look short-backed and short-coupled because of a rather long rib cage and a short loin. Their strong, straight back slopes only slightly from the withers to the root of the tail.[2] Their height at the withers should be 20 1/2 inches for dogs and 19 1/2 inches for bitches. Adult dogs should weigh about 55 pounds and bitches should weigh about 48 pounds.[3]

The breed's black prick ears of good leather are high-set and very mobile. The head is broad and wedge-shaped, with a black, medium-length muzzle that tapers to a blunt nose. The stop is clearly defined, and the nose is straight. The male head must appear strong and masculine. The bitch may have a more feminine appearance, without being refined.[2] Their calm, friendly eyes are oval and dark brown, and should not protrude.

Their distinctive, smooth-lying gray coat has a dense, woolly undercoat and coarse, black-tipped covering hair. This coat allows them to withstand the coldest weather. The coat is longest on the back of the neck, buttocks and underside of the tightly curled tail. The tail sits high and is centered on the back. The coat should not be altered by trimming, clipping or any other artificial treatment. Whisker trimming is optional.[3]

The only disqualification is any solid overall color other than gray, such as red, brown, black or white.[3]

Norwegian Elkhounds should have no dewclaws on their back legs. Their paws are comparatively small and oval, with tightly closed toes and thick pads. The pasterns should be strong and not knuckled over, and the feet should turn neither in nor out.

BREEDING AND WHELPING

Norwegian Elkhound bitches normally come into estrus every six months, usually beginning at 6 to 10 months. Estrus lasts three weeks. Many breeders attempt to breed on the 10th day, although bitches vary as to when they will accept the dog. Generally it is better to wait until the bitch's third season to breed, since bitches mature between 1 1/2 and 2 years old. Dogs mature as late as 2 1/2 years. Norwegian Elkhounds have no unique problems in breeding and whelping. Many bitches whelp in a squatting position and lie down between births.

Litter size ranges from one to 12 puppies, averaging seven or eight. Some bitches consistently whelp large litters, while others whelp litters of varying sizes. Puppies average 10 to 12 ounces at birth. In a small litter, puppies may weigh a pound. In a large litter, 5 to 6 ounces is not an uncommon birth weight (Figure 1).

Norwegian Elkhound puppies are born black or, occasionally, dark gray. Many puppies have white tips on their feet or a small white streak on their chests. In a week or so, the puppies' coats fur out and begin to change to their characteristic gray color.

Any dewclaws on the hind legs should be removed soon after birth. The breed has no common defects that are discernible at birth.

DENTITION

The correct bite for Norwegian Elkhounds is a scissors bite. **Overshot** and **undershot** bites and missing teeth are undesirable. As in many breeds, level or undershot bites in puppies tend to worsen as the puppy grows. Since jaw structure is hereditary, animals with undesirable bites should not be bred.

RECOGNIZED PROBLEMS

The Norwegian Elkhound is generally a healthy dog. Given a balanced diet, fresh water and exercise, it tends to lead a long, healthful life.

Because of their dense coats, Norwegian Elkhounds are often plagued with **"hot spots" (moist dermatitis)**. The cause is controversial. Treatment consists of the elimination of external parasites which may incite itching, cleaning the area with hydrogen peroxide (mixing one part hydrogen peroxide to 10 parts water), applying some soothing ointment or lotion, and systemic treatment to overcome pruritus. Clipping hair from the area should be avoided. The new growth of covering hair is quite often darker in color in the affected area.

Subcutaneous cysts have been observed in Norwegian Elkhounds. These may be single or multiple. They move freely and are not painful. No treatment is necessary; however, they must be differentiated from cancerous or precancerous lesions. Such lesions are usually indurated and extend into the surrounding tissue. An excisional biopsy may be necessary to establish a diagnosis in a suspected lesion. **Keratoacanthoma** has been reported.[4]

Generalized **progressive retinal atrophy** is found in the breed. Progressive deterioration of the retina occurs as a recessive Mendelian trait.[1,3,5,6,7,8,9,10] **Cataracts** are also found.[11] A recent study concluded that there were eight breeds at higher risk of developing **glaucoma** than mixed-breed dogs.[12] The Norwegian Elkhound was one of these breeds.

There are reported cases of **drug sensitivities** but none occurring with regularity in Norwegian Elkhounds. **Seborrhea (flaky skin)** and dry coat do occur but they can usually be corrected by diet. The inclusion of unsaturated fatty acids and oil soluble vitamins augment an otherwise balanced diet and aid return of the skin to normal.

Norwegian Elkhounds are listed as having **renal cortical hypoplasia**. Signs of hypoplasia, with uremia and later, parathyroidism, begin at about one year.[13,14,15,16]

Many Elkhounds have a tendency to be overweight. Their metabolism is such that conversion of foods to fat and protein is very efficient. Therefore, intake of a balanced dog food must be limited, depending on the individual and the amount of exercise it receives. Vitamin supplement should be administered, especially for dogs receiving a limited portion of dog food.

BEHAVIOR

The Norwegian Elkhound makes a good family pet, although he adapts more readily to country life than to city dwelling. He is territorial and rarely wanders away. He is independent, affectionate, intelligent, clean and likes children.

OLD AGE

Many Norwegian Elkhounds live to 13 or 14 years of age. **Kidney conditions**, such as **interstitial nephritis**, often lead to death in the aged dog.

GROWTH CHART* (Figure 1)							
Litter Size	**Weeks of age: Birth**	**1**	**2**	**3**	**4**	**6**	**12**
1	1 LB 2 OZ	2 LB 2 OZ	3 LB 8 OZ	5 LB	6 LB	9 LB	20 LB
7	1 LB TO 1 LB 3 OZ	1 LB 4 OZ TO 2 LB 1 OZ	1 LB 8 OZ TO 2 LB 7 OZ	2 LB TO 3 LB	2 LB 10 OZ TO 3 LB 12 OZ	5 LB 4 OZ TO 7 LB	15 LB TO 16 LB
10	8 OZ TO 10 OZ	1 LB TO 2 LB 4 OZ	1 LB 1 OZ TO 2 LB 4 OZ	1 LB 13 OZ TO 3 LB	2 LB 10 OZ TO 4 LB 3 OZ	5 LB 8 OZ TO 7 LB 14 OZ	14 LB TO 17 LB

*The above are the actual weights of a small, average and large litter of Norwegian Elkhound puppies.

References

1. Wallo, Olav *The Complete Norwegian Elkhound*. (Howell Book House, Inc. New York, NY, 1970).
2. The Norwegian Elkhound Association of America: Interpretive Comments on the Norwegian Elkhound and the Standard, 1976.
3. *The Complete Dog Book*, The American Kennel Club: (Howell Book House, 18th ed. 1992); 199-202.
4. "A Catalogue of Congenital and Hereditary Disorders"
5. Cogan, D.C. "Kuwabara: Photosensitive Abiotrophy of the Retina in the Elkhound," *Path. Vet.*; 1965: 2:101-128.
6. Kirk, R.W. and Bistner, S.I. *Handbook of Veterinary Procedures and Emergency Treatment: Hereditary Defects in Dogs*. 1975: Table 124, 661.
7. Barnett, K.C. "Abnormalities and Defects in Pedigree Dogs, IV: Progressive Retinal Atro-

phy," *J. Sm. Anim. Prac.;* 4: 465-467.

8.   Barnett, K.C. "Canine Retinopathies III: The Other Breeds," *J. Sm. Anim. Prac.*; 1965: 6: 185-196.

9.   Barnett, K.C. "Genetic Anomalies of the Posterior Segment of the Canine Eye," *J. Sm. Anim. Prac.*; 10: 451-455.

10. Aguirre, C.D. and Rubin, L.F. "Progressive Retinal Atrophy (Rod Dysplasia) in the Norwegian Elkhound," *JAVMA;* 158:208-218.

11. Barnett, K.C. "Inherited Eye Disease in the Dog and Cat," 1988 29:7, 462-475; 33 ref.

12. Slater, M.R. and Erb, H.N. "Effects of Risk Factors and Prophylactic Treatment on Primary Glaucoma in the Dog," *JAVMA*; 1986: 188:9, 1028-1030; 7 ref.

13. Finco, D.R. "Congenital and Inherited Renal Disease," *JAAHA;* 1973: 9:301-303.

14. Finco, D.R., et al: "Familial Renal Disease in Norwegian Elkhounds," *JAVMA;* 156: 747-760.

15. Finco, D.R. "Familial Renal Disease in Norwegian Elkhound Dogs: Physiologic and Biochemical Examinations," *Am. J. Vet. Res.*; 37: 87-91.

16. Picut, C.A. and Leis, R.M. "Comparative Pathology of Canine Hereditary Nephropathies: An Interpretive Review," *Vet. Res. Comm.;* 1987: 11: 6, 561-581; 91 ref.

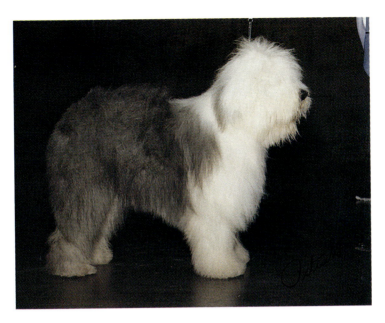

OLD ENGLISH SHEEPDOG

ORIGIN AND HISTORY

Although the origin of the Old English Sheepdog has conflicting records, it is clear they appeared about 200 years ago in England in Devon and Somerset. These bobtailed driving dogs make good house dogs, as has been found since their introduction to the United States.

DESCRIPTION

With its characteristic shuffling gait, the Old English Sheepdog presents an appearance of casual friendliness that reflects its true disposition. A soft-mouthed, adaptable dog, it is ideal as a family pet. The breed is noted for clownish antics, protectiveness and a deep-seated herding instinct. They are profusely coated, thick-set, muscular dogs with intelligent expressions.

The Old English Sheepdog is presently gaining great popularity in this country. The breed should be treated as part of the family, never kenneled alone.

A common belief that the head coat or fall covering the eyes prevents blindness is not true. The fall protects a dog's eyes while working in the fields, but the fall may be removed or brushed back without harming the eyes.

THE SHOW RING

The adult is best described by the Standard as a strong, compact-looking dog of great symmetry. The ideal dog is practically the same in measurement from shoulder to hip as in height. It is absolutely free from legginess or weaselness, and is elastic in its gallop. In walking or trotting it has a characteristic ambling or pacing movement. Its bark should be loud with a distinctive "pot-casse" ring to it. It should be free from Poodle or Deerhound characteristics. Soundness should be considered most important.

Major faults are yellowish brown eyes, narrow head, slab side, long body and brown coat. The mahogany-tipped puppy coat and young adult coat with mahogany shading at the hocks and elbows is a sunburned coat and does not indicate an adult brown coat. Examination at the base coat reveals the black, blue or gray coat.

BREEDING AND WHELPING

The pregnant Old English Sheepdog bitch should maintain her usual activity, but she should avoid hard exercise. A veterinarian should be consulted for information on diet or supplements. She will probably need smaller but more frequent meals toward the end of her gestation.

Puppies usually weigh 10 to 16 ounces. They are black and white with little or no pigmentation of the nose. Freckling of the nose will begin within 2 to 3 days after birth with complete pigmentation varying from 6 weeks to 1 1/2 years. Eyelid pigmentation is not considered important, but many prefer black eyelids to complete the expression.

GROWTH

Whelps are born with a white-tipped tail that must be docked at 2 to 3 days, depending upon size and strength of the puppy. All dewclaws are removed at the same time. THE TAIL SHOULD BE AMPUTATED AS CLOSE TO THE BODY AS POSSIBLE. The tail is washed with a disinfectant but not shaved. No anesthesia is necessary. A straight pair of scissors is used. The scissors are placed approximately 1/8 inch behind the cutaneous zone of the rectum and angled about 30 degrees in an anterior direction. Two horizontal mattress sutures are placed to approximate the skin edges and to control hemorrhage. The rectococcygeal muscle is severed in this procedure; if it is not, the tail will be too long.

Eyes will open at 12 to 14 days. Blue eyes are not uncommon, and often there is one blue eye and one steel gray eye which will turn dark brown. Dark eyes are usually preferred to blue eyes. The puppy will begin responding to loud noises about the 15th to 17th day.

In selecting a puppy, choose the square, solid, big-boned puppy with a large, square head and a big black nose.

It should have straight front legs that do not toe in or out and they should not be cowhocked. It should not be close or weak in the rear. Color markings are a matter of individual preference.

DENTITION

A level bite is ideal. **Overshot** and **undershot** are distinct faults. Often, the two mandibular central incisors are labial to the maxillary incisors while the remaining teeth will remain level in position.

RECOGNIZED PROBLEMS

The Old English Sheepdog is subject to **ear infections.** Hair must be cleaned from inside the ear.

The Old English is also one of the breeds reported with **congenital deafness.**[1]

Excessive intake of water can produce loose stools in older dogs and diarrhea in puppies. **Hip dysplasia** is a severe problem. OFA reports that hip dysplasia regressed linearly in Old English from 1974 to 1984.[2] In Norway 35% of 305 Old English x-rayed between 1972-1984 were dysplastic.[3]

Recently, **juvenile cataracts (bilateral)** have been reported, and **retinal detachment** is a problem.[4,5] Cases of **inverted eyelids (entropion)** have been reported.

Prepubertal vaginitis is commonly seen in puppies; usually no treatment is required as the condition clears spontaneously following the bitch's first estrous cycle. The breed has a higher incidence of **cryptorchidism** than most.[6]

Old English Sheepdogs are prone to **bloat.**[7]

Cervical vertebral deformity[8] **(wobbler syndrome)** has been described in Old English Sheepdogs. Clinical signs may progress from partial **paraplegia** to total **quadriplegia.** Signs usually first occur between 3 and 12 months of age. Hind legs are affected, followed in some dogs by the fore limbs. Rear limb incoordination, hypermetria (a prancing gait) or dragging of the feet may occur.

Mitochondrial myopathy, a disease causing exercise intolerance, has recently been diagnosed in two Old English. Mode of inheritance and treatment are unknown.[9]

Immune mediated **hemolytic anemia** has been reported.[10]

Coat problems usually develop at around 1 to 1 1/2 years of age. Particular care must be given the areas around the ears, neck, chest and legs that rub the body. Hair between the pads should be removed to prevent mud balls. Rear end and coat should be kept clean. **Demodicosis** has been reported in Old English.[11]

Old English Sheepdogs are seen with **ciliary dyskenesia.** These dogs will have recurring pneumonia, a nasal discharge and a productive cough.[12]

BEHAVIOR

Old English are very active and love to play with children. They are protective of their own and make excellent guard dogs. They require frequent grooming if they are to be house dogs.

OLD AGE

The Old English Sheepdog usually lives from 10 to 15 years.

References

1. Strain, George M. "Deafness in Dogs and Cats," *Proc. 10th ACVIM Forum*, May, 1992.
2. Corley, E.A. and Hogan, P.M. "Trends in Hip Dysplasia Control: Analysis of Radiographs Submitted to the Orthopedic Foundation for Animals, 1974 to 1984," *JAVMA;* 1985: 187:8, 805-809; 8 ref.
3. Lingaas, F. and Heim, P. "A Genetic Investigation of the Incidence of Hip Dysplasia in Norwegian Dog Breeds," *Norsk-Veterinaertidsskrift;* 1987: 99:9, 617-623; 22 ref.
4. Koch, S.A. "Cataracts in Interrelated Old English Sheepdogs," *JAVMA;* 1972: 160(3):299-301.
5. Koch, W. "Neue Pathogene Erbfaktoren Bei Hunden," *Z. Indukt. Astamm u-Vererb L;* 1935: 70:503-506.
6. Bell, Jerold S. DVM "Sex Related Genetic Diseases: Did Mama Cause Them?" *The American Kennel Club Gazette*, Feb. 1994; 76.
7. Old English column, *The American Kennel Club Gazette;* April, 1991.
8. Foley, J.F., et al: "Abnormalities of Companion Animals," Iowa State University Press, Ames, IA,1979: 1935.
9. *JAVMA;* Vol. 201, #5, September 1, 1992.
10. Ettinger, S.J. *Textbook of Veterinary Internal Medicine, Diseases of the Dog and Cat.* (W.B. Saunders Co. Philadelphia, PA 1989); 92.
11. Scott, D.W. and Paradis, M. "A Survey of Canine and Feline Disorders Seen in a University Practice," *Small Animal Clinic, University of Montreal, Saint-Hyacinthe, Quebec,* (1987-88) 50 ref.
12. King, L.G., DVM "Respiratory Congenital Disorders." Western Veterinary Conference. Feb.1994.

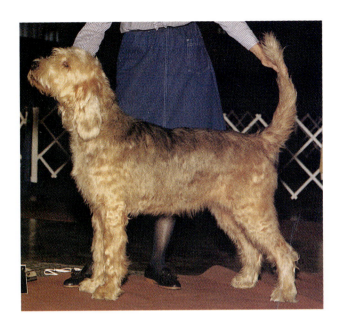

OTTER HOUND

ORIGIN AND HISTORY

This "bloodhound in sheep's clothing," the Otter Hound, is an unusually appealing breed. A hardy fellow, he celebrates cold, wet weather and voices his approval in a deep bass bay. He is rare in both England and America. Appearing in America in 1900, the Otter Hound was mentioned in the time of King John, who reigned in England from 1199 to 1216.

DESCRIPTION

Otter Hounds are amiable, boisterous and gregarious. They usually get along well with other dogs. They are remarkably gentle with puppies and children. They are extremely vocal, often rumbling and growling. Their noises signify pleasure or displeasure, according to the individual. Their bay is loud and can be heard for a mile or more.

THE SHOW RING

The Otter Hound male should weigh 75 to 115 pounds, and stand from 24 to 27 inches tall at the withers. Bitches should weigh between 65 to 100 pounds and stand from 23 to 26 inches tall at the withers. All colors are equally acceptable. Coat color changes greatly during the life of an individual hound. Black and tan, grizzle and red dogs often appear black at birth;

the tan usually appears within 2 weeks and increases with age. Liver or liver and tan are easily distinguished at birth. Puppies that carry a white spotting gene usually show some white at birth, but the white may be obscured in the adult by the length and general lightening of the coat. Tricolor puppies may darken with increasing age and appear grizzle as adults. Dark colors often lighten with age; many older Otter Hounds look blond or gray. A double coat consisting of a harsh outer coat and a woolly undercoat is an important breed characteristic.

The breed Standard does not specify any disqualifying faults.

BREEDING AND WHELPING

Otter Hounds show the usual variation in estrus and gestation. Pregnancy can be difficult to detect by palpation, and false pregnancies occur. The average litter is seven to 10 puppies. Litters as small as one puppy or as large as 13 have been observed.

Otter Hounds normally weigh about one pound at birth. At 1 month they weigh about 6 pounds. Puppies should be chosen for breeding or show according to general soundness.

Puppy color at about 1 month is usually a better indication of color genotype than adult color. Dogs carrying white spotting genes may have incomplete nose pigment, but the pigment is usually complete by maturity (1 1/2 to 2 years).

DENTITION

A scissors or **overshot** bite is preferable to an **undershot** bite. Full dentition is usual, but improperly undershot and overshot bites are common. Overshot bites often correct to a scissors bite, but a bite that becomes undershot after the permanent teeth are in usually remains so. Bites may go undershot as late as 6 to 8 months. Changes in bite can occur until a dog matures, at about 18 months.

RECOGNIZED PROBLEMS

Almost all Otter Hounds show radiographic evidence of **hip dysplasia**, but few show clinical symptoms. All breeding stock should be x-rayed and the condition of the hips considered along with all other faults and virtues in choosing a mate. OFA has reported **elbow dysplasia** in this breed.[1]

Canine thrombocytopathy is a congenital blood platelet defect carried as an incomplete dominant autosomal trait.[1,2] Both homozygotes and heterozygotes can be identified by blood testing. At one time the gene frequency of this defect was extremely high in Otter Hounds. A blood testing program and the elimination of affected hounds from breeding programs have greatly reduced the gene frequency. It is important that all Otter Hound puppies be blood tested when they reach 10 pounds at 7 or 8 weeks old. Antibiotics, vermicides and

394

inoculations should not be administered within a week to ten days before blood testing.[3]

When facilities for blood testing are not readily accessible, the following screen test may be performed.

Draw 1/2 ml fresh blood into a plastic syringe containing 4.5 ml cold buffered saline. Mix. Place 2 ml of this mixture into each of two small (10 x 75 mm) glass test tubes containing 1 unit bovine thrombin. Topical thrombin (Parke-Davis) 1000 N.I.H. units per vial. Add 10 ml saline to vial (=100 units/ml of solution). Freeze this solution in 1 ml lots. Put 0.1 ml in each glass tube for above test, i.e., 0.1 contains 1 unit thrombin. Remaining 9 ml or concentrated (100 U/ml) thrombin is frozen in 1 ml lots in small plastic tubes to be diluted and used as needed. Mix. Place the mix in an ice bath or a refrigerator for 30 minutes, then transfer the mix to a water bath or an incubator at 37°C for 1 hour. Record retraction as 1+ to 4+, or as 20 to 100% of the normal control. The length and diameter of the clot are compared to a normal control sample run simultaneously. A normal sample rapidly retracts within 1/2 hour to an hour to form a very small (approximately 1/8" wide X 3/4" long) cylindrical clot hanging downward from the top of the fluid layer. (Plastic tubes should not be used because a plastic surface is hydrophobic and this quality affects the behavior of aqueous solutions such as plasma and thrombin.)

The difficult part is grading the degree of clot retraction. The method requires comparison with a normal sample. If an Otter Hound's sample retracts to only 50% or less (i.e., 2+ or less) than that of the normal sample tested at the same time, the Otter Hound may be a carrier.

A healthy dog of another breed would be free of inherited thrombocytopathy, as would a healthy mongrel. It is unlikely that an entire litter of Otter Hound puppies would all be carriers. The litter can be tested together and any differences between puppies would suggest that some are carriers and some are clear. If the puppies with the smallest clots look like the normal dog's clot, you can safely assume those puppies are clear of thrombocytopathy. Many Otter Hounds presently living in this country were born in New York or New England and have been blood tested by Dr. W. Jean Dodds, of the New York State Department of Health. These Otter Hounds can serve as a standard for comparison of other dogs. Any Otter Hound that fails the screening test should be referred for full testing. Such a hound should not be considered for a breeding program unless cleared by more sensitive and specific platelet function tests. Otter Hounds seem to be predisposed to **dermatological cysts** and **tumors.**

BEHAVIOR

The Otter Hound makes a good family pet. He is cheerful and affectionate, and re-markably weather resistant.

OLD AGE

Otter Hounds live 10 to 12 years. The usual conditions of old age afflict the breed.

References

1.   Bodner, Elizabeth, DVM, "Genetic Status Symbols," *The American Kennel Club Gazette*; Sept. 1992.
2.   Dodds, W.J. "Inherited Hemorrhagic Disorders," *JAAHA;* 1975: 11:366-373.
3.   Dodds, W.J. and Kaneko, J.J. "Hemostasis and Blood Coagulation," (Kaneko,J.J., Cornelius, C.E. Eds) *Clinical Biochemistry of Domestic Animals 22.* Academic Press, New York, NY).
4.   Taylor and Zuckers: *Nature* 222:99: 1969. (Annotated by Harvey Pough and W.J. Dodds).

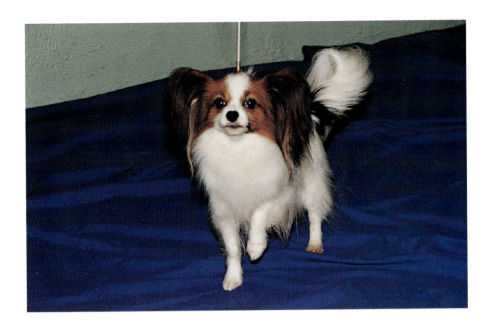

PAPILLON

ORIGIN AND HISTORY

The Papillon is a small, friendly, elegant toy dog, distinguished from other breeds by butterfly-like ears.

The breed is very old. Papillons appear in some frescoes in Italian churches dating back to the 14th century. The early Papillon was known as the Continental Spaniel and carried its ears dropped. Today two types exist: one with erect ears and one with dropped ears. The dropped-ear type is known as Phalene after the night moth that droops its wings. They are judged simultaneously in the ring in both the United States and England with a preference for neither type. In France, the Phalene is judged separately. They are also judged separately at some specialty shows in the United States.

DESCRIPTION

Although Papillons are dainty and fine-boned, they are sturdy little dogs that need no coddling. They enjoy a good romp in the snow and can tolerate moderate heat. They are easily trained and score exceptionally high in obedience. Papillons have good dispositions. Dogs and bitches are equally affectionate.

THE SHOW RING

Their height, measured to the top of their shoulder blades, is 8 to 11 inches. Their weight is in proportion to their height. A Papillon more than 11 inches tall is faulted.

White predominates in the coat, with patches of any color except liver. Some dogs are tricolor (black and white with tan spots over the eyes, on the cheeks, in the ears and under the tail). Color must cover both ears and extend over both eyes. A clearly defined white blaze and nose band along with symmetrical head markings are preferable but not essential. The size, shape and placement of patches on the body are unimportant. A saddle is permissible. None of the allowed colors is preferred. **Disqualified from the ring are dogs whose coats are all white or dogs whose coats have no white, and dogs whose height is over 12 inches.**

A pink, spotted or liver-colored nose is severely penalized. Any dewclaws must be removed from the hindlegs, and preferably from the forelegs, too. Although, according to the breed standard, the removal of dewclaws on the forelegs is optional, removal is strongly advocated for a better-looking leg. The nails on a dewclaw grow rapidly and may cause trauma. Removal of the dewclaws should be around the fifth day after birth.

BREEDING AND WHELPING

Breeding Papillons is not difficult. No brood bitch should be fat. A pregnant bitch should get regular, moderate exercise. The breeding of a small dog to a large bitch seldom produces a litter of medium sized puppies. Such a litter usually contains some small and some large puppies.

Bitches should not be bred until their second or third season. If a bitch is of show quality, she should finish her championship before being bred. Bitches throw their coats after whelping and the coat can require from 6 months to 1 year before it is back in show form.

About 3 weeks after being bred, a bitch may stop eating for a few days.

Eclampsia is a problem in the breed. The pregnant and lactating bitch should be watched carefully for early symptoms.

Most Papillon litters are whelped before the 63rd day of the gestation period, especially when the litter consists of four or five puppies. The weight of the puppies at birth varies from 2 1/2 to 7 ounces, averaging 4 to 5 ounces. A puppy weighing less than 3 ounces must be watched carefully. Puppies should be weighed at birth and again a day or two later, to be sure they are gaining.

The color of a puppy at birth often changes later. Black and white puppies can become tricolors. Dark brown puppies generally turn sable or even red. Blazes tend to narrow. A little white on the edge of an ear can disappear.

DENTITION

Papillon puppies attain their full growth by 7 or 8 months. By 7 months all temporary teeth should be shed; if not, they should be extracted. Even at 4 months, if milk teeth seem to be interfering with a good bite, they should be extracted.

Teeth in the older dog should be cleaned regularly. Because of tartar accumulation, teeth can loosen and fall out.

RECOGNIZED PROBLEMS

The breed is not afflicted with hip dysplasia or progressive retinal atrophy. Like most of the toy breeds, it often has **luxating patellas**. A dog with a loose patella should not be bred. **Entropion** has been diagnosed but it is rare.

Papillons are listed as having congenital **deafness**.[1]

BEHAVIOR

The Papillon is an excellent watch dog, and is charming and affectionate. He is clean and odorless, grooming himself like a cat. He is dedicated to his owner and can be possessive and jealous.

OLD AGE

It is best not to breed a female after 7 years of age. Most Papillons live to between 12 and 15 years.

References
1. Strain, George M. "Deafness in Dogs and Cats," *Proc. 10th ACVIM Forum*; May, 1992.

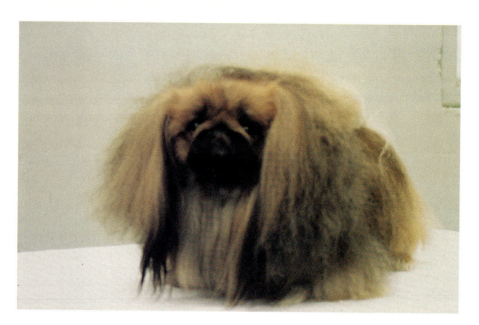

PEKINGESE

ORIGIN AND HISTORY

The origin of the Pekingese, also known as the Lion Dog of China, is lost in antiquity. Chinese objects of art dating as far back as 900 AD depict Fu Dogs and Kylins that greatly resemble Pekingese. The Pekingese may have emerged as a result of interbreeding among various types of dogs in China.

The Pekingese quickly became a great favorite of the Chinese court. During the Manchu Dynasty in 1644 they were treasured possessions of the Empress Tsu Hai and were referred to as the Imperial Pekingese. In 1860 the Imperial Palace was invaded by the British and five Pekingese were found at the Palace.

The others had been killed or taken. These five Pekingese were taken to England. One was presented to Queen Victoria and was appropriately named Looty. Others were eventually imported into England after much trouble and effort because the Chinese were loath to part with them.

Pekingese were recognized by the Kennel Club of England in 1898. In 1904 The Pekingese Club was formed in England; and the Pekingese Club of America was formed in 1909.

DESCRIPTION

Pekingese are courageous, loyal and independent. One who desires servility in a dog should not choose this breed. They are a determined breed and like to have their own way. If Pekingese are not well-trained they can become stubborn. This stubbornness has earned the breed the reputation of being bad-tempered. The breed respects discipline and quickly takes

400

advantage of indecision. Pekingese have sharp intelligence and are loyal companions.

THE SHOW RING

Pekingese weigh as much as 14 pounds, which is the maximum according to the Breed Standard. They may be cream, white, fawn, red, black, parti-colored and black or red with white predominating. A black mask or muzzle is desirable but not essential.

The dogs should be sound enough to romp and run as well as dogs of any other breed. Dewclaws need not be removed, nor tails docked. A Dudley nose is a disqualifying fault. Weight over 14 pounds is also disqualifying. Serious faults are: protruding tongue, badly blemished eye and overshot or wry mouth.

BREEDING AND WHELPING

Estrus in Pekingese usually occurs twice a year and lasts approximately 14 days. The 10th to 12th day of estrus is considered the best time for mating. Pekingese require assistance for breeding because of their coats and the shape of their bodies. Litters average three puppies, but four or five are not uncommon. Puppies weigh 4 to 6 ounces at birth. Delivery is difficult. **Cesarean section** is often necessary. Bitches should never be left unattended because they require assistance in delivering and cleaning the puppy. The flatness of their faces makes it difficult to sever the cord or to clean the puppy. Pekingese are generally good mothers and usually meticulous about keeping the puppy clean.

Umbilical and inguinal hernias are common at birth but often disappear with age. Every puppy should be checked for these conditions at birth. Delivering a litter of Pekingese requires some knowledge of the problems that can be encountered. **Cleft palates** and **cleft lips** are also more likely to occur in brachycephalic breeds.

Pekingese puppies are usually strong and quite active at 3 weeks of age. Puppies should be partially weaned when they are 4 weeks old. Once the coat begins to grow, the puppies' rectums should be checked regularly for cleanliness.

Puppies change considerably in facial properties and foreleg formations as they grow. At 10 weeks it is possible to tell whether a puppy has sound fore- and hindlegs. Weak pasterns can also be easily determined at that time. Extra long nails can affect a puppy's movement; therefore, they should be checked from the age of 5 weeks and trimmed as needed.

GROWTH

Adults should not be allowed to become overweight. The breed can stand cold better than heat and has difficulty breathing in humid weather.

The coat needs care, particularly the area behind the ears and the fringe of the hindlegs.

The coat sheds once a year. All dead hair should be removed when the dog starts to shed. This can be done with a comb or pin brush.

RECOGNIZED PROBLEMS

Since the Pekingese is a chondrodystrophied breed,[1,2,3,4,5] it is prone to formations of **uroliths** and **deterioration of intervertebral discs**.

The incidence of **urolithiasis** in dogs is about 0.5 to 1percent. Male dogs suffer from **urinary calculi** twice as frequently as bitches, whereas the latter have more urinary-tract infections. 29 percent of all dogs with urinary calculi are adipose.[6] The Pekingese is one of six breeds known to have a significantly high risk for uriolithiasis, compared with other breeds.[7]

Pinched nostrils, **short skull**, **flat chests** and **unsound fore- and hindlegs** are hereditary faults. Another fault which should be guarded against in breeding is the **elongated soft palate**. This condition prevents correct breathing. A puppy with this problem usually has difficulty breathing. Surgery to shorten elongated soft palates is very rewarding. Pekingese are listed as having **bronchial dysplasia**.[8]

Skull measurements were taken on 66 dogs of seven breeds. Using mostly data from breeders' studbooks, breed differences in reproduction were also examined. Litter size averaged 2.52 ±1.27 for Pekingese. It was concluded that **dwarfism** results in small litters and, in combination with extremely domed head shape, tends to increase the incidence of **dystocia**.[9]

In an anesthesia survey there was no evidence to suggest that some breeds were more likely than others to die under anesthesia, with the possible exception of Pekingese.[10]

Many **eye problems** in the Pekingese are related to the set and shape of their eyes. These problems include **trichiasis**, **distichiasis**,[11,12,13] **lacrimal duct atresia**, **microphthalmia**, **juvenile cataract**, **atypical pannus** and **progressive retinal atrophy**.[14] Breeders are overcoming these problems through selective breeding programs. The tear film of the Pekingese has been shown to have a reduced stability, thus enhancing the risk from factors more usually considered to initiate **corneal ulceration** in the breed.[15] **Hypoplasia of the Dens**[16] has also been reported in the Pekingese.

The wrinkle over the nose and under the eyes should be kept clean and dry with cotton wool or tissue; otherwise, it can become irritated and the dog may attempt to scratch it and injure the eye. Some breeders believe dewclaws should be removed because of this danger.

The Pekingese is not generally **allergic** or **sensitive to drugs**. **Persistent penile frenulum** is seen in the Pekingese,[17] as is **cryptorchidism**.[18]

BEHAVIOR

The Peke is a wonderful companion and lap dog. He is loyal, obedient and devoted. He can be a barking watch dog and is sensitive and courageous.

The Peke needs frequent grooming, which consists of brushing and combing his haircoat and keeping the area around his eyes clean.

OLD AGE

The Pekingese is a sturdy breed and needs little daily care. The life span averages 13 to 15 years. Although a change of diet is not necessary in old age, a dog usually appreciates it.

References

1. Kirk, R.W. and Bistner, S.I. *Handbook of Veterinary Procedures and Emergency Treatment: Hereditary Defects of Dog*s. 1975: Table 124, 661.

2. Burns, M. and Fraser, M.N. *Genetics of the Dog*. Oliver and Boyd, London, England;1966.

3. Groggin, J.E., et al: "Canine Invertebral Disk Disease Characterization by Age, Sex, Breed, and Anatomic Site of Involvement," *Am.J.Vet.Res.*; 31:1687-1692.

4. Hansen, H. "A Pathological-Anatomical Study of Disk Degeneration in the Dog," *Act. Orthop. Scand. Suppl.*; 1952: 11:1-117.

5. Hansen, H. "The Body Constitution of Dogs and Its Importance for the Occurrence of Disease," *Nord. Vet. Med.*; 1964: 16:977-987.

6. Hesse, A. and Bruhl, M. "Urolithiasis in Dogs: Epidemiological Data and Analysis of Urinary Calculi," *Kleintierpraxis*; 1990: 35:10, 505-512; 18 ref.

7. Bovee, K.C. and McGuire, T. "Qualitative and Quantitative Analysis of Uroliths in dogs: Definitive Determination of Chemical Type," *J. Amer. Vet. Med. Assoc.*; 1984: 105: 9,983-987. 18 ref.

8. King, L.G., DVM "Respiratory Congenital Disorders." Western Veterinary Conference. Feb. 1994

9. Hahn, S. "Variation of Skull Traits and Reproduction in Breeds of Small Dogs," Thesis, Tierarztliche Hochschule Hannover, Ger. Fed. Rep. 1988, 130; 111 ref.

10. Clarke, K.W. and Hall, L.W. "A Survey of Anaesthesia in Small Animal Practice: AVA/BSAVA report," *J. of the Assoc. of Vet. Anaesthetists of G.B. and Ire.*; 1990: 17, 4-10; 10 ref.

11. Bedford, P.G.C. "Eyelashes and Adventitious Cilia as Causes of Corneal Irritation," *J. Sm. Anim. Prac.*; 1971: 12:11-17.

12. Startup, G.G. *Disease of the Canine Eye*, Bailliere and Tindall, London, England,1971: 82-91.

13. Lawson, D.D. "Canine Distichiasis," *J.Sm.Anim.Prac.*; 1973:14:469-478.

14. Magrane, W.G. *Canine Ophthalmia*, (Lea & Febiger, Philadelphia, PA.,1977); 305.

15. Carrington, S.D., Redford, P.G.C., Guillon, J.P., and Woodward, E.G. "Biomicroscopy of the Tear Film: The Tear Film of the Pekingese Dog," *Vet Record*; 1989: 124:13, 323-328; 20 ref.

16. Kirk, R.W. and Bistner, S.I. *Handbook of Veterinary Procedures and Emergency Treatment: Hereditary Defects of Dogs.*1981: Table 119, 825.

17. Ettinger, S.J. *Textbook of Veterinary Internal Medicine.* (W.B. Saunders Co., Philadelphia, PA 1989); 1884.

18. Bell, Jerold S., DVM "Sex-Related Genetic Disorders: Did Mama Cause Them?" *American Kennel Club Gazette* Feb. 1994: 76.

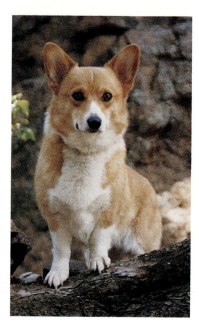

Photo by Samel

PEMBROKE WELSH CORGI

ORIGIN AND HISTORY

The Pembroke Welsh Corgi is one of the dwarf breeds. It originated from the same family as the Spitz, the Elkhound and the Pomeranian. Unlike the Cardigan Welsh Corgi, Pembrokes do not have Dachshund characteristics.

DESCRIPTION

Pembroke Welsh Corgis are intelligent, devoted family companions and guardians with little tendency to roam. Their medium-length coats need little grooming, although seasonal shedding does occur. Corgis are often possessive of their owners and property; consequently, training and discipline must begin when they are young. The unmanageable dog is the result of the owner's failure to teach restraint and acceptance of authority. Typically, such a dog is not of unsound temperament. Male Corgis are seldom compatible when housed together. Bitches are more compatible, but it is best to house one of each sex together.

THE SHOW RING

The Pembroke Welsh Corgi Standard lists no disqualifications. Very serious faults are overshot or undershot bites; mismarked, gray or smokey-red (blues) or predominantly white dogs; drop or button ears; and long coated (fluffy) dogs.

Snappish or overly shy dogs are not acceptable, and should be dismissed from the ring by the judge. Very large or extremely small dogs are heavily penalized. Such Corgis should not be bred.

BREEDING AND WHELPING

Pembroke Welsh Corgi bitches have normal periods of estrus and gestation. They are usually about 9 months old, rather than 6, when estrus begins. Corgi dams should not whelp unattended because they are sometimes slow to remove the placental sac and sever the umbilical cord, and a tendency toward **dystocia** is an unfortunate trait of this breed.[1,2,3]

An average litter consists of six or seven puppies, but can be as large as 10 or 12. Corgi puppies can be larger than those in other breeds of similar size and usually average 10 ounces at birth, with a range of 6 to 19 ounces.

Most puppies are grizzled brown or black and tan. Some are born with white markings. White puppies with patches of color or blue-gray puppies with pale gray pigmentation and yellow eyes are abberations.

GROWTH

An adult Pembroke Welsh Corgi dog should be 10 to 12 inches tall and weigh 27 or 28 pounds (not more than 30 pounds). Bitches should weigh 24 or 25 pounds (not more than 28 pounds). Dogs reach adult height and weight between 8 months and 2 years. Those that mature late go through a lanky adolescent period. Differences in age of maturation make it difficult to plot a chart showing average rate of growth.

Front and rear dewclaws should be removed when the tail is docked.

Tails at birth can be just stubs, or can be longer. The tail should be docked so it does not protrude beyond the anus, but it should not be so short as to form an indentation. A tail that is docked too short makes clean elimination difficult for the dog.

Ears usually become erect between 4 weeks and 4 months old. Drooping ears should be lightly taped for short periods (4 to 6 days) starting at about 3 months.

DENTITION

A scissors bite is preferable and normal, but a level bite is acceptable. **Overshot and undershot** bites are common, but a more serious bite problem, **"shark mouth,"** occasionally occurs. In this condition, the upper jaw grows more rapidly than the lower, and few teeth mesh properly.

RECOGNIZED PROBLEMS

The breed is subject to several serious conditions. Chief among these is **cervical disc syndrome**. **Epileptic seizures** of various types also occur, usually starting at 18 months to 2 years of age.

Some Corgis are predisposed to **bladder stones** and other **urinary-tract problems**. The Corgi has been reported as one of six breeds with a high risk for **urolithiasis**, compared to other breeds.[4]

Hip dysplasia occurs in Corgis but seldom becomes disabling. **Luxation of the lens**, **dermoid cyst of the cornea**, **progressive retinal atrophy** and **secondary glaucoma** have been reported.[5,6,7]

Swimmer puppies also occur in the breed. Some puppies are affected in only the front or hind quarters, others in both.

Cutaneous asthenia[6] **(Ehlers-Danlos Syndrome)** has been observed in the Welsh Corgi as well as in some Spaniels, Beagles, Manchester Terriers and mongrels. Clinical signs in dogs include fragility of skin and peripheral blood vessels, hyperextensibility and laxity of the skin. Subcutaneous hematomas may develop at sites of injury. Cutaneous asthenia in dogs is genetically transmitted. It is a collagen abnormality inherited as an autosomal dominant trait with complete penetrance. Animals showing the trait should be removed from the breeding program.

Allergic reactions are not considered typical of this breed. Some dogs have a tendency to **moist dermatitis** in hot, humid weather. **Von Willebrand's** disease has been reported in Pembroke Welsh Corgis in the United Kingdom.[8]

BEHAVIOR

The Pembroke Welsh Corgi is a little more gentle than the Cardigan variety. He is easily trained and makes an excellent companion dog.

OLD AGE

The Pembroke Welsh Corgi is a long-lived dog. Usually they do not show their age until about 10 years old. Their average life span is 12.5 years. Many Corgis die from kidney or heart failure, but most old dogs are euthanized simply because they can no longer live happy, ambulatory lives as a result of arthritis, incontinence, or various ailments that afflict the aged.

References
1. Freak, M.J. "The Whelping Bitch," *Vet Rec.*; 1948: 60:295-302.
2. Freak, M.J. "Abnormal Conditions Associated with Pregnancy and Parturition in the Bitch,"

Vet. Rec.; 1962: 74:1323-1335.

3. Erickson, F., et al: "Congenital Defects in Dogs: A Special Reference for Practitioners," Ralston Purina Co. (reprint from *Canine Practice*, Veterinary Practice Publishing Co., 1978).

4. Bovee, K.C. and McGuire, T. "Qualitative and Quantitative Analysis of Uroliths in Dogs: Definitive Determination of Chemical Type," *JAVMA*; 1984: 185: 9, 983-987; 18 ref.

5. Keep, J.M. "Clinical Aspects of Progressive Retinal Atrophy in the Cardigan Welsh Corgi," *Aust. Vet. J.*; 1972: 48:197-199.

6. Magrane, W.G. *Canine Ophthalmology*, 3rd ed. (Lea & Febiger, Philadelphia, Pa., 1977); 305.

7. Foley, C.W., et al: "Abnormalities of Companion Animals," Iowa State University Press, Ames, Ia.

8. Littlewood, J.D., Herrtage, M.E., Gorman, N.T., and McGlennon, N.J. "Von Willebrand's Disease in Dogs in the United Kingdom," *Vet Record*; 1987: 121:20, 463-468; 28 ref.

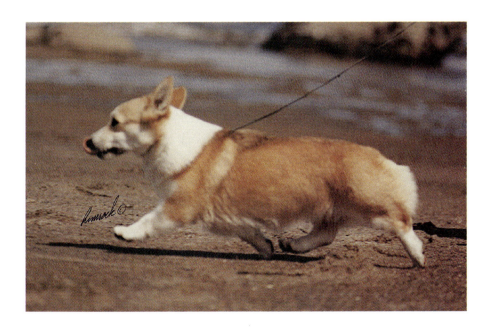

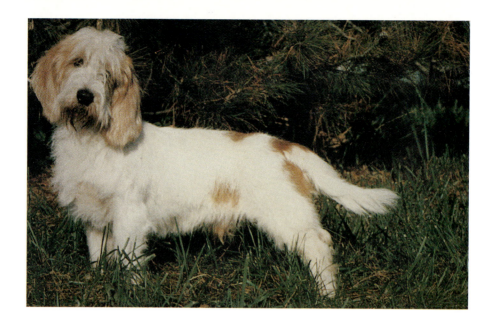

PETIT BASSET GRIFFON VENDEEN

ORIGIN AND HISTORY

The Petit Basset Griffon Vendeen is a small French hunting dog with an intriguing and charming appearance and personality. He was developed as a hound to hunt by scent on the western coast of France — the Vendee, characterized by thick underbrush, rocks, thorns and brambles. This difficult terrain demanded a hardy, alert, bold, determined, intelligent hunter with both mental and physical stamina. Originally the same Standard served both the Petit and the Grande Basset Griffon Vendeen. It wasn't until the 1950s that the "Petits" had their own standard. Not until 1975 was the interbreeding of the two sizes disallowed. As a result of the long-time practice of interbreeding, when Petits are bred today, both Petit and Grande characteristics manifest themselves and are likely to do so for generations to come. The Petit Basset Griffon Vendeen Club of America was founded in 1984. The breed became eligible to compete at licensed AKC shows on February 1, 1991.[1]

DESCRIPTION

Because both sizes can appear in the same litter, heavy emphasis is placed on type and size so that breeders and judges will learn the features unique to a Petit and encourage the right characteristics. The "PBGV" is a vocal, mellow breed, more a terrier than a lap dog.

THE SHOW RING

The most distinguishing characteristics of this bold hunter are his rough, unrefined outline and his proudly carried head. Important to the breed type is the compact, casual, rather tousled appearance with no feature exaggerated and his parts in balance. Both sexes should measure between 13 and 15 inches at the withers, somewhat longer than tall. At maturity, a female Petit will weigh from 30 to 34 pounds and a male from 38 to 42 pounds. He is white with any combination of lemon, orange, black, tricolor or grizzle markings. **Height of more than 15 ½ inches at the withers is a disqualification.**[1] Dewclaws may or may not be removed.

RECOGNIZED PROBLEMS

Petit Basset Griffon Vendeen have a low incidence of **hip dysplasia**, but some are seen with **thyroid imbalance** and **generalized allergies**. **Epilepsy** is documented in the breed. The ear problems of drop-eared hounds are seen. Breeders are currently studying a condition that has been called **Receptive Sterile Meningitis**. Dogs with this condition show elevated temperatures as high as 106°. They become rigid and arch their backs. White cell count is in excess of 45,000. There is no vascular dilation. Spinal and cerebellar fluids are normal. Twelve hours after an injection of corticosteroid, total white blood cell count returned to normal. One recovered bitch is now blind due to optic nerve swelling.[2] Young Petit Basset Griffon Vendeen are seen with **retinal folds (multifocal retinal dysplasia).**[3] They become fewer or less distinct as the dog matures.

BEHAVIOR

This is a breed that mixes well with other breeds. The PBGV makes a loyal, devoted family companion. He is intelligent and easily trained. Busy by nature, he is a happy, rustic "beater of bushes." Breeders say that life with a Petit Basset Griffon Vendeen is like living with a cartoon character.

OLD AGE

The Petit Basset Griffon Vendeen can be expected to live 13 to 15 years. They have no unique old age infirmities and succumb to the usual ills.

References
1. *The Complete Dog Book*, 18th ed. The American Kennel Club: (Howell Book House. 1992); 207-210.
2. Rand, T. and Link, V. Personal Communication. 1994.
3. Rubin, L.F. *Inherited Eye Diseases in Purebred Dogs*. (Williams & Williams. 1989); 322.

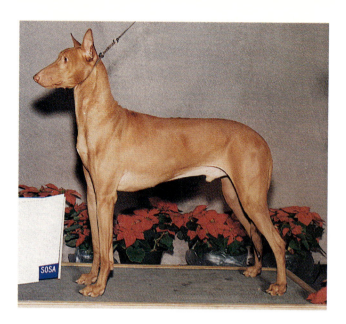

PHARAOH HOUND

ORIGIN AND HISTORY

It is fairly certain that the Pharaoh Hound lived in the Maltese Islands for thousands of years. The Pharaoh Hounds were probably brought to the Mediterranean region by Phoenicians. Protected by their island location from outside influences, the dogs bred true for centuries before being introduced to other parts of the world.

DESCRIPTION

This lightly built hound is noted for its great speed and agility. It requires a lot of exercise, but fanciers find the animal's affectionate, playful nature and exceptional intelligence well worth the effort.

The Pharaoh Hound is believed to have originated in ancient Egypt, where drawings and tomb sculptures dating to 4000 B.C. show surprisingly similar animals. A characteristic of the breed is its excellent sense of smell; it is one of the few "gazehounds" that also track quarry by scent.

This hardy dog is not daunted by low temperatures or rainy weather. It has all the skills of a good retriever. It needs frequent and long runs.[1]

410

THE SHOW RING

The Pharaoh Hound's appearance is one of grace, balance, power and speed. A screw tail is a fault. Any solid white spot on the back of the neck, shoulder or any part of the back or sides of the dog is disqualifying. Any tendency to throw the feet sideways, or a high-stepping "hackney" action is a definite fault. Dogs should be 23 to 25 inches; bitches from 21 to 24 inches.[2]

RECOGNIZED PROBLEMS

Lymphocytic-plasmolytic gastritis has been reported. It is not known yet if this disease is hereditary.[3]

Some of the breed's most common problems are **cardiovascular disease, gastrointestinal disorders** ranging from minor to major in nature and **dermatologic** conditions. According to OFA's Dr. E.A. Corley, 3.6 percent of x-rayed Pharaohs show signs of **hip dysplasia**.[4]

BEHAVIOR

The Pharoah Hound is an affectionate companion. He needs a lot of exercise and is very playful.

References
1. *Reader's Digest Illustrated Book of Dogs*. 1989.
2. *The Complete Dog Book*, The American Kennel Club. 18th edition. 1992.
3. The Pharaoh Hound column, *The American Kennel Club Gazette*; March, 1993.
4. The Pharaoh Hound column, *American Kennel Club Gazette*; November, 1990.

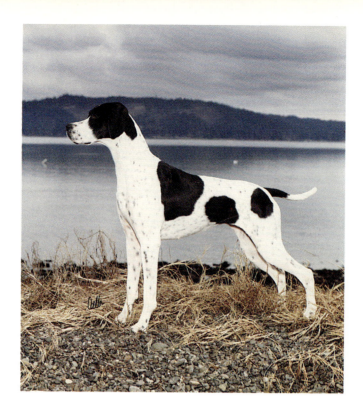

POINTER

ORIGIN AND HISTORY

Pointers were used to find and point hares for hounds to chase before guns were invented. Early in the 18th century wing shooting became popular and the Pointer became the sportsman's favorite.

Although the Pointer was established as a breed as far back as 1650, it has changed little since that time. Pointers are still lean-limbed, lithe, muscular dogs of endurance and concentration.

DESCRIPTION

Typically, Pointers are friendly, alert and eager to please. Excessive shyness or aggressiveness is not desirable. Considerable socializing is necessary to develop the proper temperament. Dogs bred from pure field strains are generally much smaller than those bred from show lines.

They carry a much higher tail set and are inclined to have less depth of flews.

Large patches or markings are evident at birth, although lemon puppies may appear all white. Ticking starts to become evident within about 2 weeks.

THE SHOW RING

The adult dog usually measures 25 to 28 inches at the withers and weighs 55 to 75 pounds. Bitches are from 23 to 26 inches in height and weigh from 45 to 65 pounds. The present AKC Standard does not list any disqualifications, but in the breed ring, light eyes, white or mottled ears, long "houndy" ears, shallowness, lack of rib spring and poor movement are extremely undesirable. The tail should have a heavy base, taper to a fine point and reach no farther than the hock. A well-balanced head with good depth of muzzle, definite stop and a pleasant, alert expression is desirable. Removal of dewclaws is desirable but not mandatory.

BREEDING AND WHELPING

Pointers, as a rule, are easy whelpers. They usually carry their litters to full term, but they may whelp as early as the 59th day. Litter size ranges from six to 16 puppies and birth weight varies from 10 to 18 ounces. Normally, body weight decreases slightly during the first 24 hours. Following this weight loss, the puppies should gain 6 to 10 ounces by the end of the first week and another 16 ounces during the second week. During the second week, puppies open their eyes. At 3 weeks of age body weight is expected to be approximately 4 pounds. The nourishment of a puppy showing slow growth may be supplemented with bottle or tube feedings, and at 3 weeks, regular supplemental feeding may be started.

DENTITION

Undershot mouths are common in Pointers. The defect may not be detected until eruption of the permanent incisors, or sometimes not until the dog is 8 or 9 months old. An even bite in a 6-month-old puppy is often the precursor of an undershot bite in the adult. Evidently, the mandible continues to lengthen for a longer time than does the upper jaw.

RECOGNIZED PROBLEMS

Pointers have only a few congenital abnormalities or inherited defects. The breed does have a fairly high incidence of **entropion**, usually of the lower eyelid. This condition irritates the cornea and causes a chronic runny eye. One or both eyes may be affected. Entropion can usually be surgically corrected, but since this is cosmetic surgery, it is not recommended for show dogs. **Bilateral cataract** with opaque lenses has been reported in the breed.[1,2]

Dr. George M. Strain lists Pointers as one of the breeds in which **congenital deafness** has been found.[3] **Hip dysplasia** in the breed is a problem, but the incidence is quite low. **Neuromuscular atrophy** is reported in Pointers.[4]

Neurotropic osteopathy is thought to be inherited recessively in Pointers.[5,6,7,8,9] Signs appear at 3 to 9 months and include toe gnawing, self-mutilation and degeneration of the spinal cord. This neurological disorder affects puppies of either sex, causing a loss of temperature with pain sensation. **Bithoracic ectromelia** is listed as a congenital defect of Pointers by Erickson, et al.[10] **Demodectic mange** is more prevalent in Pointers than in some other breeds. Onset of lesions usually begins during adolescent growth, when the dog is 4 to 10 months of age. Most lesions are self-limiting, but in about 10% of cases, they become generalized and are difficult to control. They are usually associated with secondary bacterial infection. Occasionally they are refractory to therapy.

Two problems seen in Pointers are related to the body conformation and short hair coats. The first is seen in Pointers with **very active tails**. When kept in close quarters, such as crates or runs, the tips of the tails are traumatized to bleeding. Although this seems a minor problem, it can be difficult to turn around and can result in amputation. Consequently, breeders developed the practice of docking tails. The second problem, related to the short coat, is the development of unsightly **calluses** on the lateral sides of the elbows or on the sternum. Calluses on the sternum appear more prevalent in certain dogs and certain bloodlines, because of the posture assumed by the dog at rest. This problem, like that of bleeding tails, is best managed by preventive measures. Proper bedding prevents calluses, but Pointers are notorious chewers, quickly demolishing pads and mats. Experience has shown that boxes filled with about 4 inches of straw, replenished as necessary, help prevent all types of calluses in kennels. Household dogs overcome the problem themselves if they are allowed on the furniture. Calluses can be removed surgically, but healing is slow and recurrence is common.

Umbilical hernias[11] and **progressive retinal atrophy**[12] are two other problems reported in the breed. **Calcinosis circumscripta**[13] **(calcium gout)** is found in Pointers and other large breeds of dogs. The incidence is highest in dogs up to 2 years of age. The lesions appear as firm, painless nodules in the subcutaneous tissue, most often on the limbs, and occur especially on the tarsus, foot and elbow. The average size of the nodules is 1 1/2 to 3 cm in diameter. In some cases the skin may ulcerate and discharge chalky, putty-like white fluid. Pointers are also reported to have a breed susceptibility to **eosinophilic panostitis**.

There is an **inherited dwarfism** that appears to be unique to the Pointer.[14,15] Breeders have reported **epilepsy** in the breed. Pointers have been reported to be one of several breeds at higher risk of developing **colonic disease.** A German study describes **sensory neuropathy** in Pointers, with information on symptoms, diagnosis and prognosis and treatment.[16]

BEHAVIOR

The Pointer is easily trained, intelligent, clean and affectionate. He is patient with children. He is not a good watch dog. Pointers that are house dogs develop a strong protective attitude toward their owners' homes and property, and will protect them vigorously.

OLD AGE

Pointers usually have a life span of 12 to 15 years. Dogs kept in kennels and those worked very hard in the field may not have this longevity. Older dogs still enjoy a bit of hunting or a good run and should not be deprived of these pleasures without good reason. Older dogs may be arthritic. Warm sleeping quarters in cold weather aid in keeping the dog comfortable.

Reference

1. Erickson, F., et al: "Congenital Defects in Dogs," *Canad. Pract.*; 2.
2. Host, R. and Sveinson, S. "Arvelig Katarakt hos Hunden," *Norsh Vet-tidsskr.*; 1936: 48:244-270.
3. Strain, George M. "Deafness in Dogs and Cats," *Proc. 10th ACVIM Forum*; May, 1992.
4. A Catalogue of Congenital and Hereditary Diseases.
5. Erickson, F., et al: "Congenital Defects in Dogs," *Canad. Pract.;* Oct. 1977; 56.
6. Broz, M. "New Findings on Hereditary Neurotropic Osteopathy," *Vet. Bul.;* 1966: 36:302.
7. Sanda, A. and Krizenecky, J. "Genetic Basis of Necrosis of Digits in Shortcoated Setters," *Vet. Bul.*; 1966: 36:2764.
8. Sanda, A. and Pivnik: "Necrosis of the Toes in Pointers," *Vet. Bul.;* 1964: 34:2283.
9. Sova, A. "Paw Necrosis, a Neurotropic Hereditary Osteopathy: Disease of Puppies of the Prognathous Breeds of Dogs," *Tier. Praxis*; 1974: 2:225-230.
10. Erickson, F., et al: "Congenital Defects in Dogs," *Canad. Pract.;* Aug. 1977: 60.
11. Hayes, H.M. "Congenital Umbilical and Inguinal Hernias in Cattle, Horses, Swine, Dogs and Cats: Risk by Breed and Sex from Hospital to Patients," *Am. J. Vet. Res.*; 1974: 35:839-842.
12. Magrane, W.A. *Canine Ophthalmology.* ed. (Lea & Febiger, Philadelphia, Pa., 1977); 305.
13. Kirk, R.W. *Current Veterinary Therapy, VI.* (W.B. Saunders, Philadelphia, Pa., 1977); 87.
14. Whitbread, T.J. University of Liverpool, Department of Veterinary Pathology.
15. Whitbread, T.J., Gill, J.J.B., and Lewis, D.G. "An Inherited Enchondrodystrophy in the English Pointer," *J. Sm. Anim. Prac.*; 1983: 24:7, 399-411; 20 ref.
16. Bichsel, P. "Neuromuscular Diseases of Young Dogs," *Jahresversammlung.* Schweizerische Vereinigung fur Kleintiermedizin. 2.-4.Juni 1988. Bazel. 1988, 43-50. Zool Bern, Switzerland; c/o H. Heinimann, Schweis. Serum und Impfinstitut, Postfach 2707.

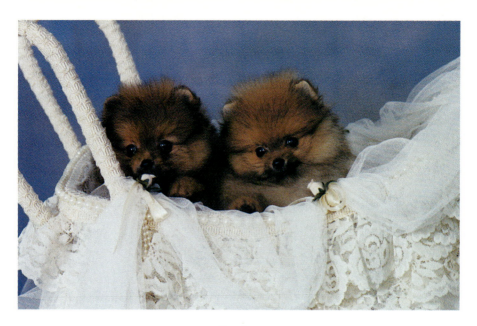
Puppies

POMERANIAN

ORIGIN AND HISTORY

The tiny Pomeranian of today strongly resembles the larger Arctic dogs and was probably bred down from them. Although their origin is northern Europe, early Greek gems and jars depict a dog much like the Pomeranian of today. In obedience trials, they are often rated top dog, displaying a sheepdog's cunning. Pomeranians come in a wide spectrum of colors. In past years there was controversy about acceptable color.

The Pomeranian is unusually intelligent and one of the most hardy of the Toy breeds. They are quite vociferous, making alert little watch dogs and companions.

DESCRIPTION

The revised (1991) Standard accepts any solid color or any solid color with lighter or darker shadings of the same color, any solid color with sable or black shadings, parti-color, sable and black and tan.

Some of the more serious faults in the breed are domed skull, too large and low set ears, undershot mouth, light eye rims, light or Dudley nose, out at elbows, down in pasterns, cow hocks, loose patellas, soft open coats and solid-color dogs with white chests or white front legs. Dewclaws on rear legs should be removed at 4 to 5 days. Removal of front dewclaws is optional.

BREEDING AND WHELPING

Pomeranian bitches follow the usual pattern of estrus and gestation, but they require more time to whelp than some breeds. Live whelps may be delivered after many hours of light to moderate contractions. Too many bitches are rushed into delivery with shots or **cesarean sections**. An average litter of Pomeranians consists of three puppies, each weighing from 3 to 5 ounces. Their color at birth ranges from a mixture of black, brown and gray to clear colors such as orange, black or white.

Some puppies may be as tiny as one ounce at birth and should be watched carefully the first few days. Sometimes they are unable to nurse because the nipples of the dam are too large for their mouths. Even though Poms are an unusually hardy breed for their size, newborns need much attention the first 2 to 4 weeks. Some breeders report the occurrence of puppies seemingly uninterested in eating. These should be checked to see if the tongue is clamped to the roof of the mouth. As they appear unable to relax enough even to nurse, hand feeding is necessary with these puppies. Some bitches will not have enough milk and the puppies should be supplemented with hand feedings.

GROWTH

Puppies vary so greatly in their rate of development that a growth chart is of little value. The average Pom probably weighs about 5 pounds at maturity; the skeletal growth is usually complete by 7 months. The weight limit for adults is from 3 to 7 pounds, with 4 to 5 pounds considered ideal.

RECOGNIZED PROBLEMS

The Pomeranian as a breed suffers from most of the same defects as other Toy breeds. These include **open skulls** (usually considered a manifestation of hydrocephalus), **patellar luxations**[1,2,3,4] (or loose knees, probably recessive polygenic), **cryptorchidism** (undescended testicles), **glycogen storage disease** (low blood sugar) and **tracheal collapse**.[5,6,7,8] Weight control is essential to control breathing problems associated with tracheal collapse.

Some breeders have reported a condition they call "elephant skin" or "black skin." The dog suffers massive coat loss and his bare skin darkens. This occurs in a symmetrical pattern, normally beginning at the base of the tail.[9]

Patent ductus arteriosus also occurs in the breed.[10,11,12,13,14,15,16] The mode of inheritance has not been determined. The condition is a persistence or nonclosure of the duct be-

417

tween the aorta and pulmonary artery with a left to right shunt.

Dislocation of the shoulder is a problem.[17,18]

Hypoplasia of dens (Odontoid process) has been reported in the breed.[19,20,21,22,23] The condition results in atlanto-axial subluxation. Onset may be at any age, and it produces signs of neck pain or, occasionally, quadriplegia.

Eye problems associated with the breed are **epiphora**, **nasolacrimal puncta atresia** and **progressive retinal atrophy**.[24]

Skull measurements were taken on 66 dogs of seven breeds. Using mostly data from breeders' studbooks, breed differences in reproduction were also examined. Litter size averaged 1.73 ± 0.82 for Poms. Pup mortality averaged 17.16% for Poms. It was concluded that **dwarfism** results in small litters and, in combination with extremely domed head shape, tends to increase the incidence of **dystocia**.[25]

BEHAVIOR

The Pomeranian is an excellent companion dog. He is lively, intelligent and affectionate. He is very clever and can be taught tricks very easily.

OLD AGE

A Pomeranian may live as long as 15 or 16 years. The senior dog slows down just as an older human being does. They are subject to heart and kidney trouble, **cataracts** and **deafness**. The dogs suffer from **prostate** problems, and the bitches from **metritis**. Their diets should be softer to compensate for loss of teeth. Teeth are lost mostly from plaque build-up. Regular dental care will help prevent this.

References

1. Knight, G.C. "Abnormalities and Defects in Pedigree Dogs III: Tibio-femoral Joint Deformity and Patella Luxation," *J. Sm. Anim. Prac.*; 1963: 4:463-464.
2. Kodituwakku, G.E. "Luxation of the Patella in the Dog," *Vet. Rec.;* 1962: 74:1499-1507.
3. Loeffler, K. and Meyer, H. "Hereditary Luxation of the Patella in Toy Spaniels," *Vet. Bull.*; 1962: 32:1703; 1962
4. Priester, W.A. "Sex, Size and Breed as Risk Factors in Canine Patellar Luxation," *JAVMA*; 1972: 160:740-742.
5. Done, S.H., et al "Tracheal Collapse in the Dog: A Review of the Literature and Report of Two New Cases," *J. Sm. Anim. Prac.*; 1970: 11:743-750.
6. Leonard, H.C. "Collapse of the Larynx and Adjacent Structures in the Dog," *JAVMA;* 1960: 137:360-364.
7. Leinard, H.G. "Surgical Correction of Collapsed Trachea in Dogs," *JAVMA;* 1971158:598-600.

8. O'Brien, J.A., et al: "Tracheal Collapse in the Dog," *J. Am. Vet. Rad. Soc.;* 1966: 7:12-19.

9. *American Kennel Club Gazette.* Pomeranian column. Dec. 1990: 132.

10. Patterson, D.F., et al: "Hereditary Cardiovascular Malformation of the Dog: Birth Defect," Original article series in XV Cardiovascular System. National Foundation,1973: 100-174.

11. Kirk, R.W. and Bistner, S.I. *Handbook of Veterinary Procedures and Emergency Treatment: Hereditary Defects of Dogs.* 1975: Table 124, 661.

12. Mulvihill, J.J. and Priester, W.A. "Congenital Heart Disease in Dogs: Epidemiologic Similarities to Man," *Teratology;* 1973: 7:73-78.

13. Patterson, D.F. "Epidemiologic and Genetic Studies of Congenital Heart Disease in the Dog," *Circ. Res.;* 1971: 23:171-202.

14. Patterson, D.F. "Canine Congenital Heart Disease:Epidemiological Hypotheses," *J. Sm. Anim. Prac.;* 1971: 12:263-2287.

15. Mulvihill, J.J. and Priester, W.A. "The Frequency of Congenital Heart Defects (CHD) in Dogs," *Teratology;* 1971: 4:236-237.

16. Patterson, D.F., et al: "Hereditary Patent Ductus Arteriosus and its Sequelae in the Dog," *Circ.Res.;* 1971: 29:1-13.

17. Campbell, J.R. "Shoulder Lameness in the Dog," *J. Sm. Anim. Prac.;* 1968: 9:189-198.

18. Vaughn, L.C. and Jones, G.D.C. "Congenital Dislocation of the Shoulder Joint of the Dog," *J. Sm. Anim. Prac.;* 1969: 10:1-3.

19. Downey, R.S. "An Unusual Cause of Tetraplegia in a Dog," *Canad. Vet.J.;* 1967: 8:216-217.

20. Geary, J.C., et al: "Altanto-axial Subluxation in the Canine," *J.Sm.Anim.Prac.;* 1967: 8:577-582.

21. Ladds, P., et al: "Congenital Odontoid Process Separation in Two Dogs," *J. Sm. Anim. Prac*; 1970: 12:463-471.

22. Parker, A..J. and Park, R.D. "Atlanto-axial Subluxation in Small Breeds of Dogs: Diagnosis and Pathogenesis," *VM/SAC;* 1973: 68:1133-1137.

23. Erickson, F., et al: "Congenital Defects in Dogs: A Special Reference for Practitioners," *Ralston Purina Co.;* (reprint from *Can. Prac.*,Veterinary Practice Publishing Co.;1978)

24. Magrane, W.G. *Canine Ophthalmology*, 3rd ed. (Lea & Febiger,Philadelphia,PA.,1977); 305.

25. Hahn, S. "Variation of Skull Traits and Reproduction in Breeds of Small Dogs," Thesis, Tierarztliche Hochschule Hannover, Ger. Fed. Rep. 1988: 130; 111 ref.

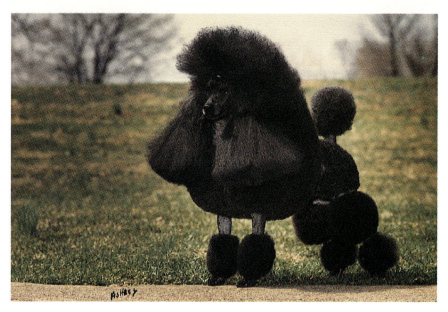
Miniature

POODLE (MINIATURE AND TOY)

ORIGIN AND HISTORY

The name Poodle comes from the German "pudel," meaning "to splash in the water."[1] Pictures of the Poodle's earliest ancestors were found on Roman coins. The coins depicted a medium-sized dog with lion-like mane and long tail.[2]

It is believed that the Poodle's ancestors were introduced into Germany about the 1st century A.D. by mercenary troops. Later, sometime before the 15th century A.D., they were taken to France in the same way. The term "French Poodle" evolved naturally from the breed's tremendous popularity in that country as water retrievers and circus trick dogs. They also were court favorites of French royalty, particularly Louis XVI.

The Poodle breed actually includes three distinct varieties—the Standard, Miniature and Toy. The smaller two, Miniature and Toy, were intentionally developed from the Standard (a major breeding achievement), in England in the 18th century during the reign of Queen Anne. The tiny "sleeve dogs" were sometimes known as White Cubans and were taught to dance to music.

The practice of clipping Poodles started as a relief from their heavy coats while swimming. Becoming fashionable all over Europe, as many as eight types of Poodle clip are popular today, although only three styles are allowed in the show ring.

DESCRIPTION

The Poodle is a highly intelligent, sensitive breed with a great willingness to learn. Poodles make playful companions.

The Miniature must stand between 10 and 15 inches at the shoulder; the Toy poodle stands 10 inches or less. There is a 1-inch difference in English Breed Standards. Any individual over 15 inches tall is classified as a Standard Poodle. The adult Miniature bitch weighs between 14 and 15 pounds; the Miniature dog, 15 to 16 pounds. The adult Toy is much smaller; the dog weighs 6 or 7 pounds while the bitch weighs 5 to 6 pounds.[1]

Poodle trimming is fashionable but also delicate. Clipping should be done professionally at least the first few times until the owner learns the procedure thoroughly.

THE SHOW RING

The Poodle's size is the characteristic that determines the breed. Although parti-colors are born, only solid colors are allowed in the show ring. The most common colors are solid black and solid white. The Poodle should be an even color at the skin. All colors should have black pigmentation of nose and eye rims except brown and brown derivatives, which may have liver. Characteristics of body shape which are crucial in correct Poodle type include the skull and muzzle, eyes, tail and legs.[1] The skull should be moderately rounded with a slight but definite stop. In contrast, the muzzle is long and straight with a definite chin. The very dark eyes are set far apart and must be oval-shaped. The ears are judged less severely, but they should be set low and close to the head.

Overall body proportions of the Poodle are deep and strong, although trimmed legs and the docked tail give a delicate appearance. A Poodle's feet should be small, arched ovals with tight pads. Faults include round, protruding or large eyes. Jaws should not be undershot or wry. Poodles' feet should not be flat or splayed. Other faults include low tail set or squirrel tail.

Disqualifications are as follows: A dog in any type of clip other than those listed under coat shall be disqualified. Parti-colored dogs shall be disqualified: the coat of a parti-colored dog is not an even, solid color at the skin but of two or more colors. A Toy Poodle over 10 inches shall be disqualified. A Miniature over 15 inches shall be disqualified.

BREEDING AND WHELPING

In breeding Poodles for the show ring, care should be taken to adhere to the Toy and Miniature size standards.[1] Miniature litters are usually three to four puppies, each averaging less than 8 ounces at birth. Healthy puppies will increase in weight quite rapidly. The Miniature rarely comes in heat before 1 year of age. Like the Standard variety, Miniature and Toy Poodles have relatively fast-growing coats. The tails should be docked at 3 to 5 days of age. Leave a little less than 2/3. All dewclaws should be removed at this time in order to give the legs a straight, clean appearance.

DENTITION

The breed Standard calls for a scissors bite, but a level bite is not unusual.

RECOGNIZED PROBLEMS

The Poodle is a highly sensitive breed whose defects include complications with the **skin**, **allergies**, **ear infections**, **achondroplasia** and **eye disorders**.

A cytogenetic analysis of 112 dogs of 28 breeds led to the detection of a new **Robertsonian translocation**, restricted to the Poodle breed.[3]

Atopic dermatitis, common in Miniature and Toy Poodles, is a hereditary condition which inhibits the ability to resist allergens inhaled from the environment. The results are **pruritus** on the feet and face, and also **seborrhea** and **pyoderma** (often seasonal).[4] Hyposensitization may relieve the symptoms through formation of blocking IgG antibodies.

The thickness of the hair inside the ear often causes another problem, that of accumulated wax and dirt with subsequent infection.

In the Miniature Poodle, **achondroplasia** is an inherited abnormality transmitted as a simple autosomal recessive trait. The characteristic of abnormally short limbs is caused by impaired ossification of long bone cartilage.

Disorders of the eye are quite common in Miniature and Toy Poodles. **Distichiasis** is one of the problems, a congenital condition of a second abnormal row of eyelashes either on the upper or lower lid[4] (extra or blepharospasm). Distichiasis can develop at any age. Recommended treatment is electroepilation.[5,6]

Another congenital eye problem is **nasolacrimal puncta atresia**, the absence of the openings to the lacrimal canal. Symptoms are **epiphora** (excessive tearing) and the ballooning of the duct. **Optic nerve hypoplasia** has been reported in Toy Poodles.[7]

Miniature Poodles have a problem with **congenital epiphora**.[8] Over-production of tears can also be caused by **trichiasis**, **entropion** and allergens as well as **distichiasis**. It results in a chronic clear discharge that stains the hair and face, a condition known as "wet eye." Successful treatment on Miniatures is surgery which removes the tear-producing gland and part of the T-shaped cartilage, at the base of the third eyelid.

Like Standards, Miniature Poodles are subject to **cataracts** transmitted as an autosomal recessive trait.[9,10] Poodles tend to develop equatorial cataracts at an early age relative to other breeds, with some individuals experiencing visual loss between 6 and 18 months.

Lens-induced uveitis is most common in Toy and Miniature Poodles.[11]

Compared with mixed-breed dogs, eight breeds have been reported at higher risk of developing **glaucoma**. "Minis" are one of these eight breeds.[12]

Retinal atrophy sometimes develops in Miniature and Toy Poodles. This cupping or depression of the optic nerve head accompanies atrophy of the optic disc, evident as a lack of visible blood vessels.[5] The Miniature Poodle with **progressive rod-cone degeneration (prcd)** is a model for human retinitis pigmentosa (RP). Since previous studies from several laboratories have shown abnormalities in plasma lipids in human RP, the plasma lipids of prcd-affected dogs were examined. Fasting blood was drawn on three separate occasions from affected and control Miniature Poodles and on one occasion from normal Irish Setters and those affected with a different inherited retinal degeneration (rod-cone dysplasia). Plasma phospholipids from prcd-affected animals had significantly lower levels of docosahexaenoic acid (22:6omega3) and cholesterol, compared to control Miniature Poodles. No differences were observed in plasma levels of phospholipids, vitamin A or Vitamin E, and no lipid differences were found between control and affected Irish Setters. The ratios of 22:5omega3 to 22:6omega3 and of 22:4omega6 to 22:5omega6 were significantly elevated in prcd-affected Poodles compared to controls. Since the conversion of 22:5omega3 to 22:6omega3 and 22:4omega6 to 22:5omega6 is catalyzed by a delta4 desaturase, it is concluded that there is a defect in desaturase activity in the prcd Poodle.[13]

Hemeralopia (day blindness) has also been reported in Miniature Poodles, as has **Von Willebrand's Disease**.[14] This disease is also known as **pseudohemophilia** and is characterized by prolonged bleeding time, low Factor VII, reduced platelet adhesiveness and abnormal prothrombin consumption time. Patients may exhibit recurrent melena, prolonged estrual bleeding, excessive bleeding after trauma and subcutaneous hematoma. **Hemophilia A** has been reported in a family of Miniature Poodles.[15]

Nonspherocytic hemolytic anemia, characterized by marked reticulocytosis, hepatosplenomegaly, hemosiderosis of reticuloendothelial organs, bone marrow myelofibrosis, and osteosclerosis, was diagnosed in five related Poodles. The unremitting anemia was clinically evident by 1 year of age, and was fatal as early as 3 years of age. Despite intense diagnostic endeavors including erythrocyte fragility studies, erythrocyte enzyme assays and hemoglobin electrophoresis, the cause of this nonspherocytic hemolytic anemia remains to be determined.[16] The incidence of **urolithiasis** in dogs is about 0.5-1%. Poodles often have **urinary calculi**.[17] Male dogs suffer from urinary calculi twice as frequently as bitches, whereas the latter have more urinary-tract infections. Twenty-nine percent of all dogs with urinary calculi were obese. In a recent study of 839 **uroliths** submitted by veterinarians for analysis, 562 (67%) were composed of at least 70% magnesium ammonium phosphate, and 57 (6.8%) at least 70% calcium oxalate. Most were found in the bladder. Uroliths occurred more frequently in females than in males, but there was little difference in prevalence between dogs aged from 1 to 12 years. The uroliths were found in 60 known breeds. Incidence in Miniature Poodles was second highest, with ten percent.[18]

Found in both the Toy and the Miniature breed are other hereditary autosomal imbalances[19] including a tendency to **ectopic ureters.**[20] As in some breeds of farm stock, a possible result of this condition is reduced fertility due to the pooling of urine in the vagina or uterus. **Patent ductus arteriosus** has been described in Miniature Poodles along with congenital **deafness**, **epiphyseal dysplasia**, **intervertebral disc degeneration**, **Legg-Perthes**[21] (the incidence is such to indicate monogenic recessive inheritance of the condition) and **patellar luxation. Demyelination of the brain stem and the spinal cord** has been reported in young Miniature poodles. Affected dogs are between 2 and 5 months of age. Clinical signs start with a progressive paraperesis followed by tetroparesis, paraplegia and tetraplegia over a period of two weeks.[22] **Epilepsy**, **amaurotic idiocy**, **ectodermal defect**, **hairlessness** and **entropion** have been reported.[23,24] **Congenital deafness** is also seen in the Toy Poodle.[25] **Persistent penile frenulum** is seen in the Miniature Poodle and **hypospadia** is common in the Toy Poodle.[26]

Pseudo-hermaphroditism, cryptorchidism and missing teeth are also considered problems in this breed. Miniature Poodles have an increased breed incidence for **hyperadrenocorticism**[27] and **bronchial esophagus fistula.**[28] Of 13,974 dogs presented at a clinic in Germany from 1977 to 1985, 699 (5%) had **neoplasms**. The commonest site was the mammary gland (31%), and the breeds most involved were the Poodle and the German Shepherd.[29]

The association between breed, sex and **canine heart valve incompetence** was investigated by an observational study of a veterinary clinic population. Odds ratio estimations from 370 affected dogs and 9028 controls of 15 breeds revealed significant associations between some small and medium-sized breeds including Miniature Poodles and heart valve incompetence, and significant negative associations between some large breeds and heart valve incompetence. The log odds, determined for each breed and sex, indicated that males were more susceptible.[30] **Renal dysplasia** has been reported in the Poodle in a Cornell study of nephropathies believed to have a genetic basis.[31]

Pyruvate kinase deficiency has been reported in Miniature Poodles (see Basenji).

Breed, sex and age distribution of **primary hypothyroidism** are discussed in a Swedish study.[32] Poodles have **narcolepsy** and are used by the Stanford University sleep disorder clinic to study the disease.[33] Poodles are one of a few breeds so far diagnosed with **adult onset growth hormone deficiency**.[34] Signs include alopecia and hyperpigmentation in a striking bilateral truncal pattern.

BEHAVIOR

Fundamentally good natured and stable, the Poodle is highly trainable, sociable and intelligent. He is animated and loves human company. Unfortunately, because of his universal popularity, indiscriminate breeding with no attention paid to genetics or temperament has provided us with too many high-strung poodles subject to many genetic faults. In a study of 245 cases of **aggressive behavior** in 55 breeds of dogs, dominance aggression was found in Toy Poodles while Miniature Poodles had a high incidence of fear-elicited aggression.[35]

OLD AGE

Even though it is a sensitive breed, the Poodle adapts well to new owners even late in life. Life expectancy is about 10 to 14 years.

References
1. *The Complete Dog Book*, American Kennel Club (Howell Book House,New York, NY.,1992); 521-528,462.
2. Jones, N.H. and Hamilton, F., Eds: *The World Encyclopedia of Dogs*. (Galahad Books, New York, NY, 1971); 168-173.
3. Mayr, B., Krutzler, J., Schleger, W., and Auer, H. "A New Type of Robertsonian Translocation in the Domestic Dog," *J. of Heredity;* 1986: 77:2, 127; 8 ref.
4. Kirk, R.W. Ed.: *Current Veterinary Therapy VI*. (W.B. Saunders, Philadelphia, PA.,1977); 541-573,664.
5. Magrane, W.G. *Canine Ophthalmology*. (Lea & Febiger, Philadelphia, PA.,1968); 59, 165,190,214.
6. Magrane, W.G. *Canine Ophthalmology*, 3rd ed. (Lea & Febiger, Philadelphia, PA., 1977); 79, 204, 264, 266.
7. Barnett, K.C. "Inherited Eye Disease in the Dog and Cat," *J. Sm. Anim. Prac.*; 1988: 29:7, 462-475; 33 ref.
8. Prendergrast, J.C. "Surgical Correction of Epiphora in a Poodle." *The Southwest. Vet.*; 1971: 238.
9. Rubin, L.F. and Flowers, R.D. "Inherited Cataract in a Family of Standard Poodles," *JAVMA;* 1972: 61(2):207-208.
10. Erickson, F., et al "Congenital Defects of Dogs," Part 1, *Canad. Prac.*; 1977: 4(4):61.
11. Woerdt, A. Van Der, Naisisse, M.P., and Davidson, M.G. "Lens-Induced Uveitis in Dogs," *JAVMA;* 1992: 201:6, 921-926; 46 ref.

12. Slater, M.R. and Erb, H.N. "Effects of Risk Factors and Prophylactic Treatment on Primary Glaucoma in the Dog," *JAVMA*; 1986: 188:9, 1028-1030; 7 ref.

13. Anderson, R.E., Maude, M.B., Alvarez, R.A., Acland, G.M., and Aguirre, G.D. "Plasma Lipid Abnormalities in the Miniature Poodle with Progressive Rod-Cone Degeneration," *Experimental Eye Research;* 1991: 52:3, 349-355;44 ref.

14. Dodds, W.J. *Current Veterinary Therapy VI: Inherited Hemorrhagic Defects*, (W.B. Saunders, Philadelphia, PA.,1977); 444-445.

15. Mansell, P.D., Parry, B.W., and Van Orsouw, P.J. "Hemophilia A in a Family of Miniature Poodles," *Aus. Vet. Jour.;* 1990: 67:11, 420-421; 10 ref.

16. Randolph, J.F., Center, S.A., Kallfelz, F.A., Blue, J.T., Dodds, W.J., Harvey, J.W., Paglia, D.E., Walsh, K.M., and Shelly, S.M. "Familial Nonspherocytic Hemolytic Anemia in Poodles," *Am. J. of Vet. Research*; 1986: 47:3, 687-695; 32 ref.

17. Hesse, A. and Bruhl, M. "Urolithiasis in Dogs: Epidemiological Data and Analysis of Urinary Calculi," *Kleintierpraxis*; 1990: 35:10, 505-512; 18 ref.

18. Osborne, C.A., Clinton, C.W., Bamman, L.K., Moran, H.C., Coston, B.R., and Frost, A.P. "Prevalence of Canine Uroliths: Minnesota Urolith Center," *Vet. Clinics of N. Amer, Sm. Anim. Prac.;* 1986: 16:1, 27-44; 6 ref.

19. Hare, W.C.D. and Bovee, K. "A Chromosomal Translocation in Miniature Poodles," *Vet. Rec.*; 1974: 7:217-218.

20. Hayes, H.M. Jr. "Breed Associations of Canine Ectopic Ureters: A Study of 217 Female Cases," *J. Sm. Anim. Prac.*; 1984: 25:8, 501-504; 12 ref.

21. Robinson, R. "Legg-Calve-Perthes Disease in Dogs: Genetic Aetiology," *J. of Sm. Anim. Prac.*; 1992: 33:6, 275-276; 7 ref.

22. Ettinger, S.J. *Textbook of Veterinary Internal Medicine, Diseases of the Cat and Dog.* (W.B. Saunders Co., Philadelphia, PA. 1989); 2383.

23. Leipold, H.W. "Nature and Causes of Congenital Defects of Dogs: Symposium on Canine Practice," *The Veterinary Clinics of North America;* 1977: 8(1):64.

24. Foley, C.W., et al: "Abnormalities of Domestic Animals," Iowa State University Press, Ames, Ia.,1979.

25. Strain, George M. "Deafness in Dogs and Cats," *Proc. 10th ACVIM Forum.* May, 1992.

26. Ettinger, S.J. *Textbook of Veterinary Internal Medicine.* (W.B. Saunders Co. 1989); 1884.

27. Brignac, Michele M. "Congenital and Breed Associated Skin Diseases in the Dog and Cat," published in *KalKan Forum;* (December 1989)

28. King, L.C., DVM "Respiratory Congenital Disorders." Western Veterinary Conference. Feb. 1994.

29. Fabricius, E.M., Schneeweiss, U., Schroder, E., Dietz, O., Wildner, G.P., Schmidt, W., Baumann, G., Benedix, A., Weisbrich, C. and Stuhrberg, U. "Serological Diagnosis of Neoplasms in Dogs With a Clostridium Butyricum Spore Preparation," *Monatshefte fur Vet.;* 1986: 41:7, 220-224; 40 ref.

30. Thrusfield, M.V., Aitken, C.G.G., and Darke, P.G.G. "Observations on Breed and Sex in Relation to Canine Heart Valve Incompetence," *J. Sm. Anim. Prac.*; 1985: 26:12, 709-717;

14 ref.

31. Picut, C.A. and Lewis, R.M. "Comparative Pathology of Canine Hereditary Nephropathies: An Interpretive Review," 1987: 11:6, 561-581; 91 ref.

32. Larsson, M. "The Breed, Sex and Age Distribution of Dogs With Primary Hypothyroidism," *Svensk-Veterinartidning*; 1986: 38:15, 181-183; 3 ref.

33. Tovfexis, Anastasia "Narcolepsy: A Neglected Area of Medicine," *Med. Trib.*; Dec. 17, 1975: 4.

34. Ettinger, S.J. *Textbook of Veterinary Internal Medicine.* (W.B. Saunders Co. 1989); 7.

35. Borchelt, P.L. "Aggressive Behavior of Dogs Kept as Companion Animals: Classification and Influence of Sex, Reproductive Status and Breed," *Applied Animal Ethology;* 1983: 10:1, 45-61; 24 ref.

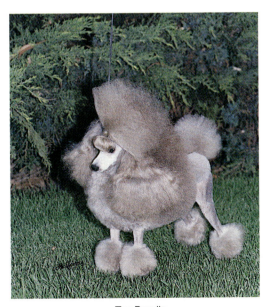

Toy Poodle

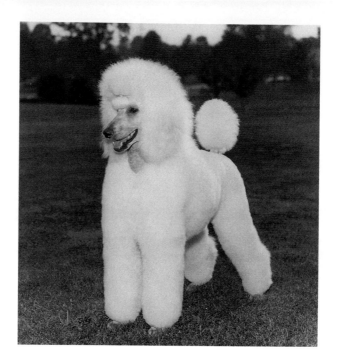

POODLE (STANDARD)

ORIGIN AND HISTORY

The Standard Poodle, the largest and possibly the oldest of the three varieties of Poodles, is believed to have originated somewhere in Europe. The name comes from the German "pudel" (meaning "to splash in the water") because of their instinctive joy and ability in swimming. When used as water retrievers, shearing their hindquarters was found desirable to facilitate their swimming. The main coat on head, neck and chest and the bracelets were retained to provide buoyancy and protection from the cold. The modern show trims are stylized variations of this tradition.

DESCRIPTION

The Poodle is gentle, alert and affectionate. Truly sharp temperaments are quite rare. The breed adapts well to changes in environment and masters even late in life. Generally, Poodles are very easy to train. The coat should be wiry with close curls. Trimming is a matter of taste, but must be done in a specified style if the dog is to be shown. The Poodle requires regular grooming to maintain a healthy skin.

THE SHOW RING

The three varieties have strict size standards. The Standard Poodle must be more than 15 inches high at the shoulder,[1] with an average of about 22 to 27 inches. Mature weight will vary from 45 to 75 pounds. For exhibiting, only solid colors are allowed.[1] Black and white are most common, with apricot, brown and cream also popular. The evenness and clearness of the color at the skin is important in judging. Colors often lighten in old age.

At maturity, browns turn cafe-au-lait. Brown Poodles may have liver-colored noses, eye-rims and tips, dark toenails and dark amber eyes. Black, blue, gray, silver, apricot, cream and white poodles should have black eye rims, noses and lips. Black and self-colored noses, eye rims and lips, self-colored toenails and amber eyes are permitted but not desirable. Although common, it is undesirable for hair color to change on scar tissue. Faults include round, protruding or large eyes. An **undershot, overshot** or wry jaw is a fault. Flat or spread feet are also faults. If the tail is set low, curled or carried over the back, points will be docked in judging.

Breed disqualifications are; height under 15 inches at shoulder; any type of clip other than those listed under coat; and parti-colors, (the coat of a parti-colored dog is not an even, solid color at the skin but is two or more colors).

BREEDING AND WHELPING

Standard Poodle puppies that will reach normal size may weigh from 8 to 16 ounces at birth. The normal litter is six to 10 puppies, but litters of as many as 15 may occur. Puppies which at maturity will be silver are usually born black, while puppies of other colors usually remain the same color as at birth. Nose and lip pigmentation may not be apparent for the first few days after whelping. Standard Poodles generally follow the norm in length of gestation, but usually do not come in heat before 12 to 15 months. Umbilical hernias in whelps are common.

GROWTH

Healthy puppies double their birth rate the first 8 days and will continue to gain the same amount weekly for the first 2 months. Removal of dewclaws is recommended but not required. Tails should be docked at approximately 1/2 their length at birth, but tail length at birth varies. Docking should be done so the tail, on the mature dog, is shorter than the top of the head. This is longer than veterinarians generally allow. A tail docked too short can spoil the show prospects of a Poodle.

DENTITION

Missing teeth are undesirable. Overshot bites of as much as 2 1/2 cm will sometimes correct as late as 14 months. The scissors bite is required, but level bites are not unusual.

RECOGNIZED PROBLEMS

Hip dysplasia is a definite problem in Standard Poodles and breeding should be done only with stock judged to be normal. Many eye problems have been reported in the Poodle and a comprehensive examination should be done on each dog. These conditions include **iris atrophy, distichiasis (an abnormal extra row of eyelashes)**,[2,3,4,5,6,7] **microphthalmia (small eyes)**,[7] **juvenile cataracts**,[5] **entropion** and **epiphora (excessive tearing)**,[3,4] resulting in a stained face.[2] **Progressive retinal atrophy,** a problem in the other varieties, has been documented in the Standard Poodle but is not considered a common problem.

Classic **epilepsy** is reported by breeders in standard Poodles. **Patent ductus arteriosus**, a genetic-influenced failure to close the left aortic arch, has been diagnosed in the breed.[2,8,9] A Poodle's ears can be a problem if not cleaned regularly. The breed seems to have more wax build-up than others, and a regimen of care must be followed, including wax and hair removal.

Osteogenesis imperfecta[10] is a condition representing a deficient or delayed-developmental formation of bone believed to result from a deficiency of osteoblast. It has also been found in Norwegian Elkhounds and Bedlington Terriers. Clinical manifestations are skeletal abnormalities usually of the spinal column and posterior extremities. Numerous fractures result from minor injury, but heal rapidly. Abnormalities are apparent at 6 to 8 weeks of age and abnormal characteristics usually improve at puberty. **Bloat (gastric torsion)** is a problem in the Standard Poodle. Poodles are susceptible to **inhalant allergies.**[11]

Sebaceous adenitis has become more evident, particularly in Standard Poodles. The Poodle Club of America has given a grant to Michigan State University for study of a test breeding to determine the mode of inheritance of this skin disease.[12,13,14] For more information about this skin disease, contact the Genodermatosis Research Foundation (GRF) at 1635 Grange Hall Rd., Dayton, Ohio 45432. The **alopecia** associated with dilute colors is reported in Standard Poodles.

The Poodle is one of several breeds reporting a significantly higher disposition for **malignant neoplasms**.[15] In a Swedish study of **hypothyroidism**, there was a higher than average incidence of the disorder in Standards.[16] **Renal dysplasia** has been reported in the Poodle as an hereditary nephropathy.[17] **Adult onset growth hormone deficiency** has been described in Poodles.[18] Signs include alopecia, hyperpigmentation in a striking bilateral truncal pattern.

BEHAVIOR

The Standard Poodle is an excellent family companion. He is cheerful, obedient and easily trained. He can also be hunted over as he is an excellent swimmer and retriever if properly trained. The breed does need frequent grooming.

OLD AGE

Life expectancy of the Poodle is about 10 to 14 years.

References

1. *The Complete Dog Book*, The American Kennel Club (Howell Book House, New York,NY, 1992).
2. Kirk, R.W. Ed: *Current Veterinary Therapy VI.* (W.B. Saunders, Philadelphia, PA,1977); 537-541.
3. Helper, L.C. and Geiser, D.F. "A Surgical Treatment of Epiphora," *Ill.Vets*; Nov. 1971: 10-12.
4. Prendergrast, J.C. *Surgical Correction of Epiphora in a Poodle*, 1971.
5. Rubin, L.F. and Flowers, R.D. "Inherited Cataract in a Family of Standard Poodles," *JAVMA*; 1972: 161:207-208.
6. Magrane, W.G. *Canine Ophthalmology*. 3rd Ed. (Lea & Febiger, Philadelphia, PA., 1977); 79, 204, 264-266.
7. Leipold, H.W. "Nature and Causes of Congenital Defects of Dogs: Symposium on Canine Pediatrics," *The Veterinary Clinics of N. Am*; Feb. 8:64.
8. Patterson, et al: "Hereditary Cardiovascular Malformation of the Dog—Birth Defects," *Nat. Found.;* 1972: 15: 100-174.
9. Jubb, K.J.F. *Pathology of Domestic Animals*. (Academic Press, New York, NY.,1964).
10. Foley, C.W., et al: *Abnormalities of Companion Animals*, Iowa State University Press, Ames, Ia., 1979: 157.
11. Ackerman, Lowell, DVM. "Allergic Skin Diseases," *American Kennel Club Gazette*; September, 1990.
12. Poodle column *American Kennel Club Gazette*; October, 1990.
13. Laratta, Diane "Identifying Sebaceous Adenitis," *The American Kennel Club Gazette*; January, 1991.
14. Rosser, E.J., Dunstan, R.W., Breen, P.T., and Johnson, G.R. "Sebaceous Adenitis with Hyperkeratosis in the Standard Poodle: A discussion of 10 Cases," *JAAHA*; 1987: 23:3, 341-345; 12 ref.
15. Kusch, S. "Incidences of Malignant Neoplasia in Dogs Based on PM Statistics of the Institute of Animal Pathology, Munich, 1970-1984," Inaugural Dissertation,Tierarztliche Fakultat, Ludwig Maximilians Universitat, Munchen, German Federal Republic. 1985: 21 pp. of ref.
16. Larsson, M. "The Breed, Sex, and Age Distribution of Dogs With Primary Hypothyroidism," *Svensk-Veterinartidning*; 1986: 38:15, 181-183; 3 ref.
17. Picut, C.A. and Lewis, R.M. "Comparative Pathology of Canine Hereditary Nephropathies: An Interpretive Review," *Vet. Res. Comm.*; 1987: 11:6, 561-581; 91 ref.
18. Ettinger, S.J. *Textbook of Veterinary Internal Medicine*. (W.B. Saunders Co., 1989) 7.

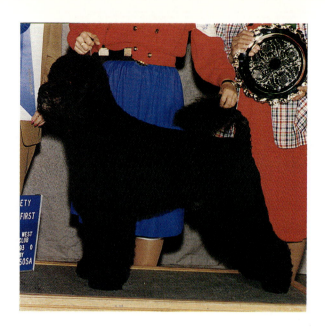

PORTUGUESE WATER DOG

ORIGIN AND HISTORY

In 1960 there were only 11 Portuguese Water Dogs in America. Deyanne and Herb Miller imported a bitch from Portugal in 1968, which they named Renascenca, Portuguese for "renaissance," and that's what happened to the breed. Her first litter was born in 1971 and the Millers kept importing puppies from Portugal.

In 1972 the Portuguese Water Dog Club of America was formed. On the club's 8th anniversary the PWDCA boasted of 339 dogs distributed in 30 states. The breed became eligible to compete in the Working group on January 1, 1984.

DESCRIPTION

In Portugal, the breed is called Cao de Agua (pronounced Kown-d'Agwah) which means "dog of water." It was taught to herd fish into the nets, to retrieve lost tackle and to act as a courier from ship to ship, or from ship to shore.

This is an intelligent breed—calm, rugged and robust, with a profuse non-allergenic, non-shedding, waterproof coat and webbed feet.

He has two coat types, curly or wavy.

THE SHOW RING

Males are 20 to 23 inches high at the withers—the ideal is 22 inches. Females are 17 to 21 inches—the ideal is 19 inches. Weight for males is 42 to 60 pounds, for females weight is 35 to 50 pounds. The dog comes in black, white and various tones of brown, also in combinations of black or brown with white.

DENTITION

Bite should be scissors or level with canines strongly developed. Teeth should not show when the mouth is closed.

RECOGNIZED PROBLEMS

Reported in this breed are **gangliodosis or GMI (storage disease), puppy eye syndrome, sudden puppy death syndrome, congenital kidney disease, Addison's disease and progressive retinal atrophy.**[1] Dr. Bell cites a case of PRA diagnosed in a PWD at 7 years of age that had a normal CERF exam at 5 1/2 years of age. It's very important to have your dogs CERF-examined for the duration of their lives. A full sibling to an affected animal has a 25% chance of being affected and a 66.7% chance of being a carrier if not affected. Pedigree-coefficient and PRA-relevant analyses are available from Dr. Bell. Requests can be made by the AKC-registered owner or breeder of any Portuguese Water Dog.

Researchers all agree that PRA in the PWD is controlled by a single, simple autosomal recessive gene and that there are no "kindreds" of dogs that have an earlier or later onset or course of the disorder. Studies show that in almost all instances, PRA in PWDs is a mild, late onset, slowly progressive disorder.

Dr. Riis (Cornell) feels that 2 years could be considered a safe preliminary cutoff of PWDs with normal ERGs (electroretinograms). Dr. Aguirre stresses that anyone who gets a CERF diagnosis of PRA must ask the examiner to state the disease on the form as early, middle or late progression.

Electroretinographic examinations, while able to identify affected dogs earlier than CERF examinations, are not considered a viable screening test for PRA. The procedure requires general anesthesia, specialized computerized equipment, and can only be performed at a handful of institutions in the country. Remember that a normal CERF or ERG exam only shows that the dog is not affected at the time of the examination. It proves nothing about the possible carrier status of the dog.

Some breeders are advocating test breedings to affected PWDs to statistically clear a breeding dog of the gene for PRA. The logic is that if seven or more resultant pups have a normal ERG at 2 years of age, the tested parent has a 99% chance of being normal for the PRA gene. While this procedure is scientifically sound when using proper protocols, the time and financial and emotional expense involved in test breeding each breeding dog makes this an option for few individuals.[2]

Hip dysplasia has been studied quite extensively in the PWD due to a greater total percentage of OFA evaluations compared to other breeds. The study showed a decrease from 24% dysplastic PWDs evaluated between 1962 and 1982 to 17% dysplastic PWDs in 1987.[3] Dr. Corley of OFA reports that the trend continues, although not at the rate hoped for. The study of litters of PWDs from parents of known hip status generated the following data:

PARENTS	DYSPLASTIC OFFSPRING
Both dysplastic	55%
1 OFA clear/1 dysplastic	30%
Both OFA clear	19%

These figures tell us two things. Firstly, breeding from only OFAed parents can reduce the risk of hip dysplasia. But secondly, observing the hip status of the parents *alone* will not satisfactorily control hip dysplasia.[4]

Puppy eye syndrome has been found in PWDs. It presents with multiple ocular and congenital abnormalities. The ocular abnormalities include: microphthalmia (small globe), microphakia (small lens), corneal dysplasia and persistent pupillary membranes. These pups also have other congenital abnormalities which cause them to be unthrifty. In 1989 Dr. Padgett (Michigan State U.) reported to the PWD club on seven litters with 14 of 54 affected (26%), and no significant sex difference. Dr. Aguirre (U. Pa) reported to the club that he had studied approximately 10 to 15 dogs over a six-year period. He was unable to get two affected dogs to reproduce due to low fertility.

Both researchers suspect a recessive mode of inheritance. Some dogs may have been included in both studies, so a total number of affected dogs is not available.

Addison's disease (Hypoadrenocorticism) is a shutdown of the functioning of the adrenal glands in adult dogs. There are 26 confirmed cases (as of Dec. 1992) in Portuguese Water Dogs, and seven additional suspected or unreleased cases. This disorder is well known and not uncommon in purebred and crossbred dogs. There have been genetic studies performed on this disorder. One study was done in Poodles, where a major autosomal recessive gene seemed to be involved, but it did not appear to be a simple one-gene system.

The PWD parent club is currently investigating the incidence of **cardiomyopathy (sudden puppy death).** Cardiomyopathy is usually a breed-specific disorder of adult dogs, most typically seen in Doberman Pinschers, Boxers and Great Danes. Congenital cardiomyopathy is seen in cats and humans. Canine parvo virus Type 1(CPV-1) is rarely seen now, but used to

434

cause heart damage in young dogs. The heart lesion for CPV-1 is reported to be classical and not similar to the findings in these PWDs.[5]

Congenital kidney disease is reported in this breed. Six cases of chronic kidney failure have been documented in PWDs between the ages of 6 months and 2 years. There are no clinical or pathological signs of toxins or infectious agents reported in these cases. Most cases originally present with increased thirst and urination around 6 to 9 months of age. The condition progresses slowly, with weight loss and loss of appetite, ending in kidney failure and death by 2 to 3 years of age.

Other breeds have reported individuals with congenital kidney disease (also reported as **congenital kidney dysplasia** or **juvenile renal failure).** There are no well-worked-out genetic studies in the veterinary literature. Reports on the Soft Coated Wheaten, Shih Tzu and Miniature Schnauzer breeds suggest a recessive, but not simple recessive mode of inheritance. Many other breeds have sporadic cases reported.[6]

A disease being called **follicular dysplasia** has been identified in PWDs by Dr. William Miller at Cornell and appears to be similar to sebaceous adenitis.[7] For a number of years there have been young adult PWDs reported with a progressive-patterned permanent hair loss. This syndrome is not associated with allergies, itching or endocrine disease. Dr. William Miller of Cornell has been studying this disorder, funded by the PWDCA. Dr. Miller has studied skin biopsies from young and old, affected and non-affected PWDs. Of 56 dogs biopsied, 22 had hair loss. The sexes of the affected dogs were 14 female and eight male (no statistical difference). The coat type of the affected dogs was 21 curly and one wavy (statistically significant; and there is some question on confirming the coat type of the reported wavy). Signs include: decreased hair follicle activity, increased keratin in follicles, abnormal keratinization of hairs, abnormal melanin, dysplastic hairs and abnormal hair bulbs. The biopsies conclude that this is not an endocrine, allergic or nutritional disease. The disease starts with weak hairs that break more easily (hair loss), regrowth of hair with an abnormal texture, and later, follicles that shut down (permanent hair loss). The progression of the hair loss in affected dogs will vary from dog to dog.

The genetic data seen shows a biopsy diagnosis in 16 litters with 20 affected (plus three additional littermates that were not biopsied). There are an additional seven litters with 12 reported affected PWDs. Some of the later dogs may have been biopsied by Dr. Miller since the report was compiled. The genetic data shows that the biopsied and clinically reported affected dogs are all curly, from curly-to-curly matings.

Dr. Miller feels that the early signs of follicular dysplasia are the weak, fragile hairs. He has suggested that a screening test on groomed hairs may be possible for an early diagnosis.[8]

BEHAVIOR

The Portuguese Water Dog makes an excellent companion dog. He is protective of children, lively, intelligent and good company. He adapts equally well to city or country living.

References
1.   Bell, Jerold, Genetic Consultant to the Portuguese Water Dog Club of America. *American Kennel Club Gazette*; January 1993.
2.   "Progressive Retinal Atrophy," *The Courier*; Dec.1992/Jan.1993: 52-53.
3.   Keller, G., et al: "Progress in the Control of Hip Dysplasia," *AKC Gazette*, November, 1991: 55.
4.   "Hip Dysplasia," *The Courier*; Dec.1992/Jan.1993: 50.
5.   "Sudden Puppy Death: Cardiomyopathy," *The Courier*; Dec.1992/Jan.1993: 50.
6.   "Congenital Kidney Disease," *The Courier*; Dec.1992/Jan.1993: 50-51.
7.   Veterinary News, *American Kennel Club Gazette*; April, 1993: 38.
8.   "Hair Loss," *The Courier;* Dec. 1992/Jan.1993: 51-52.

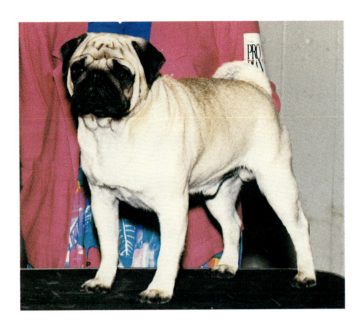

PUG

ORIGIN AND HISTORY

The Pug is an ancient Oriental breed that originated from the Lion dog. The latter were used as temple guards.

DESCRIPTION

Pugs are outgoing, friendly house dogs. The snoring sound from their short noses is sometimes confused for growling, but bad tempers are rare. Some breeders refuse to sell Pugs to families with children, but the breed is a good choice for a family looking for a sturdy dog with a toy temperament. It is imperative to prevent small children from injuring the dog. Pugs are especially susceptible to eye injuries.

THE SHOW RING

The Pug is the largest toy breed. Although the Standard of the breed is 14 to 18 pounds, they may weigh up to 22 pounds without being obese.

Black Pugs should be raven black; rusty or white patches on a black coat are faults.

No disqualifying faults are specified in the breed Standard. The general AKC disqualifications of blindness, deafness, lameness, bilateral or unilateral cryptorchidism or illegal operative procedures to change appearance also apply to the Pug.

BREEDING AND WHELPING

Bitches usually have their first season between 9 and 12 months of age—late for a toy dog. Dogs can be used at stud as early as 6 months.

Gestation commonly lasts 58 to 60 days. Most strains can whelp naturally, although some strains have a tendency towards uterine inertia. Birth weight ranges from 4 to 9 ounces.

The nose and foot pads are pink at birth and pigment is evident by the time the dog is 10 to 14 days old. Patches of white on the chest or toes are allowable, but large white areas, such as an entire leg, are not likely to leave.

In fawn-colored puppies, the face mask and ears are dark and turn to black with age. The trace on the back is dark and prominent at birth, but tends to spread and fade as the puppy gets older. Very light fawns may lose their trace entirely. Fawn color that is smutty at 6 months is unlikely to clear, but occasionally fades as late as the second year. Fawn color that is clear when the dog is young tends to remain clear.

The tail is straight or slightly curved at birth and sickle-shaped by 6 weeks. It may not be tightly curled until 5 or 6 months old.

The pattern of head wrinkles can be seen in a wet newborn puppy. The pattern fades away during puppyhood but returns at 3 to 6 months. Overtone wrinkles are present from birth and do not fade.

GROWTH

A puppy reaches its maximum linear growth by 10 to 12 months, but full weight and maturation may not be complete until 24 to 36 months. The head may continue to grow after maximum linear growth is achieved; it reaches maximum size by 20 to 24 months.

The front legs of puppies should be straight and not bowed. The straightness of a puppy's legs is best observed while the puppy is sleeping or completely relaxed.

Disturbances of bone growth are very rare in the Pug.

A puppy's eyes should be examined for **entropion** and signs of infection or injury. Puppies with large white markings are undesirable for show but make fine pets. A puppy should be lively, outgoing, curious and unafraid.

DENTITION

Although the Standard does not specify bite, it is important for facial appearance. Puppies with **undershot** bites tend to be up-faced as adults, and the problem does not correct. A puppy with a scissors bite is likely to be short in chin and lippy as an adult. **Overbites** in puppies may not correct themselves by adulthood. An overbite is associated with a weak lower jaw and a lippy look. But a small amount of undershot (1/8 inch or less) is desirable, as long as the dog is not up-faced. A large number of missing teeth is unusual.

RECOGNIZED PROBLEMS

A Pug's foot should be compact. The combination of the breed's long nails against smooth floors in runs tend to splay the feet and to break down the pasterns.

Pugs are subject to some hereditary defects. Newborn puppies should be checked for **cleft lips and palates**. **Pinched nostrils** are seen with increasing frequency. This defect can be repaired surgically, but such dogs should not be bred. **Elongated soft palates** cause poor eating and intolerance to heat in an older dog.

The stifles and hips of a Pug puppy should be checked carefully. While **hip dysplasia** is seen infrequently, the condition becomes evident at 6 to 12 months. **Slipped stifles (medial luxating patellas)** are more commonly seen than hip dysplasia and are thought to be an incomplete dominant trait.

Intertrigo of the head wrinkles, particularly over the nose, occurs frequently. It can be prevented by daily cleaning and application of petroleum jelly to the wrinkles and the tip of the nose. Intertrigo can be treated by wiping the wrinkles daily with moistened cotton. If infection occurs, it can be treated with an antibiotic-steroid ointment.

Intolerance to heat is a frequent trait of Pugs, especially those dogs with large soft palates. Pugs should be protected from the sun and from exertion in the hot weather. Pugs are subject to **delayed heat prostration**, and recurrences are possible after the first spell.

The breed is able to withstand most forms of anesthesia. Because of the breed's soft palate, proper airway should be assured by intubation.

Eye injuries are common. Many breeders keep a tube of ophthalmic ointment available. Eyes should be examined daily for excessive tearing, irritation or milkiness of the cornea. Some **pannus formation** of the medial cornea occurs frequently in adults. The breed is subject to a congenital form of **pigmentary keratitis.**[1] **Trichiasis** and **distichiasis**[2] often develop, irritating the cornea further.[3,4]

Entropion occurs more frequently in black Pugs than fawn Pugs and can cause serious, chronic eye irritation.

Pugs have been reported to have a significantly higher risk for **urolithiasis** than most other breeds.[5] They are also at higher risk for generalized **demodectic mange.**[6]

Obesity, a result of improper diet and lack of exercise, is often accompanied by **arthritis** and **heart disease**. Male **pseudohermaphroditism**[7] has been reported. This condition is characterized by the presence of undescended abdominal testicles and external manifestation of a vulva containing an os penis. **Encephalitis** has been seen in Pugs.[8]

Legg-Calve-Perthes[2] disease has been described in the breed and incidence is such to indicate monogenic recessive inheritance of the condition.[9]

BEHAVIOR

The Pug is very clever and mischievous. He is affectionate and lovable. He can also be sulky and hostile with strangers. He can be an amusing companion.

OLD AGE

Older Pugs are subject to the same conditions of old age as other breeds. Pugs commonly live 12 to 14 years if they are guarded from obesity and given regular health care and exercise. They can easily walk one or two miles, except in hot weather.

References
1. Magrane, W.G. *Canine Ophthalmology*, 3rd ed. (Lea & Febiger, Philadelphia, PA. 1977); 305.
2. Foley, J.F. and Osweiler, G.D. *Abnormalities of Companion Animals*. Iowa State Univ. Press, Ames, Iowa,1969.
3. Startup, F.G. *Disease of the Canine Eye*, Baliere and Tindall, London, Eng., 1969.
4. Host, P. and Sveinson, S., "Averlig Katarhat has Hunder," *Norsk Vet*; 1936: 48: 244-270.
5. Bovee, K.C. and McGuire, T. "Qualitative and Quantitative Analysis of Uroliths in Dogs: Definitive Determination of Chemical Type," *JAVMA*; 1984: 105: 9, 983-987; 18 ref.
6. Griffin, C., Kwochka, K., and McDonald, J. *Current Veterinary Dermatology, the Science and Art of Therapy*; Mosby Yearbook, St. Louis, Mo. 1993.
7. Stewart, R.W., et al: "Canine Intersexuality in a Pug Breeding Kennel," *Cornell Vet.;* 62: 464-473.
8. Ettinger, S.J. *Textbook of Veterinary Internal Medicine: Diseases of the Dog and Cat.* (W.B. Saunders Co., Philadelphia, Pa 1989); 608-609.
9. Robinson, R. "Legg-Calve-Perthes Disease in Dogs: Genetic Aetiology," *J. Sm. Anim. Prac.*; 1992: 33: 6, 275-276; 7 ref.

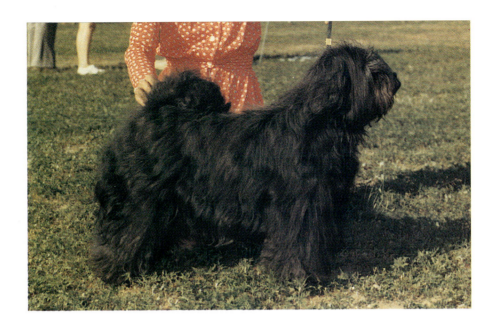

PULI

ORIGIN AND HISTORY

The Puli (plural Pulik) has played an important part in the lives of Hungarian shepherds for more than 1,000 years. Black Pulik were used for day herding and white for night work. The breed is quick and agile and has been reported to jump upon the back of a straying sheep and return it to the flock. The Puli's unique coat is best described as unkempt. The breed shares its ancestry with the Kuvasz and Komondor, and owes part of its lineage to the Tibetan Terrier.

DESCRIPTION

Adult Pulik have outgoing, happy temperaments. They are extremely intelligent, devoted to their owners, active and healthy. They are tireless workers. If given the chance, they will destroy any raccoons, woodchucks or porcupines on their owners' land.

Only the white Puli is born white; black and gray Pulik are born jet black. The puppies' coats are smooth like those of Labrador Retriever puppies.

THE SHOW RING

The Puli is a compact, square-appearing, well-balanced dog of medium size. His original function was as a herder of flocks in Hungary. Agility, combined with soundness of mind and body, is of prime importance for the proper fulfillment of this centuries-old task.

Ideally, males are 17 inches, measured from the withers to ground; bitches, 16 inches. An inch over or under these measurements is acceptable.

Only the solid colors of rusty black, black, all shades of gray and white are allowable. On the chest a white spot no bigger than 2 inches is allowed. The Puli may be shown either corded or brushed. **There are no breed disqualifications.**

BREEDING AND WHELPING

The length of gestation for a Puli differs from that of most breeds. Whelping is more likely to occur from the 65th to the 67th day of gestation, instead of the usual term of 62 to 63 days. The Puli is usually easy to breed and whelps without difficulty. Pregnant bitches often revert to the wild and seek seclusion for whelping. Great care should be taken to prevent Puli bitches from straying outside to make their own nests under a building or woodpile.

GROWTH

Puli puppies are born vigorous and hardy. Birth weights vary greatly, but Puli puppies normally weigh 6 pounds at 6 weeks of age.

Dewclaws should be removed 4 to 5 days after birth. Neither ear cropping nor tail docking is required. The breed Standard mentions that a bob-tail Puli has been known to be whelped abroad, but so far none have been whelped in the United States.

RECOGNIZED PROBLEMS

Missing teeth are rare in this breed. **Hip dysplasia** is common. Only dogs that have x-rays showing that they are free of hip dysplasia should be bred.

The coat requires daily care to prevent the hair from matting.

BEHAVIOR

The Puli does not make a good indoor pet because of its coat. He does not like strangers or children. He has a tendency to wander. He is protective of his territory and his master's possessions.

OLD AGE

Pulik have long life spans. Many remain active up to 17 years of age. Minor arthritis and skin problems are sometimes seen.

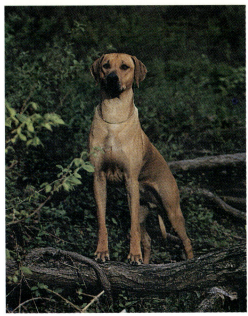
Kerrin Winter

RHODESIAN RIDGEBACK

ORIGIN AND HISTORY

Although the Rhodesian Ridgeback was developed in Africa, the breed is not native to that continent. Only one of the "Ridgeback's" ancestors was a native African dog. It was also the only ancestor having a ridge. This was a small, prick-eared dog found with Hottentot tribes. It was described by Jan Van Riebeek when he arrived at the Cape of Good Hope in 1652. He also described a variety of European dogs that, when crossed with this native dog, produced dogs with ridges.

Other breeds that comprise the Ridgeback's genetic makeup are the Mastiff, the Greyhound, the Pointer, the Labrador Retriever, the Boer Hound (probably a mixture of European dogs brought to Africa by the early settlers), and other dogs brought from various parts of Europe.

The name of the breed is not completely accurate, because the breed originated in the Cape Area. It almost became extinct there, but a small group in Rhodesia revitalized the breed and popularized it to some extent. In 1922 this group wrote the Standard for the breed and it is used today in both the United States and Africa.

The first Rhodesian Ridgeback was brought to the United States from Africa in the late

443

1930s or early 1940s. Soldiers returning from Africa brought more Rhodesian Ridgebacks over during and after World War II. The breed was recognized by the American Kennel Club in 1955.

DESCRIPTION

Ridgebacks are extremely intelligent. They have definite minds of their own and need much individual attention and affection to mature in the proper direction. Otherwise, they may become overly shy or aggressive. Ridgebacks that are raised properly become loyal friends and companions, and courageous defenders of property and charges. Their size and the sound of their bark are sufficient to deter a potential intruder.

THE SHOW RING

The Rhodesian Ridgeback is a large, clean-lined, handsome dog. The adult dog stands 25 to 27 inches at the withers. His desirable weight is 85 pounds. The bitch stands 24 to 26 inches and her desirable weight is 70 pounds.

The color of the coat varies from light to dark red-brown. The breed presents two distinct color varieties: black-nosed with dark eyes, and liver-nosed with amber eyes. Neither variety has an advantage in the show ring.

A Ridgeback must have the ridge, and it must be correct. The ridge should have no more nor less than two crowns or swirls. These crowns should be exactly opposite each other near the shoulder. The crowns should not be multiple; that is, they should not occur at points along the ridge other than near the shoulder.

The only disqualification in the breed is ridgelessness.

BREEDING AND WHELPING

Ridgebacks are usually easy whelpers and frequently have large litters. Litters as large as 15 have been reported. Puppies in a litter may vary considerably in size. The mean weight of puppies of nine litters from various parts of the United States was 465 gm for dogs, n=38, range 325 to 595 grams and for bitches 452 grams, n=32 and range 290 to 560 grams.[1] Dew-claws should be removed shortly after the puppies are born.

Liver-nosed dogs should not be repeatedly mated to each other because color in succeeding generations will fade. The same is true of the black-nosed variety; eventually their color becomes muddied and their faces become too black.

Since pigment on the nose and footpads does not fill in until a puppy is about 2 weeks old, newborn puppies that will have black noses can easily be mistaken for liver-nosed puppies. As liver is a recessive color factor, livers will appear, as does any other recessive trait.

The ridge from which the breed derives its name is considered a dominant genetic

444

factor coupled with incomplete penetrance. This must be concluded because the ridge is the distinctive mark of the breed although it was possessed by only one dog in the breed's background. Mating a Ridgeback to a dog of any other breed can produce a puppy with a ridge; yet mating two purebred Ridgebacks occasionally produces puppies lacking the ridge.

RECOGNIZED PROBLEMS

Dermoid sinus is a serious condition related to the ridge.[2,3,4,5] Sinuses do not, however, occur in the area of the ridge but in the midline anterior to the ridge (neck) or posterior to the ridge (rump). This condition consists of a funnel of outer skin that has grown inward from the surface down to and frequently patently connected with the dura mater (covering of the spinal cord). This funnel usually contains hair, sebum and cellular debris as if it were a normal part of the coat.

There is no means of eliminating debris, so it provides a path of contamination between the external environment and the spinal cord. Consequently contamination, inflammation and infection are likely.

Although surgical removal of the sinus is possible, its proximity to the spinal cord in the lumbar area sometimes makes surgery difficult. The problem becomes greater when multiple sinuses occur.

The frequency with which the sinus occurs indicates that it is not due to a simple recessive factor of inheritance, but to a gene complex. Therefore, most Ridgebacks probably carry some of the factors, so the condition could appear in any breed line.[6] Instead of surgical correction, the more logical and humane course is to euthanize affected puppies as soon as potential cyst-producing sinus cords are found. The sinus can be detected by raising the skin at the midline with one hand and palpating with the other hand, allowing the subcutaneous tissues to slip back and forth between thumb and forefinger.

Diagnosis can be confirmed by clipping and revealing the skin which exposes the external opening with a tuft of hair sometimes projecting from it. In old dogs, the structure is thick-walled and easier to palpate.

Cervical vertebral deformity,[7] **lumbosacral transitional vertebrae,**[8,9] and **hypothyroidism**[8] have been described in the breed. Excluding dermoid sinus, Rhodesian Ridgebacks are not more or less prone to medical problems than other breeds of similar size and structure. **Hip dysplasia** and **aggression** occur but can be controlled with good breeding and management.

Rhodesian Ridgebacks are one of the breeds reported to have congenital **deafness**.[10]

BEHAVIOR

The Ridgeback is trainable, good-natured, tranquil and obedient. He makes a good family house dog.

OLD AGE

Rhodesian Ridgebacks have a life span that averages 10 to 14 years.

References

1. Clough, E. *The Ridgeback. Newsletter of the Rhodesian Ridgeback Club of the U.S.,Inc.*, in press.
2. Kirk, R.W. and Bistner, S.I. *Handbook of Veterinary Procedures and Emergency Treatment.* 1975: Table 124, 661.
3. Hoare, T. "A Congenital Abnormality of Hair Follicles in Dogs," *J. Path. and Bact.*; 1932: 35:569-571.
4. Hofmeyer, C.F.D. "Dermoid Sinus in the Rhodesian Ridgeback," *J. Sm. Anim. Prac.*; 1963: 7: 631-642.
5. Clinical Item: "Dermoid Sinus in the Rhodesian Ridgeback Dog," *JAVMA;* 1970: 157:961-962.
6. Lord, L.H., et al: "Mid-Dorsal Dermoid Sinuses in Rhodesian Ridgeback Dogs," A Case Report. *JAVMA*; 1957: 515-518.
7. Lane, J.S. *J. Am Radiological Society;* XVIII, 1977: 76-79.
8. Clough, E. Unpublished Personal Data.
9. Winkler, W. "Transitional Lumbosacral Vertebrae in the Dog," Dissertation: Fachbereich Veterinarmedizin der Freien Universitat Berlin. 1985: 143;50 ref.
10. Strain, George M. "Deafness in Dogs and Cats," *Proc. 10th ACVIM Forum.* May, 1992.

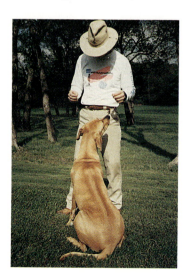

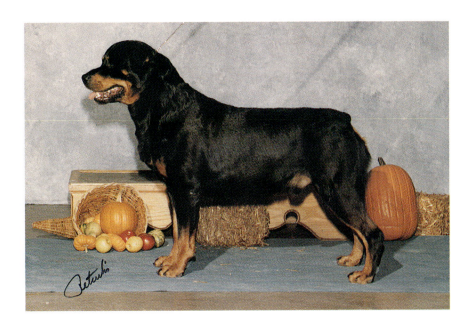

ROTTWEILER

ORIGIN AND HISTORY

The Rottweiler is a very old breed. Some historians claim Rottweilers were used by the Roman legions to drive cattle. Later they were used by German farmers to drive cattle to market and guard both money and master on the journey home. They have been used successfully as military and police dogs and as "eyes" for the blind, both in Europe and the United States. The breed as we see it today was developed by the German Breed Club, which wrote the Standard and established the breeding rules for Rottweilers.

DESCRIPTION

The Rottweiler is a highly intelligent dog and responds well to training; many hold obedience degrees. It is a dog devoted to its family, and its dependable and unexcitable nature makes it an ideal household companion in a small or large home. It is powerful but gentle, excellent with children, and yet a determined and courageous guard against intruders. Essentially a working dog, its qualities make it an excellent guard and companion. Not all families are suited to the ownership of a Rottweiler. While the breed is adaptable to varieties of climate and living quarters, like any large breed it needs adequate exercise. Unlike some breeds it is most happy when allowed to be a part of the family activities. A fenced yard or confinement when the

447

Rottweiler cannot be with the family will protect it from the hazards of motorized urban life.

THE SHOW RING

The Rottweiler is a large dog, though not a giant breed. The dog averages 24 to 27 inches at the shoulder. The bitch stands from 22 to 25 inches at the shoulder. Rottweilers weigh from 90 to 130 pounds. The coat is black, of medium length, coarse and flat, with a soft undercoat which insulates in cold climates and in the water, which it loves. The coat is accented with mahogany-tan markings above each eye, on the cheeks, under the tail, on the muzzle, throat and chest, and on all 4 legs. It requires no special grooming beyond a weekly brushing.

Breed disqualifications are: entropion; ectropion; overshot; undershot; wry mouth; two or more missing teeth; unilateral cryptorchid or cryptorchid males; long coat; any base color other than black; absence of all markings; a dog that, in the opinion of the judge, attacks any person in the ring.

BREEDING AND WHELPING

Rottweilers are late-maturing dogs, and the first estrus season rarely occurs before a bitch is 8 months old. A bitch carrying a very large litter is likely to whelp early, especially with the first litter. With an older bitch and a small litter, late whelping is not at all unusual. Average litter size is seven puppies. Weight of puppies at birth is from 12 to 18 ounces. A puppy whose birth weight is less than 7 ounces has slim chances of survival. Most Rottweiler bitches whelp normally.

Some males are reported to be **"lazy breeders"** and an Artificial Insemination is required.[1] Most bitches produce milk and are good mothers, providing they have been well nourished and allowed to exercise during gestation. Occasionally with a first litter, the bitch may take a few hours to settle down and accept the puppies. The bitch that does not instinctively care for her puppies is a rarity. She is protective of her puppies, especially during the first week or two, and most particularly toward strangers from outside the family circle.

Cleft palates in newborns have been reported.

GROWTH

If the litter is larger than average, it may be advisable to offer supplemental feedings to the puppies. For bottle feeding, a standard baby nursing bottle and nipple are essential, but the Rottweiler puppies may be easily and quickly fed with a tube and a syringe. They should gain 1/2 to 1 ounce per day at first, then gain more rapidly as they get older. A typical 7- to 8-week-old puppy should weigh 12 to 15 pounds.

As the Rottweiler reaches maturity it profits from a good maintenance diet which is, again, a good commercial dog food. Regular exercise and proper weight ensure the hard, fit look of the working dog and prolong the life of the animal.

Although **gastric torsion** is not a common problem in younger Rottweilers, the owner who has an "eager eater" or a "food gulper" might be well advised to split the normal daily ration of food into two feedings—also a good recommendation for a bitch in whelp.

Puppies are most successfully weaned directly onto a commercial puppy chow mixed with water in a blender to the consistency of thick malted milk. By the time they are ready to go to their new homes at 7 to 8 weeks, puppies are usually eating regular puppy food, soaked in warm water.

Puppies should be kept on a puppy food for the first year, with minimal vitamin and mineral supplements. Average growth should be aimed for, not maximum. Rottweilers have usually reached their full height by the time they are 1 year old, but do not reach the full bloom of maturity until 3 or 4 years old. Two things that often alarm new puppy owners unnecessarily are that the distal end of the radius in the area of the growth plates looks larger than it should, and the occipital process is very often quite pronounced in appearance.

DENTITION

Rottweilers should have a scissors bite. Less than full dentition (42 teeth) in an adult dog is a serious fault. More than two missing teeth is a breed-ring disqualification, as are over-shot, undershot or wry mouths.

RECOGNIZED PROBLEMS

The Rottweiler is a very "natural" dog. Through the years, selection for breeding has been based on working qualities. Canine **hip dysplasia** is the one developmental problem found in the breed with any statistical frequency. All of the Rottweiler Specialty breed clubs in the United States recommend that Rottweilers should not be bred until 2 years of age and proven radiographically free of **hip dysplasia** by the Orthopedic Foundation for Animals, Inc. (University of Missouri-Columbia, Columbia, Missouri 65201). As with any other large, heavy breed, **shoulder injuries** may result from too much rough play with older dogs, or forced exercise, such as jumping, during the formative months of the first year.[2]

Of 408 Rottweilers x-rayed in Norway in 1972-1984, 22% were dysplastic.[3]

Elbow dysplasia has been reported.[4,5]

An American study has concluded that there is no sex predilection for unilateral hip dysplasia.[6] Analysis of data collected over a 5-year period from 616 dogs, of which 52.1% were females, on the incidence of the condition **Arthrosis of the elbow joint**, revealed that the relative risk of males developing the disease was 1.5 times that of females. The heritability of the condition was 0.26 when based on full-sib analysis and 0.32 when based on regression of parent on offspring.[7]

A study was made of 335 dogs (Labradors, Rottweilers, Golden Retrievers) with **elbow osteochondrosis** that had been seen at the Royal Veterinary College in 1977 to 1987. Males were affected more often than females. The condition was bilateral in 50% of cases and the peak age for the onset of lameness was 4 — 6 months. In Rottweilers, the lesions found at exploratory arthrotomy were predominantly abnormalities of the coronoid process,[8] while in Retrievers lesions most commonly affected the medial humeral condyle or the coronoid process.[9]

Osteochondrosis in the lateral trochlear ridge of the talus was diagnosed in seven Rottweiler dogs (four male and three female, aged 6 — 15 months). Each dog had a history of hindlimb lameness of 2 to 5 months duration. Defects in the lateral trochlear ridge and osteochondral fragments arising from the dorsal and proximal margins of the ridge were visible radiographically. Four dogs had lesions in both legs. The dorsal 45 degrees lateral-plantaromedial oblique (D45° L-P1MO) projection was the most useful in identifying the lesions. Exploratory arthrotomies were performed in six affected tarsi of five dogs, and all osteochondral fragments were removed. In three cases, histological examination revealed mineralized osteochondral fragments consistent with a diagnosis of osteochondrosis. In two dogs examined 8 weeks after surgery, the lameness was still evident but had improved. Two years later, one dog was intermittently lame.[10]

A group of 55 Rottweiler pups was studied from 3 to 12 months of age to assess the incidence and clinical significance of disease involving the palmar-metacarpal sesamoid bones. It was concluded that **sesamoid disease** can result in clinical lameness in young Rottweilers, but that subclinical disease is common.[11,12]

The presence and the result of **ossification centers** in the radius have been reported in a German study.[13]

Neuroaxonal dystrophy (NAD) and **leukoencephalomalacia (LEM)** are two neurological disorders of the Rottweiler that initially present as ataxia of all four limbs. Disorders to be included in the differential diagnosis are caudal-cervical spondylomyelopathy, canine distemper virus, meningoencephalomyelitis, other nervous-system infections or inflammations and spinal cord neoplasia. All diagnostic tests including myelography, cerebrospinal fluid analysis, electrodiagnostic testing and serum and cerebrospinal fluid titres for canine distemper virus are normal in NAD and LEM. There is no treatment for either disease and neurological signs progressively deteriorate. Eventually neurological deficits develop besides ataxia, and these help differentiate NAD from LEM. Dogs with NAD develop head tremors and nystagmus while dogs

450

with LEM develop conscious proprioceptive deficits and quadriparesis; the short-term prognosis for NAD is better than for LEM. Most dogs with LEM are euthanized because of non-ambulatory tetraparesis within one year. The histopathological lesions associated with NAD include axonal spheroids in many spinal cord and caudal brainstem nuclei and reduced numbers of Purkinje cells in the cerebellum, while in LEM, multifocal areas of demyelination and malacia of the spinal cord and brainstem are the primary histopathological lesions. Both NAD and LEM are suspected to have an autosomal recessive genetic transmission.[14,15,16,17,18]

Ectropion and **entropion**[19] have been controlled in the Rottweiler by careful breeding so it is a possible, but not a significant, factor.

Rottweilers are identified as one of the breeds with congenital **deafness**.[20]

Inherited forms of **muscular dystrophy** linked to the "X" chromosome are being studied and have been identified in Rottweilers.[21]

Familial kidney failure attributable to **atrophic glomerulopathy** has been reported in Rottweilers. The congenital renal failure reported in Doberman Pinschers and Samoyeds is histologically different from that which has been identified in Rottweilers.[22]

There appears to be some predisposition to **parvovirus** infection in Rottweilers.[23,24] In the opinion of the authors incidence may be no higher, but manifestation of symptoms is more pronounced. **Diabetes mellitus** has been reported.[25]

Vitiligo is an asymptomatic depigmenting disease of skin, mucosa and haircoat, especially of the nose, lips, eyelids, claws and trunk. A questionnaire was included in a publication sent to 1500 members of the American Rottweiler Club. Fourteen questionnaires and thirteen pedigrees were returned of dogs affected with vitiligo. Analysis of this data showed that the majority of dogs developed clinical signs between 1.5 and 5 years of age, and large areas of the body were involved in seven dogs. While a current theory of immune-mediated destruction of melanocytes explains the pathogenesis of vitiligo, the author suggests further research in the prevalence, genetics, and role of immune-mediated mechanisms in the disorder.[26]

BEHAVIOR

The Rottweiler is a formidable guard dog if properly trained. If he is to be a house pet he must have a master who trains by earning his obedience and respect. He is naturally aloof and wary of strangers but should not be vicious. If trained as a family companion he will be gentle with the children.

OLD AGE

The life span of a Rottweiler is 10 to 11 years. Problems that appear most often in old age are the same ones that other breeds and human beings finally succumb to—cancer, heart ailments, bloat and other geriatric debilities.

References
1. Walkowicz, Chris "The Mechanics of Breeding." *The American Kennel Club Gazette*; May, 1990: 68.
2. Kirk, R.W. and Bistner, S.I. *Handbook of Veterinary Procedures and Emergency Treatment.* 1975: Table 124, 661.
3. Lingaas, F. and Heim, P. "A Genetic Investigation of the Incidence of Hip Dysplasia in Norwegian Dog Breeds," *Norsk-Vetrinaertidsskrift*; 1987: 99:9, 617-623; 22 ref.
4. Veterinary News, *American Kennel Club Gazette*; June, 1990.
5. Bodner, Elizabeth, DVM, "Genetic Status Symbols," *The American Kennel Club Gazette*; September, 1992.
6. Keller, G.G. and Corley, E.A. "Canine Hip Dysplasia: Investigating the Sex Predilection and the Frequency of Unilateral CHD," *Vet.Med.*; 1989: 84:12, 1162, 1164-1166; 13 ref.
7. Grondalen, J. and Lingaas, F. "Arthrosis of the Elbow Joint Among Rottweiler Dogs: Results From Investigations into Hereditary Disposition," *Tijdschrift-Voor-Diergeneeskunde*; 1988: 113: Supplement, 49S-51S.
8. Read, R. "Fragmented Coronoid Process in the Rottweiler—A Review of 35 Cases," *Australian Vet. Prac.*; 1987: 17:3, 140-141.
9. Guthrie, S. "Use of a Radiographic Scoring Technique for the Assessment of Dogs With Elbow Osteochondrosis," *J. Sm. Anim. Prac.;* 1989: 30:11, 639-644; 5 ref.
10. Wisner, E.R., Berry, C.R., Morgan, J.P., Pool, R.R., Wind, A.P., and Vasseur, P.B. "Osteochondrosis of the Lateral Trochlear Ridge of the Talus in Seven Rottweiler Dogs," *Vet.-Surgery;* 1990: 19: 6, 435-439; 9 ref.
11. Read, R.A., Black, A.P., Armstrong, S.J., MacPherson, G.C. and Peek, J. "Incidence and Clinical Significance of Sesamoid Disease in Rottweilers," *Vet. Record.*; 1992: 130:24, 533-535; 12 ref.
12. Vaughan, L.C. and France, C. "Abnormalities of the Volar and Plantar Sesamoid Bones in Rottweilers," *J. Sm. Anim. Prac.*; 1986: 27:9, 551-558; 6 ref.
13. Zenses, W., Schreiber, and Kupper, W. "Ossification Centers in the Radius as a Cause of Lameness in Rottweilers," *Praktische-Tierarzt.*; 1989: 70:12, 40, 42-43; 6 ref.
14. Chrisman, C.L. "Neurological Diseases of Rottweilers: Neuroaxonal Dystrophy and Leukoencephalomalacia," *J. Sm. Anim. Prac.*; 1992: 33:10, 500-504; 15 ref.
15. Wonda, W. and Van Nes, J.J. "Progressive Ataxia Due to Central Demyelination in Rottweiler Dogs," *Vet Quarterly;* 1986: 8:2, 89-97; 13 ref.
16. Gamble, D.A. and Chrisman, C.L. "A Leukoencephalomyelopathy of Rottweiler Dogs," *Vet-Path.;* 1984: 21:3, 274-280; 28 ref.
17. Chrisman, C.L., Cork, L.C. and Gamble, D.A. "Neuroaxonal Dystrophy of Rottweiler Dogs," *JAVMA*; 1984: 184:4, 464-467; 9 ref.
18. Ettinger, S.J. *Textbook of Veterinary Internal Medicine: Diseases of Dogs and Cats.* (W.B. Saunders Co., Philadelphia, PA 1989); 599.

19. Magrane, W. *Canine Ophthalmology*, 3rd ed. (Lea & Febiger, Phildelphia, PA.,1977); 305.
20. Strain, George M. "Deafness in Dogs and Cats," *Proc. 10th ACVIM Forum*. May, 1992.
21. "Veterinary News," *The American Kennel Club Gazette*; October, 1991.
22. *JAVMA*; Volume 202, No. 1, January 1, 1993.
23. Seton, R. and Seton, J. "Canine Parvovirus in Rottweiler Pups," *Australian Vet. Practitioner;* 1990: 20:4, 231.
24. Glickman, L.T., Domanski, L.M., Patronek, G.J., and Visintainer, F. "Breed-Related Risk Factors for Canine Parvovirus Enteritis," *JAVMA*; 1985: 187:6, 589-594; 12 ref.
25. Catalogue of Congenital and Hereditary Diseases.
26. Scott, D.W. "Vitiligo in the Rottweiler," *Canine Practice*; 1990: 15:3, 22-25; 8 ref.

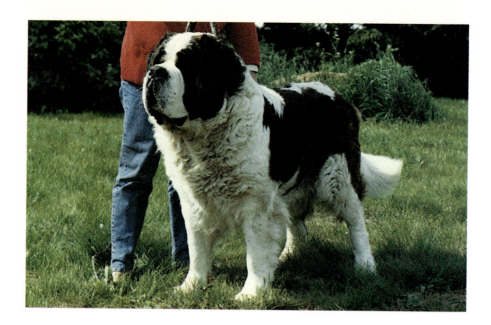

SAINT BERNARD

ORIGIN AND HISTORY

The St. Bernard is thought to have descended from the Asian Mollossian type dog, which was brought to Switzerland during various invasions. The Hospice of St. Bernard de Menthon in the Swiss Alps began to keep these dogs in the 1660s. These large, hardy dogs accompanied the monks as they searched the mountains for travelers trapped by storms. The dogs soon proved valuable at pathfinding and locating lost travelers. The St. Bernard dogs of the Hospice are credited with saving over 2,500 lives during their work in the mountains. In 1830, Newfoundlands were bred to the Hospice dogs to increase the latter's size and vigor. This outcross also resulted in a long-haired variety of St. Bernards.[1]

DESCRIPTION

In addition to its courage and stamina, the St. Bernard's gentle spirit and devotion to man have made it a valued companion. Because of the danger of an avalanche from loud noises, the monks bred quieter dogs.[2] In a survey of canine behavioral complaints by breed, St. Bernards ranked slightly lower than the all-breeds norm. The two leading complaints were of unruliness and disobedience.[3]

THE SHOW RING

Mature St. Bernards weigh 160 pounds and may get as large as 200 pounds.[2] The minimum height at the shoulder is 27 1/2 inches for the dog, but more often is 30 to 31 inches. The bitches are slightly smaller, the minimum height being 25 1/2 inches.[1,2] St. Bernards may be of red or brown-yellow color with white marks on the chest, feet and tip of tail, noseband, collar or spot on the nape; the latter and blaze are very desirable. The coat is very dense, short-haired, smooth and tough. The thighs and tail are bushy. A St. Bernard should be powerful, proportionately tall, strong and muscular, with powerful head and intelligent expression. The more common faults include long or sway back, bent or cowhocks, out at the elbows, and weak pasterns. Dewclaws sometimes appear on the hindlegs.[1]

There are no breed disqualifications.

BREEDING AND WHELPING

St. Bernard bitches have an estrous pattern typical of most breeds. Their first heat generally occurs at about 9 months of age, but can vary from 6 to 15 months. After the first heat they have an estrous cycle that averages 6 months in length so that they come into heat twice a year. The gestation length also runs near the average of 63 days. Whelping difficulties are seldom encountered, but **uterine inertia** and **eclampsia** are occasionally seen.[4] The litter size may vary from three to 17, but eight to 10 is the more usual size. At birth the puppies weigh just less than a pound.[2]

GROWTH

St. Bernard puppies have an extremely rapid rate of growth.[5] During the first few months of life they gain 20 to 26 pounds per month and then growth slows until they reach full size at 2 years.

An uncoordinated puppy, and especially one with a large, heavy body, puts undue mechanical stress on his developing skeleton. In the giant puppy, this stress can cause problems. Because of their rapid growth and degree of weight bearing, the radius and ulna are usually the first bones to show signs of growth abnormalities. Before the growth plates close, bone diameter increases proportionately to the rate of growth. Since the distal ulnar growth plate is responsible for 85% of the ulna's growth and the distal radial growth plate contributes only 70% of the radial length, the distal ulna must grow faster than the distal radius and therefore increases its diameter more. At 4 to 5 months, the diameter of the ulna is 50% larger than that of the radius. By 7 to 9 months, the diameters are about equal, and in the adult the ulna is only about half the size of the radius. At 5 to 6 months, because the radius and ulna are growing so rapidly, their growth plates are vastly enlarged. Since the bones overlie each other, at this time a very noticeable enlargement normally occurs above the carpus. The enlargement should not be mistaken for metabolic bone disease or abnormal bone growth.[6,7]

It is important to feed a balanced diet to the growing puppy. If a good-quality dog food is fed, supplementation is seldom necessary. Dogs of the giant breeds have large nutritional requirements during their extremely rapid period of growth. The total requirement is larger than that of other dogs, but is in the same proportions.[5] A problem may occur when St. Bernard puppies are fed a poor-quality dry dog food. The food's low digestibility makes it impossible for the puppy to consume enough digestible nutrients to meet his needs.[5] Conversely oversupplementation can result in certain growth abnormalities. Feeding the giant puppy a highly palatable and energy-rich diet, free choice, results in maximal growth, which is not compatible with optimal skeletal development. In feeding trials, Hedhammer showed that giant puppies fed a complete and balanced diet, free choice, had a greater number of skeletal diseases than their littermates fed restricted amounts. Skeletal problems encountered due to overfeeding include **coxa valga**, **enostosis**, **hip dysplasia**, **hypertrophic osteodystrophy, osteochondrosis dissecans** and **"wobblers syndrome."** Hedhammer recommended that growing puppies be fed restricted amounts of a complete and balanced diet with no supplementation.[8]

RECOGNIZED PROBLEMS

The St. Bernard's large size creates problems in three ways: 1) the factor (growth hormone) size, when present in excess, has undesirable effects on many tissues, 2) rapid growth is not conducive to optimal development, 3) the large adult size puts additional mechanical stress on bones and skeleton and predisposes to anatomical abnormalities not seen in smaller dogs. St. Bernards are also subject to some hereditary problems which are unrelated to size.

The St. Bernard is an acromegalic breed. The pituitary gland of the St. Bernard resembles **neoplastic pituitaries** of other breeds. The pituitary gland of the St. Bernard shows frequent abnormalities which include **epithelial lined cysts** in the anterior pituitary,[9] especially many eosinophilic cells which produce growth hormone. The results of excess growth hormones are seen mostly in skin and bone. The long bones have enlarged diameters and all the bones are rough with frequent **exostosis**.[9] The sternum is enlarged to produce a "keel."[10] **Acromegaly** also produces excess skin generally seen over the head, chest and shoulders where it lays in folds.[9,10]

One condition which results from excess skin is **lip fold pyoderma**, an infection develops in the deep fold of the lower lip. Treatment may be medical or surgical depending on the

456

severity of the infection.[11,12] Acromegaly and consequent excess skin on the head contribute to **entropion** and **ectropion**, both seen in the St. Bernard as congenital conditions. **Distichiasis**, seen more frequently in St. Bernards than in other breeds, may complicate lid problems. Surgical treatment is preferred for both entropion and ectropion and should be performed when the dog is near maturity. **Eversion of the membrana nictitans** also occurs in St. Bernards.[13]

Osteochondrosis dissecans is seen in St. Bernards and other large breed dogs.[14,15] In St. Bernards acromegaly may be a contributing factor to this condition. Growing dogs that were treated with somatotropin and thyrotropin were found to have thick subchondral bone trabeculae especially in the humeral head, irregular arrangements of cells lacking nuclei in the thick articular germinative zone and epiphyseal cartilage with cells in clusters on only a few cells in places. The changes in the treated dogs resembled those seen in clinical cases of osteochondrosis dissecans.[14]

Acromegaly in the St. Bernard may be the reason that **diabetes mellitus** is seen more frequently in this breed. Krook et al (1960) found that an association may exist between the increased secretion of somatotropin in the giant breed dogs and the development of diabetes.[16,17] The anterior pituitary has been shown experimentally to be involved in the initiation and the maintenance of diabetes. Growth hormone particularly has been shown to be responsible for this effect. When crude extracts of the anterior pituitary gland are injected into certain animals they produce a diabetic state. Alternately, diabetes caused by pancreatectomy can be relieved by hypophysectomy.[15]

St. Bernards have a greater incidence of **hip dysplasia** than any other breed.[18,19] Dogs and bitches are affected equally.[20] Forty-three percent of St. Bernard pelvic radiographs submitted to the Orthopedic Foundation for Animals showed dysplasia. The incidence is certainly much higher than this as radiographs of obviously affected animals are not submitted. Acromegaly and subsequent rapid growth rate may underlie most of the etiologies suggested for hip dysplasia. A metabolic defect, pelvic muscle mass, pectineus muscle spasm, shallow acetabulum, slanting pelvis and a rapid growth rate have all been cited as causes.[21] **Elbow dysplasia** has been reported in the breed.[22]

Genu valgum is a deformity seen in giant dogs in which the knees are bowed medially. The first signs are usually seen when the dog is 3 to 4 months of age and consist of reluctance to move. Pain is seen on hindleg extension. Usually when the period of rapid growth is over the dog accommodates to the limb deformity and is able to ambulate reasonably well. The degree of deformity seen at 8 to 11 months of age is permanent. Genu valgum is felt to occur when the bone growth rate exceeds the capacity of the circulation to transport sufficient nutrients to the lateral distal femoral metaphysis and proximal tibial metaphysis. Growth is slowed on the ischemic lateral sides of the growth plates and medial bowing results. Oversupplementation of the diet predisposes to genu valgum.[23]

Retained cartilage cores in the distal ulnar metaphysis may occur during the period of rapid growth in which the bone grows faster than its blood supply and causes lack of vascularization in the center of the metaphyseal ulnas and lack of normal cartilage ossification. Clinically this is seen as a cranial bowing of the radius, a rotated carpus and an abducted foot.[7]

Osteosarcoma is a neoplastic condition seen primarily in large dogs, especially St. Bernards and Great Danes.[24,25,26] In a study of breed distribution of 130 dogs with osteosarcoma, only six weighed less than 30 pounds. Within various breeds, the tumor seems to have a predilection for specific sites. St. Bernards tend to have osteosarcomas which originate primarily from the forelimbs at the metaphyseal region. Hindlimb osteosarcoma is less common and origin from flat bones is very rare.[27] Trauma is suspected to play a role in the etiology of osteosarcoma, as often owners will report some sort of previous injury to the tumor-affected leg.[28,23] Also large dogs, whose bones must bear much mechanical stress, are more affected than smaller dogs. The continuous mechanical trauma to which the forelegs (which bear most of the animal's weight) are subjected may explain why the distal radial metaphysis is the most common site for osteosarcoma in the St. Bernard.[24,25] Diagnosis is usually made radiographically. Biopsy and histopathologic exam provide positive diagnosis. The prognosis for osteosarcoma is generally grave, but not hopeless. If there is no metastasis to the lungs, amputation of the affected limb is recommended. Improvement may be seen immediately following surgery, but the average survival time postoperatively is only six months. Dogs having undergone surgery to remove an osteosarcoma were found, at necropsy, to have more metastasis than dogs with osteosarcoma that did not have surgery. The former group also lived longer, allowing more time for metastasis. (Note: some dogs are too heavy and arthritic to be ambulatory after amputation, so a careful preoperative evaluation of their general health is recommended.) When metastasis occurs it is by invasion of the veins. Local lymph node involvement is rare.[24] Drug treatment has been used with some success.[29]

St. Bernards are one of a group of dogs at high risk for **canine lymphoma**.[30,31,32]

Hemophilia A has been reported in St. Bernards.[33] Other problems associated with large breeds are **gastric or splenic torsion**,[34] **cardiomyopathy**, **hygroma**, **hypertrophic osteodystrophy** and **idiopathic degenerative joint disease**. These problems are not specific in the St. Bernard, but are seen generally in the large and giant breeds.[35,36,37,38]

Although rarely seen today because of selective breeding, several hereditary problems have been reported in St. Bernards. The first is **Stockard's Paralysis**, an inherited defect causing a fatal loss of function in certain motor neurons and preganglionic sympathetic neurons of the lumbar region of the spinal cord. At least three mutant, dominant genes control the trait. Onset of signs may be sudden or gradual with paralysis in certain groups of thigh and leg muscles at 11 to 14 weeks of age. Puppies may show only minor changes in gait or in severe cases may lack all motor control of the hind legs. The initial prostration may last a few days to a month. During this time the puppy is not in pain, and urination, defecation and tail movement are normal. Priapism may be observed due to paralysis of vasoconstrictors to the penis. Eventually the puppy learns to rotate and twist his legs to lift and support the posterior region of the body and assumes an awkward and rolling gait. There is no treatment for this condition and owners should be cautioned against breeding affected animals.[9,39]

Another hereditary disease which has been reported in St. Bernards is **Hemophilia B (Factor IX, PTT Deficiency or Christmas Disease)**.[40] The inheritance mechanism is through an X-linked recessive gene and therefore most signs are seen in the males.[21,41] An affected dog may have less than 1% of the normal factor nine level and female carriers have 40 to 60% of the normal level. Bleeding problems are due to defective intrinsic clotting which is seen in long whole blood clotting, plasma recalcification, partial thromboplastin times and very short prothrombin consumption or serum clotting times.[42,32]

Signs of a bleeding problem include listlessness, anorexia and melena or fresh blood in the feces. Signs tend to be especially severe in St. Bernards because of their size. It is unusual to see epistaxis or hematemesis. Umbilical bleeding at birth is usually not a problem and the first signs in puppies are frequently seen during the period of vaccination with live virus vaccines, which can aggravate their hemostatic defect by superimposing thrombocytopenia or thrombocytopathy.

Treatment should be instituted when the packed cell volume falls below 20%, and consists of transfusions of fresh-frozen homologous plasma every 12 hours. It is important to cross match the blood since dogs with hemophilia B will require repeated transfusions throughout their lives.

Medications to avoid include aspirin, promazine-type tranquilizers, phenylbutazones, sulfonamides, nitrofurans or any other drugs that interfere with hemostasis. Dogs with bleeding problems should not be given intramuscular injections. Medications should be given orally, intravenously or subcutaneously with a 25-gauge needle. General care should include separate housing, a soft diet, and control of internal and external parasites.[9]

Epilepsy is reported more frequently in St. Bernards than in other breeds and may have a hereditary basis.[16] **Corneal dermoids** occur occasionally in the large breed dogs, and have been reported to be hereditary in the St. Bernard.[43] The St. Bernard is predisposed to **acute moist dermatitis (hot spots)** due to its thick hair coat and commonly develops **acral**

lick dermatitis (acral lick granulomas).[44] **Uveodermatologic Syndrome** has been reported in the Saint Bernard.[45]

Saint Bernards are one of the Breeds reported to have congenital **deafness**.[46]

BEHAVIOR

Cheerful, loyal and patient with teasing children, the Saint makes an excellent family companion, but is not suited to apartment life and does not always relate well to small dogs.

References

1. American Kennel Club: *The Complete Dog Book*. (Howell Book House, New York, NY 1992); 303-307.
2. Kay, H. *Man and Mastiff*. (MacMillan, New York, N.Y. 1976).
3. Campbell, W.E. *Behavior Problems in Dogs*. (American Veterinary Publishing, Inc., Santa Barbara, Ca.,1975).
4. Migliorina, M. *St. Bernards*. (Arco Pub. Co., New York, NY, 1976).
5. Morris, M.L., Jr., *Canine Dietetics*. (Mark Morris Assoc.,Topeka, KS 1972).
6. Riser, W.H. "Radiographic Differential Diagnosis of Skeletal Diseases of Young Dogs," *J. Amer. Vet. Rad. Soc.*; 1965: 6:50-64.
7. Riser, W.H. and Shirer, J.F. "Normal and Abnormal Growth of the Distal Foreleg in Large and Giant Dogs," *J. Amer. Vet. Rad. Soc.*; 1965: 6:50-64.
8. Hedhammer, A., et al "Overnutrition and Skeletal Disease," *Cornell Vet.*; April 1974: 64 Supplement 5:1-160.
9. Stockard, C.R. "A Hereditary Lethal for Localized Motor and Preganglionic Neurones with a Resulting Paralysis in the Dog," *Amer. J. Anat.*; May 1936: 59:1-53.
10. Smythe, R.H. "The Anatomy of Dog Breeding," (Chas. C. Thomas Publ. Co., Springfield, Ill.,1962).
11. Archibald, J. *Canine Surgery*, 2nd Ed. (American Publ. Co. Santa Barbara, CA. 1974).
12. Muller, G.H. and Kirk, R.W. *Small Animal Dermatology*, 2nd ed. (W.B. Saunders, Philadelphia, PA. 1976).
13. Magrane, W.G. *Canine Ophthalmology*, 2nd ed. (Lea & Febiger, Philadelphia, PA, 1974).
14. Paatsama, S., et al "Somatoropin, Thyrotropin, and Corticotropin Hormone-induced Changes in the Cartilages and Bones of the Shoulder and Knee Joint in Young Dogs," *J. Sm. Anim. Prac.*; 12:595-601.
15. Bergsten, G. and Nordin, M. "Osteochondrosis as a Cause of Claims in a Population of Insured Dogs," *Svensk-Veterinartidning*; 1986: 38:15, 97-100.
16. Cameron, M.P. and O'Connor, M. Eds *Aetiology of Diabetes and its Complications*, Little, Brown, & Co., Boston, Ma.1964.
17. Ettinger, S.J. Ed *Textbook of Veterinary Internal Medicine*. (W.B. Saunders, Philadelphia, PA. 1975).
18. Larsen, J.S. "Report on Canine Hip Dysplasia," *JAVMA;* 162: 662-668; April 15, 1973.

19. Lingaas, F. and Heim, P. "A Genetic Investigation of the Incidence of Hip Dysplasia in Norwegian Dog Breeds," *Norsk-Vetrinaertidsskrift*; 1987: 99:9, 617-623; 22 ref.

20. Riser, W.H. and Larsen, J.S. "Influence of Breed Somatotypes on Prevalence of Hip Dysplasia in the Dog," *JAVMA;* July 1, 1974: 165:79-81.

21. Priester, W.A. and Mulvihill, J.J. "Canine Hip Dysplasia: Relative Risk by Sex, Size, and Breed, and Comparative Aspects," *JAVMA;* March 1, 1972: 160:735-738.

22. Veterinary News, *American Kennel Club Gazette*; June, 1990.

23. Riser, W.H., et al: "Genu Valgum: A Stifle Deformity of Giant Dogs," *J. Amer. Vet. Rad. Soc.*; 1969: 10:28-37.

24. Brinkhous, K.M. et al "Expression and Linkage of Genes for X-Linked Hemophilias A and B in the Dog," *Blood;* April, 1973: 41:577-583.

25. Hansen, J. "The Body Constitution of Dogs and its Importance for the Occurrence of Disease," *Nord. Vet. Med.*; 1964: 16:977-987.

26. Owen, L.N. "The Differential Diagnosis of Bone Tumors in the Dog," *Vet. Rec.;* April 14, 1962: 74:439-446.

27. Brodey, R.S., et al "Canine Bone Neoplasms," *JAVMA;* Sept. 1, 1963: 143:471-495.

28. Nielsen, S.W. et al "The Pathology of Osteogenic Sarcoma in Dogs," *JAVMA*; Jan.1964: 28-34.

29. Owen, L.N. and Stevenson, D.E. "Observations on Canine Osteosarcoma," *Res. Vet. Sci.;* 1961: 2:117-129.

30. Madewell, Bruce R. VMD, MS, "Canine Lymphoma," *Vet. Clinics of N. Amer.: Sm. Anim. Prac.*; July 1985: Vol. 15, #4.

31. McCaw, Dudley, DVM, "Canine Lymphosarcoma," AAHA's 56th Annual Meeting Proceedings, 1989.

32. Rosenthal, Robert C., DVM, MS, PhD, "The Treatment of Multicentric Canine Lymphoma," *Vet Clinics of N. Amer., Sm. Anim. Prac.*; July 1990: Vol.20, #4.

33. Catalogue of Congenital and Hereditary Disease.

34. Betts, C.W., et al: "A Retrospective Study of Gastric Dilation Torsion in the Dog," *J. Sm. Anim. Prac.;* 1974: 15:727-733.

35. Holling, H.E., et al "Pulmonary Hypertrophic Osteoarthropathy," *Lancet*; Dec. 9 1961: 1269-1274.

36. Howenstein, J.R. et al "Torsion of the Splenic Pedicle in a St. Bernard," *VM/SAC*; May 1975: 548-550.

37. Johnston, D.E. "Hygroma of the Elbow in Dogs," *JAVMA;* Aug. 1 1975: (3):213-219.

38. Wingfield, W.E., et al "Pathophysiology of the Gastric Dilation-Torsion Complex in the Dog," *J. Sm. Anim. Prac.*; 1974: 15:735-739.

39. Hoerlein, B.F. *Canine Neurology*, 2nd ed. (W.B. Saunders, Philadelphia, PA., 1971).

40. Ettinger, S.J. *Textbook of Veterinary Internal Medicine: Diseases of the Dog and Cat.* (W.B. Saunders Co., 1989); 2259.

41. Mustard, J.F., et al "Canine Hemophilia B (Christmas Disease)," *Brit. J. Haemat.;* 1960:

6:259-260.

42. Dodds, W.J. "Inherited Hemorrhagic Disorders," *Amer. Anim. Hosp. Assoc. J.*; May/June 1975: 11:366-373.

43. Gellat, K.N. "Bilateral Corneal Dermoids and Distichiasis in a Dog," *VM/SAC;* July 1971: 66:658-659.

44. Brignac, Michele M. "Congenital and Breed Associated Skin Diseases in the Dog and Cat," published in *Kalkan Forum;* Dec. 1989: 9-16.

45. Griffin, C., Kwochka, K., and McDonald, J. *Current Veterinary Dermatology,: The Science and Art of Therapy.* Mosby Yearbook, St. Louis, MO. 1993: 218.

46. Strain, George M. "Deafness in Dogs and Cats," *Proc. 10th ACVIM Forum*; May, 1992.

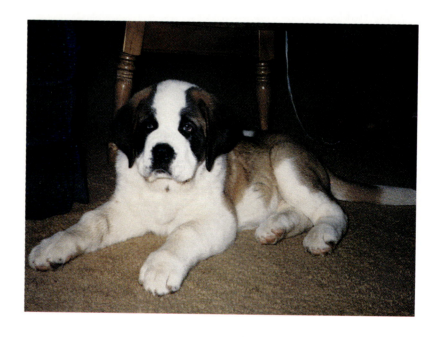

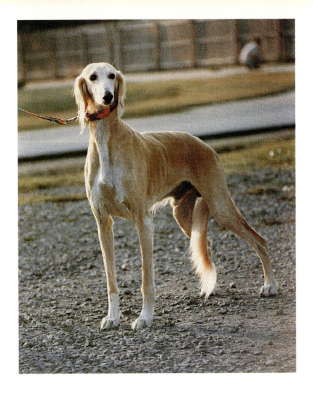

SALUKI

ORIGIN AND HISTORY

The Saluki is probably the oldest breed of dog known to man. Pictures of Salukis have been found on the walls of Egyptian tombs. They are among the fastest breeds; they were used by the sheiks to hunt gazelle. The Saluki is the only dog mentioned with honor in the Koran. Originally there were two strains, one Arabian in origin, the other Persian.

DESCRIPTION

The breed tends to be aloof and cautious, even shy with strangers, but they make strong commitments to their owners or trainers. An extended period of grieving, with physical symptoms, may be anticipated when a Saluki between 8 months and 2 years changes homes. Because of this commitment to a limited family and a distrust of strangers, owners should be present when the dog is recovering from anesthesia. With the support of its owner, a Saluki will stand patiently, even for a complicated repair, with only a local anesthetic. Because of the dangers inherent in general anesthesia with Salukis, local anesthetic is recommended for all but the most radical repairs.

Height varies between various Saluki strains. Dogs from Persian strains are heavier and taller at maturity than dogs from Arabian desert strains.

THE SHOW RING

The Standard for the breed allows a 5-inch leeway (23 to 28 inches at the shoulder) for mature dogs. Bitches are proportionately smaller. In the United states the average dog is usually at least 26 inches at the shoulder. Twenty-three inch dogs are seldom encountered. They should be proportionately smaller, not small because of malnourishment. The majority of bitches range from 24 to 27 inches at the shoulder.

BREEDING AND WHELPING

The estrous cycle of Saluki bitches rarely follows the norm. The first estrus may occur from 8 months to 2 years of age. Intervals between estrus may vary from 5 months to more than a year. Once established, the estrus cycle is fairly regular, but ovulation is highly irregular and may occur from the 5th to the 28th day of estrus. Vaginal smears can be helpful to predict ovulation. Also, change of color, flagging, and the beginning of withering in the vulva are usually reliable signs.

Most Saluki studs function well, but it is generally advisable to hold the bitch. Because of the difficulty of determining when ovulation will occur, several breedings are recommended. As a result of the slow maturation of the breed, first litters can be planned as late as 6 or 7 years without incurring difficulty. A loss of libido in a usually competent Saluki male often can be traced to developing **hypothyroidism**.

Saluki bitches often do not show in whelp until far along in gestation. A marked increase in appetite and changes in temperament, such as laziness or irritability with other dogs can be clues. Usually Salukis are easy whelpers. They need and appreciate the presence of a familiar human being; without this presence, they may become distraught, especially in a first whelping. But once they settle down, they are wise, devoted, protective mothers.

Saluki bitches lose their tail feathering within several months of whelping. The feathering requires nearly a year to grow back.

Because Salukis bear extreme pain with great fortitude, signs of infection are easily overlooked until too late. Uterine smears taken during heat and after whelping in Saluki dams that have already born several litters may improve detection of uterine infection.

The breed is not particularly subject to **eclampsia**. Generally, Saluki bitches produce sufficient milk but some large-breasted bitches have deceptively little milk and their puppies should be checked for regular weight gains.

Removal of dewclaws is recommended but not required. Removal eliminates the danger of a dewclaw tearing while the dog is coursing or running.

GROWTH

Growth rates differ, but in general most puppies double their birth weight by a week or 10 days, triple their birth weight in another 10 days, and gain steadily at the rate of about 2 ounces per day. Body weight increases rapidly between 6 to 8 and 10 to 12 weeks of age. Daily gains may average 4 to 8 ounces for a short period. Because of their rapid growth, Salukis sometimes appear poorly coordinated. Their front and rear legs appear to grow at different times and at different rates.

Puppies that have a red coat at maturity appear black with a brownish cast at birth. Colors usually change during the first year. Ticking often does not appear until after the seventh week. Differentiation of the smooth variety cannot be made with certainty until about the fifth week.

Saluki puppies need other puppies as sparring partners to properly develop their fronts, rears and temperaments. They spend many hours sleeping on the softest surfaces available, but also need room to run, preferably with a companion.

Salukis have a long adolescence. They do not mature until 4 years of age. During adolescence, Salukis need careful education and guidance and suffer more than most breeds from neglect, harshness or spoiling. The breed's extreme sensitivity demands corresponding sensitivity on the part of the owners, and a willingness to protect and guide the young dog for several years. As a breed, Salukis show amazing patience and tolerance of children.

Small **umbilical hernias** are not unusual. These may need surgery eventually, but can often be corrected by taping a coin over the hernia as the walls of the opening begin to harden, at about 8 to 9 weeks.

DENTITION

Full dentition is normal, but not required by the Standard. **Undershot** bites are occasionally seen. **Overbites** occur in about 1/3 of all puppies, appearing as early as 2 months when the top and bottom jaws are growing at uneven rates, and usually correcting by 9 months. Permanently overshot bites are occasionally found in lines with extremely long muzzles. Teeth last well but should be watched for tartar.

RECOGNIZED PROBLEMS

Black hair follicle dysplasia has been studied in black and white Salukis.[1]

Cryptorchidism appears only rarely, and there is little evidence that it is directly inherited. **Hip dysplasia** is practically unknown in the breed.

Broken legs occur in Salukis as a result of their great speed and love of running and coursing. Plating is highly recommended for repair, because the usual methods of splinting and

465

pinning seldom result in a correct repair.

Because they have been selectively bred for thousands of years, Salukis have few inherited vulnerabilities or defects. However, the breed is unusually susceptible to physical problems with a **psychosomatic etiology**. For instance, a transfer at a crucial age may set off **skin problems** or **coccidiosis**. Otherwise, skin problems are rare, with the exception of some susceptibility to mange or ear mites. Salukis' ears are especially susceptible to mites and infections and should be frequently checked.

Progressive retinal atrophy has been described in the breed.

Salukis need soft beds. Without a soft bed, they may develop long **calluses** under their breast bones. These calluses sometimes must be removed surgically. Salukis often bump their elbows, ankles, hip bones or ribs, so that trauma to the bursas occurs. These injuries usually disappear in a few weeks without treatment.

The Saluki's **response to barbiturates** is unpredictable. Violent recovery, extremely long sleeping time, and death frequently occur. Because Salukis have little fat, thiobarbiturates should be avoided. No barbiturate should be used with a preanesthetic, and they should always be given only to effect. A minimal dose of preanesthetic followed by an inhalant is the safest method, although it is not without risk. When possible, as in repair of wounds, cleaning of ears and teeth and minor surgery, local anesthesia should be used.

Salukis may be sensitive to **choline-esterase inhibitors**—those drugs used orally or topically to rid a dog of parasites. A flea collar should be removed from packaging and exposed to the air for several days before it is put on a dog, and should be removed several days before any treatment or surgery.

After its long childhood and adolescence, the Saluki emerges as a dependable, contributing family member with few problems other than the need to be protected from cars. A course in obedience in a dog's younger years greatly enriches the dog by developing its capacity to willingly respond to its family's needs.

BEHAVIOR

Salukis cannot be kept as kennel dogs. If left for long periods without human companionship, they become withdrawn, spooky, dull or destructive. Salukis are also social among themselves and do not do well without companions. When left alone, they tend to dig, tear or chew. The solitary Saluki usually becomes sedentary. However, formal coursing or sustained running should not be initiated until the dog is at least a year old.

Most Salukis have no car sense and, with their capacity for speeds of more than 40 miles an hour, are readily struck by cars if they are allowed to roam. They require constant protection in the form of locked gates and high, sturdy fences.

The Saluki adapts readily to the life of a house dog, but he needs lots of running room and exercise. He is sensitive and friendly with children.

OLD AGE

The breed grows old gracefully and very slowly, seldom having problems in hearing or sight. Care should be taken that the older dog, with his sedentary habits, does not become overweight.

Salukis are often potent studs after 12 years of age. Bitches can produce nearly as long, if they have already had at least one litter, and have been well cared for. Salukis enjoy hunting and coursing well after 10 years. They can live about 16 years, but are usually killed by cars. Cancer is rare in this breed.

The final years of a Saluki are usually characterized by health, energy and a mellow contentment. The Saluki that lives out its years is apt to die in its favorite chair, without a history of degenerative difficulties.

References

1. Hargis, A.M., Brignac, M.M, Al-BagDadi, K., Muggli, F., and Mundell, A. "Black Hair Follicle Dysplasia in Black and White Saluki Dogs," *Veterinary Dermatology*; 1990: 1:181-187.

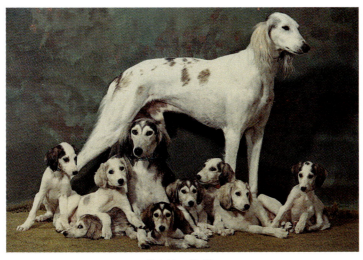
Salukis with litter.

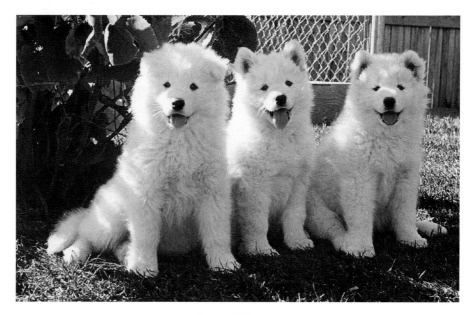

Samoyed Puppies

SAMOYED

ORIGIN AND HISTORY

The most numerically popular of the arctic shepherd dogs, the Samoyed hails from Siberia. A hardy sled dog, it also herded reindeer and guarded the huts of the Samoyed people. Registered in England in 1909, it has proved to be an eye-arresting show contender.

DESCRIPTION

Samoyed temperament is one of the breed's most highly prized qualities. They are "people dogs" and derive their happiness from being near their master. They do not make good yard dogs and often become prone to excessive barking when deprived of human companions. Samoyeds are excellent diggers and chewing may result from sheer boredom. Their nature is to be "talky," engaging in vocal communication with kennelmates and people. Their paws are frequently used to communicate their willingness to play or to be petted. This sort of "body language" is used to express themselves not only to human beings but to other dogs as well.

The Samoyed is keenly intelligent and friendly with other dogs. Even an adult male will sometimes care for a new puppy in the household. Some males live together, in complete harmony, for a lifetime and most seem to enjoy the company of other dogs. They are extremely sensitive to the moods of the household and react with obvious concern.

Some bloodlines have a predisposition toward weak hocks or cowhocks. Also seen are some light boning and "snipy" muzzles, more Spitz-like than Samoyed. Light or liver colored noses may be the result of heredity, age or climate. Noses often lighten during winter months, becoming darker with exposure to more sunshine.

THE SHOW RING

Today's Samoyeds are generally at the top of the breed Standard, with dogs standing from 21 to 23 1/2 inches at the shoulder, and bitches from 19 to 21 inches. Dogs may weigh 60 to 75 pounds, bitches 50 to 60 pounds.

Noses and lips are usually dusty pink at birth; with color beginning to show after the second or third day. Pigmentation is slow to develop in some lines, and lip "breaks" may fill in as late as 2 to 3 years. Incomplete eye rims, however, if not completely colored at an early age, will not fill in later. Most coats are white, but biscuit and cream shadings are not infrequent and tend to produce the very desirable silver tips in the coat. **Any coat color other than white, cream, biscuit or white and biscuit is disqualifying. Blue eyes are a disqualification and, since this is an inherited factor, dogs with such faults should not be used for breeding.** The blue-eyed Samoyed usually shows **albino** characteristics and is lacking in proper pigmentation of lips and nose as well, with generally pink eye rims, lips and eyes. The eyes are extremely sensitive to light.

BREEDING AND WHELPING

Most Samoyed breedings are accomplished without difficulty. Bitches are normally bred on the 10th or 12th day, but successful matings may occur as early as the 7th day or as late as the 20th. First seasons may not occur until the bitches are a year, or older; thereafter they generally occur at regular 6-month intervals.

Occasionally bitches suffer from postpartum infections, sometimes resulting in a loss of milk and making it necessary to tube-feed puppies. Samoyeds take their maternal duties seriously and with enthusiasm and spend much time nuzzling their whelps affectionately.

The average litters of six or seven are usually full term, being born 61 to 62 days after mating. Whelps weigh from 10 to 18 ounces at birth, and birth defects, such as cleft palate, missing limbs, etc. are exceedingly rare. Eyes open at approximately 9 days and are a dark slate blue at birth, changing to the characteristic brown at about 8 to 10 weeks. A profuse, short, white coat covers puppies within a week after birth. Dewclaws are usual on rear legs and should be surgically removed when the pups are 4 to 5 days of age.

GROWTH

Puppies develop rapidly and by 2 weeks are often on their feet for short periods. Ears are up by 6 weeks, but may be up and down until the teething process has been completed. Shaving an ear that is slow to erect frequently results in the ear becoming erect almost immediately.

Their white coats belie how easily they may be kept clean, although frequent and thorough brushing, at least weekly, is a necessity. Mature dogs shed profusely, usually once a year, and bitches twice yearly, approximately 4 months after their estrus. Particular care is necessary in keeping the dog well brushed at this time, for shedding frequently produces matting, especially in the heavily coated areas over the back, under the tail and around the neck. The Samoyed coat is odor free when dry, but can pick up undesirable odors from other sources. When wet, the coat smells like damp wool. Frequent bathing is unnecessary if sufficient care is taken in maintaining a regular brushing routine, and the coat can be cleaned quite well by the use of grooming powder or chalk, worked into a dry, or barely damp, coat and carefully removed by brushing. Incidence of bathing is influenced by coat texture, some lines having coats that almost never require baths. Samoyeds are not immune to the usual "hot spots" seen in the heavily coated breeds. Often persons who are allergic to other breeds are able to tolerate the Samoyed. The Samoyed coat combing may be spun into yarn and knit or woven into garments.

DENTITION

Scissors bite or level bite is correct and usual and generally the breed does not tend to have missing teeth.

RECOGNIZED PROBLEMS

The incidence of **progressive retinal atrophy** is low, and the Samoyed owners are kept constantly alert against the threat of PRA, **dysplasia** and other conditions through a concerned national breed club.

The iridocorneal angle of the left eye was investigated in 203 Samoyeds. Comparison was made of judgements of the width of the anterior opening of the ciliary cleft when performing gonioscopy with an objective method of estimation based on measurements on goniophotographs. Results indicated high degree of correlation. Various degrees of narrowness of the iridocorneal angle width were revealed and clinical **glaucoma** with total-angle closure was found in six of 203 dogs. The intraocular pressure was higher in eyes with closed iridocorneal angles than in eyes with any other width of the angle. Appearance of the structures of the iridocorneal angle, particularly the pigment bands, indicated extensive individual variation. In approximately 25% of the eyes, **dysplasia of the pectinate ligaments** of variable degree existed, indicating that

470

this anomaly is common in the Samoyed breed. There were no differences in intraocular pressure between eyes with different degrees of dysplasia of the pectinate ligaments.[1]

Hip dysplasia is found in the breed. Current practice is to breed only dysplasia-free adults certified by the Orthopedic Foundation For Animals. Many breeders x-ray at 1 year and again at the age of two. A collection of over 14,000 radiographs of the spine of 10 breeds of dogs were examined for abnormal vertebrae in the lumbosacral region, which were manifested by different types of fusion (sacralization and lumbalisation). There was some link between these abnormalities and hip dysplasia.[2] Such abnormalities were seen in 4% of 73 Samoyeds.

Six Samoyeds with short limbed **dwarfism** and ocular defects from five litters were examined. The most prominent abnormalities were small stature and valgus deformity of the carpi. Radiographic evidence of retarded growth at the distal ulnar physis was apparent by 12 weeks of age. Ocular defects included **cataracts** and **retinal detachment**. Family studies and limited breeding experiments were consistent with an autosomal recessive mode of inheritance.[3] Samoyeds are listed as being predisposed to **Hemophilia A** and **pulmonic stenosis**,[4] although these conditions are rarely seen. The Samoyed may occasionally develop **tonsillitis**, **impacted anal glands**, **urinary infections** and **non-specific dermatitis**. The coat is subject to sunburn, resulting in harsh, brown spots. There is no treatment. Although rare, **diabetes** in older, overweight dogs is reported. Relatively infrequent are **spinal disc problems**, particularly in the cervical area. Inherited forms of **muscular dystrophy** linked to the "X" chromosome are being studied and have been identified in Samoyeds.[5]

Over three years a breeder had six litters in which one or more pups at 3 weeks of age showed generalized tremors and was unable to stand. One affected male pup (5 weeks old) was examined for clinical and pathological lesions. Gross and microscopic studies, including immunocytochemical demonstrations of myelin basic protein, showed a lack of myelin throughout the central nervous system. Ultrastructurally a total absence of normal myelin was associated with oligodendrocyte which were immature in appearance, greatly reduced in number, and incapable of forming compact myelin. Astrocytosis and an increase in the third type of neurological cells were observed. The changes differed from those reported in other canine forms of hypomyelinogenesis and were compared with hypomyelinating diseases in other species. The findings suggested that this hypomyelination was the result of **retarded gliogenesis**.[6]

Affected male (AM) Samoyed dogs with **x-linked hereditary nephritis** (HN) show splitting of all their glomerular basement membranes (GBM) and rapidly develop renal failure within the first year of life; features are similar to those seen in male patients with x-linked HN. In contrast, carrier female (CF) dogs with x-linked HN show only isolated foci of splitting of GBM, and renal failure is never seen at such an early age. The present study assessed whether a diet designed for dogs in renal failure could modify the changes seen in GBM of AM and CF dogs and improve the clinical outcome in the AM dogs. Beginning at 35 days of age, one group of dogs (seven unaffected, seven AM and six CF) was fed on a normal diet, while a second group (seven unaffected, nine AM, six CF) was fed a modified diet (low in protein, lipid, calcium and phosphorus). AM dogs fed the modified diet showed a smaller reduction in glomerular filtration rate than AM dogs fed the normal diet, indicating a delay in the onset and a decrease in the severity of renal damage. All of the AM dogs died of renal failure regardless of diet. However, the onset and progression of renal failure were delayed and the severity of splitting of GBM was reduced in AM dogs fed the modified diet; these dogs lived 53% (362±17 vs. 239±14 days) longer than AM dogs fed the regular diet. CF dogs fed the modified diet also showed a reduced severity of splitting of GBM. In addition, when two CF dogs on the modified diet were changed to the normal diet, splitting of their GBM increased, indicating that continual administration of the modified diet was required to maintain the reduced rate of splitting. These studies indicate that the modified diet was beneficial in canine x-linked HN, and suggest that similar benefits (reduction in severity of splitting of GBM and delayed development of renal failure) might be observed in patients with HN who are treated with an appropriately modified diet.[7]

The inheritance pattern of **glomerulopathy** among 140 dogs (74 male, 66 female) descended from a single pair of purebred Samoyeds was consistent with a dominant gene carried on the x-chromosome. It appeared that a gene mutation in a daughter of the original pair was perpetuated in such a way that the severe disease occurred in about half of the male offspring, with a much less severe form in females (variable heterozygotes), regardless of the relationship between sire and dam. Affected males are infertile. There is a close similarity with hereditary nephritis in man.[8,9]

A **uveodermatological syndrome** has been reported in the Samoyed.[10] Growth-hormone-responsive **dermatosis** has been seen in Samoyeds, as has **sebaceous adenitis.**[11]

BEHAVIOR

The Samoyed is gentle, loyal, obedient and cheerful. He loves playing with the children. He is clean, but he is a frequent barker.

OLD AGE

The average lifespan is approximately 10 to 12 years, although today's better nutrition and care frequently extend the lifespan to 15 or more years of age. Older Samoyeds tend toward obesity and should be diet-controlled to produce less strain on older hearts and other organs. **Benign skin tumors** and **sebaceous cysts** are occasionally seen. **Kidney disease** has been found in older males. **Malignancies** may occur in older dogs of both sexes and

arthritis is not uncommon. The aging Samoyed is one of the finest of all canine companions, and the relationship developed between man and Samoyed through years of association is a gentle, comfortable and very strong bond of mutual love and understanding which is beautiful to behold. The greatest gift the master of a Samoyed can give to his dog is the privilege of spending his declining years at his master's side. The Samoyed earns such a reward by a lifetime of intense and faithful devotion.

References

1. Eke sten, B; Narfstrom, K. "Correlation of Morphologic Features of the Iridocorneal Angle to Intraocular Pressure in Samoyeds." *Am. J. of Vet. Research.* 1991, 52:11, 1875-1878; 16 ref.
2. Winkler, W. "Transitional Lumbosacral Vertebrae in the Dog." Dissertation, Fachbereich Veterinarmedizin der Freien Universitat Berlin. 1985, 143pp.; 50 ref.
3. Meyers,VN; Jezyk,PF; Aguirre, GD; Patterson, DF. "Short-Limbed Dwarfism and Ocular Defects in the Samoyed Dog." *JAVMA.* 1983, 183:9, 975-979; 12 ref.
4. Foley, C.W., et al. *Abnormalities of Companion Animals.* Iowa State University Press, Ames, Iowa. 1979; p 35
5. Veterinary News, *The American Kennel Club Gazette*; October, 1991
6. Cummings, J.F.; Summers, B.A.; De Lahunta, A., and Lawson, C.; "Tremors in Samoyed Pups with Oligodendrocyte Deficiencies and Hypomyelination." *Acta-Neuropathologica.* 1986, 71:3/4, 267-277; 38 ref.
7. Valli, V.EO., Baumal, R., Thorner, P., Jacobs, R., Marrano, P., Davies, C., Qizilbash, B., and Clarke, H. "Dietary Modification Reduces Splitting of Glomeruler Basement Membranes and Delays Death Due to Renal Failure in Canine x-linked Hereditary Nephritis." *Lab. Investigation.* 1991, 65:1, 67-73; 44 ref.
8. Jansen, B., Tryphonas, L., Wong, J., Thorner, P., Maxie, M.G., Valli, Ve., Baumal, R., and Basrur, P.K. "Mode of Inheritance of Samoyed Hereditary Glomerulopathy: An Animal Model for Hereditary Nephritis in Humans." *J. of Lab. and Clinical Med.* 1986, 107:6, 551-555; 35 ref.
9. Picut, C.A. and Lewis, R.M. "Comparative Pathology of Canine Hereditary Nephropathies: An Interpretive Review." *Vet. Res. Comm.* 1987, 11:6, 561-581; 91 ref.
10. Romatowski, J. "A Uveodermatological Syndrome in an Akita Dog." *JAAHA.* 1985, 21:6, 777-780; 7 ref.
11. Griffin, C., Kwochka, K., and McDonald, J. *Current Veterinary Dermatology: The Science and Art of Therapy.* Mosby Yearbook, St. Louis, MO. 1993: 171, 289.

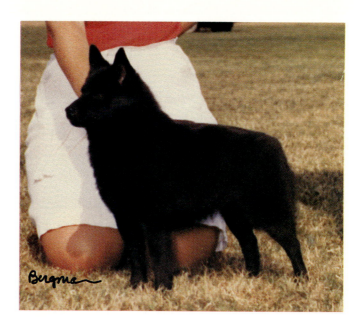

SCHIPPERKE

ORIGIN AND HISTORY

The exact origin of the Schipperke was never documented. Early Belgian authorities believe the Schipperke originated in Flanders and the provinces of Antwerp and Brabant. The known history of the breed begins about the year 1690, in Brussels. It first came to the United States in 1889, but practically disappeared following World War I.

In 1924 Miss Isabel Ormiston imported a young bitch from Belgium, and continued to import Schipperkes. Miss Ormiston's Kelso Kennels provided the foundation for the breed in this country, and the Schipperke Club of America is a member of the AKC due primarily to the efforts of Miss Ormiston.

DESCRIPTION

The Schipperke is tremendously loyal to its owners, and protective of its owners' possessions.

By nature, the Schipperke is suspicious of strangers. Once its friendship is won, it is close to unshakable. The dog's curiosity is insatiable — a trait which helps make it the perfect watch dog.

THE SHOW RING

The Schipperke's preferred heights are 11 to 13 inches from the highest point of the withers to the ground for males and 10 to 12 inches for bitches. The coat is jet black, and a dense undercoat raises the neck hairs in a ruff with a jabot between the front legs. The coat over the body is flatter, with a rounded rump and culottes on the rear legs, meeting between the hindlegs, and being as long as the ruff hairs. The undercoat may be grayish, brownish or black, but appears to be a black dog. Shedding time, sunburning or poor health may cause browning of the coat. No other coat is acceptable, with no white markings allowable.

The Schipperke, with a sloping topline, tailless rear, ruff, culottes and fox-like head and expression, has a unique silhouette.

Disqualifications are any coat color other than solid black, drop ear or ears.

BREEDING AND WHELPING

Estrus in the Schipperke bitch seems to present a wide variance in age of first appearance. The first estrous cycle usually occurs when the bitch is 1 year to 14 months old. It is not unusual for a bitch to be 2 years old before the first season is noted. Silent seasons are common, with very little or no spotting. The Schipperke bitch is extremely clean, and this makes spotting less evident. The use of white bedding in her crate or sleeping quarters is of considerable help in noting her season.

The three-week season is normal and gestation is usually 63 days. Delivery is usually normal with a reasonable labor time. The typical litter is four puppies. However, litter sizes have been noted ranging from one to eight puppies. At birth Schipperke puppies usually weigh from 4 to 5 ounces. Considerable variation exists and puppies of two ounces have been successfully raised to normal-sized dogs. Weights over 9 ounces do occur. Birth defects are uncommon. An occasional **cleft palate** or random deformity is possible but unusual. Tail length is perhaps the most peculiar birth variance in the Schipperke. In some lines entire litters are born with stub tails of varying lengths.

GROWTH

Growth rate is quite varied. In general the Schipperke has reached about 60% of its growth at 6 months of age. Schipperkes do not reach full maturity until they are approximately 5 years of age.

Early care of puppies has few requirements. The most important thing is seeing that the puppy eats enough. Schipperkes are not fussy eaters; they simply do not want to take the time to eat. Feeding several times a day seems to be the best solution to this problem. In later life the Schipperke becomes as obese as any house dog that is too close to the pantry, and must be watched carefully. Selection of a puppy under 6 to 8 months of age for show is speculative. Selection for temperament is no different from that of any other puppy. At 6 to 10 weeks, adult size is undetermined.

Dewclaws, which appear only on the front legs, and tails are removed at 3 to 5 days of age in the normal, healthy puppy. The tail is properly removed to the last possible joint, leaving no stub, despite the Standard which allows up to 1 inch of tail. The Schipperke that appears in the ring with an inch of tail will place last in the class, no matter what other good points it might possess. The SCA has complete instructions for tail docking in its book, *The Schipperke Anthology*, available from SCA.

Tail docking is major surgery, requiring expert handling, stitching of the wound, and attention to serious bleeding. Veterinarians should keep puppies in their care for at least an hour after surgery to watch for bleeding. A small dose of local anesthetic seems to give considerable comfort to puppies, which can cry and fuss for 12 to 18 hours after surgery.

DENTITION

A level bite or a tight scissors bite is desired in the Schipperke. Bites seem to be very unpredictable. An excellent puppy bite may become bad with the second teeth. The opposite can occur, but is unlikely.

Common bite defects in Schipperkes are **undershot** jaw or bite. Another problem is having one or two incisors at one side of the mouth slightly protruding. The most individual problem the Schipperke has is the late maturing of the jaws, which causes the level bite at a year, or older. Teeth are normally strong and of good size. Tartar is easily formed and Schipperkes seem to need professional cleaning frequently. There is little loss of teeth, if properly cared for, until extreme old age.

RECOGNIZED PROBLEMS

The Schipperke is remarkably free of breed abnormalities. **Entropion** and **narrow palpebral fissure** have been reported in the breed.[1] There is some **dermatitis** that may appear in the fall, caused by allergy, but it responds to treatment well. **Pemphigus foliaceous** has been reported. (See Akita) A **hay fever asthma** occasionally appears in the fall in some individuals.

The one problem that is serious and is occasionally seen is **Legg-Perthes disease**. Even it is not common enough to be known and recognized by all Schipperke breeders.

An extremely high incidence of **hypothyroidism** has been reported.[2]

BEHAVIOR

An excellent watch dog, the Schipperke is trainable, intelligent, curious and good with the children, but is very suspicious of strangers.

476

OLD AGE

The Schipperke adult requires no great attention peculiar to the breed. Good basic health care is adequate.

The Schipperke, given proper care, should attain the age of 16 to 17 years in relatively good health. At that age, sight or hearing may diminish, but an age of 18 or 19 years is not unusual. Proper exercise and attention to weight and diet suitable for any older dog seem to be all that is required for an active old age.

References
1. Quinn, A.J., Personal Communication, 1982
2. Schipperke column, *The American Kennel Club Gazette*; February, 1993

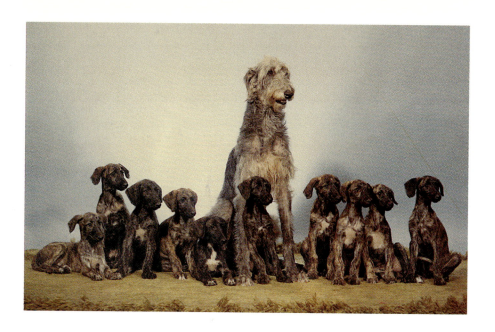

SCOTTISH DEERHOUND

ORIGIN AND HISTORY

Scottish Deerhounds were well known in the British Isles during the 16th century. Sir Walter Scott called the breed "the most perfect creature of the heaven." These stately, yet rugged, hounds coursed the stag by day and lay at the feet of lords by evening. They are sensitive and are said to remember "with accuracy both benefit and injury."

DESCRIPTION

Deerhounds are gentle and loving. A sharp temperament is a rarity and usually the result of extreme stress, poor handling or illness. Deerhounds are not good watch dogs, and they do not bark. Removal of dewclaws is optional. Ears are not trimmed, nor tails docked.

THE SHOW RING

General conformation is that of a Greyhound of larger size and bone and with harsh, wiry hair. Desired height of males—from 30 to 32 inches and weight from 85 to 110 pounds. Desired height of bitches—over 28 inches and weight from 75 to 95 pounds.

A white blaze on the head or a white collar are disqualifying.

BREEDING AND WHELPING

Deerhound bitches begin estrus at 12 to 14 months of age or later. Thereafter, estrus occurs at 8- to 10-month intervals. In some bitches, it occurs as often as every 6 months. Ovulation usually occurs around the 13th day. The length of gestation is normal or sometimes slightly longer.

Bitches need normal amounts of exercise during gestation. Their appetite may increase for 2 to 3 weeks, then decrease for about 2 weeks and then increase again. The breed experiences no particular problems during gestation or whelping.

Puppies are usually born in pairs at 20- to 30-minute intervals. The average litter is eight to nine puppies that average 1 to 2 pounds. Puppies are black with small amounts of white on their toes and chest. White is not required but is usually present. The puppies resemble Labrador Retrievers.

Few puppies are born with abnormalities. An occasional puppy will have a broken tail.

GROWTH

The Scottish Deerhound's growth rate is usually sporadic. Dogs mature at 3 years, bitches at about 2 1/2 years. Adult dogs weigh about 100 pounds and stand above 30 inches; bitches weigh about 75 pounds and stand 28 inches or more. Some lines are taller and heavier than the average. Deerhounds attain most of their height by 12 to 18 months. Growth patterns depend upon the individual, the line, diet and exercise.

RECOGNIZED PROBLEMS

The breed has little problem with teething or bite.

Deerhounds are susceptible to disturbances of growth and development typical of the giant breeds. **Hip dysplasia** is not a common problem.

Two Scottish Deerhound puppies were presented with clinical and pathological features consistent with the diagnosis of congenital **non-goitrous hypothyroidism**. The study suggests that possible mechanisms include either **primary thyroid hypoplasia** or an **unresponsiveness to thyroid-stimulating hormone**.[1]

Deerhounds are prone to **bloat** and **gastric torsion**. They should be watched carefully. Strenuous exercise immediately before or after eating is not recommended. Water should be limited after strenuous exercise. Feeding should be on demand (dry kibble always available) and the main meal should be soaked (soft).

Torsion of the lung, torsion of the spleen and **osteochondritis (OCD)** have been diagnosed in Scottish Deerhounds.[2]

BEHAVIOR

Deerhounds do not make good kennel dogs. They prefer the home environment and being with human companions. They are usually gentle with other animals and seldom start quarrels, although they do play aggressively. They are not fighters and will submit to older, more aggressive dogs. If kenneled, they should have an area no less than 100 feet by 10 feet for exercise.

OLD AGE

Older dogs sleep more and require less exercise. However, they do need room to run. Feedings can be cut almost in half for dogs of 7 or 8 years. Fat dogs are unhealthy. Because Deerhounds are generally healthy, they require no more than the usual geriatric care.

The lifespan of the breed is 10 to 12 years. Bloat and heart problems are the usual causes of death in dogs older than 10 years.

References
1. Robinson, W.F., Shaw, S.E., Stanley, B., and Wyburn, R.S. "Congenital Hypothyroidism in Scottish Deerhound Puppies." *Australian Vet. Journal.* 1988, 65:12, 386-388; 10 ref.
2. Scottish Deerhound column, *The American Kennel Club Gazette*; May, 1990

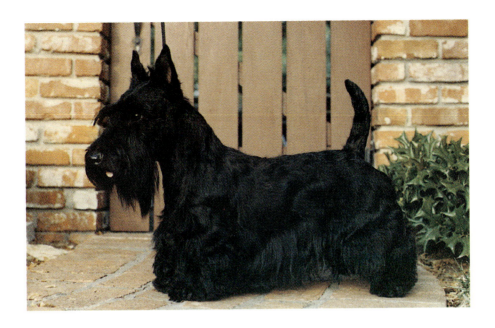

SCOTTISH TERRIER

ORIGIN AND HISTORY

Staunch little Scottish Terriers are believed to be one of the oldest breeds of dogs in Britain. They are dedicated to their family and friends. Scottish Terriers are good watch dogs but accept strangers admitted by the family.

DESCRIPTION

A puppy can be black, brindle or wheaten, but it may be difficult to determine whether a puppy is black or dark brindle in the first few weeks. A small spot of white on a puppy's chest or chin generally blends into the coat at maturity.

Dewclaws may be removed if desired, but removal is not required by the Standard.

THE SHOW RING

A Scottish Terrier generally weighs 18 to 22 pounds and stands 10 inches high at the shoulders. Major faults in the breed are soft coat, round or very light eye, over or undershot bite, shyness and failure to show. The Breed Standard states that no judge should put to Winners or Best of Breed any Scottish Terrier not showing real terrier character in the ring.

There are no disqualifying faults.

481

BREEDING AND WHELPING

Scottish Terrier bitches usually follow normal seasons and should be bred between the 10th and 14th day of estrus. The large heads of the puppies can cause problems in delivery; occasionally a **cesarean section** is required. Scottish Terrier puppies generally weigh 6 to 8 ounces at birth. Puppies are occasionally born with kinks in their tails, but with massage and muscle development the kinks usually straighten by maturity.

DENTITION

Full dentition is usual. A scissors bite is preferred, but an even bite is acceptable. To ensure proper alignment, milk teeth should fall out or be removed before permanent teeth come in.

RECOGNIZED PROBLEMS

Craniomandibular osteopathy is seen in Scottish Terriers (see West Highland White Terriers). Scottish Terriers are also susceptible to **Scottie cramp.**[1,2] It is a hyperkinetic disorder that is apparently inheritable as a recessive trait.[3] It may first appear in a dog at 6 weeks. The syndrome is characterized by intermittent spasms of rigidity of the limbs, back, and tail muscles or generalized paralysis. The spasms consist of abduction of the forelimbs, excessive flexion of the hindlimbs, arching of the back and tucking of the head. The spasms last for about 15 seconds. They may be induced by physical or psychic stress or by the administration of amphetamines. The elicitation of an episode is highly dependent upon psychic factors. By identifying those situations in which an episode will predictably be elicited, an owner may reduce the incidence of episodes by not exposing the dog to the stimulus or, if this is not possible, by behaviorally training the dog to accept the stimulus. Potent inducers of an episode may be events such as feeding or going for a walk, which make the dog excited. Fear is also a potent inducer. There have been several reports of dogs with Scottie Cramp exhibiting signs when confronted with stairs. In one case the veterinarian sedated the dog and, through repetitive exposure to stairs, was able to eliminate them as an initiator of cramp. On the other hand, anxiety inhibits the manifestation of the disorder and may explain the difficulty in eliciting clinical signs when a dog is taken to a veterinarian.

Dogs may suppress the elicitation of clinical signs by modifying their activity. Young puppies often exercise freely until clinical signs become evident. Thereafter, the dogs may stop exercising or may modify the intensity of exercise when they feel the beginning of clinical signs. It is, therefore, not uncommon to find clinical signs more prevalent in younger dogs. The owner may think that the adult dog showing fewer clinical signs has outgrown the disease.

The environment of the dog may also influence the expression of the disease. Most, if not all, stressful conditions have the potential to modify the clinical signs of Scottie Cramp. This means that dogs with Scottie Cramp raised in a quiet home may exhibit fewer clinical signs than dogs raised with other dogs or placed in a more intense environment. Thus the dog may again appear to *grow out* of the disorder when taken from the kennel at a young age to a home environment.

If the health status of the dog with Scottie Cramp deteriorates, the clinical signs become more severe. The increase in clinical signs can be marked. When presented with a mature dog that *suddenly* exhibits clinical signs of Scottie Cramp, it must be realized that the dog was born with Scottie Cramp, that the owner did not recognize the dog to have Scottie Cramp, and that some other event is increasing the severity of clinical signs. The owner and the veterinarian should direct their efforts toward defining these other events. In some cases, if an infectious cause is suspected, the dog may be placed on penicillin-containing antibiotics. This will further increase the severity of clinical signs. With the correction of the primary problem and cessation of treatment, the severity of clinical signs will dissipate and the signs will return to the predisease and pretreatment state. This waxing and waning have been incorrectly interpreted to mean that the clinical signs observed were due to a drug idiosyncrasy and that the dog does not have Scottie Cramp.

Nutritional factors are also important in determining the severity of clinical signs, and altering the diet can be very effective in reducing the clinical signs. Methods that increase the availability of tryptophan may be beneficial in reducing the likelihood that an episode will occur. Glucose administration, for example, will increase the function of serotonergic neurons in affected dogs. Giving the dog a small amount of glucose, such as a candy bar, may reduce the clinical signs if given 1 hour prior to exposure to a stressful situation.

Unfortunately, there is no laboratory test for Scottie Cramp and diagnosis is made on observation of clinical signs. The original diagnostic criteria for Scottie Cramp included a clinical history indicating abnormal locomotion or seizure-like activity during excitement or exercise, exacerbation of the condition following administration of amphetamine, and remission of signs following the administration of diazepam or promazine derivatives. The familial history and the clinical history are still highly significant. Pharmacological challenge to elicit an episode of Scottie Cramp is more appropriately performed with drugs that will selectively affect serotonergic neuronal activity, and is recommended only if excited exercise is not effective in eliciting clinical signs. Parachlorophenylalanine at 100 mg/kg/day, over a three-day period, is very effective in increasing the signs of Scottie Cramp. Subclinical, or minimally affected, animals are easily detected by p-CPA treatment because the clinical signs become proportionately more increased than in severely affected dogs. Unfortunately, p-CPA is not readily available for use in veterinary practice and therefore is not useful in clinical situations. Methysergide offers great potential for diagnostic testing for Scottie Cramp. Following oral administration of a single dosage of Methysergide, the clinical signs of Scottie Cramp will be increased within a 2-hour period. The effects of Methysergide disappear after an 8-hour period. With the exception of some transient nausea and gastrointestinal irritation, side effects are not obvious. Experimentally, clinical signs are easily seen at dosages of 0.1 mg/kg to 0.6 mg/kg. The dose at which there is a 50% increase in clinical signs is 0.3 mg/kg. Exceeding 0.6 mg/kg does not increase the effect of Methysergide upon cramp behavior, but does increase the severity of its side effects. The authors recommend starting at a dosage of 0.3 mg/kg, increasing the dosage to 0.6 mg/kg if clinical signs are not seen. If the signs become excessive, treatment with diazepam should decrease them accordingly.

Clinical signs are the most prominent at the end of the daily light cycle and less prevalent from midnight to early morning. This and other findings lead to the suggestion that serotonergic neuronal function modulates the expressions of Scottie Cramp. Treatments that increase the CANS levels of serotonin provided a beneficial effect. Nialamide, a relative selective monoamine oxidase inhibitor, improved the clinical rating by preventing the catabolism of serotonin. Treatment consists of avoiding stimuli that elicit episodes, and injecting intramuscularly a tranquilizer such as chlorpromazine (1.0-1.75 mg/kg or diazepam (0.50-1.50 mg/kg). Oral diazepam given at doses of 0.5 mg/kg three times daily has effectively controlled episodes. Vitamin E at doses above A/kg given once per day is very effective in elevating the threshold for the elicitation of clinical signs.[4]

Recent work with Scottie pups affected by **Splayleg** (motor disorder) has led to belief that this disorder is caused by hereditary abnormality in the frontal and parietal bones, but the mode of inheritance of Splayleg is yet to be established.[3] Scottish Terriers are prone to **hematomas of the ears**. Special attention should be given to keeping their ears clean. Male Scotties can be prone to **uroliths**. After the uroliths are removed the dog should be placed on medication permanently to prevent recurrence. As they grow older, both sexes have a tendency to develop **histiocytomas**, especially on the head. These can be removed surgically.

The Scottish Terrier is one of the breeds with a hereditary predisposition of **atopic hypersensitivity** to certain pollen antigens. This condition appears spontaneously at 2 or 3 years of age. It manifests itself as urticarial lesions and areas of self-trauma that occur during the blooming seasons of certain weeds. Females have a greater incidence of this condition. Scotties are highly susceptible to **inhalant allergies**[5] and may be predisposed to food allergy.[6]

A blood disorder reported in this breed is **Von Willebrand's disease (pseudohemophilia)**. The condition is hereditary, transmitted as an autosomal, incomplete dominant trait.

Thyroid problems have recently been seen in the Scottie. This condition responds well to medication.

Other defects known to Scotties are **cystinuria, primary uterine inertia, achondroplasia (dwarfism), deafness, luxation of the lens** and **melanoma.**

Because of their shortened legs they are predisposed to **elbow dysplasia** and **intervertebral disc syndrome.**[7]

Scotties are one of a group of breeds at high risk for **canine lymphoma.**[8,9,10]

A unique, presumably hereditary, **pyogranulomatous** and **vasculitic disorder of the nasal planum,** nostrils and nasal mucosa is described in five Scottish Terriers.

The initial symptom was a bilateral nasal discharge at 3 to 4 weeks of age or a bilateral ulcerative and destructive process of the nasal planum, nostrils and nasal mucosa at 5 to 6 months of age. Histopathological findings included nodular-to-diffuse pyogranulomatous inflammation with concurrent leukocytoclastic vasculitis.

Special stains were negative for microorganisms. Therapy was unsuccessful and all pups were euthanized.[11,12]

Alexander's disease was detected in a 9-month-old Scottish Terrier with progressive tetraparesis. Results from this case and previous reports suggest that this disease may have a congenital or genetic basis.[13]

Bladder cancer has been reported.[14]

Scottish Terriers are basically hardy, stoic animals, so illness is often undetected for some time. Older bitches can develop **pyometra,** so spaying is recommended if the animal is not going to be bred.

BEHAVIOR

The Scottie is lively, independent and intelligent. He is devoted to his family and indifferent to strangers.

He readily reacts to both criticism and praise. He does not bark a lot and plays well with children.

OLD AGE

The Scottish Terrier retains its terrier spirit and bounce as it ages. The breed's life expectancy is about 12 years. They generally die of kidney problems or carcinomas of various origins.

References
1. Meyes, K.M., et al: "The Genetic Basis of Kinetic Disorder of Scottish Terrier Dogs." *Jour-*

485

nal of Heredity, 1971; pp189-192.

2. Hoerlein, B.F. *Canine Neurology*. W. B. Saunders, Philadelphia, PA., 1971:266-267.

3. Andersson, B. and Andersson, M. "Scottie Cramp and Splayleg-Clinical Signs, Probable Mode of Inheritance and Causes." *Svensk-Veterinartidning*. 1986, 38: 15,166-171; 16 ref.

4. Clemmons, R.M., DVM, PhD., Peters, R.R., PhD., and Meyers, K.M., PhD. "Scottie Cramp: A Review of Cause, Characteristics, Diagnosis, and Treatment." *The Compendium of Cont. Educ.*, Vol.II, No. 5, May, 1980: pp 385-388.

5. Ackerman, Lowell, DVM. "Allergic Skin Diseases," *American Kennel Club Gazette*; September, 1990

6. Werner, A. "Aspects of Food and Food Supplements in Skin Disease." *Pedigree Breeder Forum*. 1993, Vol.2 #1.

7. Ettinger, S.J. *Textbook of Veterinary Internal Medicine*. W.B. Saunders Co., Philadelphia, PA. 1989: 2383

8. Madewell, Bruce R., VMD, MS. "Canine Lymphoma," *Vet. Clinics of N. Amer; Sm. Anim. Prac.*,Vol. 15, #4, July, 1985

9. McCaw, Dudley, DVM. "Canine Lymphosarcoma," AAHA's 56th Annual Meeting Proceedings, 1989

10. Rosenthal, Robert C.., DVM, MS, PhD. "The Treatment of Multicentric Canine Lymphoma," *Vet. Clinics of N. Amer.: Sm. Anim. Prac.*, Vol. #4, July, 1990

11. Pedersen, K and Scott, D.W. "Idiopathic Pyogranulomatous Inflammation and Leukocytoclastic Vasculitis of the Nasal Planum, Nostrils and Nasal Mucosa in Scottish Terriers in Denmark." *Veterinary Dermatology*. 1991, 2:2, 85-89; 9 ref.

12. Pedersen, K. "Vasculitis in Scottish Terriers—A New Disease Complex" *Dansk-Veterinaertidsskrift*. 1990, 73:11, 601; 4 ref.

13. Sorjonen, D.C., Cox, M.R., and Kwapien, R. "Myeloencephalopathy With Eosinophilic Refractile Bodies (Rosenthal Fibers) in a Scottish Terrier" *JAVMA*. 1987, 190:8,1004-1006; 18 ref.

14. *A Catalogue of Congenital and Hereditary Diseases*.

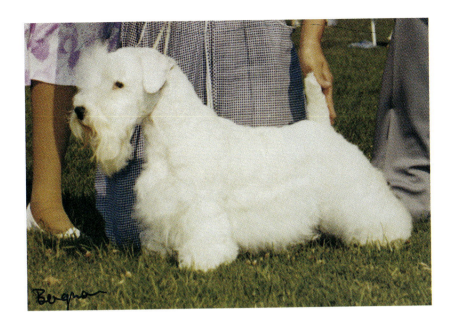

SEALYHAM TERRIER

ORIGIN AND HISTORY

The Sealyham Terrier takes its name from the country home of its developers, Sealyham House, in Haverfordwest, Wales.[1] Its earliest ancestors can be traced to the 15th century, when the Tucker family bred a small white terrier. The probable stock was Welsh Pembroke Corgi, Dandie Dinmont and West Highland White Terrier.[2] Between 1850 and 1891, Captain Edwardes of Sealyham bred his Terrier into a hunting dog, known for skill in ratting and digging badgers. His relative, Fred Lewis, known as the father of the breed, started classes, showed the dog in 1903 and founded the Sealyham Terrier Club in 1908. The Sealyham Terrier was first recognized by the British Kennel Club in 1911. The American Kennel club also recognized separate breed status in 1911. Since that time, the Sealyham's popularity has produced specialty shows of American-bred dogs.

DESCRIPTION

The Sealyham Terrier is lively and strong willed. For this reason it makes a devoted companion if given firm discipline and training when young.

THE SHOW RING

Sealyham Terriers should be longer from the shoulder to the tail than from the shoulder to the ground. English and American Standards differ, but all clubs agree that size is more important than weight. In Britain, the dog should measure something less than 12 inches at the shoulder. The Sealyham Terrier is a white breed with any other color allowed only on the head and ears. These secondary colors include lemon, tan and badger. Skin should have even pigmentation to avoid blotchy appearance of the coat.

The Sealyham Terrier has a weather-resistant double coat; a short, dense undercoat and a hard, wiry overcoat. The breed sheds relatively little.

The head, skull and neck have definite specifications. The American Standard calls for about 10 1/2 inches for either sex. The dog's weight limit is 23 to 24 pounds. The limit for the bitch is slightly less.[2] The long, broad head must balance the body length (roughly three-quarters the height at the shoulder).[3] The head should be about 1 inch longer than the neck. Slightly domed, the skull should have a moderate but definite stop.

In all clubs except Britain, dark eye rims are specified. The dark oval eyes should be set wide apart and fairly deep; any deviation in the eyes is a major fault.

The ears should be folded level to the top of the head. They should be rounded at the tip.[3] Tulip-shaped, prick or hound ears are also judged as bad faults.

There is a definite contrast between forelegs and hindlegs. The forelegs should be strong and heavy-boned, with the hindlegs longer and lighter boned.

Because the Sealyham Terrier is highly developed, there are some characteristics which are very strictly judged. For example, any black ticking in the body coat or a silky or curly coat may disqualify an individual. **Overshot** or **undershot** jaws are major faults.

The carriage should be straight, so that feet point absolutely forward and forelegs should not be knuckled or out at the elbow.

There are no disqualifying faults in this breed.

BREEDING AND WHELPING

Tails are docked at 3 to 5 days of age, leaving 1/3 to 1/2.

RECOGNIZED PROBLEMS

As in light-colored breeds, the Sealyham Terrier has trouble with **allergies** and other **skin ailments**.[2] Indications are swelling of the face, itching, flaking and possible loss of hair.

Sealyham Terriers are one of the breeds reported to have **congenital deafness**.[4]

Two eye disorders common in the Sealyham Terrier are **retinal dysplasia**[5] and **lens luxation**.[6,7,8] In common with the Bedlington Terrier, Labrador Retriever and Australian Shep-

488

herd, Sealyham Terriers may have **congenital retinal dysplasia**. The abnormality affects the layers of the retina, causing detachment and reduced intraocular tension. The condition usually results in blindness. Cataracts are a secondary finding. It is a developmental defect which may not be noticeable in newborns; reduced vision often begins at several weeks of age. Mode of inheritance is simple recessive.

The **glaucoma** found in many Sealyhams is the result of **lens luxation**. This condition is a disruption of the ligament attachment of the lens and vacated patella fossa. The results are **uveitis** and/or secondary glaucoma. Although the mode of inheritance has not been determined,[9] there is a definite genetic instability in the breed which allows **luxation from trauma** that would not develop in other animals. Because of the Sealyham's excitability and head-shaking habits, this condition is particularly common. Both clipping and stripping (about twice a year) are necessary for the adult because of this breed's double coat.

BEHAVIOR

The Sealyham has become a quiet, affectionate, well-behaved lapdog. He needs frequent grooming.

OLD AGE

Sealyham Terriers usually live an average of 13 years.

References

1. Jones, A.F. and Hamilton, F., Eds *The World Encyclopedia of Dogs*. Galahad Books, New York, NY, 1971; p 473
2. Johnson, N.H. *The Complete Puppy and Dog Book*. Atheneum, New York, NY, 1973; pp 70-71, 200, 258, 320.
3. *The Complete Dog Book*, The American Kennel Club, Howell Book House, New York, NY. 1992; 18th ed: 399-401.
4. Strain, George M. "Deafness in Dogs and Cats" *Proc. 10th ACVIM Forum*; May, 1992.
5. Wikstrom, B. "Retinal Dysplasia." Svensk-Veterinartidning. 1986, 38: 15, 129-130; 10 ref.
6. Magrane, W.G. *Canine Ophthalmology*. Lea & Febiger, Philadelphia, PA,1977; p 206,259
7. Hoskins, H.P., et al *Canine Medicine*, Am. Vet. Publ., Inc., Santa Barbara, CA, 1959: 532, 528, 543.
8. Kirk, R.W. Ed. *Current Veterinary Practice*. W.B. Saunders, Philadelphia, PA, 1977: 590, 632, 635.
9. Erickson, F., et al: "Congenital Defects of Dogs, Part 1," *Canad. Pract*. 4 (4); 61; August, 1977

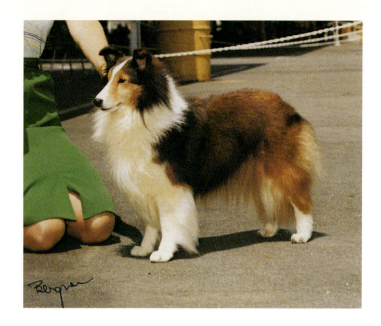

SHETLAND SHEEPDOG

ORIGIN AND HISTORY

"Like a Scottish Collie of the best kind seen through the wrong end of a telescope"—this is an apt description of this nimble dog, native of the isles northeast of Scotland. Designed to guard both cottage and flock, the Shetland Sheepdog is thought to be of Collie, Spaniel and small dog crosses.

DESCRIPTION

The "Sheltie" is an intelligent, sensitive dog and is ideally suited to a family. It is permissible and not unusual for them to be reserved toward strangers.

Shetland Sheepdog puppies range from 4 to 10 ounces at birth, but average around 7 ounces. Newborn puppies are similar in coat color to the adult. Golden and mahogany sable are easily recognized, although in some lines, puppies are born very dark and lighten as they mature. Tricolors and blue merles may have few if any sable markings at birth. These can show up in 2 or 3 weeks, but in some strains, if bicolors are prevalent, the tan will not develop.

In blue merles, the grayish-blue with black marbling is present at birth. White markings change very little at maturity, although a wide blaze will tend to look smaller and a pencil blaze generally disappears. Dewclaws are often found on the rear legs and must be removed. Dewclaws on the front legs may be removed if desired.

THE SHOW RING

The breed has two disqualifications: a height under 13 inches or over 16 inches, and brindle color. The Standard heavily penalizes a dog with conspicuous white spots, and one with more than 50% white.

BREEDING AND WHELPING

Shelties are often irregular in their heat pattern, with the first estrus appearing as early as 7 months and as late as 17 months. However, the average is at 10 months to 1 year. Subsequent heats vary with individuals but generally there is a period of 7 to 8 months between them. Some bitches can go from 10 months to 1 year between seasons. Although most Shelties ovulate on the 11th to the 13th day, there is quite a percentage that must be bred as early as the 8th day or as late as the 20th day. Generally, they are not willing breeders, especially when sent away to be bred. The gestation period is usually 61 to 63 days. The litter usually consists of four to six puppies. They whelp normally, as a rule.

GROWTH

At birth, a Sheltie's head is short and blocky with the muzzle square and full. At 6 weeks the head is wedge-shaped but the muzzle is still short. The head and muzzle start to lengthen at about 3 months so that at 6 months the dog should have the longer adult head.

At 6 weeks, the puppy is a ball of fuzz; sables are a much lighter buff shade than the adult color, with a dark streak down its back. From 3 to 5 months, the puppy fuzz is lost, and they are almost smooth coated. At 6 months, the new coat has partly grown out, so they look more like the adults.

Oversize was once a major problem in the breed, and it still is in some lines. Generally, a puppy that is obviously larger than its littermates and has larger feet will go oversize (over 16 inches).

RECOGNIZED PROBLEMS

One of the peculiarities of the breed is the late descent of the testicles. They are very hard to find at 6 weeks. Often, one can be found at 3 to 4 months while the second does not descend until 7 to 12 months. If neither is present at 4 months, they probably will not descend.

Because eye problems such as **central progressive retinal atrophy, choroidal hypoplasia, coloboma, walleye, trichiasis** and **cataracts**[1] sometimes occur, the eyes should be examined at an early age. **Walleye (heterochromia iritis)** is thought to be inherited as an

491

incomplete dominant trait, while cataract is thought to be autosomal recessive.[2] Walleye occurs in dogs that have dappling (or merling) in their coats such as Collies, Shetland Sheepdogs and Great Danes.

Ectasia syndrome[3,4] is a recessive hereditary problem in this breed. It is character-ized by excessive tortuosity of retinal vessels, excavation of the optic disc, or retinal detach-ment. **Intraocular hemorrhage** and **vermiform streaks of the fundus** may occur in young dogs. Shelties are a breed in which **Hemophilia A (Factor VIII deficiency),** inherited as an x-linked recessive, has been diagnosed.[2]

Shetland Sheepdogs have the recessive form of **Von Willebrand's** disease.[5]

Collies and Shetland Sheepdogs have **ulcer conditions of apocrine glands**, rare in other breeds, that cannot be treated at this time.[6]

Hip dysplasia has been found in Shetland Sheepdogs.[7]

Nasal solar dermatitis[6] is seen in this breed, though the mode of inheritance has not been determined. Hereditary lack of pigmentation probably predisposes a dog to this condition.

A skin disease closely resembling **familial dermatomyositis** of Collies is described in one male and two female Shetland Sheepdogs, all sired by the same father. **Dermatitis** first developed at 8-10 weeks of age. The two females had **myositis**, but it was prominent in only one. The male was infertile. A tentative diagnosis of epidermolysis bullosa was discounted because of the absence of large skin vesicles.[8] **Muscular dystrophy**, a rare x-linked recessive disease that is fatal, has been identified in Shetland Sheepdogs.[9]

Disproportionate dwarfism is generally referred to as **achondroplastic dwarfism**, although this term is not totally accurate, and may refer to any one of several conditions which are superficially similar. Disproportionate dwarfism occurs in many animal species, although it frequently presents itself as a mutation. In some breeds of dogs where the condition is consid-ered "normal" (e.g., Basset Hounds, Dachshunds, Corgis) the heterozygous state appears as an intermediate condition. A "short-legged mutant" has been reported in Cockers, and it is reported that achondroplasia has occurred in Miniature Poodles with a single recessive gene as mode of transmission.

Dr. Fletch and Dr. Frasier at the University of Toronto have determined that the affected Shetland Sheepdogs do not show abnormal blood findings and thus confirmed that the Sheltie dwarfism is not the same as that observed in the Alaskan Malamute.[10]

It is important to note that the parents of the affected animals are all normal, and there is no reason to assume that there is an intermediate condition affecting the carriers.

Patent ductus arteriosus has also been reported in the breed.[11]

In a Swedish study it was found that the Sheltie had a higher-than-average incidence of

hypothyroidism.[12] Shetland Sheepdogs are one of the breeds that are reported to have **congenital deafness.**[13]

Two cases of **bilateral renal agenesis** (one pup from each of two related bitches) were observed in a purebred Shetland Sheepdog breeding colony. Gross and histopathological examinations confirmed a diagnosis of bilateral renal agenesis as the cause of death. Limited available data strongly suggest an inherited etiology for bilateral renal agenesis. [14]

Shelties are predisposed to developing a **yeast dermatitis** caused by Malessezia. They appear to be predisposed to **discoid lupus.**[15]

Two female Sheltie littermates simultaneously developed **pemphigus foliaceous** at 6 months of age. Three other littermates were not affected. One bitch (tricolored) was not treated and the disease remained active for 2 years. The other bitch (blue merle) was successfully managed with glucocorticoids and gold salts.[16]

Uveodermatologic syndrome has been recognized in a Shetland Sheepdog.[15]

Polyartharitis of the hoc joint has been reported in Shetland Sheepdogs.[17]

BEHAVIOR

The Sheltie is lively, suspicious with strangers, but affectionate with its family, especially the children. Intelligent and trainable, the Sheltie has become one of the most popular obedience-competition dogs.

OLD AGE

Members of this breed have been known to live to 17 years of age, but 14 to 15 is more common. Arthritis is fairly common in the older dog, and kidney failure and cancer are two common causes of death.

References
1. Magrane, R.G. *Canine Ophthalmology*, 3rd ed. Lea & Febiger, Philadelphia, PA.,1977
2. Kirk, R.W. and Bistner, S.I. *Handbook of Veterinary Procedures and Emergency Treatment*, 2nd ed. 1975; p 683
3. Mason, T.A. and Cox, K. "Collie Eye Anomaly." *Aust. Vet. J.* 47: 38-40.
4. Erickson, F., et al "Congenital Defects in Dogs, A Special Reference for Practitioners." Ralston Purina (reprint from *Canine Practice, Vet. Prac.Publ. Co.*)
5. Bell, J.S., DVM: "Identifying and Controlling Defective Genes." *AKC Gazette*, July, 1993; 85.
6. Lorenz, M. Lecture Notes, Oklahoma State Convention, Tulsa, OK 1974.
7. Muller, G.H. and Kirk, R.W. *Small Animal Dermatology*. W.B. Saunders, Philadelphia, PA.
8. Hargis, A.M., Haupt, K.H., Prieur, D.J., and Moore, M.P. "A Skin Disorder in Three Shetland Sheepdogs: Comparison With Familial Canine Dermatomyositis of Collies." *Com-*

pendium on Continuing Education for the Practicing Veterinarian. 1985, 7: 4, 306-315; 24 ref.

9. Bell, Jerold S., DVM "Sex-Related Genetic Disorders: Did Mama Cause Them?" *American Kennel Club Gazette* Feb. 1994: 75.

10. Miller, W.H., Jr. *Sheltie Disease.* DVM, June, 1979

11. Kirk, R.W. and Bistner, S.I. *Handbook of Veterinary Procedures and Emergency Treatment*, 3rd ed. 1981; p 827

12. Larsson, M. "The Breed, Sex and Age Distribution of Dogs with Primary Hypothyroidism." *Svensk-Veterinartidning.* 1986, 38:15, 181-183; 3 ref.

13. Strain, George M. "Deafness in Dogs and Cats" Preced. *10th ACVIM Forum*; May, 1992.

14. Brownie, C.F., Tess, M.W., and Prasad, R.D. "Bilateral Renal Agenesis in Two Litters of Shetland Sheepdogs." *Vet. and Human Toxicology.* 1988, 30:5, 483-485; 8 ref.

15. Griffin, C., Kwochka, K., and McDonald, J. *Current Veterinary Dermatology: The Science and Art of Therapy.* Mosby Yearbook, St. Louis, Mo. 1993 p 45, 150, 218.

16. Noxon, J.O. and Myers, R.K. "Pemphigus Foliaceous in Two Shetland Sheepdog Littermates." *JAVMA.* 1989, 194: 4, 545-546; 4 ref.

17. Alexander, Joe. *Personal Communication.* June 1994

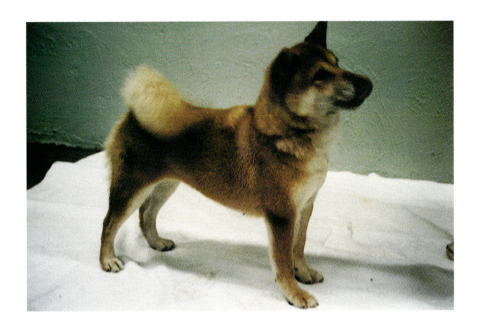

SHIBA INU

ORIGIN AND HISTORY

Originally, Shibas were bred to flush birds and small game, and were occasionally used to hunt wild boar. Now they are primarily kept as pets, both in Japan and the United States.

There were three main varieties of Shiba, each named for its region of origin: the Shinshu Shiba, from the Nagano Prefecture; the Mino Shiba, from the Gifu Prefecture; and the Sanin Shiba, from the northeastern part of the mainland. Although similar, the Shibas from each area contributed to differences in breed type seen today. From the original Japanese "native" dogs, six breeds in three different sizes evolved. They are the Akita (large size); Kishu, Hokkaido, Shikoku, Kai, (medium size); and the Shiba, (small size). There are several theories about the origin of the name "Shiba." One theory is that the word *shiba* means "small"; another theory is that the word *shiba* means "brushwood," and the dogs were named for the brushwood trees where they hunted; yet another theory is that the fiery red color of the Shiba is the same as the autumn color of the brushwood leaves. These theories are often combined and the Shiba Inu is called "the little brushwood dog."[1]

DESCRIPTION

It is a medium-boned, moderately compact and well-muscled dog. Because of its

495

hunting heritage, it should be quick and agile. At birth it is difficult to tell exactly how the coat will look at maturity. The Shiba's dense coat and rugged constitution enables him to enjoy outdoor life. He prefers the company of humans and is reserved with strangers. He makes an excellent house pet.[1]

THE SHOW RING

The Shiba Inu should have a height-to-length ratio of 10 to 11. Males are from 14 1/2 to 16 1/2 inches tall, with females ranging from 13 1/2 to 15 1/2 inches. **Height over upper limits is a disqualification.** Weight varies according to height up to about 28 pounds. All colors are acceptable, but red, red sesame and black-and-tan are preferred.[1]

BREEDING AND WHELPING

First estrus in the Shiba is usually seen from 6 to 8 months with 6-month cycles following. The bitches are free whelpers and often deliver four puppies in one or two hours. Average litter size is three or four whelps, and they are rather large for so small a breed, often weighing 9 or 10 ounces. Front dewclaw removal is optional.

DENTITION

Missing teeth are seen in some strains, as are wry mouths.

RECOGNIZED PROBLEMS

Reflex regurgitation has been reported in the Shiba. The breed has a low incidence of **hip dysplasia**, but **luxated patellas** are seen. An **uveodermatological syndrome** has been reported in the Shiba Inu.[2] It is a breed remarkably free from allergies and eye problems.

BEHAVIOR

There is a large range of temperament in this breed, ranging from skittish with strangers to total acceptance. They are not effusive. The normal Shiba is neither a barker nor a biter. It is a breed that can be kept together in groups. Veterinarians should be forewarned that Shibas have a piercing scream unlike any heard from other breeds.

References
1. Holden, Jacey "Konnichiwa, Shiba Inu." *The American Kennel Club Gazette*: June, 1992.
2. Romatowski, J. "A Uveodermatological Syndrome in an Akita Dog." *JAAHA*. 1985, 21: 6, 777-780; 7 ref.

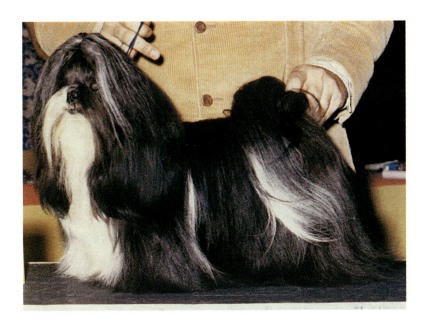

SHIH TZU

ORIGIN AND HISTORY

The Shih Tzu is a breed with a fashionable history. It takes its name from the Chinese Shih Tzu Kou "Lion Dog."[1] Its ancestors appeared in Tibetan recorded history as holy dogs as early as the 7th century A.D. During the Chinese Chi'ng (Manchu) dynasty (1642-1912), Shih Tzus were preferred gifts to monarchs and the subject of carvings, embroidery and other decorative art. Empress Tsu-hsi was particularly interested in dog breeding and received several of the Shih Tzus as gifts.

After 1908, smugglers introduced Shih Tzus to visitors from Great Britain. A controversy over its name and form was not resolved until the 1930s. Called Tibetan Poodle or Lhasa Lion Dog by the Chinese Kennel Club, the Shih Tzu was soon distinguished from the Lhasa Apso by English breeders. Its popularity continued in the United States in the 1960s; the American Kennel Club first recognized Shih Tzu in 1969.

DESCRIPTION

Originally intended as a house pet, the Shih Tzu makes an intelligent companion. This energetic breed is highly adaptable and suited for both rural and town dwelling.

497

THE SHOW RING

Weight of mature dogs is 9 to 16 pounds, with 12 to 15 pounds preferred. An important test of proportion is that the length from withers to tail should be slightly longer than the height at the withers. Height is less critical, but it should be between 9 and 10 1/2 inches, and no more than 11 nor less than 8 inches.

All colors are permissible, but best markings include a white badge on the forehead and a white tip to the tail. Noses should be black 1 to 1 1/2 inches up from the tip. Dogs with liver markings may have liver noses and slightly lighter eyes.

Critical points of judgement include the tail, legs and head. All of the coat, as well as the coat on the tail, should be heavy and straight. Also the tail should be curled over the back. Short, muscular legs are emphasized by the dense coat. The head shape distinguishes the Shih Tzu: it is broad and round (unlike the Lhasa Apso's squarer head), and the nose is flat with upturning hair (distinguishing it from the Pekingese's wrinkled nose).

Characteristics considered faults are those that detract from a generally heavy, arrogant appearance. For example, a narrow head, long legs, pig jaws and "snipyness" are faults. Sparse coats or curly coats are also faults. Since a black nose is preferred, breeders judge any pinkness on the nose or eye rims as a negative marking. Dewclaws should be removed from back feet if they are present. Front dewclaw removal is optimal but preferred by most exhibitors.

There are no breed disqualifications.

BREEDING

Litters average three to four puppies, each puppy weighing an average of 6 ounces.

DENTITION

The bite of a Shih Tzu should be slightly undershot.

RECOGNIZED PROBLEMS

In a recent study of 839 **uroliths** submitted by veterinarians for analysis, 562 (67%) were composed of at least 70% magnesium ammonium phosphate, and 57 (6.8%) at least 70% calcium oxalate. Most were found in the bladder. Uroliths occurred more often in females than in males, but there was little difference in prevalence between dogs aged 1 to 12 years. The uroliths were found in 60 known breeds of dog; Shih Tzu, 5%.[2]

The Shih Tzu shares with the Lhasa Apso, Norwegian Elkhound and Cocker Spaniel the problem of hereditary **renal cortical hypoplasia**.[3,4] The condition occurs as a bilateral syndrome and leads to **uremia** and **hypoparathyroidism**. Signs of the hypoplasia, which

498

begin in dogs about 1 year old, are **polydipsia** and **polyuria**. A genetic study in Sweden suggests a simple recessive mode of inheritance.[5] Hereditary nephropathies in dogs represent multiple, complex clinicopathological entities which cause renal failure in juvenile, adolescent and young adult dogs. To date, nephropathies believed to have a genetic basis have been described in 11 breeds. These disorders represent a variety of developmental, degenerative and metabolic defects. Many canine hereditary nephropathies are analogous to childhood nephropathies in man. The diseases reviewed include **renal dysplasia** in Shih Tzus.[6]

     Hypospadia is reported in this breed.[7]

     Skull measurements were taken on 66 dogs of seven breeds. Using mostly data from breeders' studbooks, breed differences in reproduction were examined. Litter sizes averaged 3.28±1.50 for Shih Tzus. Pup mortality averaged 10.49 percent for Shih Tzus. It was concluded that dwarfism results in small litters and, in combination with extremely domed head shape, tends to increase the incidence of dystocia.[8]

     Achondroplasia characterized by limb shortening, flared metaphyses, depressed nasal bridge, shortened maxilla, wedge or hemivertebra, elbow luxation and patella luxation is found in this breed. The mode of inheritance is incompletely dominant autosomal trait.[9]

     The Shih Tzu also has problems with hereditary **cleft lip and palate**.[2,10] The mode of inheritance is recessive. They are also highly susceptible to **inhalant allergies**.[11]

     Von Willebrand's Disease (VWD) has been reported in this breed.[12]

     In a study of dogs with chronic **hypertrophic pyloric gastrophy**, Shih Tzus were one of the two breeds most commonly affected.[13] The Shih Tzu has a number of diseases of the eye. They include **medial canthal entropion,** various **trichiasis** problems, **dermoids,** third eyelid **gland prolapse, chronic keratitis,** and **corneal ulcers, progressive retinal atrophy, vitriol syneresis** and **retinal detachment.** Most are inherited or of suspected genetic origin.[14]

BEHAVIOR

     The Shih Tzu adapts easily to the life of a pampered companion animal. He loves to romp and play. He is good with quiet, well-mannered children. The Shih Tzu needs frequent grooming.

OLD AGE

     Shih Tzus are hardy dogs that live 12 to 14 years.

References

1. Jones, A.F. and Hamilton, F. *The World Encyclopedia of Dogs*. 1971; 190-193. 195,545.
2. Osborne, C.A., Clinton, C.W., Bamman, L.K., Moran, H.C., Coston, B.R. and Frost, A.P.

"Prevalence of Canine Uroliths: Minnesota Urolith Center." *Vet. Clinics of N. Amer., Sm. Anim. Prac.* 1986, 16:1, 27-44; 6 ref.

3. Erickson, F., et al: "Congenital Defects of Dogs, Part 1." *Canad. Prac.* 4(4):58-61; 1977

4. Hoppe, A. "Progressive Nephropathy. Congenital Kidney Disease in a Number of Dog Breeds." *Svensk-Veterinartidning.* 1990, 42:10, 399-402; 19 ref.

5. Hoppe, A, Swenson, L., Jonsson, L., and Hedhammar, A. "Progressive Nephropathy Due to Renal Dysplasia in Shih Tzu Dogs in Sweden: A Clinical Pathological and Genetic Study." *J. Sm. Anim. Prac.* 1990, 31:2, 83-91; 39 ref.

6. Picut, C.A. and Lewis, R.M. "Comparative Pathology of Canine Hereditary Nephropathies: An interpretive Review." *Vet. Res. Comm.* 1987, 11:6, 561-581; 91 ref.

7. Ettinger, S.J. *Textbook of Veterinary Internal Medicine: Diseases of the Dog and Cat.* W.B. Saunders Co., Philadelphia, PA. 1989: p 1884

8. Hahn, S. "Variation of Skull Traits and Reproduction in Breeds of Small Dogs." Thesis, Tierarztliche Hochschule Hanover, German Fed. Rep. 1988, 130pp.; 111 ref.

9. Ettinger, S.J. *Textbook of Veterinary Internal Medicine: Diseases of the Cat and Dog.* W.B. Saunders Co., Philadelphia, PA. 1989; P 2383.

10. Cooper, H.K. and Mattern, C.W. "Genetic Studies of Cleft Lip and Palate in Dogs." *Birth Defects.* Series 7: 98-100; 1971.

11. Ackerman, Lowell, DVM. "Allergic Skin Diseases," *American Kennel Club Gazette*; September, 1990

12. Shih Tzu column, *American Kennel Club Gazette*; August, 1990.

13. Ballenger, C.R., Maddison, J.E., MacPherson, G.C., and Ilkiw, J.E. "Chronic Hypertrophic Pyloric Gastrophy in 14 Dogs," *Australian Vet. Jour.* 1990, 67:9 317-320; 19 ref.

14. Christmas, R.E. "Common Ocular Problems of Shih Tzu Dogs," *Can. Vet. Journal.* 1992, 33: 6, 390-393; 12 ref.

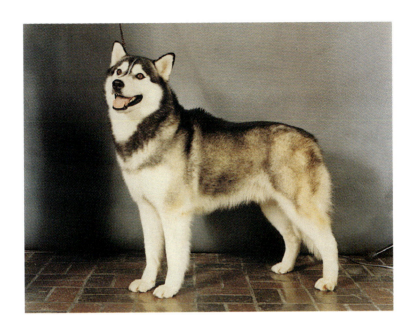

SIBERIAN HUSKY

ORIGIN AND HISTORY

Siberian Huskies have been bred by the Chukchis of Northeastern Asia for thousands of years. The Chukchis needed a sled dog with a conformation designed to provide maximum speed and strength over great distances with a minimum expenditure of energy. They required a dog capable of such endurance on a small amount of food. From the Chukchi breeding, a sturdy but graceful dog gradually evolved, having moderate bone structure, medium length of leg, and fairly close coupling. This same capable, solid appearance and easy grace characterizes the Siberian Husky today.

DESCRIPTION

The breed's temperament is very gentle; an aggressive temperament is undesirable. Any Siberian that is overly aggressive should not be used for breeding and should be disciplined. The characteristic temperament of the Siberian is friendly, gentle, alert and outgoing. They do not display the possessive qualities of guard dogs, nor are they overly suspicious of strangers or aggressive with other dogs. Some measure of reserve and dignity may be expected in mature dogs. Their intelligence, tractability and eager disposition make them agreeable companions and willing team workers. As their instinct to run can endanger them, they should usually be leashed or confined in pens.

All colors are permissible in the breed. Puppies of all colors and markings occur to-gether in a litter. The color red is a simple recessive trait. A breeding of two red dogs will produce all red puppies with liver points and either blue or hazel eyes. Breeding a red dog to a black or grey dog produces puppies of any color.

Eye color is neither a true recessive nor a dominant trait. Blue-eyed dogs do not always produce blue-eyed dogs. This is one of the few breeds in which blue, brown and hazel eyes all occur, as well as different-colored eyes in the same animal. On some dogs the eyes may not be a solid color, for example, a blue eye can have a wedge of brown in it.

THE SHOW RING

Being oversize is the only breed disqualification. Dogs taller than 23 1/2 inches and bitches taller than 22 inches at the withers are disqualified from the show ring. Mature dogs weigh 45 to 60 pounds and bitches weigh 35 to 50 pounds.

Any rear dewclaws should be removed. Removal of front dewclaws is optional.

BREEDING AND WHELPING

Many Siberian Husky bitches are extremely difficult to breed. A good muzzle and an assistant are recommended to protect the stud owner. They have few problems during gesta-tion, but a bitch that has gone beyond the 65th day should be watched very closely. This breed whelps naturally and easily. Bitches take a long time to deliver. Consequently, some breeders mistakenly rush Siberians into a **cesarean section**. Bitches normally rest 1 or 2 hours between puppies. In the middle of a large litter, a rest of 5 or 6 hours is not unusual. A litter of six puppies may take the bitch 10 to 12 hours to deliver.

Siberian Husky puppies weigh 12 to 16 ounces at birth. The size of a litter averages three to seven puppies. Bitches do not seem to have the ability to digest the huge quantities of food required to provide enough milk for extremely large litters.

These bitches are subject to prolonged diarrhea during the entire period of lactation. By the time a large litter is weaned, the bitch is in extremely poor condition and requires special attention to rebuild her stamina.

With smaller litters, bitches can complete a normal lactation of 6 weeks with little loss of weight.

Bitches usually shed their coats completely between 7 and 10 weeks after whelping. During this period a bitch should be groomed at least twice a week.

GROWTH

Growth patterns vary greatly. Some strains are slow to mature and grow in stages that include an awkward or gangly period at 4 to 10 months. Other strains grow at an even pace. Some strains mature as late as 3 years. Some puppies eat lightly and are quite lean after 4 months. When these dogs are healthy and free of parasites, they may be exhibiting the breed's characteristic of surviving on little food.

Loose stool syndrome in Siberian Husky puppies and lactating bitches can usually be corrected by feeding a high-protein, chicken-based dry dog food in a self-feeder.

Small amounts of food often are more easily digested by the Siberian. Most puppies should be taken off self-feeding at 4 months of age so they do not become overweight. Feed a sufficient amount of food twice a day to insure proper growth.

They have relatively few birth problems or defects.

DENTITION

Full dentition and a scissors bite are normal.

RECOGNIZED PROBLEMS

Serious breeders of Siberian Huskies became concerned with **hip dysplasia** in the early 1960s and started an extensive campaign of x-raying all breeding stock. As a result the breed now has fewer problems with this condition.[1] OFA rates them the fifth-least-affected of all breeds. All Siberian Husky breeding stock should be certified as free of hip dysplasia by the OFA.

Over 14,000 radiographs of the spine of 10 breeds of dogs were examined for abnormal vertebrae in the lumbosacral region, which were manifested by different types of fusion. Such abnormalities were seen in 4% of 486 Siberian Husky dogs. There was some link between these abnormalities and hip dysplasia.[2]

Hemophilia A is reported in Siberian Huskies, as is **ventricle septal defect**.[3]

Progressive retinal atrophy is also found in the breed and **corneal dystrophy,**[4] **cataracts** and **heterochromia of the iris** have been reported.[1,5] According to a report there are eight breeds at higher risk of developing **glaucoma** than mixed-breed dogs. Siberians are one of these eight breeds.[6]

A full ophthalmic examination was performed on 40 Siberian Husky dogs using direct and indirect ophthalmoscopy, gonioscopy and nasolacrimal cannulation. [**Eight (20%) of the dogs were found to have distichia, 10 (25%) had excessive median caruncular hairs, eight (20%) had absence, displacement, or narrowing of the nasolacrimal puncta and two (5%) had unilateral areas of lateral corneal lipidosis. Fifty percent of the dogs had**

some abnormality of the iridocorneal (drainage) angle.] However, in only one of these was the deformity severe enough to require glaucoma prophylaxis. An association between blue iris color and malformation of the iridocorneal angle was noted. [7]

A syndrome of **uveodermatosis**, associated with uveitis and depigmentation and erosion of areas of skin and mucous membrane on the head and, in one dog, on the scrotum, was observed in two male Siberian Huskies. These clinical signs are similar to the Vogt-Koyanagi-Harada syndrome in man.[8]

Siberian Huskies appear to have a predisposition for **discoid lupus.**[9] A castration-responsive **dermatosis** has been reported in this breed.[9]

Alaskan breeds are more susceptible to **zinc deficiency**.[10,11] A dermatosis in a Siberian Husky (4 yrs old) was completely resolved clinically and histopathologically, after one month of oral treatment with zinc sulphate (250 mg/day: 50 mg essential Zn). Skin lesions, which recurred when treatment was discontinued after a year, healed completely when treatment was resumed.[12]

Congenital laryngeal paralysis has been reported in Siberian Huskies. It causes dyspnea and coughing in very young puppies.[13,14]

Ectopic ureter was diagnosed in 228 dogs. The female to male ratio was 217:11. Siberians were one of six breeds identified with greater frequency of diagnosis than expected. The strength of association in certain purebred dogs suggests a familial relationship.[15] **Epilepsy** has been reported in the breed.[16]

BEHAVIOR

The Siberian Husky is sociable, affectionate, good company and easily bored. He is the most docile of all the sled dogs, but still needs proper training to be an acceptable family companion.

References

1. Keller, G.G. and Corley, E.A. "Canine Hip Dysplasia: Investigating the Sex Predilection and the Frequency of Unilateral CHD." *Vet. Med.* 1989, 84: 12, 1162, 1164-1166; 13 ref.
2. Winkler, W. "Transitional Lumbosacral Vertebrae in the Dog." Dissertation, Fachbereich Veterinarmedizin der Freien Universitat Berlin. 1985
3. Foley, C.W., et al: *Abnormalities of Companion Animals.* Iowa State University Press. Ames, IA., 1979:37.
4. Waring, G.O., MacMillan, A., and Reveles, P. "Inheritance of Crystalline Corneal Dystrophy in Siberian Huskies." *JAAHA.* 1986, 22: 5, 655-658; 9 ref.
5. Quinn, A.J. Personal Communication, 1982.
6. Slater, M.R. and Erb, H.N. "Effects of Risk Factors and Prophylactic Treatment on Pri-

mary Glaucoma in the Dog." *JAVMA.* 1986, 188:9, 1028-1030; 7 ref.

7. Stanley, R.G. and Blogg, J.R. "Eye Diseases in the Siberian Husky Dog." *Aust. Vet. Jour.* 1991, 68:5, 161-162; 10 ref.

8. Vercelli, A. and Taraglio, S. "Canine Vogt-Koyanagi-Harada-Like Syndrome in Two Siberian Husky Dogs." *Vet. Dermatology.* 1990, 1: 3, 151-158; 18 ref.

9. Griffin, C., Kowchka, K., and McDonald, J.: *Current Veterinary Dermatology: The Science and Art of Therapy.* Mosby Yearbook, St. Louis, Mo. 1993:p 150, 218, 299.

10. Samuelson, Marvin, DVM, Personal Communication, 1992.

11. Meyer, H, Rodenbeck, H., Zentek, J., Grubler, B., Kienzle, E., and Carlos, G.M. "Contribution to the Clinical Picture and Aetiology of a Dermatosis in Siberian Huskies." *Effem-Forschung-fur-Heimtiernahrung.* 1989, No. 29, 1-11; 15 ref.

12. Degryse, A.D., Fransen, J., Van Cutsem, J., and Ooms, L. "Recurrent Zinc-Responsive Dermatosis in a Siberian Husky." *J. Sm. Anim. Prac.* 1987, 28: 8, 721-726; 17 ref.

13. Neuhoff, Kathleen, Personal Communication.

14. O'Brien, J.A. and Hendriks, J. "Inherited Laryngeal Paralysis: Analysis in the Husky Cross." *Vet. Quarterly.* 1986, 8: 4, 301-302; 4 ref.

15. Hayes, H.M., Jr. *Breed Associations of Canine Ectopic Ureter: A Study of 217 Female Cases.* 1984, 25:8, 501-504; 12 ref.

16. Bell, Jerold S., DVM, "Sex-Related Genetic Disorders: Did Mama Cause Them?" *American Kennel CLub Gazette,* Feb. 1994: 76.

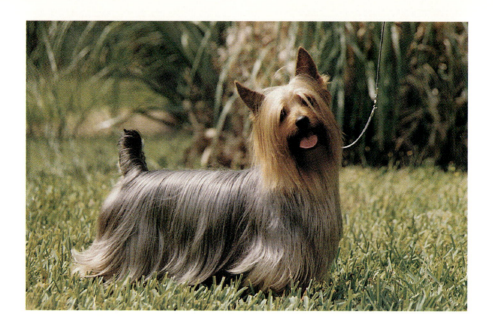

SILKY TERRIER

ORIGIN AND HISTORY

The Silky Terrier, formerly known as the Sydney Silky Terrier, originated from cross-breeding the Yorkshire Terrier and the Australian Terrier.[1] The Silky Terrier was accepted in the United States as a separate breed in 1959.[1]

DESCRIPTION

The Silky Terrier is a high-spirited little dog with aggressive tendencies. It is very alert and makes an excellent watch dog.

THE SHOW RING

The Silky weighs from 8 to 10 pounds and stands approximately 9 to 10 inches at the withers. The colors are blue and tan and gray-blue and tan, with a silver or fawn topknot. The coat should be fine and glossy with a silky texture, and should be 5 to 6 inches in length; it should not approach floor length.[1] Faults include any nose color other than black; curly, woolly, wavy, short or harsh coat; any body color other than blue and tan or gray-blue and tan (puppies excepted); undershot or overshot mouth; overweight or underweight dog; white or flesh colored toenails; ewe neck; weediness; coarseness or unsoundness.[2] The American Kennel Club lists these added faults: (1) toeing in or out, and (2) a body either too long or too short.

Its gait should be light-footed and lively. The ears are naturally pricked to a V-shape. At 5 days of age or less, dewclaws should be removed and tails docked to leave one-third (about 1/2 inch).

BREEDING AND WHELPING

Pregnancy does not present any unusual problems and usually lasts 60 to 62 days. **Dystocia** is not uncommon, especially with the first pregnancy in older bitches. **Cesarean sections** are often necessary. Usual litter size is three to four puppies. **Cleft palates, imperforate anus** and some other defects are occasionally found at birth. During gestation, **eclampsia** is not an uncommon problem.

RECOGNIZED PROBLEMS

Storage disease has been well characterized in the Silky Terrier.[3,4] The disease is rare and has been shown to have a recessive mode of inheritance, so only certain littermates are affected.[5] Affected individuals are normal at birth, but fail to grow normally. They are usually presented with multifocal neurological disease which is progressive and fatal.

The disease can be confirmed antemortem by assessment of flucocerebroside levels of the peripheral blood leukocytes or cultured cells such as skin fibroblast. Storage cells can be identified in biopsy material.

Three Silky Terriers were presented with non-pruritic **alopecia** and hyperpigmentation. Alopecia had been evident when affected dogs were purchased as pups and was non-progressive. Skin changes were bilaterally symmetrical and most severe over the dorsal and lateral portions of the trunk, sparing the head and distal limbs. Affected animals were normal in other respects. Histopathological features of **color dilutant alopecia** were evident in skin biopsies from all three cases.[6]

This breed is predisposed to **yeast dermatitis** caused by Malassezia.[7]

Due to their shortened limbs they are predisposed to **intervertebral disc disease** and **elbow dysplasia**.[8]

The Silky unfortunately develops all the problems of most Toy breeds such as **tracheal collapse, cryptorchidism, odontoid process dysplasia, hydrocephalus, occipital dysplasia, patella luxation, avascular necrosis of the femoral head (Legg-Perthes disease), congenital cardiovascular abnormalities** and **diabetes mellitus.**

BEHAVIOR

The Silky is extremely vocal and makes an excellent watch dog for the apartment dweller.

He is active, demanding, cheerful, sociable and intelligent.

OLD AGE

Old dogs usually develop moderate to severe **dental problems**. Occasionally, **cataracts** develop. The life span is 11 to 13 years, with some individuals living to 20 years.

References

1. Burnell, R.B. *The World Encyclopedia of Dogs.* World Publishing Co., New York, NY. 1971
2. RAS Kennel Club: Australian Breed Standards
3. Hartley, W.J. and Blakemore, W.F. *Veterinary Pathology.* 10:191;1973
4. Blakemore, W.F. *Vet. Ann.* 1975; p 242.
5. Farrow, B.R.H. *Proc. 4th Ann. Conf. Aus. Sm. Anim. Vet. Assoc.* 1977
6. Malik, R and France, MP. "Hyperpigmentation and Symmetrical Alopecia in Three Silky Terriers." *Australian Vet. Practitioner.* 1991, 21: 3, 135-136, 138; 7 ref.
7. Griffin, C., Kowchka, K. and McDonald, J. *Current Veterinary Dermatology: The Science and Art of Therapy.* Mosby Yearbook, St. Louis, Mo. 1993: 45.
8. Ettinger, S.J. *Textbook of Veterinary Internal Medicine.* W.B. Saunders Co., Philadelphia, PA. 1989: p 2383

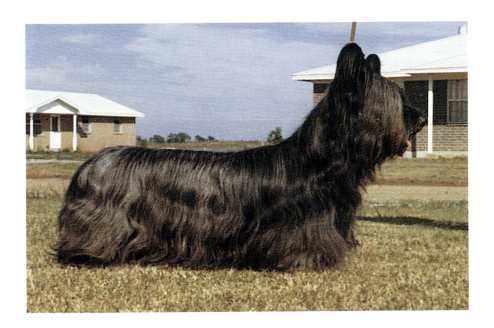

SKYE TERRIER

ORIGIN AND HISTORY

The Skye Terrier takes its name from the Island of Skye off the northwest coast of Scotland. The breed is an old one, and proponents who claim it is as old as any other Terrier have some basis for their claims. There is evidence that the Skye Terrier has been known for at least 300 years. The Skye was included in the first volume of the English Kennel Club Stud Book. Shortly after 1840 the breed became popular during the reign of Queen Victoria. She owned many outstanding specimens and kept both varieties—the prick-eared and the drop-eared—as constant companions. The American Kennel Club Studbook first listed five Skyes for the year 1887. The Skye Terrier Club of America was founded in New York on January 17, 1938. The first Skye Terrier was shown in the United States over 100 years ago in 1878.

DESCRIPTION

The Skye Terrier is a dog of style, elegance and dignity. It is agile and strong, with sturdy bone and hard muscle. Long, low and lank, twice as long as it is high, it is covered with a profuse coat that falls straight down either side of its body. It stands with its head high and long tail hanging. Of suitable size for its hunting work, it is strong in body, quarters and jaw. It is fearless, good-tempered, loyal and canny. Friendly and gay with those it knows, reserved

509

and cautious with strangers, the Skye Terrier is not a breed for everyone.

Parti-colored Skye Terriers that are white, grey and black, fawn, dark gray and almost white do occur, but their origin is not precisely understood. A study of color genetics of the breed is needed.

There are two varieties of Skye Terriers, differing only in ear carriage: the prick and the drop-ear. Both may appear in the same litter, and offspring do not always follow the carriage of their parents. The best breeding method is to breed drop-to-drop and prick-to-prick. The drop ear was more popular in the original working terrier. The prick-ear became more fashionable in the mid-1800s. Skye Terriers were divided into two varieties in England in 1904, remaining divided until 1922 when registrations dropped. After 1922, the breed was not divided and ear problems arose, such as weak-eared prick, low-placed ears, semi-prick ears, soft or tulip or drop ears carried with a lift, and ears not symmetrical in carriage.

The German breeding rules are special and important. Since 1932 it has been prohibited to cross the prick-eared variety with the drop-eared variety. The offspring by prick-eared parents or offspring by drop-eared parents that do not have the same ear carriage of their parents are disqualified from breeding and show ring.

THE SHOW RING

The Skye is distinguished by a long head with powerful jaws, prick or drop ears, dark eyes, elegant neck, long level back, deep chest and well-sprung ribs, broad shoulders, short, straight and muscular legs, and sound movement. The average height at the shoulder is 10 inches for dogs, and 9 1/2 inches for bitches. The average length, chest bone over tail at rump, is 20 inches for dogs. The ideal ratio of body length to shoulder height is 2 to 1.

Acceptable colors in the breed are black, blue, dark or light gray, silver, platinum, fawn or cream. The coat must be an allowed color with black points of ears, muzzle and tip of tail.

The most common fault in cream-colored Skyes is lack of black points. Breeding cream to cream seems to cause loss of pigmentation in the black points of the ear feathering, muzzle, and tail. **A Dudley, flesh-colored, or brown nose is a disqualification.**

DENTITION

The bite is very important in this terrier breed. The jaw is strong. The incisor teeth close even in a level bite or the upper teeth slightly overlap the lower in a scissors bite. The **undershot** or **overshot** bite is a handicap in a working terrier because it prevents the dog from gripping game. Missing premolars or molars is a common fault.

RECOGNIZED PROBLEMS

A fairly common genetic fault is a **kink tail**, conspicuous at birth. When examined, vertebrae appear to be fused, or a decided hook at the end is noticed. Altering the tail disqualifies the dog from the show ring.

Ulcerative colitis has been reported as a breed problem in Germany.[1] **Laryngeal collapse** has also been reported.[2,3]

Enlarged foramen magnum is reported in the breed.[4,5] Some dogs have no symptoms, while others appear to have pain over the occipita-cervical region. Scratching of the ear is common. The tongue may protrude from the mouth, with loss of pain sensation in the tongue. Pawing at the face is also noted. In puppies, the sign of dorsal spinal cord involvement may be observed with unsteadiness of forelegs. Sudden, temporary changes in the dog's temperament may occur. Signs may be observed in the young puppy or may not appear until the dog is fully mature.

Skyes are susceptible to **inhalant allergies.**[6] In a recent survey of Skye breeders conducted by Dr. Donald Brown, chairperson of the health committee, it was found that 45% of the dogs represented in the survey had some type of **allergy**; 22% of the dogs with allergies also had **autoimmune thyroid disease.**[7]

Also discussed by breeders was a condition called **Skye hepatitis**, a fatal disease generally affecting young dogs. Symptoms include lethargy, loss of appetite and abdominal swelling. Diagnosis is by liver biopsy which shows intra-hepatic destruction.[7]

The orthopedic problem most often reported was **premature closure of the distal radius** (**PC**) which occurs when the radius prematurely stops growing. The ulna continues to grow and is ultimately displaced from its socket. Current thinking is that the tendency for PC is expressed by the interaction of several genes.[7] **Piddling** or **wet puppies** are ones with weak bladders. They are always wet around the tail. Some breeders claim the condition improves in time.

A front limp called **juvenile limp** sometimes occurs in heavier puppies between 3 and 8 months of age. It usually disappears without treatment. Most veterinarians suggest limiting exercise.

Megaesophagus has been reported in the breed.[8,9]

BEHAVIOR

The Skye Terrier has a strong sense of property and is stand-offish with strangers. He is an ideal companion dog for the city. He is polite and affectionate with his family.

References

1. Adler, Von R. and Troup, S. "Psychischse Faktorenbeienem Coitis-Ulcerosaahnlichen Krankheitsbild Eines Kerry-Blue-Und Eines Skye Terriers." Ver: Dialog Search Files, *Bio. Reviews*: 72-76

2. Sounders: *Catalog of Genetic Disorders. In Current Therapy VI*. Kirk, R.W., Ed. 1977; p 86

3. Koch, W. "Neue Pathogene Erbfaktoren bei Hunden 2." *Indukt Astann u-Vererb-L* 70:503-506; 1935

4. Foley, C.W., et al *Abnormalities of Companion Animals*. Iowa State University Press, Ames, IA., 1979: 37

5. Bardens, J.W. "Congenital Malformation of the Foramen Magnum in Dogs." *Southwest Vet.* 18: 295-298; 1965

6. Ackerman, Lowell, DVM. "Allergic Skin Diseases," *American Kennel Club Gazette*; September, 1990

7. Kuczynski, L.A., *AKC Gazette*, Dec. 1993; pp115-116.

8. Veterinary News, *The American Kennel Club Gazette*; May 1991

9. The Skye Terrier column. *The American Kennel Club Gazette*; Sept. 1992

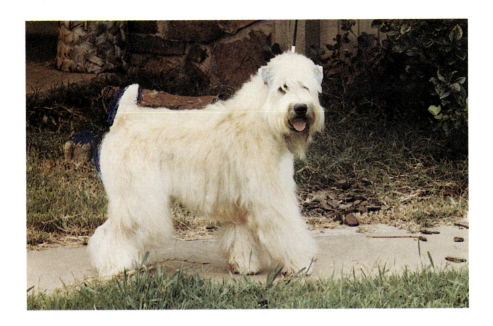

SOFT-COATED WHEATEN TERRIER

ORIGIN AND HISTORY

The Soft-coated Wheaten Terrier has been known for over 200 years in Ireland. The Wheaten is probably an important ancestor of the Kerry Blue.[1] It was originally a working dog, used to hunt small game and to guard its master.

DESCRIPTION

The Soft Coated Wheaten Terrier whelp is generally between 5 and 8 ounces in weight. Usually brown or red, color at birth may vary from gray to almost black, and some puppies are wheaten or golden. A black mask and black stripe down the back are often present. Color gradually lightens during the first year, sometimes becoming very light, but color should deepen again with maturity. Nose pigment may be pink or black at birth, but noses and pads should be black by 3 weeks.

New coats often appear deeper in color and rougher in texture at the tips. Matting is a problem during the period of change from puppy to adult coat.

Lack of pigment and yellow or green eyes have been seen. These dogs should not be used in a breeding program. Breeders feel there is a dilution factor in the breed, and puppies born blonde whose pigment is not complete by 3 weeks should be suspect as carriers.

The Wheaten is not a typical terrier in temperament. It is calmer and steadier, easier to train. Alert and intelligent, it is not a "yappy" dog. The Soft-coated Wheaten Terrier is very affectionate, needing close family relationships. Playfulness is a trait that lasts its entire adult life.

THE SHOW RING

Major faults are **overshot** and **undershot** bites, coat-texture deviation, nose color other than black, timid or overly aggressive dogs, and any adult color other than Wheaten. The coat must be single-layered and soft; there is specific shading on the ears and muzzle.

There are no breed disqualifications.

BREEDING AND WHELPING

Bitches are best bred when they reach their third season, or no earlier than 20 months of age. Generally they are easy breeders and free whelpers. An occasional **resorbed pregnancy** can be directly attributed to immaturity or poor condition. Ovulation generally occurs between the 11th and 15th day, although some are receptive as early as the eighth day. Litters average five to seven puppies, and as many as 12 whelps have been reported in a single litter. Pregnancy is often hard to detect, and care should be taken to deliver all the whelps, since the last birth can be somewhat delayed. Newborn mortality is low.

GROWTH

Dewclaws must be removed when tails are docked at 3 days. One-third to 1/2 of the tail (the lesser amount for the shorter-backed whelps) is removed. Thin tails should be docked slightly shorter than thick ones. The Wheaten is a slow-maturing breed. Full height may not be achieved until after a year of age, and dogs may not fill out until they are 3 years old.

The Breed is an easy keeper and a moderate eater. Diet of the young dog should be based on high-quality proteins. Care must be taken throughout life not to overfeed. Ears must be kept free of excess hair to prevent infection.

DENTITION

Undershot and open bites are currently major problems, as are missing teeth.

RECOGNIZED PROBLEMS

There is evidence of **heart disease** in older animals. The breed has a low incidence of **hip dysplasia** and many have been x-rayed "good" and "excellent."

Cataracts have been described in aged dogs. **Progressive retinal atrophy** has been reported recently.

Experience with older Wheatens in the United States has been limited. However, reports from Ireland of adult Wheatens imply that **congenital heart problems** lead to adult weaknesses in some lines.

Wheatens often have **dermatitis.** This is a result of sensitivity to grass and fleas.

Hereditary nephropathies in dogs represent multiple, complex clinicopathological entities which cause renal failure in juvenile, adolescent and young adult dogs. **Renal dysplasia** is reviewed in Soft-Coated Wheatens.[2,3]

In two litters of Soft-Coated Wheaten Terriers, with the same parents, chronic renal failure developed in five of 10 dogs. The dogs died or were destroyed at 30 months of age. Clinical signs were inappetence, weight loss, vomiting, depression, and, in two cases, polydipsia and polyuria. The laboratory data revealed isosthenuria, non-regenerative anemia, extremely high serum area nitrogen and creatinine values. Pathology included small kidneys with an irregular and pale external surface. Cortical lesions were mostly segmental in distribution, and consisted of loss of glomerular elements and increased interstitial connective tissue. Medullary lesions were severe, diffuse in distribution, and consisted of loss of tubules and proliferation of connective tissue. The clinical, laboratory and pathological findings show similarities to renal diseases seen in young dogs in other breeds.[4]

BEHAVIOR

The Soft-Coated Wheaten Terrier is an all-round animal. He is a guard dog, a shepherd, a hunter and a good companion for the house or yard. He is active, enterprising and versatile.

References
1. *The Complete Dog Book*, American Kennel Club: Howell Book House, New York, NY. 18th Ed. 1992; pp 406-412
2. Picut, C.A. and Lewis, R.M. "Comparative Pathology of Canine Hereditary Nephropathies: An Interpretive Review." *Vet. Res. Comm.* 1987, 11: 6, 561-581; 91 ref.
3. Nash, A.S., Kelly, D.F., and Gaskell, C.J. "Progressive Renal Disease in Soft-Coated Wheaten Terriers: Possible Familial Nephropathy." *J. Sm. Anim. Prac.* 1984, 25:8, 479-487;6 ref.
4. Eriksen, K and Grondalen, J. "Familial Renal Disease in Soft-Coated Wheaten Terrier." *J. Sm. Anim. Prac.* 1984, 25: 8, 489-500; 32 ref.

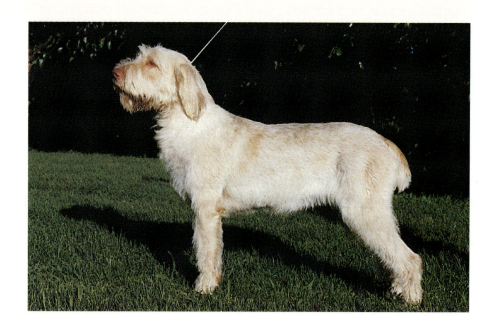

SPINONI ITALIANI

ORIGIN AND HISTORY

The Spinoni Italiani or Italian Pointer is one of the oldest griffon varieties in existence and is descended from an ancient hunting breed found in the Piedmont region of Italy. He is Italy's all-purpose hunting dog.

A dog similar to the Spinoni was painted by Mantegna in the fifteenth century. Popular with both commoners and nobility in the 1700s, it was used for all types of hunting until the French Revolution. After a long decline it returned to popularity in the late nineteenth century.[1]

DESCRIPTION

This is a solid, sturdy dog with strong bones and well-developed muscles.

Its name Spinoni comes from the word "spino" which means "thorn." It refers to the dog's coat, which is hard like thorns, and thick and tight to its body. Longer hair covers the arched eyebrows, cheeks and lips, giving the dog a characteristic beard. He is sociable, patient, affectionate, courageous, equally adaptable to stable life or apartment life.

The breed is extremely robust and untiring, with an immediate point, an excellent sense of smell, and oily, leathery skin that allows it to hunt in water without ever becoming ill. At the end of the hunting season, the Spinoni is perfectly adaptable to the house. He is clean, polite and tranquil.[2]

BREEDING AND WHELPING

The average litter size is ten. Bitches usually have their first estrus between 9 and 12 months of age. In the United States most tails are docked leaving 2/5, although in Italy they leave 3/5.

THE SHOW RING

Height should be from 20 to 26 inches at the shoulder. Weight should be about 56 pounds. The total length of the head should be 2/5 of the height at the withers. Its large nose is meat red or brown, depending on the color of its coat. Its jaws are strong with an arched dentition that meets perfectly. The eyes are yellow or light brown. Ears are typical hound ears, large, dropped and hanging close to the cheeks, although set fairly high. They can be white, white with yellow or light brown patches.[3]

RECOGNIZED PROBLEMS

Breeders report some Spinoni Italiani have **thyroid imbalances. Hip dysplasia** is seen. **Vaginal prolapse** has been seen in the breed.

BEHAVIOR

The Spinoni Italiani is intelligent, sociable and affectionate. He happily adapts from hunting life to family life and adores children. He will brave any danger to defend his master. He is a mellow, docile dog and not suitable for a heavy-handed hunter.

References
1. *Reader's Digest Illustrated Book of Dogs.* 1989
2. *Guide to Dogs,* Simon and Schuster
3. *Breed Standards for Miscellaneous Class Breeds,* American Kennel Club. June, 1993.

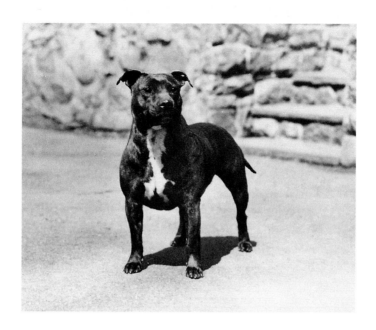

STAFFORDSHIRE BULL TERRIER

ORIGIN AND HISTORY

The Staffordshire Bull Terrier is a small descendant of the infamous bull-baiting dog and the Bulldog. In the early 19th century, the 30- to 45-pound Staffordshire was developed.

Although the Staffordshire Bull Terrier is a cousin of the (usually) all white English Bull Terrier, the Staffordshire was associated with dog fighting for years. Therefore, the Staffordshire was denied purebred registration in England until 1935. By that time, it had evolved as a pet and a show dog.

This terrier was first recognized by the American Kennel Club in 1974.[1]

DESCRIPTION

Although small, the Staffordshire Bull Terrier is a strong, muscular dog. It should be of great strength for its size and, although muscular, should be active and agile.

THE SHOW RING

It is smooth-coated with a square shape, weighing between 28 and 38 pounds; the bitch weighs between 24 and 34 pounds. Both the dog and bitch are between 14 and 16 inches tall. The head should be short and broad with a definite stop.

518

Any nose color other than solid black, e.g., pink or Dudley, is a fault.

The eyes are dark and round and set straight ahead. Ears other than rose-shaped or half-pricked are faulted.[1]

Black-and-tan or liver colors are disqualifications.

BREEDING AND WHELPING

This breed requires **cesarean section** more than the average, but not as often as might be expected in a large-headed breed.

RECOGNIZED PROBLEMS

Problems found in Staffordshire Bull Terriers are **bilateral cataract (recessive)** [2,3] **persistent hyperplastic primary vitreous**[4,5] and **clefts of the lip or palate**.[6]

BEHAVIOR

The Staffordshire Bull Terrier is a companion animal that exhibits great devotion to its owners and is kind with children. It is courageous and intelligent and is not belligerent with humans unless provoked or encouraged to attack.

References

1. *The Complete Dog Book,* American Kennel Club: Howell Book House, New York, NY. 18th ed. 1992: 410-412.
2. Barnett, K.C. "The Diagnosis and Differential Diagnosis of Cataract in the Dog." *J. Sm. Anim. Prac.* 1985, 26:6, 305-316; 20 ref.
3. Petrick, S.W. "Genetic Eye Disease Diagnosed in Staffordshire Bull Terriers." *J. of the So. African Vet. Assoc.* 1988, 59:4, 177; 1 ref.
4. Barnett, K.C. *Inherited Eye Disease in the Dog and Cat.* 1988, 29:7, 462-475; 33 ref.
5. Leon, A., Curtis, R., and Barnett, K.C. "Hereditary Persistent Hyperplastic Primary Vitreous in the Staffordshire Bull Terrier." *JAAHA.* 1986, 22: 6, 765-774; 27 ref.
6. Kirk, R.W. and Bistner, S.I. *Handbook of Veterinary Procedures and Emergency Treatment,* 3rd ed. 1981; p 827

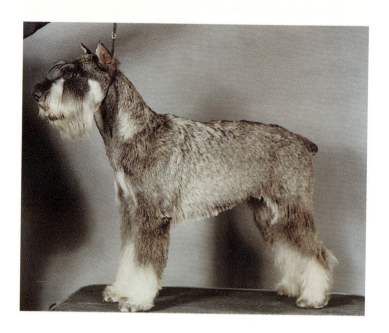

STANDARD SCHNAUZER

ORIGIN AND HISTORY

The Standard Schnauzer is the prototype for the Giant and the Miniature Schnauzer. The breed originated in Germany, where their breeding is strictly controlled. Breeding stock is selected not only for appearance, but also for skill as guard dogs and ratters. The breed is second to none in sagacity and has been described by owners as the dog with the human brain.

DESCRIPTION

This high-spirited dog is fundamentally a guard dog. Aloofness or wariness when confronting a stranger should not be considered unusual. **Shyness and aggressiveness** do occur, especially in Schnauzers that have not been constantly exposed to varied social situations. Administering a mild tranquilizer is often advisable before the dog visits the veterinarian.

THE SHOW RING

Adult dogs ideally measure 18 1/2 to 19 1/2 inches, bitches 17 1/2 to 18 1/2 inches. To predict adult size, breeders must rely on knowledge of the sire and dam and their progenitors. **Any dog that measures under 18 inches or over 20 inches in height or any bitch that measures under 17 inches or over 19 inches will be disqualified. Viciousness is also a**

disqualification.

BREEDING AND WHELPING

Bitches have normal intervals of estrus, times of ovulation, and lengths of gestation. They are easy whelpers, delivering an average of six to eight puppies in a litter, although large litters are not rare. Lactation problems are uncommon. The puppies are generally hearty and have no common birth defects. Standard Schnauzer puppies usually weigh 7 to 12 ounces at birth and gain 5 to 10 ounces during the first week. However, size at birth and rate of early development are not reliable indications of adult height. Growth patterns are highly individual. A small puppy may become an oversized adult.

Puppies are usually black at birth. Those that will be light salt-and-pepper at maturity often show some gray, particularly on the paws and sides of the body. Within a few days the characteristic lighter markings on the legs and muzzle begin to appear and spread rapidly.

GROWTH

All dewclaws should be removed and tails should be docked by 3 days. The tail of the adult should not be less than 1 inch nor more than 2 inches long. Although experienced veterinarians dock the tails proportionately by eye, the tail can usually be docked at the end of the light markings, which extend from the rectal area up the underside of the tail.

Ears may be left natural but are customarily cropped at 6 to 10 weeks. Although the crop should be tailored to the size and shape of the individual puppy's head, all crops should leave the ears medium height with a minimum of bell.

Standard Schnauzer puppies should not be raised in an impersonal environment if they are to mature into steady, reliable adults. From 3 to 4 weeks old they require individual socialization with people. After their ears are cropped, they should be exposed to a variety of persons and situations.

DENTITION

Full dentition is usual but **undershot** bites do occur. Adults should have a true scissors bite. Puppies with a tight scissors bite or a level bite are apt to develop an undershot bite when the adult teeth arrive. **Overshot** bites in puppies usually correct themselves.

RECOGNIZED PROBLEMS

Hip dysplasia occurs in this breed. The breed is also subject to a specific **follicular dermatitis**, (Schnauzer Comedo Syndrome; see Miniature Schnauzers). Plucking the hard, wiry coat every 4 to 6 months may help prevent this condition. Eruptions respond to Panalog®

(Squibb) and/or alcohol applied to affected areas daily.

Pulmonic stenosis has been reported in the breed and is thought to be inherited as a polygenetic trait.[1] **Conjunctivitis** is sometimes a problem due to the irritation of facial hair. It can be corrected and prevented from recurring by cutting away the standing hair in front of the eyes in an inverted V that runs from the inner corner of the eye and blends into the whiskers.

Benign fatty tumors and **perianal adenomas** often appear in older dogs.

In a Swedish study the Standard Schnauzer was described as having a higher-than-average incidence of **hypothyroidism**.[2]

BEHAVIOR

Although not the ideal pet for every family, Standard Schnauzers are extremely intelligent, trainable and totally devoted to their families. They do not have a doggy odor. After reaching adulthood, many do not change homes readily. A person who acquires an adult dog should be prepared for a fairly long period of adjustment.

OLD AGE

This hearty breed stays active and high-spirited throughout its long life.

Life expectancy is 13 to 15 years. Death is usually due to heart failure.

References
1. Foley, C.W., et al *Abnormalities of Companion Animals*. Iowa State University Press, Ames, IA.,1979.
2. Larsson, M. "The Breed, Sex and Age Distribution of Dogs with Primary Hypothyroidism," *Svensk-Veterinartidning*. 1986, 38:15, 181-183; 3 ref.

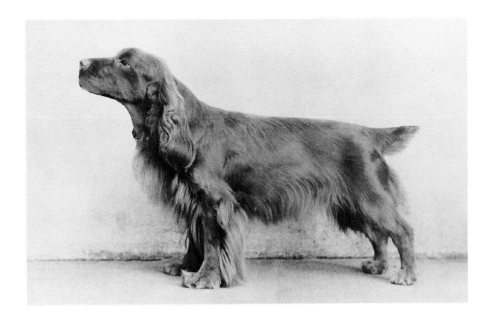

SUSSEX SPANIEL

ORIGIN AND HISTORY

This breed is closely bred, originating from the kennel of a Mr. Fuller in Sussex, England, in the 19th century.

DESCRIPTION

Sussex Spaniels differ from other small Spaniels in that they are slower, have a keen nose and are inclined to give voice on scent. Adults weigh 35 to 45 pounds; bitches generally weigh less than dogs. They often do not reach full weight until 3 or 4 years of age. Their height is 13 to 15 inches. Sussex Spaniels are brownish at birth and do not lighten to their characteristic golden-liver color until 9 months or older. Nose and other pigmentation are brownish-pink at birth and gradually darken to liver.

THE SHOW RING

The Standard ranks features of the breed into three categories. The most important features of the breed are color and general appearance. The features of secondary importance are the head, ears, back and back ribs, legs and feet. Features of lesser importance are the eyes, nose, neck, chest and shoulders, tail and coat. **There are no disqualifications in the**

Sussex Spaniel standard.[1]

BREEDING AND WHELPING

Bitches often skip estrus. Some have estrus only once a year, the time of ovulation varying with the individual. Some ovulate as early as the 8th day of estrus, others as late as the 18th or 20th day. Many breedings are unsuccessful because of this variation in time of ovulation and also because of disinterest on the part of the male.

Often a male Sussex shows absolutely no interest in a bitch in full season. The bitch should be kenneled with the dog before estrus begins. This practice seems to help, as does an injection of testosterone two to four days before breeding.

Bitches should never be left alone at whelping, for they often make no effort to open the sacs or cut the cord. Once puppies are clean and breathing well, the mothers generally take over. They are excellent mothers and are reluctant to wean puppies until 8 weeks old.

The Sussex Spaniel has been considerably inbred during the past 60 years because of the breed's small base. Puppies often die as a result of genetic abnormalities. It is not unusual to lose half of each litter within the first two weeks of life.

Sussex Spaniel puppies should weigh 4 to 6 ounces at birth, but many females are smaller. A 2-ounce puppy has little chance of survival. A normal litter is two to eight pups, although litters of nine or 10 occur occasionally.

Male puppies are generally much stronger than female puppies. All are subject to **respiratory problems**. Eyes do not open until 3 weeks of age in many cases. They should not be forcibly opened.

GROWTH

Sussex Spaniel puppies grow slowly at first, often weighing only 3 pounds at 5 weeks. The puppies are much slower to crawl, walk and mature than puppies of most other breeds.

Tails should be docked at 3 to 4 days.

Slightly less than 2/3 of the tail should be removed. The tail should be about 5 inches long at maturity for a balanced look.

Dewclaws may be removed when the tail is docked.

DENTITION

The breed has a high incidence of **undershot** bites. The puppy teeth are usually perfect, but often with the permanent teeth the bite will become undershot.

RECOGNIZED PROBLEMS

Hip dysplasia has not been described in the Sussex. However, many of these dogs have **heart murmurs** and **enlarged hearts**. Sussex Spaniels are subject to **intervertebral disc syndrome** and many breeding problems. Ears must be kept extremely clean to discourage ear mites and external ear-canal infections. Since the ears are heavily covered with feather, parasites and infections thrive if careful treatment is not followed.

BEHAVIOR

Although excellent with people, they are rather snappy and jealous of other dogs, especially those of the same sex. They are strong minded and will "talk back." They are intelligent and trainable.

OLD AGE

The Sussex is a very sensitive and loving dog and responds best as a member of the family. Life expectancy is 12 to 14 years, but **carcinomas** are common, especially in unneutered dogs and bitches.

Reference
1. *Breed Standard.* The American Kennel Club; April, 1992.

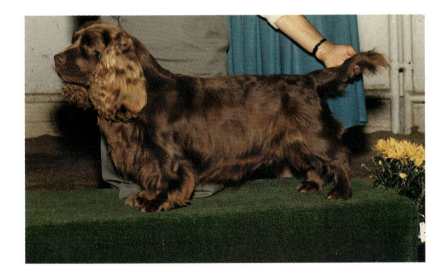

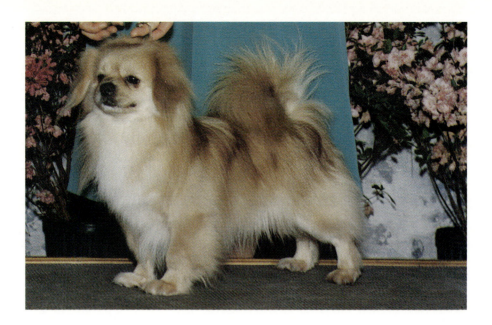

TIBETAN SPANIEL

ORIGIN AND HISTORY

Little is known about the Tibetan Spaniel except that it is of ancient lineage. Whether it was the father of the Pekingese or whether the Pekingese was its forebear, most authorities do agree that the two breeds are linked in some way.

Some experts maintain that Tibetan Spaniels were introduced into China as tributes to noblemen. These animals then mated with Pugs to produce the Pekingese. Others believe that Pekingese presented to Tibetan officials were cross-bred with Lhasa Apsos and Japanese Chins, eventually developing into the Tibetan Spaniel known today. Actually, the dog is not a spaniel; its name was selected to distinguish it from the Tibetan Terrier.

Although the presence of the Tibetan Spaniel was first noted in Britain in 1905, the breed did not become established there until the mid-1940s. Since that time the Tibetan Spaniel has achieved great popularity in the West, both as a show dog and as a pet. The breed became eligible to compete in AKC events in 1984.

DESCRIPTION

The true Tibetan Spaniel is the only one of all Tibetan breeds to have a hare foot instead of a round or cat foot.

The Tibetan Spaniel possesses a unique personality, described by many as "cat-like." The breed is known to be extremely intelligent, sweet-natured and affectionate, family oriented and very trusting of other dogs and people.

THE SHOW RING

The Tibetan Spaniel should be about 10 inches tall with its body slightly longer than tall. Ideal weight is 9 - 15 pounds.

Faults: Large, full eyes; light eyes; mean expression; very domed, or flat, wide skull; accentuated stop, long, plain down face without stop; broad, flat muzzle; pointed, weak or wrinkled muzzle; liver or putty-colored pigmentation; overshot mouth; protruding tongue; very bowed or loose front; cat feet; straight stifles; cow hocks; nervousness.

There are no disqualifications in this breed.

RECOGNIZED PROBLEMS

Progressive retinal atrophy has been reported in Tibetan Spaniels.[1]

A Norwegian study reports severe **oxalate nephropathy** with end-stage kidney lesions in two pups of a litter of three Tibetan Spaniels. This histopathological finding strongly suggests a primary hyperoxaluria, since there was no exposure to agents capable of producing secondary hyperoxaluria. Primary hyperoxaluria has not been reported as a spontaneous disease in the dog, although it is a well-known, but rare, inherited metabolic disease of man.[2]

BEHAVIOR

The "Tibbie" is a devoted companion dog, lively and affectionate with its owners, but distrustful toward strangers. He is a good watch dog.

References
1. Barnett, K.C. " Inherited Eye Disease in the Dog and Cat." *J. Sm. Anim. Prac.* 1988, 29:7, 462-475; 33 ref.
2. Jansen, J.H. and Arnesen, K. "Oxalate Nephropathy in a Tibetan Spaniel Litter. A Probable Case of Primary Hyperoxaluria." *J. Comp. Pathology.* 1990, 103:1, 79-84; 12 ref.

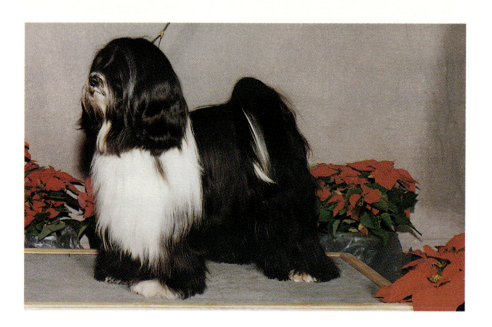

TIBETAN TERRIER

ORIGIN AND HISTORY

Tibetan Terriers were accepted by the American Kennel club on March 13, 1973, and first shown in the United States in October, 1973. The Canadian Kennel Club accepted the breed in April, 1974. Both countries placed the breed in the non-sporting group.

Dr. A.R.H. Greig of England introduced the Tibetan Terrier to the world outside Tibet. Dr. Greig was a physician and surgeon employed by the British government in India. In 1892, she was given a Tibetan bitch puppy, one of a pure breed known in Tibet as the Holy Dog. When she showed the dog, the judges told her they had never seen that breed of dog before. At a later show, the secretary of the Indian Kennel Club agreed with a panel of judges that the dog was a Tibetan Terrier, a breed that was purebred in the monasteries of Tibet.

DESCRIPTION

Tibetan Terriers do not have the usual temperament of a terrier. They are much quieter than other terriers, and are less likely to start or enjoy fights. Several can be kept together, both dogs and bitches, and they all get along well.

The dogs are true friends and devoted companions. They are great travelers and enjoy riding in cars.

The colors of the sire and dam do not indicate the color of the puppies. Two black parents may produce a litter of golden puppies. A black bitch bred to a white dog may produce a litter of puppies with white and black markings. The colors in the backgrounds of the sire and the dam will be repeated in the litters. A dog's adult color is usually the same as its color at birth. Occasionally a black puppy turns silver at about a year of age, and some puppies that are light cream become white.

The breed is free of odor. Frequent bathing is not necessary because the breed's long coat sheds dirt. The outer coat's texture is similar to human hair. Too much bathing has a tendency to soften the outer coat. Frequent brushing and combing keep the coat in good condition. The undercoat is very fine and has a texture like wool. This loosens when the seasons change and becomes matted in the long hairs of the outer coat if not combed out promptly. The undercoat should never be removed, and the coat should never be parted down the back. Sometimes a natural part occurs in a coat. A natural part does not make the coat appear to hang close to the dog, as does an artificial part.

THE SHOW RING

Tibetan Terriers should have square bodies, and their legs should be in proportion to their bodies. They should not exceed the Standard size of 15 to 16 inches at the shoulders for dogs, slightly smaller for bitches.

Faults in the breed are poor coat or no undercoat, "snipy" foreface, badly **overshot** or **undershot** bite, a nose any color other than black, wry mouth, lack of fall over eyes and foreface, any height over 17 inches or under 14 inches, and extreme shyness.

There are no breed disqualifications.

Dewclaws on both front and back legs should be removed at 4 or 5 days old.

BREEDING AND WHELPING

Bitches do not have unusual problems during gestation. They usually do not eat for 24 hours before whelping. About a week before they are due to deliver, they will nest in a broodbox provided for them. **Cesareans** are rarely necessary.

Puppies usually weigh 4 or 5 ounces at birth. They are more loosely built than other breeds, and have no arch to their feet.

DENTITION

The breed can be slow in cutting teeth. Sometimes a puppy older than 9 months still lacks some teeth.

RECOGNIZED PROBLEMS

In 18 years of breeding Tibetan Terriers, one breeder has seen only two malformed puppies, and has found the breed to be free of congenital abnormalities. Careful breeding probably has eliminated weak individuals. Also, the breed's conformation does not require the exaggeration of anatomy that create problems in many other breeds.

Hypothyroidism is being reported more frequently in the breed.[1] **Progressive retinal atrophy** has been documented in the breed.[2,3]

Neuronal ceroid lipofuscinosis has been seen in the breed.[4]

BEHAVIOR

The Tibetan is a companion dog, and his unusual deep bark makes it an excellent watch dog. It is lively and playful, but like most Tibetan guard dogs, it is wary of strangers.

OLD AGE

The breed ages gracefully. The first sign of old age is usually a dog's inability to jump up and sit beside the owner without assistance. Failing eyesight is usually the next sign of age, but this does not occur until about 10 or 11 years old. Their hearing stays acute for many years, but they are susceptible to kidney failure, although they do not become incontinent for many years. Tibetans live to about 15 or 16 years old. Some have lived to 22 years.

References
1. Tibetan Terrier column, *American Kennel Club Gazette.* May, 1993
2. Barnett, K.C. "Inherited Eye Disease in the Dog and Cat." *J. Sm. Anim. Prac.* 1988, 29:7, 462-475; 33 ref.
3. Millichamp, N.J., Curtis, R., and Barnett, K.C. "Progressive Retinal Atrophy in Tibetan Terriers." *JAVMA.* 1988, 192:6, 769-776; 21 ref.
4. Cummings, J.F., de Lahunta, A., Riis, R.C., and Loew, E.R. "Neurological Changes in a Young Adult Tibetan Terrier with Subclinical Neuronal Ceroid Lipfuscinosis." *Progress in Vet. Neurology.* 1990, 1:3, 301-309; 36 ref.

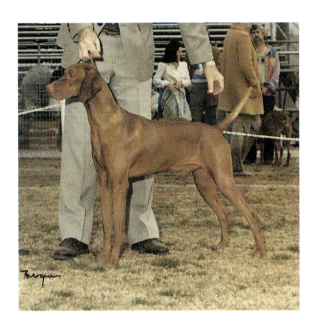

VIZSLA

ORIGIN AND HISTORY

The origin of the Vizsla, or Hungarian Pointer, is obscure. The breed descends from dogs that were companions and hunters of Magyar hordes who swarmed over Europe 1000 years ago and settled in what is now known as Hungary.[1]

DESCRIPTION

The Vizsla temperament must be regarded as more hypersensitive than other breeds in the sporting group.

THE SHOW RING

Dogs should measure 22 to 24 inches and bitches 21 to 23 inches at the shoulder. **Any male over 25 1/2 inches or under 20 1/2 inches and any female over 24 1/2 inches or under 19 1/2 inches will be disqualified.** Bitches should weigh 42 to 46 pounds, dogs 45 to 50 pounds. Colors should be solid, rusty gold, or dark sandy yellow in different shades with darker shades preferred. Dark brown and pale yellow are undesirable. Small white spots on chest or feet are not faulted. Yellow eyes and rabbit-like feet are objectionable. The nose should be brown. **A completely black nose is a disqualification. Massive areas of white** on chest, white anywhere else on body or solid white extending above the toes are dis-qualifications.

BREEDING AND WHELPING

Rear dewclaws, if present, should be removed. Front dewclaws are usually removed but it is not required for the show ring. When docking the tail, 2/3 should remain.

Puppies normally weigh 10 to 14 ounces at birth. Litter average is six to eight puppies.

RECOGNIZED PROBLEMS

A hereditary defect described in the breed is **Hemophilia A**,[2] which is an inherited x-linked recessive syndrome. **Hip dysplasia** occurs in the breed but incidence is low. **Craniomandibular osteopathy**[3,4] and **facial nerve paralysis** have also been reported in this breed. **Sebaceous adenitis** has been documented in Vizslas. The reference discusses two case histories.[5]

BEHAVIOR

The Viszla is stable, trainable and affectionate. He is calm and sensitive with a keen sense of smell. He is not a suitable dog for urban living. He has too much energy to burn up and if confined will become a nuisance. The Vizsla Club of America reports that this breed does not hunt well if kenneled away from the family members.

OLD AGE

The Vizsla is a healthy breed and usually lives 10 to 14 years.

References
1. *The Complete Dog Book,* American Kennel Club: Howell Book House. New York, NY; 1992: 124-127.
2. Buckner, R.G,.et al "Hemophilia in the Vizsla." *J. Sm. Anim. Prac.* 8: 511-519; 1967
3. Kirk, R.W. and Bistner, S.I. *Handbook of Veterinary Procedures and Emergency Treatment: Hereditary Defects in Dogs.* 1975; Table 124: 661.
4. Erickson, F., et al "Congenital Defects in Dogs: A Special Reference for Practitioners." Ralston-Purina Co.(reprint from *Canine Practice*, Veterinary Publishing Co.), 1978.
5. Stewart, L.J., White, S.D., and Carpenter, J.L. "Isotretinoin in the Treatment of Sebaceous Adenitis in Two Vizslas." *JAAHA.* 1991, 27:1, 65-71; 22 ref.

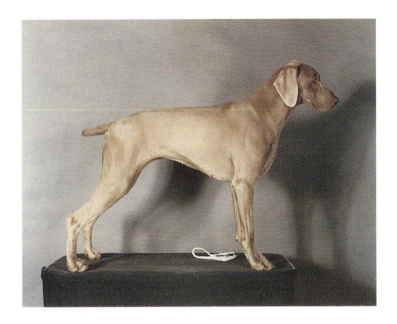

WEIMARANER

ORIGIN AND HISTORY

Nicknamed "The Grey Ghost" as much for its quiet movement when working as for its color, this breed is a fairly recent addition to the American show ring, having first been exhibited in 1941. The Weimaraner originated in Germany, where it was used to trail the wolf, bear and mountain lion and to point and retrieve birds.

DESCRIPTION

Weimaraner puppies are a buckskin tan to gray with dark stripes running the length of their body at birth. These stripes will disappear by 1 week of age in normal-size puppies but may remain up to 3 weeks in large puppies. Novice breeders have been known to destroy an entire litter because of these stripes.

Two silvers produce only silvers, a blue and a silver or two blues will produce a mixed litter of blues and silvers. Blue puppies are readily identifiable at birth. White toes, pasterns and genitals are not unusual, although they are undesirable. A distinctly white outline around the toes will usually not show in the adult silver. White on the abdomen will remain. White on the chest diminishes with growth, appearing proportionately smaller in a grown dog than it did in the puppy. All white on the blue dogs will remain very definite because of contrast.

The Weimaraner is an extremely fine-coated breed, and loss of hair is often seen in a bitch nursing whelps. The adult Weimaraners tend to hyperactivity and are extremely sensitive. They do not kennel well but thrive when treated as members of the family. Two males when grown will rarely tolerate each other and will fight viciously. They are natural guard dogs and good (although possessive) with children.

They are a soft-skinned breed and tear easily if hunted in a bushy area. Boots are often used to protect the feet.

THE SHOW RING

A distinctly long coat or a distinctly blue or black coat are disqualifications.

This rather uniquely colored dog is penalized in the show ring if it has a pink nose or eyes other than gray, blue-gray or light amber. A black-mottled mouth is a very serious fault. A small, white marking on the chest is permitted.

When running in Weimaraner Club of America field trials beyond the puppy class, they are required to have at least three digits of their AKC number tattooed in their right ear.

Dogs are 25 to 27 inches at the withers; bitches 23 to 25 inches. **Deviation in height of more than one inch from the Standard either way is a disqualification.**

GROWTH

Dewclaws should be removed and tails docked at 3 to 5 days of age. In very weak or tiny puppies, this may be delayed up to the 10th day. The tail is docked to between 1 and 1 1/2 inches measured from the underside. There is a natural taper point which can be felt by running the fingers down the tail. The tail should be tucked between the legs, making sure that the genitals are covered. All three measurements should coincide or be rechecked until they do. Because of various sizes and tail sets, each puppy should be checked individually. A too long tail is much preferred to one that is too short. After clipping the tail, one small piece of bone should be removed to provide padding at the tip. The tail should be sutured as excessive scar tissue will cause white-hair growth.

Whelps weigh approximately 10 to 16 ounces and have a rapid growth rate. There is not as much weight variance in the bitches. Weight is not as important a factor as height. There should be an appearance of overall balance.

RECOGNIZED PROBLEMS

Reported problems include **undershot** bites, **hip dysplasia, bloat, double eyelashes, entropion, cryptorchidism** and **Hemophilia A (factor VII deficiency).**[1,2,3]

Eversion of nictitating membrane is an eye problem of this breed.[4,5]

Dermoid cyst of the cornea and **ununited anconeal process** are documented as occurring in Weimaraners.[6]

Spinal dysraphism[7] **(syringomyelia)**[6,7] is an incomplete closure of the primary neural tube and was studied by McGrath in 78 purebred Weimaraners. The classic clinical sign is an abnormal gait in the hindlimbs in which the animal hops symmetrically like a rabbit. The dog stands peculiarly in a crouching position. Unilateral stimulation usually induces bilateral flexor and scratch reflexes in the hindlimbs. Once the clinical signs are established, there is typically no progression or retrogression. This spinal abnormality is not a sex-linked inherited defect since both sexes are equally involved. The first signs appear at 4 to 6 weeks of age. Diagnosis can probably be aided by careful radiography, considering age and breed, and typical history. There is no treatment.

Three of eight and one of seven pups from two separate litters of Weimaraners developed tremors by 3 weeks of age. Light and electron-microscopic findings in one dog from each of the litters were compared to those of two age-matched controls. Many axons in the brain and spinal cord were either thinly myelinated or nonmyelinated in the affected dogs relative to the controls, while the peripheral nervous system was normally myelinated.

The degree of **hypomyelination** was particularly severe at the periphery of the lateral and ventral funiculi of the spinal cord. In all areas of white matter examined, astrocytes outnumbered oligodendrocytes in the Weimaraners, while the reverse was true in the controls. This discrepancy in oligodendrocyte and astrocyte numbers was confirmed quantitatively in the spinal cord. These findings suggested that abnormal glial differentiation was responsible for the **hypomyelination**. Clinical signs in two affected littermates of one of the dogs gradually resolved, suggesting that the underlying lesion was reversible.[8]

A study of 18 related Weimaraners in Australia that developed recurrent and persistent infections led the researchers to suspect an inherited **defect in the host defense mechanisms**.[9]

Growth-hormone therapy (0.1 mg/kg of body weight/dose, 14 doses) during a 1-month period in two immunodeficient **dwarf** pups resulted in clinical improvement and a marked increase in the thickness and cellularity of the cortex of the thymus.[10] Weimaraners have been reported as predisposed to **cutaneous mast cell tumors,**[11] **melanoma** and **fibrosarcoma**. Hereditary **XX sex reversal** has been documented in the Weimaraner.[12]

Weimaraners with **blue hair coats** are prone to dry hair and skin resulting in alopecia. They should not be bred.

BEHAVIOR

The Weimaraner makes an excellent guard dog. He is lively, cheerful, affectionate and stubborn. He needs too much exercise to make a good city dog. He is basically a hunting dog.

OLD AGE

A Weimaraner's life expectancy is about 13 years. They are known for their awkward walk, which becomes a smooth stride when gaited. This seeming awkwardness often increases with age.

References

1. Kirk, R.W. and Bistner, S.I. *Handbook of Veterinary Procedures and Emergency Treatment: Hereditary Defects of Dogs,* 1975; Table 124, p 661
2. Kaneko, J.J., et al "Canine Hemophilia Resembling Classic HemophiliaA." *JAVMA* 150:156-21; 1967
3. Erickson, F., et al: "Congenital Defects in Dogs: A Special Reference for Practitioners." Ralston Purina Co. (reprint from *Canine Practice*, Veterinary Practice Publ. Co.) 1978
4. Magrane, W.G. *Canine Ophthalmology,* 2nd ed. Lea & Febiger, Philadelphia, PA 1971
5. Priester, W.A. "Congenital Ocular Defects in Cattle, Horses, Cats, and Dogs." *JAVMA* 160: 1504-1511;1972
6. Folly, C.O., et al *Abnormalities of Companion Animals.* Iowa State University Press, Ames, IA., 1979; 37-38
7. Hoerlein, B.F. *Canine Neurology: Diagnosis and Treatment,* 2nd ed. W.B.Saunders, Philadelphia, PA.,1971; pp 266, 271.
8. Kornegay, J.N., Goodwin, M.F.A., and Spyridakis, L.K. "Hypomyelination in Weimaraner Dogs." Acta-Neuropathologica. 1987,72:4, 394-401; 33 ref.
9. Studdert, V.P., Phillips, W.A., Studdert, M.J., and Hosking, C.S. "Recurrent and Persistent Infections in Related Weimaraner Dogs." *Aust. Vet. Jour.* 1984, 61:8, 261-263; 21 ref.
10. Roth, J.A., Kaeberle, M.L., Grier, R.L., Hopper, J.G., Spiegel, H.E., and McAllister, H.A. *Improvement in Clinical Condition and Thymus Morphologic Features Associated With Growth Hormone Treatment of Immunodeficient Dwarf Dogs.*
11. Veterinary News. *The American Kennel Club Gazette;* April, 1990: 44.
12. Bell, Jerold S., DVM "Sex-Related Genetic Disorders: Did Mama Cause Them?" *American Kennel Club Gazette* Feb. 1994: 76-77.

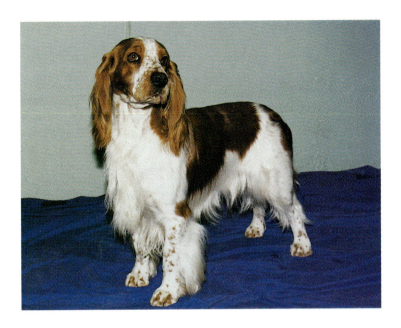

WELSH SPRINGER SPANIEL

ORIGIN AND HISTORY

The Welsh Springer Spaniel has been bred for centuries in the isolated mountains and valleys of Wales as a combination gun dog and household companion. It has been selected for health and working ability and therefore has few hereditary defects.

DESCRIPTION

The breed is gentle and peace loving and very alert to strange noises. When kept as house pets, they are excellent watch dogs. They tend to become attached to one person. They are not demonstrative with strangers but will accept them with quiet dignity.

Welsh Springers are in their natural habitat in the field, even if only out for an occasional romp. They are excellent bird dogs.

THE SHOW RING

The average adult weight is 40 to 50 pounds for dogs and slightly less for bitches.

The Standard calls for a medium-sized dog between a Cocker and an English Springer in size. The height at the shoulders should be 18–19 inches for dogs and 17—18 inches for bitches.

There are no breed disqualifications.

BREEDING AND WHELPING

Breeding and whelping are normally done with little help needed other than watching that the bitch doesn't accidentally lie on a puppy. The bitch usually comes in season the first time at about 1 year of age.

Puppies average 8 to 12 ounces at birth and are white, with markings ranging from light beige to red. Noses are pink but begin to darken in a day or two. Color darkens and freckles and spots develop. Pigmentation may continue to appear up to 6 months. Weaning should be complete by the 5th to 6th week.

GROWTH

Tails should be docked 1/3 to 1/2 and dewclaws removed at 3 to 5 days. Removal of dewclaws is not required by the Standard but is usually done.

The teeth begin to come in at 3 weeks, when the pups are ready to begin their supplementary feedings. The second teeth begin to come in at about 4 months. **Undershot** bites are occasionally seen.

RECOGNIZED PROBLEMS

Several cases of **epileptic type seizures** have been attributed to different causes (distemper, encephalitis or trauma), but they appear more prevalent in certain strains.

Spermatogenic arrest with azoospermia[1] is reported. The incidence of spermatogenic arrest in the dog can only be conjectured because testicular biopsies are infrequently performed in this species. In a survey of 200 dogs presented with a history of infertility,[2] 158 were proven stud dogs that had become infertile, usually suddenly, at about 3 1/2 years of age. Of the 200 cases, 160 yielded no sperm when a semen sample was examined. In one study[3] it was found that the ancestors of the proven, but now infertile, sires had often shown a similar trend to early, sudden sterility. The occurrence of the condition here in both father and sons leads to belief in a hereditary factor.

The clinical appearance of **hereditary cataract** is described in this breed.[4]

A study of **primary glaucoma** finds that females are more often affected than males, 2.4:1. The age of onset ranges from 10 weeks to 10 years. The mode of inheritance appears to be dominant, which should make elimination of the trait through breeding control more straightforward.[5] **Hip dysplasia** is found in the breed, but does not seem to present a severe problem at this time. In a Swedish study it was reported that the Welsh Springer had a higher-than-average incidence of **primary hypothyroidism**.[6]

538

BEHAVIOR

The Welsh Springer is an ideal housepet. He is adaptable to either city or country as long as he gets exercise. He is amiable with children and other animals. Intelligent and cheerful, he is easily trainable for field, show or obedience work.

OLD AGE

There are no particular problems found in old age that are not related to the general aging process found in all dogs.

Welsh Springers are long lived and with good care can be healthy, active companions for 12 to 15 years.

References

1. Hadley, J.C. "Spermatogenic Arrest with Azoospermia in Two Welsh Springer Spaniels." *J. Sm. Anim. Prac.* 13:135-138; 1972
2. Horrop, A.E. *J. Sm. Anim. Prac.* 7:723; 1966
3. Horrop, A.E. *Vet. Rec.* 72:362; 1960.
4. Barnett, KC. "The Diagnosis and Differential Diagnosis of Cataract in the Dog." *J. Sm. Anim. Prac.* 1985, 26: 6, 305-316; 20 ref.
5. Cottrell, B.D. and Barnett, K.C. "Primary Glaucoma in the Welsh Springer Spaniel." *J. Sm. Anim. Prac.* 1988, 29:3, 185-199; 23 ref.
6. Larsson, M. "The Breed, Sex and Age Distribution of Dogs with Primary Hypothyroidism." *Svensk-Veterinartidning.* 1986,38: 15, 181-183; 3 ref.

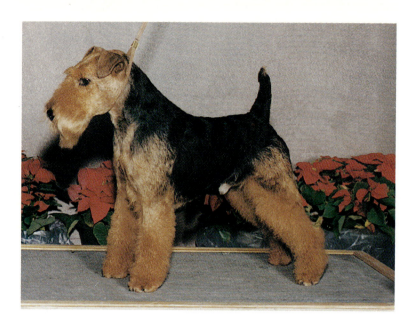

WELSH TERRIER

ORIGIN AND HISTORY

Although Welsh Terriers resemble miniature Airedales, their personality is uniquely their own. They are calm, well-mannered terriers with a gift for winning friends. Bred in England, they are pictured in early prints. Welsh Terriers were known as Kennel Terriers to the fox hunters because they lived in kennels with the hounds, ran with the pack, and climaxed the chase by going underground after the fox.

DESCRIPTION

Adult Welsh Terriers are loyal, intelligent, clean pets. They are good with children and adapt well to most family situations. They do not shed much but do require grooming. For showing, their coats should be entirely hand plucked, but a pet's coat may be clipped. Welsh Terriers are quick, graceful dogs. They run very fast and may jump or climb a 6-foot fence with little difficulty. They have proved to be capable in obedience training as well as in terrier field trials.

THE SHOW RING

Their coats should be wiry, hard, abundant and close fitting with a short undercoat of soft hair. They should be black and tan, or black grizzle and tan, with no black below the hocks or black penciling on toes.

Their ears should be V-shaped, small, not too thin, with the fold above the level of the skull, carried to the side and forward close to the cheek. Puppies usually reach their completed height by 9 months. Adult dogs should measure between 15 and 15 1/2 inches at the shoulder, bitches proportionately less. At maturity, dogs should weigh around 20 pounds, varying only a pound or two either way. The Welsh Terrier's bite should be tight-lipped with strong teeth. Upper teeth should barely overlap the lower teeth, like the blades of scissors.

BREEDING AND WHELPING

Welsh Terriers are generally easy breeders and rarely experience difficulties whelping.

Dewclaws should be removed and tails docked on the 3rd to 5th day after birth. Tail docking is important in this breed, because a dog whose tail is too short will be incorrect for show. The only way to ensure proper tail length is to measure and evaluate each puppy's tail proportionately. The tip of the tail must be in a direct line with the top of the head. A fat tail that is thick at the base will not grow as long as a thin, whip-like tail. Thus, a fatter tail should be docked a fraction higher than the top of the head. Litter sizes vary, averaging five or six. Puppies are mostly black at birth. Typical birth weight ranges from 4 to 9 ounces; bitch puppies are sometimes smaller and lighter than dogs.

RECOGNIZED PROBLEMS

To date, few congenital abnormalities have been observed in Welsh Terriers. The one exception is **luxated lens**.[1]

BEHAVIOR

The Welsh Terrier was bred as a hunting dog and he will tackle almost anything that will run and fight. He varies in his acceptance of other animals...some will live peacefully with another house dog and some won't. If trained to behave he makes a great child's companion and house dog. He is warm and affectionate and a natural watch dog.

OLD AGE

The average life span of the breed is 10 years, although many live longer. Typical geriatric diseases appear in old age.

Reference
1. Quinn, A.J. Personal Communication.

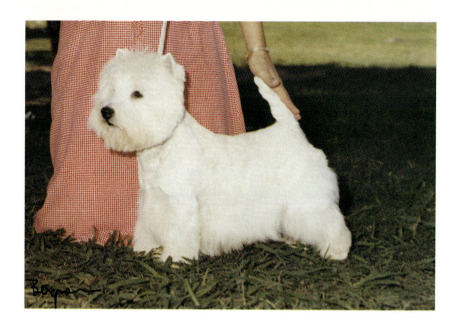

WEST HIGHLAND WHITE TERRIER

ORIGIN AND HISTORY

Like the Scottish Terrier, Cairn Terrier and Dandie Dinmont, the West Highland White Terrier is of Scottish descent.

DESCRIPTION

These Terriers are happy dogs and make wonderful pets. They are generally devoted to one member of the family but are outgoing and loving to all.

The breed is not prone to fighting and may run in packs. A Highlander will stand up for its rights against any other dog. West Highland White Terriers, like all terriers, are healthy, hardy and active. They are well-structured dogs with white double coats that protect them from all kinds of weather and are easily kept clean by wiping with a damp cloth and by daily brushing. The top coat should be stripped off (never clipped) about twice a year, and the undercoat thinned by periodic combing. Excessive bathing is not recommended.

THE SHOW RING

The ideal size is 11 inches at the withers for dogs and 10 inches for bitches. A slight deviation is acceptable. The body between the withers and the root of the tail is slightly shorter

542

than the height at the withers.

The Westie is to be a small, game, well-balanced, hardy-looking terrier, possessed of no small amount of self-esteem.

BREEDING AND WHELPING

The breed offers no special problems at birth or during early life. The puppies are usually whelped between the 60th and 62nd days of gestation. Generally they arrive rather slowly, because the Highlander is a lazy whelper.

Some males are known to be "**lazy breeders**" and an AI may be required.[1] Because of the heavy pigmentation inherent in the breed, noses and pads turn black at an early age, and normally the skin appears dirty. Dewclaws should be removed by 3 days of age. Tails should never be docked. Ears are dropped or folded over in early life but should stand erect (pricked) in adult dogs. The ears begin to lift from the folded position at 3 or 4 months and should be stiffly erect by about 6 months. To aid lifting of the ears, superfluous hair should be removed. During teething, ears may sometimes droop. If the ears have not begun to lift by 5 months, they should be taped. They will usually stand if kept reasonably free of hair.

DENTITION

Teeth require close observation during early life. The 28 milk teeth begin erupting at about 2 weeks of age. The first of the 42 permanent teeth erupt at 3 or 4 months of age. It is important to check whether the milk teeth are shed as the permanent teeth erupt. Never permit a permanent tooth to come in alongside a milk tooth; extract the milk tooth to prevent interference. Close observation of the mouth, particularly the canine and incisor teeth, is vitally important and eliminates most poor bites. Usually the breed has an acceptable bite.

RECOGNIZED PROBLEMS

Three rare diseases have been seen occasionally in young Highlanders and in several other breeds of small terriers. **Legg-Perthes disease (aseptic necrosis of the femoral head)** results from interference in the blood supply to the articular portion of the head of the thigh bone. This causes softening of the head of the bone. The first sign of the disease may be irritability, which progresses to a chronic hindlimb lameness of apparent sudden onset. Pain is elicited when the hip joint is manipulated.[2] The problem sometimes corrects itself but often requires surgical correction. The thigh muscles of the affected leg often atrophy. The femoral head is often misshapen when it heals.

In mild cases, rest allows the head to heal and it returns to normal within 3 months. In severe cases, portions of the bone disintegrate and surgical removal of the femoral head is recommended. A false joint forms after the affected head is removed, with satisfactory results. This disease generally affects dogs 6 to 8 months old. The disease is found in all breeds weighing 20 pounds or less. Breeding studies of this disease in Westies, Poodles, Yorkies and Pugs have shown the mode of inheritance to be monogenic recessive.[3]

Craniomandibular osteopathy (CMO),[4,5,6,7] sometimes called Lion Jaw, is a disease of low incidence. This is a noncancerous growth of bone on the lower jaw bone or over the angle of the mandible and tympanic bulla. In most instances it is bilateral, but not always. The bony growth can occasionally occur on other parts of the cranium, and the radius and ulna may also be involved. The disease is painful to the puppy and is usually first recognized when a puppy shows discomfort while chewing or when his mouth is being examined. By casual examination, the jaw may not appear enlarged or abnormal.[8] CMO is similar to a children's disease called infantile cortical hyperostosis (Caffey's disease).

The disease is most often recognized between the ages of 4 and 7 months, but it can occur as early as 3 to 4 weeks and rarely as late as 9 –10 months. Experienced breeders and veterinarians usually recognize it earlier than 4 months of age by clinical signs or by palpation. The disease is most often diagnosed by clinical signs and palpation with definitive confirmation by radiographs. Not all cases exhibit clinical signs of pain, so radiographs at an appropriate age are required to determine that a puppy does not have the disease.[8]

The swelling may continue until the affected dog has great difficulty opening the jaws. If not fed through a tube, these puppies may die of malnutrition. The disease can be treated with most anti-inflammatory drugs. The disease recedes when the growth plates close at 9 to 11 months. The swelling diminishes at that time. Slight abnormality of the jaw may result, but if the upper and lower jaws do not fuse, the dog is not adversely affected. If the jaws fuse, chances for recovery are poor because the dog cannot eat. Dogs nearly always recover, but the length of treatment may vary from 4 to 10 months. The disease is inherited as a simple autosomal recessive trait. [8]

Globoid cell leukodystrophy (Canine Krabbe-type),[3,9,10] another rare disease, is the most serious of the three discussed here. Similar symptoms have been observed in human beings when a genetically determined degeneration of the myelin in the central and peripheral nervous system occurs. Since the initial report in 1963, the clinical, pathological, genetic and chemical aspects of the disease in the Cairn and the West Highland White Terrier have become well defined.[3] In affected dogs, the disease manifests itself between 6 weeks and 6 months of age. It is characterized by hindlimb paresis, paraplegia, incoordination, and head, body and tail tremors. It is a diffuse disease of the nervous system, with no treatment and a fatal outcome. In the dog the disease has autosomal recessive inheritance and, like the human disease, is asso-

544

ciated with a deficiency of the enzyme B-galactocerebrosides, an enzyme that degrades or breaks down a lipid portion of myelin cerebrosides.

Carriers can be detected by measuring the mean galactocerebroside b-galactosidase enzyme activity in white blood cells.[11] **Atopic Dermatitis**[12] is also reported in Westies. The main clinical sign is pruritus, most often shown by licking or chewing feet and inguinal areas and rubbing and scratching the face, ears and axillary regions. They may also reverse sneeze, develop conjunctivitis, and have hair loss. Intradermal skin tests and radioallergosorbent test (RAST) and enzyme-linked immunosorbent assay (ELISA) tests may be useful in diagnosing the allergies. Hyposensitization can be effective but requires a long course of treatment. Atopic dermatitis is clearly inherited but the exact mode of inheritance has not been determined.[13,14]

Copper toxicosis in Westies is a disease due to an inborn error in copper metabolism which allows copper to accumulate in the liver, resulting in cirrhosis of the liver. It is fatal if not treated. The disease is usually well advanced before the first clinical signs are observed. Elevated alanine aminotransferase (ALAT) and alkaline phosphatase (AP) levels may be noted early in the disease. As copper continues to accumulate, hepatic necrosis occurs. Most dogs will recover, but occasionally one may die. The dogs show weight loss, listlessness, anorexia, vomiting, abdominal pain and jaundice. They may also develop ascites. Usually clinical signs are first noted in dogs 4 years of age or older. The only way to diagnose the disease is by liver biopsy. Treatment involves reducing the amount of copper deposited in the liver by using one of the cupruretic agents such as penicillamine or cuprid tetramine. Zinc acetate has also been shown to be effective. The definitive mode of inheritance has not been determined for Westies.[15,16,17] One study indicates that copper toxicosis may be a dominant trait.[18]

Fatty liver syndrome has been reported in several lines.[19] According to a Swedish study the high incidence of **chronic liver disease** and **liver cirrhosis** in certain breeds indicate that hereditary factors may be important in the development of these diseases.[20] **Epidermal dysplasia**, or armadillo syndrome, is a disorder that begins with erythema and pruritus of the skin, especially the feet, legs and ventral parts of the body. The skin becomes thickened, greasy, malodorous and hyperpigmented with hair loss.

There seem to be two forms of the disease. In one, all treatment fails; in the other, high doses of systemic corticosteriods for a short period of time brings a favorable response.[17] Another study on the "armadillo syndrome" suggests that Evening Primrose Oil is a successful treatment for atopy in dogs and humans. The canine dosage is 5ml per 10kg of weight.[21]

Westies have also been reported to have **cardiomyopathy, cleft palates, luxating patellas** and **hip dysplasia**.[10,11,22,23,24]

Myotonia has been seen in this breed.[25] West Highland White Terriers are one of the breeds known to have a **variation in blood serum proteins.**[26] Some were tested to have TFA type, which is the expression of a rare allele. **Inguinal hernia** is considered to be a greater risk in this breed.[27] One report states that Westies have a 38% greater risk of developing this disease than do all other breeds of dogs combined.[28]

    Pyruvate kinase deficiency in red blood cells causes a severe hemolytic anemia as a result of premature destruction of PK-deficient red blood cells. Pyruvate kinase is a key enzyme in a pathway that generates almost all energy from glucose in red blood cells. Affected dogs have pale mucous membranes, exercise intolerance and weakness. The density of all bones, especially long bones and skull appear radiographically increased. The disease is most often recognized between 4 months and 1 year, but may not be detected until later in life if a dog is not very active. After excluding more common causes of hemolytic anemia, PK deficiency should be considered, especially in animals with increased radiographic bone density. The disease is definitively diagnosed by the absence of R-type pyruvate kinase isoenzyme by cellulose acetate paper electrophoresis and clinical disease. There is no simple treatment. Experimentally, bone marrow transplantation has been shown to cure the disease. The disease is inherited as an autosomal recessive trait. Carriers can be detected by measuring PK activity in erythrocytes.[29] **Juvenile cataracts** have been reported in West Highland Terriers. A slit lamp is required to diagnose cataracts of the type reported in Westies. The mode of inheritance has not been positively determined, but it is thought to be autosomal recessive.[30] **Keratoconjunctivitis sicca (KCS)** has also been reported in Westies.[31]

    West Highlands are one of the breeds listed as having **congenital deafness.**[32]

    Westies also are reported to have **seborrhea.** Most of the cases are secondary seborrhea, often caused by underlying diseases. A primary seborrhea sometimes occurs, usually in very young puppies.[33] Westies are predisposed to developing yeast dermatitis caused by **Malassezia.**[34] **Ectopic ureter** was diagnosed in 228 dogs. The female to male ratio was 217:11. Six breeds were identified with greater frequency of diagnosis than expected, including the Westie.[35]

BEHAVIOR

    The Westie loves family life and will tolerate children, even though he would rather not. He is very adaptable as long as his family is with him. He needs daily brushing and combing.

OLD AGE

    Throughout life the breed requires little but a clean, dry place to sleep, adequate, nourishing food and plenty of human companionship. Highlanders have a normal life span of 12 to 14 years and generally die of old age without a long period of decline. They are grand dogs to own and cause a minimum of trouble because of their adaptability.

References

1. Walkowicz, Chris. "The Mechanics of Breeding," *The American Kennel Club Gazette*; May, 1990: 68.
2. Paatsama, S., Rissanen, P., and Rokkanen, P. "Legg-Perthes Disease in the Dog: An Experimental Study Using the Histological and Histochemical Methods, Oxytetracycline Bone Labeling Techinique, Autoradiography and Microradiology." *J. Sm. Anim. Prac.* 1967, 8, 215-220.
3. Robinson, R; "Legg-Calve-Perthes Disease in Dogs: Genetic Aetiology". *J. Sm. Anim. Prac.* 1992, 33: 6, 275-276; 7 ref.
4. "Canine Craniomandibular Osteopathy." *JAVRS* V:22-31; 1967.
5. Kirk, R.W. and Bistner, S.I. *Handbook of Veterinary Procedures and Emergency Treatment: Hereditary Defects of Dogs,* 1975; Table 124: 661.
6. Jubb, K.V.F. and Kennedy, P.C. *Pathology of Domestic Animals,* 2nd ed. New York, Academic Press, 1970.
7. Smith, H.A., et al: *Veterinary Pathology,* 4th ed. Lea & Febiger, Philadelphia, Pa., 1972; p 1073.
8. Padgett, G.A. and Mostosky, U.V. "Animal Model: The Mode of Inheritance of Craniomandibular Osteopathy in West Highland White Terrier Dogs." *Am. J. of Med. Gen.* 1986, 25, 9-13.
9. Fankhouser, R., et al: "Leukodystrophie Vom Typus Krabbe beim Hund." *Schweiz Arch Tierheilk* 105:198-207; 1963.
10. McGrath, J.T.: Personal Communication, 1977.
11. Selcer, E.S. and Selcer, R.R. "Globoid Cell Leukodystrophy in Two West Highland White Terriers and One Pomeranian." *Compendium of Cont. Ed.* 1984, 6, 621-624.
12. Muller, G.H. and Kirk, R.W. *Small Animal Dermatology.* W.B. Saunders, Philadelphia, Pa., 1974; 1969.
13. Ackerman, Lowell, DVM. "Allergic Skin Diseases," *American Kennel Club Gazette*; September, 1990
14. Willemse, T. "Atopic Skin Disease: A Review and Reconsideration of Diagnostic Criteria." *J. Sm. Anim. Prac.* 1986, 27, 771-778.
15. Brewer, G.J. and Yuzbasiyan-Gurkan, V. "Fighting Disease with Molecular Genetics." *American Kennel Gazette.* Jan. 1989, 106:1, 66-75.
16. Cook, C.S., Haray, R.M., Heyman, L., Thurnberg, L.P., and Twedt, D.C. "Understanding Copper Toxosis." *American Kennel Gazette.* March 1987, 25, 9-13
17. Muller, G.H., Kirk, R.W., and Scott, D.W. Ed. *Sm. Anim. Dermatology,* 4th Ed., 730-731, 1989. W.B. Saunders Co., Philadelphia, PA.
18. Thornburg, L.P. and Crawford, S.J. "Liver Disease in West Highland White Terriers." *Vet. Record.* 1986, 118:4, 110; 5 ref.
19. Van der Linde-Sipman, J.S, Van den Ingh, TSGAM and Van Toor, A.J. "Fatty Liver Syn-

drome in Toy Breeds." *Tijdschrift-voor-Diergeneeskunde.* 1988, 113:Suppl. 1, 102S-103S.

20. Andersson, M. and Sevelius, E. "Breed, Sex and Age Distribution in Dogs With Chronic Liver Disease: A Demographic Study." *J. Sm. Anim. Prac.,* 1991, 32:1, 1-5; 20 ref.

21. Scott, A.W. and Miller, W.H., Jr. "Epidermal Dysplasia and Malassezia Pachydermatitis Infection in West Highland White Terriers." *Veterinary Dermatology.* 1989; 1:25-36.

22. Corley, E.A. and Hogan, P.M. "Trends in Hip Dysplasia Control" Analysis of Radiographs Submitted to the Orthopedic Foundation for Animals 1974-1984." *JAVMA,* 1985, 187, 805-809.

23. Copper, H.K. and Mattern, G.W. "Genetic Studies of Cleft Lip and Palate in Dogs." *Birth Defects: Original Article Series,* June 1971, VII-7.

24. Denny, HR. "The Canine Stifle I. Developmental Lesions." *British Vet. Jour.,* 1985, 141, 109-113.

25. Hutt, F.B. *Genetics for Dog Breeders.* W.H. Freeman and Co., 1979; p 118.

26. Ibid, 141-142.

27. Ag Resources *Veterinary Values.* 15 West 44th Street, New York, N.Y., 10036, 1981; p 208.

28. Smeak, D.D. *Caudal-Abdominal Hernias in Small Animal Surgery, Vol.1.* Slater,DH. Ed., Ch.58, 862-869, 1985 W.B. Saunders Co., Philadelphia, PA.

29. Chapman, B.L. and Giger, U. "Inherited Erythrocyte Pyruvate Kinase Deficiency in the West Highland White Terrier." *J. Sm. Anim. Prac.,* 1990, 31, 610-616.

30. Narfstrom, K. "Cataract in the West Highland White Terrier." *J. Sm. Anim. Prac.,* 1981, 22, 467-471.

31. Sansom, J. and Barnett, K.C. "Keratoconjunctivitis Sicca in the Dog: A Review of Two Hundred Cases." *J. Sm. Anim. Prac.,* 1985, 26, 121-131.

32. Strain, George M. "Deafness in Dogs and Cats" *Proc. 10th ACVIM Forum;* May, 1992.

33. Muller, D.H., Kirk, R.W., and Scott, D.W. Ed. "Seborrheic Syndromes." *Animal Dermatology,* Ch. 15, 605-613, 1983, W.B. Saunders Co. Philadelphia, PA.

34. Griffin, C., Kwochka, K., and McDonald, J.: *Current Veterinary Dermatology: The Science and Art of Therapy.* Mosby Yearbook, St. Louis, Mo. 1993 p 45

35. Hayes, H.M., Jr. "Breed Associations of Canine Ectopic Ureters: A Study of 217 Female Cases." *J. Sm. Anim. Prac.* 1984, 25:8, 501-504; 12 ref.

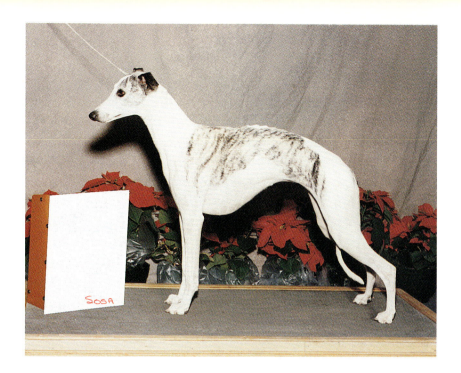

WHIPPET

ORIGIN AND HISTORY

The Whippet was developed in England as a racing dog during the middle of the last century. The sensitive, light-boned dog is one of the fastest breeds and a great racing favorite in England.

DESCRIPTION

Whippets make excellent house dogs. Although as puppies they are very active and destructive, with proper care and training they mature into delightful companions. They are smart, obedient, and responsive to training. They belie their delicate appearance. Colors are darker at birth than at maturity. Brindling is apparent at birth but clears as the base color lightens. Proper eye rim and nose pigmentation can be lacking in white or parti-color Whippets that do not have color covering the eyes. In this color pattern, nose pigmentation should begin to appear by 6 weeks. Sometimes pigmentation of the eye rims is not complete until the dog is a year old. Breeders have strong opinions as to color inheritance and preference in this breed.

THE SHOW RING

The Whippet Standard allows much leeway in size. Allowable adult size ranges from

18 to 21 inches for bitches and 19 to 22 inches for dogs. Adults in good condition can weigh from 20 pounds for an 18-inch bitch to 35 pounds for a 22-inch dog. The ideal is in the middle of the range.

All colors defined by Little in his *Coat Inheritance of the Dog* are found in Whippets. The Standard states "color is immaterial."

Disqualifications in the breed are: 1/2 inch above or below stated height limits, blue or wall eyes, undershot or overshot 1/4 inch or more, any coat other than short, close, smooth and firm in texture.

BREEDING AND WHELPING

Whippets are slow to mature. Bitches rarely have their first estrus before 1 year of age, and often not until they are past 2 years old. They breed easily and gestate normally. By the fourth week of gestation, the nipples show enlargement, and by the fifth week the underline begins to fill. Many bitches stop eating around the fourth week, for a few days to a week, but there is no cause for alarm. The average litter size is six to eight puppies, but nine, 10 and even 11 are not uncommon.

Whippet bitches normally whelp early with a minimum of difficulty. They generally have adequate milk. Whippet puppies average 8 to 12 ounces at birth and grow very quickly thereafter. When they are 4 weeks old they average 3 1/2 to 4 pounds.

Whippet puppies are very active and can be rough in play. They are also destructive chewers. Stool eating can be a problem.

GROWTH

Whippets need plenty of meat and other high-protein foods. They must be kept lean, strong, and in hard muscle to look well, particularly if they are getting the exercise they need.

DENTITION

Undershot bites, which are a disqualification in the show ring, are rarely seen. **Overbites** are more common, and a bad overbite is also a disqualification. However, puppies sometimes have overbites that correct as they mature.

RECOGNIZED PROBLEMS

The plague of the Whippet is **cryptorchidism**. It is carried in virtually every line. Unfortunately, it seems to be the most beautiful male puppy in a litter that lacks one or both testicles. Whippets seldom have hip dysplasia or the tendency to bloat. They are not usually susceptible to skin problems. However, it seems that some outbreaks of **demodectic mange** occur in pink-skinned, white dogs and parti-color dogs. Blue Whippets sometimes have the alopecia associated with the gene for color dilution.

Congenital alopecia has been reported in Miniature Poodles and one Whippet. Affected animals are usually males. Loss of hair is first observed at about 5 weeks of age. Affected puppies have dry, dull, coarse coats, with hair loss initially on the ear, nose and tail. The condition is progressive over the remainder of the body.

Whippets of all ages are inclined to have **weak digestive tracts**. Diarrhea is frequently a problem. A change to a low-fat diet of boiled rice and ground beef and sometimes more specific treatment with an antibiotic is needed to control the diarrhea.

Whippets have **variable tolerance for anesthetics**. Veterinarians should use them with caution because of Whippets' high muscle-to-fat ratio.

BEHAVIOR

The Whippet makes an ideal family pet. He does not shed, is neat and clean and easy to house-train. He doesn't like to be kenneled. He likes to sleep on a blanket, which means he will be in your bed unless you give him his own blanket. He is gentle with children and is never mean. He is adaptable to city or country as long as he gets plenty of exercise.

OLD AGE

Whippets that are well cared for live 12 to 16 years. As they pass middle age, they have a tendency to **sebaceous cysts** and **sebaceous adenomas** which, although unsightly, are usually benign and cause no problems.

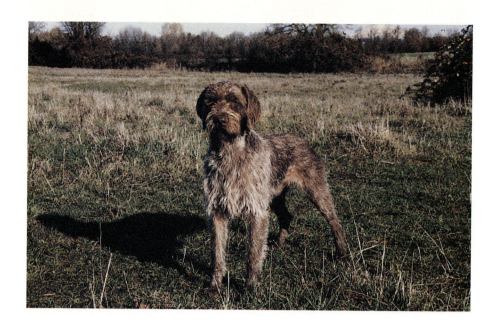

WIREHAIRED POINTING GRIFFON

ORIGIN AND HISTORY

In 1874, E. K. Korthel bred an Otterhound, a Setter, possibly a Pointer and some larger Spaniels in an attempt to produce a new sporting breed. He experimented for several years, first in Holland, then in Germany, and finally in France. The Wirehaired Pointing Griffon was the result. The first of these dogs was brought to America in the 1900s. When Griffons were first registered with the American Kennel Club, they were called Russian Setter Griffons. At first, people did not accept them because of their unkempt look.

DESCRIPTION

Griffons are possessive of their owners, not allowing other dogs near. They like to stay as close as possible to their owners and are loving pets. While at play, they are high spirited. In the field these dogs are excellent hunters for bird or for game. They are slow but very thorough. Griffons will point and retrieve, and therefore are all-purpose hunting dogs.

THE SHOW RING

The height at the shoulder is 22 to 24 inches for a dog, and 20 to 22 inches for a bitch. They have slender heads with a good stop. The hair on the head is short and thin; in the winter it is longer and fluffy. They have moustaches and eyebrows. The eyes are round with a yellow iris and with eyelashes 1/2 to 1 1/2 inches long. The Wirehaired Pointing Griffon has a dense, down-like undercoat. The outer coat is longer and coarse, with a slight wave to it. The color is a shade of brown mixed with a shade of silver, white or gray, e.g. liver with steel gray or gray, liver with platinum, liver with silver, liver with white, or chestnut with one of the other colors. The nose and lips are brown. **Breed disqualifications are: nose any other color than brown and black coat.** Breeders fault many Griffons for having too much coat on the chest, a trait of French bloodlines. There have been oversized dogs from the German bloodlines.

BREEDING AND WHELPING

Problems sometimes occur with early care of puppies in this breed. Griffons have had problems with delivery and **eclampsia** is seen in this breed. Some of the problems are due to the bitches' temperament; no disturbance during the first few days is helpful. If the owner is close to the bitch, the chance of difficulty is lessened. Litters range from four to 12 puppies. When they are born, they are mostly white with a brown head. At 1 week they develop brown specks over their body. At 3 weeks the spots blend in, giving a frosted appearance. At this time the coat will be a little wiry, with a powder-puff type moustache. The dewclaws are removed. The tail should be docked, with approximately 1/3 remaining. There has been controversy on this point because there have been Griffons with too-short tails, cut at the third joint. Some breeders stated that originally 1/3 was taken off. Docking should be discussed between the breeder and the veterinarian.

In picking a puppy, one should look for a slender head and one with an undercoat.

RECOGNIZED PROBLEMS

Wirehaired Pointing Griffons may develop **hip dysplasia**. Routine removal of hair inside the ear is recommended to prevent **otitis externa**.

BEHAVIOR

This dog is too restless to make a good house dog. If it lives in the country, where it has plenty of room to exercise, it will adapt to family living. It is good with children and needs their energy to use up some of his own. He does not confine well. The Wirehaired Pointing Griffon is patient and gentle and a good watch dog.

OLD AGE

They enjoy an average life span of 10 to 11 years.

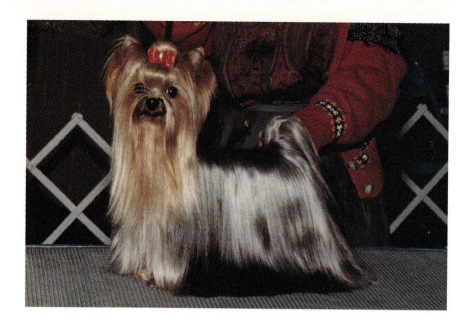

YORKSHIRE TERRIER

ORIGIN AND HISTORY

The earliest ancestors of the Yorkshire Terrier were kept by Scottish weavers for ratting.[1] Although not an ancient breed, this toy breed has changed considerably over its history. In its early years, the Yorkie was bigger and heavier than today's toy breed. Some of the Terriers who were crossbred in the 1800s to produce the Yorkshire Terrier of today include the Waterside, Black and Tan, Paisley and Clydesdale Terriers.[2] This breed was first shown in England in 1861; it was recognized by the Kennel Club of England in 1886. At that time, Yorkies weighed as much as 12 to 15 pounds. Now they must weigh 7 pounds or less. Five pounds is the most desired size.

DESCRIPTION

The Yorkshire Terrier is a lively and robust toy breed which could be called a "toy terrier." It is often the aggressor against large dogs; therefore, many are seen needing surgical repair. Yorkshire Terriers kept for show (long hair to the floor) require a great deal of grooming.

THE SHOW RING

The Yorkshire Terrier is a long-haired toy breed that must be dark blue with tan head and forequarters. The head, held high and jaunty, has a short muzzle, flat skull, and forward-looking eyes with dark rims. The bite should be either scissors or level.[1] In proportions, the back should be level and short, above straight forelegs and only slightly bent hindlegs. The docked tail is carried higher than his back, but it should not be too gay.

The coat is the Yorkshire's most important feature, and it is judged accordingly. Color must be a steel blue (not mixed with black or tan) on the body from the neck back to the tip of the tail. A clear tan must show on the head, chest, legs and underside of tail. The coat is very long and requires a great deal of care to keep it ideal — glossy, silky and perfectly straight. The long, tan fall of hair on the head and face should have dark roots, but it should not be mixed with black. The fall may be groomed in one ribbon or parted and held with two ribbons.

Although there are no disqualifications, the most common fault is deviation from the color Standard.

BREEDING AND WHELPING

First estrus onset is between 8 and 16 months of age; 8 months is the most common. About 20% of Yorkshire Terrier bitches require **cesarean section**. Puppies that become the correct steel blue with tan color are always born black with small tan markings.

Eviscerated puppies and **inguinal hernias** are problems in this breed. Any dew-claws are removed. Tails should be docked. If the tail is shaved, dock 1/4 inch out past the tan hair; if not shaved, dock 1/8 inch out beyond the tan hairline (leave about 1/2 inch).

DENTITION

Retention of primary teeth is a common problem.

RECOGNIZED PROBLEMS

Hypoglycemia occurs, especially in smaller puppies. It has often been mistakenly diagnosed as epilepsy. The Yorkshire Terrier and other toy breeds are predisposed to **juvenile hypoglycemia**, sometimes fatal.[3] **Patella luxation** is a continuing problem in Yorkshire Terriers.[4,5,6,7] Proposed as recessive polygenic and multifocal in inheritance, the luxation may be either medial or lateral. Most cases are medial and accompanied by tibial rotation. This condition may also be accompanied by bending of the distal end of the femoral shaft. Lameness often begins by 4 to 6 months of age. Another problem in this breed is **hypoplasia of dens (Odontoid process)**.[8,9,10,11,12] The result of the hypoplasia is atlantoaxial subluxation. Onset may be at any age; signs include all forms of paralysis from back pain to quadriplegia. **Legg-Perthes syndrome** is found in Yorkshire Terriers. The incidence of Legg-Calve-Perthes disease with affected individuals is such to indicate monogenic recessive inheritance of the condition.[13] Eye problems of the Yorkshire include **keratitis sicca** and **distichiasis**.

Many veterinarians have found that Yorkies are predisposed to **diarrhea** and **vomiting** at a much higher incidence than other toy breeds. A prescription diet is usually successful in controlling the problem. Skull measurements were taken on 66 dogs of seven breeds. Using mostly data from breeders' studbooks, breed differences in reproduction were also examined. Litter size averaged 2.99±1.40 and pup mortality averaged 13.59% for Yorkies. It was concluded that **dwarfism** results in small litters and, in combination with extremely domed head shape, tends to increase the incidence of **dystocia.**[14] **Congenital hydrocephalus** has been seen frequently in Yorkies.[15,16,17] Clinical signs are variable, but most are attributable to pathology of the cerebral hemisphere. The **alopecia** associated with the gene for dilution has been reported in the Yorkshire Terrier. The dog had dilute coat color, abnormal hair shafts and a patchy coat.[18]

Melanoderma and **alopecia** of Yorkshire Terriers is believed to be inherited. Signs appear at 6 months to 3 years of age. **Symmetrical alopecia** and **hyperpigmentation of** the bridge of the nose, ears, tail and feet occur. The skin is smooth and shiny. Most dogs are affected for the rest of their lives.[19] **Calcium oxalate stones** are more prevalent in Yorkshire Terriers than in many other breeds. Yorkies have been reported to be one of six breeds to have a significantly higher risk for **urolithiasis** than other breeds.[20] **Portocaval shunt** is listed as occurring in this breed. [21] **Fatty liver syndrome** has been reported in several toy breeds, including the Yorkie, as has **cryptorchidism**.[22,23]

BEHAVIOR

Like all terriers, the Yorkshire Terrier is lively, lovable and affectionate with its master and suspicious with strangers. He loves the outdoors when it's not too cold and is an excellent watch dog. He needs frequent grooming because of his long coat.

OLD AGE

Yorkshire Terriers often live 12 to 14 years.

References
1. *The Complete Dog Book,* American Kennel Club: Howell Book House, New York, N.Y., 1992: 473-475.
2. Jones, A.F. and Hamilton, F., Eds. *The World Encyclopedia of Dogs.* Galahad Books, New York, N.Y., 1971: 413-415, 498, 559, 564.
3. Van Toor, A.J., Van der Linde-Sipman, J.S., Van den Ingh, TSGAM, Wensing, T., Mol, J.A. "Experimental Induction of Fasting Hypoglycemia and Fatty Liver Syndrome in Three Yorkshire Terrier Pups." *Veterinary Quarterly.* 1991, 13:1, 16-23; 13 ref.

4. Knight, G.C. "Abnormalities and Defects in Pedigree Dogs, III: Tibio-femoral Joint Deformity and Patella Luxation." *J. Sm. Anim. Prac.* 4:463-464; 1963.

5. Kodituwakku, G.E.: "Luxation of the Patella in the Dog." *Vet. Rec.* 74: 1499-1507; 1962.

6. Koeffler, K. and Meyer, H. "Hereditary Luxation of the Patella in Toy Spaniels." *Vet Bull.* 32: 1703; 1962.

7. Priester, W.A.: "Sex, Size, and Breed as Risk Factors in Canine Patella Dislocation." *JAVMA* 160: 740-742; 1972.

8. Downey, R.S. "An Unusual Cause of Tetraplegia in a Dog." *Canad. Vet. J.* 8:216-217; 1967.

9. Geary, J.G., et al: "Atlanto-axial Subluxation in the Canine." *J. Sm. Anim. Prac.* 8: 577-582; 1967.

10. Ladds, P., et al: "Congenital Odontoid Process Separation of Two Dogs." *J. Sm. Anim. Prac.* 12: 463-471; 1970.

11. Parker, A.J. and Park, R.D. "Atlanto-axial Subluxation in Small Breeds of Dogs; Diagnosis and Pathogenesis." *VM/SAC* 68:1133-1137.

12. Erickson, et al: "Congenital Defects in Dogs, A Special Reference for Practitioners." Ralston Purina Company (reprint from *Canine Practice,* Veterinary Practice Publ. Co.).

13. Robinson, R. "Legg-Calve-Perthes Disease in Dogs: Genetic Aetiology" *J Sm. Anim. Prac.* 1992, 33: 6, 275-276; 7 ref.

14. Hahn, S. "Variation of Skull Traits and Reproduction in Breeds of Small Dogs." Thesis, Tierarztliche Hochschule Hannover, Ger.Fed. Rep. 1988: 130, 111 ref.

15. Selby, L.A. et al: "Epizootiologic Features of Canine Hydrocephalus." *Am J. Vet. Res.* 40: 411-413; 1979.

16. Hoerling, B.V.: *Canine Neurology,* 3rd ed. W. B. Saunders, Philadelphia, Pa., 1978: 733-760.

17. Morgan, J.P. *Radiology in Veterinary Orthopedics.* Lea & Febiger, Philadelphia, Pa., 1972: 330-334.

18. Miller, W.H., Jr. "Alopecia Associated With Coat Color Dilution in Two Yorkshire Terriers, One Saluki, and One Mix-Breed Dog." *JAAHA.* 1991, 27:1, 39-43; 12 ref.

19. Brignac, Michele M., "Congenital and Breed Associated Skin Diseases in the Dog and Cat" published in *KalKan Forum* (December 1989):9-16.

20. Bovee, K.C. and McGuire, T. "Qualitative and Quantitative Analysis of Uroliths in Dogs: Definitive Determination of Chemical Type". *JAVMA.* 1984: 105: 8, 983-987.

21. Yorkshire Terrier column, *American Kennel Club Gazette;* August, 1990

22. Van der Linde-Sipman, J.S., Van Toor, A.J., and Van den Ingh, TSGAM "Fatty Liver Syndrome in Toy Breeds." *Tijdschrift-voor-Diergeneeskunde.* 1988, 113:Suppl. 1, 102S-103S.

23. Bell, Jerold S. DVM "Sex Related Genetic Diseases: Did Mama Cause Them?" *American Kennel Club Gazette*, Feb. 1994; 76.

PART II

CHARTS

BREED	LENGTH AT LESS THAN 7 DAYS OF AGE
Affenpinscher	Leave 1/3 inch. Dock close to body.
Airedale	Leave 2/3.
Australian Terrier	Leave 2/5. Cut 1/16 of an inch beyond tan hair on ventral surface.
Australian Cattle Dog	Tails are not docked.
Australian Kelpie	Tails are not docked.
Australian Shepherd	Leave 4 to 5 vertebrae.
Boston Terrier	If tail is too long, dock, leaving enough for a normal appearance.
Bouvier des Flandres	Leave 1/2 to 3/4.
Boxer	Leave 3/4 inch.
Brittany Spaniel	Leave 3/4 inch.
Brussels Griffon	Leave 1/4 to 1/3.
Cavalier King Charles Spaniel	Optional[1]. Leave at least 2/3. Always leave white tip in broken-color dogs. (This may preclude docking)
Cocker Spaniel	Leave 1/3 (about 3/4 inch).
Clumber Spaniel	Leave 1/4 to 1/3 (dock at taper). Should be 4 inches long in adult.
Doberman Pinscher	Leave 1/2 inch.
English Cocker Spaniel	Leave 1/3 (4 to 5 vertebrae).
English Springer Spaniel	Leave 1/3.

English Toy Spaniel	**Leave 1/3.**
Field Spaniel	**Leave 1/3.**
Fox Terrier (smooth and wirehaired)	**Leave 2/3. The tip of the docked tail should be even with the top of the skull when the puppy is in show position.**
German Shorthair Pointer	**Leave 2/5.**
Giant Schnauzer	**Leave 1 1/4 inches (2 or 3 hours).**
Irish Terrier	**Leave 2/3. The tip of the docked tail should be even with the top of the skull when the puppy is in show position.**
Kerry Blue Terrier	**Leave 1/2 to 2/3. The tip of the docked tail should be even with the top of the skull when the puppy is in show position.**
Lakeland Terrier	**Leave 2/3. The tip of the docked tail should be even with the top of the skull when the puppy is in show position.**
Miniature Pinscher	**Leave 1/2 (two vertebrae). Enough to cover anal triangle.**
Miniature Schnauzer	**Leave 3/4 inch. Cut at demarcation of white and gray hair on ventral surface of the tail. Make sure the anus is covered.**
Norwich Terrier	**Leave 1/3. Should be long enough for a man to grasp and pull dog from a fox hole.**
Old English Sheepdog	**As close to the body as possible.**
Poodle Toy	**Leave 60%.**
Miniature	**Leave 60%.**
Standard	**Leave 60%.**
Rottweiler	**Leave 1 vertebrae.**

Schipperke	As short as possible. Leave no stub.
Sealyham Terrier	Leave 1/3 to 1/2.
Silky Terrier	Leave 1/3 (about 1/2 inch).
Soft Coated Wheaten Terrier	Leave 1/2.
Spinoni Italiani	Leave 3/5.
Standard Schnauzer	Leave 1 inch (just beyond light markings on underside of tail).
Sussex Spaniel	Leave 1/3.
Vizsla	Leave 2/3.
Weimaraner	Leave 3/5 (about 1 1/2 inches. Tuck tail between legs so genitals are covered.
Welsh Corgi Pembroke	Natural bob tail. If not, tail should be docked. Should not protrude beyond covering anus.
Welsh Springer Spaniel	Leave 1/3 to 1/2.
Welsh Terrier	Leave 2/3.
Wirehaired Pointing Griffon	Leave 1/3.
Yorkshire Terrier	Leave 1/3 (about 1/2 inch). If hair is shaved, dock 1/4 inch beyond tan hair. If not, dock 1/8 inch beyond tan hair.

This chart has been prepared from official breed standards and information obtained directly from breeders, veterinarians and professional handlers. Because opinions vary as to the most desirable length of tails in some breeds, it is always advised that these figures be used only as guidelines. Veterinarians and neophyte breeders should always seek advice from experienced breeders and handlers in their part of the country.

References
1. Deubler, M.J.: *Current Veterinary Therapy VI: Table of Standards of Tail Docking.* Kirk, R.W. (Ed.) (W.B. Sanders, Philadelphia, PA., 1977) 1363-1364.

Opthalmological Problems
Compiled by Art Quinn, D.V.M., Dipl. ACVO

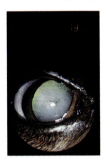

Afghan: Developmental cortical cataracts of right and left eyes.

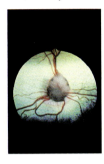

Basenji: Coloboma of the optic disc of the right eye at 5:30-9:30.

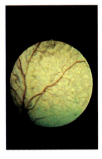

Black Labrador: Retinal dysplasia, causing streaks and irregular areas.

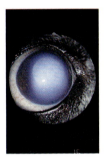

Boston Terrier: Endothelial degeneration causing cloudiness of the central cornea.

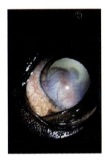

Boxer Ulcer, recurrent corneal erosion: Chronic type with neovascularization.

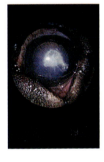

Cocker Spaniel: Cataract involving primarily the nuclear (central) portion of the lens.

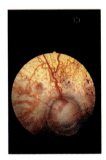

Collie Eye Anomaly: Pale area adjacent to optic disc and coloboma of optic disc of a right eye.

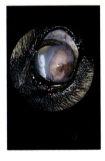

Collie Granuloma: Elevated fleshy mass invading lateral cornea with corneal degeneration adjacent.

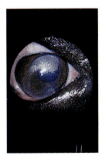

Corneal Dystrophy: The disposition of lipid or calcium in the cornea.

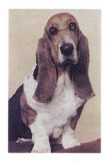

Ectropion: Note sagging of lower eyelids.

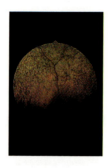

English Setter: Moderately advanced progressive retinal atrophy.

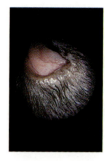

Entropion: Rolling in of lower eyelids.

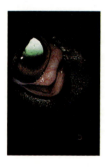

Eversion of the cartilage of the membrana nictitans (third eyelid)**:** Note the similarity to the prolapse of the gland.

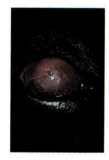

German Shepherd Pannus: Severe pigmentation and granulation tissue covering the cornea.

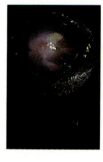

German Shepherd Pannus (three-week treatment): Note reduction of granulation tissue; patient is becoming visual.

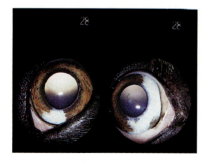

Iris Heterochromia: Blue and brown right and left irides of an Australian Shepherd.

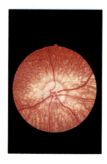

Normal Fundus Variations: Albinoid fundus (blue-eyed dog) tapetal color and pigment absent.

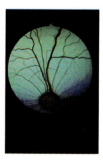

Normal Fundus Variations: Green tapetal color.

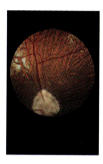

Normal Fundus Variations: Tigroid tapetum, only minimal tapetal color, also choroid vessels are visible.

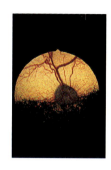

Normal Fundus Variations: Yellow tapetal color.

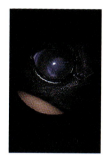

Persistent Pupillary Membranes: White strands breaching the pupil and attachment to cornea in ventral-lateral aspect causing cloudiness.

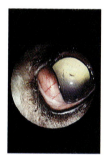

Prolapse of membrana gland, cherry eye, haws.

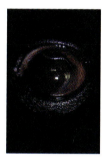

Pug: Corneal melanosis (pigmentation) covering the medial (nasal) aspect of the left cornea.

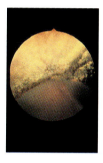

Retinal Detachment: The retinal has detached superiorly and has settled as a translucent veil over the optic disc.

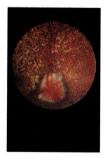

Shelty Eye Anomaly: Colomba of optic disc of the left eye at 1:00.

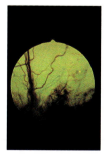

Springer Spaniel: Retinal dysplasia, streaking as in the Black Labrador.

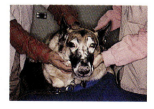

Uveodermatologic Syndrome (V-K-H) in German Shepherd: Note the loss of pigmentation of the skin and hair coat.

565

Following are the hereditary and congenital diseases common to purebred dogs listed according to breed. The condition as well as description and signs for each disease are included for easy identification. A detailed bibliography follows each chapter to assist in further research.

BREED	CONDITION/ MODE OF INHERITANCE	DESCRIPTION/SIGNS
Affenpinscher (Monkey Terrier; Monkey Pinscher)	**Elongated soft palate**	
	Oligodontia	**Missing teeth**
	Cleft palate	**Median fissures due to nonclosure of bones. Environmental and/or genetic factors may be involved.**
	Anasarca	**Walrus or rubber puppies**
	Patent ductus arteriosus	**Persistence and nonclosure of ductus areriosus between aorta and pulmonary artery with left to right shunt**
	Patella luxation (proposed are recessive polygenic and multi-focal inheritance)	**Medial or lateral. Most common are medial, accompanied by tibial rotation on the long axis, bending of the distal end of the femoral shaft and shallow femoral trochlea. Lameness at 4-6 months of age**
	Legg-Perthes disease	**Avascular necrosis of femoral head**
	Cushing's disease	
	Keratoconjunctivitis sicca (dry eye)	**Decreased tear production**
Afghan Hound	**Cataract, bilateral (R)**	**Juvenile cataract**
	Susceptible to hepatitis	**Blue eye from older forms of HLV-Hepatitis vaccine**

BREED	CONDITION/INHERITANCE	DESCRIPTION/SIGNS
Afghan Hound (continued)	Elbow joint malformation	Bilateral malformation of articular surfaces of proximal radius and ulna
	Corneal dystrophy	
	Hypothyroidism	
	Necrotizing myelopathy (R)	
Airedale Terrier (Bingley Terrier; Waterside Terrier; Wharfedale Terrier)	Cerebellar hypoplasia	Ataxia and hypermetria at about 12 weeks of age
	Umbilical hernia	Protrusion of abdominal contents through umbilicus
	Trembling of hindquarters	Seen in animals over 6 months
	Lymphoma	Cancer of lymph system
	Colonic disease	Diarrhea, sometimes intermit-tent with mucous
	Primary hypothyroidism	
Akita (Japanese Deerhound; Nippon Inu)	Umbilical hernias	Protrusion of abdominal contents through umbilicus
	Entropion	Inward rolling lids
	Progressive retinal atrophy	Dilated pupils react sluggishly to stimuli; night blindness progressing to blindness; atrophy of retinal vessels and increased reflectivity of tapetum lucidum
	Juvenile onset polyarthritis (inherited)	Incapacitating pain; fever; cyclical occurrence
	Harada's disease	Anterior uveitis; dermatitis; CNS involvement

BREED	CONDITION/INHERITANCE	DESCRIPTION/SIGNS
Akita (continued)	Pemphigus foliaceous	Scaling; crusting; alopecia; footpad lesions
	Deafness	
	Hip dysplasia	
	Elbow dysplasia	
	Hypo and Hyperthyroid	
Alaskan Malamute	Hip dysplasia	
	Recessive hemerlopia	Cannot see in bright light.
	Anemia in conjunction with chondrodysplasia	Macrocytic anemia associated with hereditary dwarfism
	Factor VII deficiency (R)	No clinical signs.
	Chondrodysplasia with coexisting anemia	Stunted forelegs, lateral deviation of paw, carpal enlargement, lateral bowing of forelegs, topline sloping forward.
	Renal cortical hypoplasia (autosomal recessive)	Polydipsia, polyuria
	Hemophilia A, Factor VIII or AHF deficiency (sex-linked recessive)	Prolonged bleeding, hemorrhagic episodes, prolonged PTT, reduced AHF and Factor VIII
	Corneal dystrophy	Deposition of calcium and cholesterol crystals in the cornea
	Hereditary polyneuropathy	Progressive muscle weakness
	Dwarfism (R)	

BREED	CONDITION/INHERITANCE	DESCRIPTION/SIGNS
American Foxhound (American Hound)	Microphthalmia (result of homozygous merle to merle matings) Deafness Osteochondrosis of the spine Thrombocytopathy	Small eyes Runners: unable to gallop properly Moderate to severe bleeding diathesis; Glanzmann's disease
American Staffordshire Terrier (Half & Half; Pit Bull; Bull Terrier;) usually have ears trimmed	Cataract, bilateral Clefts of lip and palate. Cutaneous mast cell tumors Persistent hyperplastic primary vitreous Deafness False Pregnancy	Juvenile cataract Median fissures due to nonclosure of bones; environmental and/or genetic factors may be involved.
American Water Spaniel (Brown Water Spaniel)	Hermaphroditism	Ovarian and testicular tissues as separate gonads or ovotestes; external genitalia may be immature or intermediate.
Australian Cattle Dog (Australian Heeler; Queensland Blue Heeler)	Congenital portosystemic encephalopathy. Lysosomal storage disease Deafness Eczema	

BREED	CONDITION/INHERITANCE	DESCRIPTION/SIGNS
Australian Kelpie (Kelpie;Australian Sheepdog)	Recessive microphthalmia/ multiple colobomas	Associated with microcornea, retinal detachment, equitorial staphyloma and heterochromia iridis
	Hereditary cerebellar abiotrophy	
Australian Shepherd	Umbilical hernia	Protrusion of abdominal contents through umbilicus
	Hip dysplasia	
	Microphthalmia	Small eyes
	Multiple ocular colobomas (inherited syndrome)	
	Collie eye anomaly (autosomal recessive)	
	Hereditary deafness	Associated with merle and piebald genes
	Cataracts	
	Retinal detachment	
	Progressive retinal atrophy	Dilated pupils react sluggishly to stimuli; night blindness progressing to blindness; atrophy of retinal vessels and increased reflectivity of tapetum lucidum
	Dwarfism	
	Cleft palate	Median fissures due to nonclosure of bones; environmental and/or genetic factors may be involved.
	Spina bifida	Nonclosure of the spinal canal
	Nasal solardermatitis	

BREED	CONDITION/INHERITANCE	DESCRIPTION/SIGNS
Australian Terrier	Legg-Perthes disease	Avascular necrosis of the femoral head
	Diabetes mellitus	Inability to oxidize carbohydrates due to faulty pancreatic activity; results in hypoglycemia with symptoms of thirst, hunger, emaciation and weakness
Basenji (One of the sight hounds. Belgian Congo Dog; Congo Bush Dog; Congo Hunting Terrier)	Inguinal hernia considered high risk in this breed; hereditary factors not determined	Defective formation of linea alba causing protrusion of abdominal contents through inguinal canal; usually disappears by 12 weeks of age.
	Umbilical hernia	
	Pyruvate kinase deficiency, non-spherocytic hemolytic anemia	Shortened RBC life span; reticulocytosis splenomegaly
	Coliform enteritis (R)	Genetic and behavioral factors
	Persistent pupillary membrane (autosomal dominant)	
	Intestinal malabsorption	
	Corneal leukomas	
	Renal tubular dysfunction.	
Basset Hound (Artesian Basset; Artois dog)	Inguinal hernia (a condition considered high risk in this breed; hereditary factors not determined)	Defective formation of linea alba causing protrusion of abdominal contents through inguinal canal
	Primary glaucoma	Increased intraocular pressure associated with lens luxation.
	Anomaly of third cervical vertebra (SLR)	Deformed vertebral body resulting in pressure necrosis of overlying cord; incoordination from birth to six months of age.

BREED	CONDITION/INHERITANCE	DESCRIPTION/SIGNS
Basset Hound (continued)	Platelet disorder (ID)	Mild to moderately severe bleeding; prolonged bleeding time, abnormal platelet aggregation and adhesiveness and poor clot retraction
	Achondroplasia (D)	Foreleg lameness due to unusual anatomy
	Ectropion	Outward rolled eyelids.
	Secondary glaucoma, lens luxation	
	Osteochondritis dissecans	Defect or necrosis of articular cartilage in shoulder causing distinct favoring of affected limb
	Osteodystrophy	Radial carpal joints
	Patella luxation (proposed are recessive polygenic and multi-focal inheritance.)	Medial or lateral. Most common are medial, accompanied by tibial rotation on the long axis, bending of the distal end of the femoral shaft and shallow femoral trochlea. Lameness at 4-6 months of age
	Torsion of lung	
	Gastric torsion	
	Torsion of Spleen	
	Lafara's disease	Seizures; retarded growth; susceptibility to viral and bacterial infections
	Interdigital inclusion cysts	
	Otisis externa	
	Immunodeficiency	

BREED	CONDITION/INHERITANCE	DESCRIPTION/SIGNS
Beagle	Epilepsy (RP)	Seen after 1 year of age. EEG may detect it at an early age
	Factor VII deficiency (IAD)	No clinical signs
	Hemophilia A, Factor VIII or AHF deficiency (SLR)	Prolonged bleeding, hemorrhagic episodes prolonged PTT, reduced AHF and Factor VIII
	Lymphocytic thyroiditis	Nonprogressive autoimmune disease with no clinical signs or glandular enlargement. Spontaneous occurrence.
	Primary glaucoma (R)	Increased intraocular pressure with lens luxation
	Cataract, unilateral	Most commonly seen in posterior portion of lens of left eye
	Cataract with microphthalmia (D)	Opaque lenses with small eyes associated with retinal folds
	Mononephrosis (lethal in homozygous state) (R)	Cystic degeneration of one kidney
	Clefts of lip and palate (P)	Median fissures due to nonclosure of bones. Environmental and/or genetic factors may be involved.
	Umbilical hernias	
	Ectasia syndrome	Excessive tortuosity of retinal vessels, chorioretinal dysplasia, excavation of the optic disc, retinal detachment, intraocular hemorrhage, veriform streaks of the fundus in young dogs
	Otocephalic syndrome (R)	Low grade characterized by partial agnathia, hydrocephalus and parietal fontanelles defects. High grade characterized by agenesis of all cranial structures anterior to the medulla.
	Necrotizing panotitis (genetic predisposition)	Severe inflammation of all the structures of the ear

BREED	CONDITION/INHERITANCE	DESCRIPTION/SIGNS
Beagle (continued)	Pulmonic stenosis (P)	Narrow pulmonary artery at its origin
	Unilateral kidney aplasia	Absence of one kidney with compensatory hypertrophy of the remaining kidney
	Intervertebral disc disease	Predisposition possibly due to breed conformation and other factors.
	Multiple epiphyseal dysplasia (R)	In puppies, the hind leg joints sag, causing swaying gait of hindquarters. Radiographically, "stippling" from defective ossification of epiphyseal site with several fine foci of bone
	Atopic dermatitis	Possibly hereditary immuno-logic disorder
	Distemper	Hereditary predisposition
	Brachury (AR)	Short tail
	Renal hypoplasia	Polydipsia, polyuria
	Amyloidosis	
	Hypercholesterolemia	
	Pyruvate kinase deficiency, nonspherocytic hemolytic anemia	Shortened RBC lifespan, reticulocytosis and splenomegaly
	Progressive retinal atrophy	Dilated pupils react sluggishly; night blindness progressing to blindness; atrophy of retinal vessels and increased reflection of tapetum lucidum
	Deafness	
	Epilepsy	
	Bladder cancer	
	Bundle branch block	

BREED	CONDITION/INHERITANCE	DESCRIPTION/SIGNS
Bearded Collie (Highland Collie; Mountain Collie; Highland Sheepdog) Dogs over 50% white are disqualified from shows. Smooth coats should not be registered.	Persistent pupillary membrane. Subvalvular aortic stenosis. Progressive retinal atrophy	Narrow aorta below its valve Dilated pupils react sluggishly to stimuli; night blindness progressing to blindness; atrophy of retinal vessels and increased reflectivity of tapetum lucidum
	Hip dysplasia Fading pigmentation Epilepsy Pemphigus foliaceus Colonic disease	
Bedlington Terrier (North Counties Terrier, Royhbury Terrier)	Retinal dysplasia (R)	Jumbled, abnormally formed layers of the retina with detachment, causing blindness
	Renal cortical hypoplasia (suspected of having inherited renal disease)	Polydipsia, polyuria
	Osteogenesis imperfecta	
	Copper toxicosis (AR)	Liver unable to metabolize copper
	Lacrimal duct atresia	Congenital absence of openings to lacrimal canal
	Distichiasis	A second, abnormal row of eyelashes or a few ingrowing eyelashes
Belgian Malinois (Chien de Berger; Beige Malinois)	Hip dysplasia	Deformed coxofemoral joints with clinical signs from none to severe hip lameness. Radiographically, there may be shallow acetabulum, flattened femoral head, subluxation and/or secondary degenerative joint disease.
	Epilepsy	

575

Breed	Condition/Inheritance	Description/Signs
Belgian Sheepdog	Epilepsy	
	Hip dysplasia	Deformed coxofemoral joints with clinical signs from none to lameness. Radiographically, there may be shallow acetablulum, subluxation and secondary degenerative joint disease
	Neoplasia	
Belgian Tervuren	Epilepsy	
	Hypothyroid	Hypothyroid
	Pancreatic Problems	
Bernese Mountain Dog	Clefts of lip and palate (D)	Median fissures due to non-closure of bones. Environmental and/or genetic factors may be involved.
	Blue eyes are considered a major fault and should not be bred.	
	High incidence of hip dysplasia	
	Osteochondritis dissecans	Saucer shaped necrosis or flap in the posterior central portion of humeral head, causing very distinct favoring of the affected limb
	Umbilical hernias	Protrusion of abdominal contents through umbilicus
	Cerebellar degeneration	
	Elbow dysplasia	
	Tremors in head and limbs (AR)	First noticed at 2-8 weeks. May persist through life but become less severe.

BREED	CONDITION/INHERITANCE	DESCRIPTION/SIGNS
Bichon Frise	Epilepsy Medial luxating patella. Heavy tartar formation Pemphigus	
Black and Tan Coonhound	Hemophilia B, Factor IX deficiency (SLR)	Prolonged bleeding, abnormal prothrombin consumption and thromboplastin generation and reduced Factor IX. Heterozygotes with hemophilia B bleed more than heterozygotes with Hemophilia A.
	Hip dysplasia (high incidence)	Deformed coxofemoral joint(s) with clinical signs from none to severe hip lameness. Radiographically, there may be shallow acetabulum, flattened femoral head, subluxation, and/or secondary degeneration joint disease.
	Ectropion	Outward rolling lids
	Polyrediculoneuritis	Coondog paralysis
Bloodhound (Sleuth Hound; Slot Hound)	Ectropion	Outward rolling lids
	Entropion	Inward rolling lids
	Uterine inertia	
	Malocclusion	
	Bloat	
	Bone growth disturbance	
	Elbow and hip dysplasia	
	External ear infections, hematoma and moist dermatitis	

BREED	CONDITION/INHERITANCE	DESCRIPTION/SIGNS
Border Collie	Central progressive retinal atrophy (suggested to be dominant with incomplete penetrance)	Mottling and increased reflecting of area centralis resulting in loss of central vision; difficulty in seeing stationary objects and sight is best in dim light; affecting dogs 3-5 years of age
	Corneal dystrophy	
	Patent ductus arteriosus	Persistence and non-closure of ductus arteriosus between aorta and pulmonary artery with left to right shunt
	O.C.D.	
	Ceroid lipofuscinosis	Behavioral changes; hyperactivity followed by aggression at 16 to 23 months; motor abnormalities and blindness
	Cryptorchidism	
	Deafness	
Border Terrier	Oligodendroglioma	
	Primary uterine inertia	Noncontraction of uterine muscle with an unobstructed birth canal.
	Aortic and carotid body tumors	
	Cryptorchidism (suggested recessive)	
	Hemivertebrae	
	Congenital ventricular, septal defects.	
	Mastocytoma	
	Cataract (bilateral)	
	Craniomandibular osteopathy	

BREED	CONDITION/INHERITANCE	DESCRIPTION/SIGNS
Border Terrier (continued)	Patellar luxation Pituitary tumor Hip dysplasia, P.R.A.	
Borzoi: One of the sighthounds (Russian Greyhound; Russian Wolfhound)	Missing teeth are common Bloat Hygromas Calcinosus circumscripta Aspermatogenesis Hypothyroidism Retinal dysplasia	
Boston Terrier (Boston Bull Terrier; Round-Headed Terrier)	Recessive cataract, bilateral Mastocytoma Pituitary tumor Oligodendroglioma Hemivertebra Luxating patella (proposed as recessive polygenic and "multi-focal" inheritance)	Juvenile cataract Dermal tumor of mesenchymal origin; accumulated mast cells Tumor of CNS. Asymmetric abnormal development of vertebrae, which may result in neonatal death or cord compression in older puppies. Individually, vertebrae become wedge-shaped due to underdevelopment of one half, causing scoliosis or kinked tails and crowding of ribs is found in the thoracic area. Medial or lateral. Medial more common, accompanied by tibial rotation on its long axis, bending of the distal end of the femoral shaft, and shallow femoral trochlea. Lameness at 4-6 months of age.

BREED	CONDITION/INHERITANCE	DESCRIPTION/SIGNS
Boston Terrier (continued)	Craniomandibular osteopathy	Irregular osseous proliferation of mandible and tympanic bulla. Discomfort from eating. Malnutrition may result. Intermittent fever to 104°F beginning at 4-7 months of age. Progressive until 11-13 months of age. May then regress or stop.
	Aortic and carotid body tumors	
	Distichiasis	Two rows of eyelashes (usually upper lid) resulting in irritation and epiphora
	Anasarca	Walrus or rubber puppies born with large, edematous bodies and limbs. May be due to dysplasia of lymphatic system or to multiple heart defects.
	"Swimmers"	Characterized by inability to stand at 4-6 weeks of age and flattened chest
	Hydrocephalus	Dilation of ventricles of brain with increased cerebrospinal fluid pressure
	Deafness	
	Esophageal achalasia	
	Heterochromia iridis "walleye"	Blue and white iris
	Cushing's syndrome	Polydipsia, polyuria, alopecia and weakness
	Lymphopenia eosinophilia	Increase of 17 ketosteroids and 17 hydroxy corticoids

BREED	CONDITION/INHERITANCE	DESCRIPTION/SIGNS
Boston Terrier (continued)	Clefts of lip and palate	Median fissures due nonclosure of bones. Environmental and/or genetic factors may be involved.
	Patent ductus arteriosus	Persistence and non-closure of ductus arteriosus between aorta and pulmonary artery with left to right shunt
	Endothelial dystrophy	Degenerative corneal changes in mesenchymal layer
	Hypertrophy of the nictitans gland	
	Dystocia	Difficult labor.
	Crossed eyes	
	Stenotic nares	
	Scrotal and inguinal hernias	Defective formation of linea alba associated with protrusion of abdominal contents through inguinal canal
	Intussusception	Invagination or indigitation of a portion of the intestine
	Pseudocyesis and pyometra	False pregnancy and sometimes subsequent pus-filled uterus
	Glaucoma	
	Inhalant allergies	
	Vascular ring anomaly (genetically transmitted)	Persistent aortic arch.

BREED	CONDITION/INHERITANCE	DESCRIPTION/SIGNS
Bouvier de Flandres (Belgian Cattle Dog) should receive an ear trim resembling that of the Giant Schnauzer.	Dystocia	Difficult labor.
	Umbilical hernia	Protrusion of abdominal contents through umbilicus
	Cleft palate	Median fissures due to nonclosure of bones. Environmental and/or genetic factors may be involved.
	Cystic ovaries	
	Endometritis	
	Lymphosarcoma	
	Gastric Torsion	
	Entropion	Inward rolling lid
	Ectropion	Outward rolling lid
	Elbow dysplasia	
Boxer (German Bulldog)	Gingival hyperplasia	Described in related animals; thought to be of odontogenic origin.
	Dermoid cysts	Encapsulated masses lined by epidermis, usually in the head region
	Mastocytoma	Dermal tumor of masenchymal origin; accumulated mast cells.
	Histiocytoma	Tumor primarily of hystocytes
	Oligodendroglioma	Tumor of CNS
	Abnormal dentition, extra incisor	
	Unilateral cryptorchidism	
	Cystinuria (SLR)	Excess cystine in urine, predisposing to calculi

BREED	CONDITION/INHERITANCE	DESCRIPTION/SIGNS
Boxer *(continued)*	Multiple cardiac defects in one litter	
	Pulmonic stenosis	Narrow pulmonary artery at origin
	Endocardial fibroelastosis	
	Atrial septal defects and other cardiac defects	Frequently valvular aortic stenosis and secundum-type atrial septic defects. Also persistence of right venous valve. No chromosomal abnormalities found.
	Intervertebral disc degeneration	
	Ulcerative keratitis "Boxer ulcer"	Corneal ulcer highly resistant to treatment. More than 80% occur in spayed females and estrogen therapy appears to help.
	Granulomatous colitis	Soft, bloody stools
	Factor II hypopothrombinemia	Severe epistaxis
	Vaginal hyperplasia	
	Distichiasis	An abnormal row of eyelashes
	Esophageal dilatation	
	Gastric torsion	
	Spondylosis deformity	
	Sinus arrhythemia	
	Dilated cardiomyopathy	
	Hyperadrenocorticism	
	Hypothyroidism	
	Central-peripheral neuropathy	
	Deafness	
	Aortic and carotid body tumors	
	Fibrosarcoma	
	Melanoma	
	Atopy	

BREED	CONDITION/INHERITANCE	DESCRIPTION/SIGNS
Briard (French Sheepdog) For showing double dewclaws are required on each rear leg, ears are usually trimmed.	Hypothyroidism Progressive retinal atrophy Hip dysplasia Gastric torsion Renal dysplasia	Dilated pupils react sluggishly to stimuli; night blindness progressing to blindness; atrophy of retinal vessels and increased refectivity of tapetum lucidum
Brittany (Breton Spaniel; Epagneul Breton)	Hemophilia A, Factor VIII or AHF deficiency (SLR) *Luxating patellas* Hip dysplasia Epilepsy Lip fold dermatitis Unilateral cryptorchidism	Prolonged bleeding, hemorrhagic episodes, prolonged PTT, reduced AHF and Factor VIII
Brussels Griffon	Dislocation of the shoulder Distichiasis Short skull Hydrocephalus Leaker puppies	An abnormal row of eyelashes

BREED	CONDITION/INHERITANCE	DESCRIPTION/SIGNS
Bull Terrier (White and Colored)	Deafness (AR)	Often associated with white coat color, but unrelated in the instance of the Bull Terrier.
	Recessive umbilical hernia	Protrusion of abdominal contents through umbilicus.
	Inguinal hernia	Defective formation of linea alba associated with protrusion of organs through inguinal canal.
	"Spinning Syndrome" form of epilepsy	
	Photo induced	Sunburn progressing to
	Acrodermatitis (autosomal recessive)	A lethal trait; retardation, severe skin disease
Bulldog Old English (Bull-baiting Dog; Bulldog)	Hydrocephalus several recessive genes	Dilation of ventricles of brain with increased cerebrospinal fluid pressure
	Predisposition to dystocia	Anatomical pecularities, fetal death or nervousness of the dam
	Anasarca	Generalized subcutaneous edema and fluid in abdominal and thoracic cavities; sometimes accompanied by cleft palate. Puppies are born with edema tous bodies or limbs. Must be delivered by cesarean section.
	Clefts of lip and palate (D)	Median fissures due to nonclosure of bones. Environmental and/or genetic factors may be involved.
	Hereditary abnormal dentition	Presence of one extra incisor
	Hypoplasia of trachea	Small, rigid cartilaginous rings with free ends in apposition; cough, abnormal respiratory sounds, dyspnea and decreased exercise tolerance in first 2 months of life; cannot be surgically corrected.

BREED	CONDITION/INHERITANCE	DESCRIPTION/SIGNS
Bulldog (continued)	Pulmonic stenosis	Narrow pulmonary artery at its origin
	Mitral valve defects	
	Arteriovenous fistula	Communication between an artery and a vein.
	Spina bifida	Ununited neural arches; may result in herniation of meniges and/or cord (spina bifida manifesta) or may not (spina bifida occulta) Hemivertebra Asymmetric, abnormal development of vertebrae which may result in neonatal death or cord compression in older puppies; affected vertebrae become wedge-shaped due to underdevelopment of one half, resulting in scoliosis or kinked tails and crowding of ribs if in the thoracic area
	Oligodendroglioma	Tumor of CNS
	Brachury (AR)	Short tail
	Short skull	
	"Swimmers"	Characterized by inability to stand at 4-6 weeks of age and flattened chest
	Hemophilia A, Factor VIII or AHF deficiency (SLR)	Prolonged bleeding, hemorrhagic episodes, prolonged PTT, reduced AHF and Factor VIII
	Vaginal hyperplasia	
	Ectropion	Outward rolling lid
	Entropion	Inward rolling lid
	Keratitis sicca	Dry cornea due to inefficient lacrimal secretion

Breed	Condition/Inheritance	Description/Signs
Bulldog (continued)	Predisposed to facial fold dermatitis	
	Elongated soft palate is common	
	Distichiasis	Abnormal row of eyelashes
	Open urethra	
	Cranial bifida	
	Extra incisor	
	Muzzle pyoderma	Localized infectious dermatitis
	Wrinkle dermatitis	
	Arrested uterine development	
	Follicular conjunctivitis	Round and pinkish bodies in the retrotarsal fold
	Stenotic nares	
	Hip dysplasia	Deformed coxofemoral joints with clinical signs from none to severe hip lameness. Radiographically, there may be shallow acetabulum, flattened femoral head, subluxation, and/or secondary degenerative joint disease.
	Prolapsed male urethra	
	Haws	Orbital gland hypertrophy
	Wry mouth	
	Flacid shoulder joints	
	Reflex regurgitation	
	Pyloric stenosis	Hypertrophic obstruction of the pyloric orifice of the stomach
	Schistosomus reflexes	
	Canine lymphoma	
	Cutaneous mast cell tumors	

BREED	CONDITION/INHERITANCE	DESCRIPTION/SIGNS
Bulldog (continued)	Elbow dysplasia	
	Hypothyroidism	
	Deafness	
Bullmastiff	Abnormal dentition	Presence of extra incisor
	Vaginal hyperplasia	
	Entropion	Inward rolling eyelid
	Brachury	Short tail
	Screw tail	
	Cleft palate	Median fissures due to non-closure of bones. Environmental and/or genetic factors may be involved.
	Progressive retinal atrophy	Dilated pupils react sluggishly to stimuli; night blindness progressing to blindness; atrophy of retinal vessels and increased reflectivity of tapetum lucidum
	Glaucoma	Increased intraocular pressure resulting in hardness, atrophy of the retina, cupping of optic disk and possible blindness
	Hip and elbow dysplasia	Deformed coxofemoral joints with clinical signs from none to severe hip lameness. Radiographically, there may be shallow acetabulum, flattened femoral head, subluxation, and/or secondary degeneration joint disease.
	Contact dermatitis, alopeccia and eczema	
	Bloat	
	Cervical vertebral malformation.	

BREED	CONDITION/INHERITANCE	DESCRIPTION/SIGNS
Cairn Terrier	Inguinal hernia (condition considered high risk in this breed; hereditary factors not determined)	Defective formation of linea alba associated with protrusion of abdominal contents through inguinal canal
	Craniomandibular osteopathy	Irregular osseous proliferation of mandible and tympanic bulla. Discomfort from eating and intermittent fever up to 104°F beginning at 4-7 months of age, then may regress or stop; malnutrition may result.
	Cystinuria (SLR)	Excess cystine in urine, predisposing to calculi
	Hemophilia A, Factor VIII or AHF deficiency (SLR)	Prolonged bleeding, hemorrhagic episodes, prolonged PTT, reduced AHF and Factor VIII.
	Hemophilia B, Factor IX deficiency (SLR)	Prolonged bleeding, abnormal prothrombin consumption and thromboplastin generation and reduced Factor IX; heterozygotes with Hemophilia B bleed more than heterozygotes with hemophilia A.
	Globoid cell leukodystrophy (Krabbe's disease) (R)	Progressive signs beginning at 3-6 months of age are either pelvic stiffness or cerebellar disturbance. CSF total protein is elevated. Enzyme deficiency of globoid cells in the CNS.
	Von Willebrand's disease; pseudohemophilia, vascular hemophilia (IAD)	Prolonged bleeding time, low Factor VIII, reduced platelet adhesiveness and abnormal prothrombin consumption time. May exhibit recurrent melena, prolonged estrual bleeding, excessive bleeding after trauma, subcutaneous hematomas.
	Secondary glaucoma	
	Aberrant cilia	
	Cerebellar hypoplasia	Defective or incomplete development.

BREED	CONDITION/INHERITANCE	DESCRIPTION/SIGNS
Canaan Dog	Epilepsy Hip dysplasia P.R.A. Hypo and Hyperthyroid Diabetes Unilateral cryptorchid	
Cardigan Welsh Corgi (Cardiganshire)	Generalized progressive retinal atrophy Cystinuria (SLR) Predisposition to dystocia Secondary glaucoma, lens luxation Luxated lumbar intervertebral disc	Attenuation of retinal vessels, increased reflectivity of tapetum lucidum affecting young dogs; characterized initially by night blindness leading to blindness Excessive cystine in urine predisposing to calculi. Anatomical peculiarities, fetal death, over-nervousness of the dam
Cavalier King Charles Spaniel	Diabetes Mellitus (hereditary predisposition) "Fly biting syndrome" Patellar luxation Cataract (hereditary) Episodic weakness and collapse (rare inherited disorder)	As in humans Onset at 8-18 months characterized by frequent and persistent non-existent fly-catching episodes Develops after exercise; walks stiff-legged, followed by collapse; remains conscious

BREED	CONDITION/INHERITANCE	DESCRIPTION/SIGNS
Chesapeake Bay Retriever (American Duck Retriever; Ducking Dog)	Progressive retinal atrophy	Dilated pupils react sluggishly to stimuli; night blindness progressing to blindness; atrophy of retinal vessels and increased reflectivity of tapetum lucidum
	Entropion	Inward rolling eyelid
Chihuahua (Mexican Dwarf Dog; Ornament Dog; Pillow Dog).2 varieties— Smooth Coat and Long Coat	Hydrocephalus (R)	Dilation of ventricles of brain with increased cerebrospinal fluid pressure. Hypoglycemia may follow stress in young puppies.
	Pulmonic stenosis	Narrow pulmonary artery at its origin.
	Mitral valve defects.	
	Hemophilia A, Factor VIII or AHF deficiency (SLR)	Prolonged bleeding, hemorrhagic episodes, prolonged PTT, reduced AHF and Factor VIII
	Dislocation of the shoulder.	
	Patella luxation (proposed are recessive polygenic and "multifocal inheritance")	Medial or lateral. Most common are medial accompanied by tibial rotation on the long axis, bending of the distal end of the femoral shaft and shallow femoral trochlea; lameness at 4-6 months of age.
	Collapsed trachea	Decreased rigidity, elongated elastic membrane and increased circumference of trachea. Occurs most commonly in obese dogs with dome-shaped heads, well developed necks and narrow thoracic inlets at an average of 7 years. May be surgically corrected.
	Hypoplasia of dens (odontoid process)	Either hypoplasia of dens or its non-union with C_2 produces atlantoaxial subluxation. Onset at any age producing signs ranging from neck pain to quadriplegia.

BREED	CONDITION/INHERITANCE	DESCRIPTION/SIGNS
Chihuahua (continued)	Keratitis sicca	
	Secondary glaucoma	
	Corneal edema	
	Iris atrophy	
	Cleft palate	Median fissures due to non-closure of bones. Environmental and/or genetic factors may be involved.
	Hypoglycemia	Concentration of glucose in the blood below the normal limit
	Fatty liver syndrome	
Chinese Crested	Sunburn	
	Skin allergies	
	Blackheads	
Chinese Sharpei	Stenotic Nares	
	Parrot Mouth	
	Entropion	
	Photophobia	
	Blepherospasm	
	Keratitis Sicca	
	Luxating Patella	
	Hip and elbow dysplasia	
	Interdigital erythema	
	Staphylococcus dermatitis	
	Inguinal hernia	
	Hyatal hernia	

BREED	CONDITION/INHERITANCE	DESCRIPTION/SIGNS
Chinese Sharpei (continued)	Primary megaesophagus Idiopathic mucinosis Fevers of unknown origin Swollen hock syndrome (SHS) Renal amyloidosis Ciliary dyskenesia	
Chow Chow (Cantonese Butcher Dog; Edible Dog; Oriental Spitz) Straight hindlegs desirable. No angulation at hocks or stifle.	Brachury Hypothyroidism Entropion Distichiasis Narrow palpebral fissure Elongated soft palate Cleft palate Hip dysplasia Elbow dysplasia Keratoconjunctivitis Cerebellar hypoplasia Bloat Cataract (inherited)	Short tails Alpecia, thickening of the skin, hperpigmentation Inward rolling lids An abnormal row of eyelashes Median fissures due to non-closure of bones. Environmental and/or genetic factors may be involved. Deformed coxofemoral joints with clinical signs from none to hip lameness. Radiographically there may be shallow acetabulum, flattened femoral head subluxation and secondary degenerative joint disease. Defective or incomplete development of the cerebellum

BREED	CONDITION/INHERITANCE	DESCRIPTION/SIGNS
Chow Chow **(continued)**	**Persistent pupillary membrane** **Nystagmus** **Retinal folds** **Microphthalmia**	
Clumber Spaniel	**Ectropion (diamond eye)** **Uterine inertia** **Hip dysplasia** **Missing adult teeth** **Undershot jaw**	**Outward rolling lids** **Deformed coxofemoral joints with clinical signs from none to severe hip lameness. Radiographically, there may be shallow acetabulum, flattened femoral head, subluxation, and secondary joint disease.** **Abnormal relative growth of the mandible**
Cocker Spaniel **(Cocking Spaniel; Woodcock Spaniel; three varieties: solid black, any solid color other than black (ASCOB), particolor.)**	**Distichiasis** **Cataract, bilateral** **Cataract with microphthalmia** **Primary glaucoma** **Hydrocephalus internal (R)** **Renal cortical hypoplasia (autosomal recessive)**	**Two rows of eyelashes (usually upper lid) resulting in irritation and epiphora** **Juvenile cataract** **Opaque lenses with small eyes, associated with retinal folds** **Increased intraocular pressure associated with lens luxation. Acute attacks are most common from October to May.** **Dilation of brain ventricles with increased cerebrospinal fluid pressure** **Polydipsia, polyuria**

BREED	CONDITION/INHERITANCE	DESCRIPTION/SIGNS
Cocker Spaniel (continued)	Factor X deficiency (dominant and more severe in homozygote).	Severe bleeding in newborn and young adults, mild bleeding in mature adults; prolonged prothrombin time, PTT and Russell's viper venom time
	Patent ductus arteriosus	Persistence and nonclosure of ductus arteriosus between aorta and pulmonary artery with left to right shunt.
	Clefts of lip and palate	Median fissures due to nonclosure of bones. Environmental and/or genetic factors may be involved.
	Over and undershot jaw	Abnormal relative growth of mandible and/or maxilla
	Cranioschisis (lethal recessive)	Soft spot in cranium
	Umbilical Hernia	
	Tail abnormalities (recessive)	Anury (absence of tail) and brachury (short tail).
	Hip dysplasia (polygenic)	Deformed coxofemoral joint(s) with clinical signs from none to severe lameness. Radiographically, there may be shallow acetabulum, flattened femoral head, subluxation, and/or secondary degenerative joint disease.
	Intervertebral disc disease	Predisposition possibly due to breed confirmation and other factors
	Inguinal hernia	Defective formation of linea alba causing protrusion of abdominal contents through inguinal canal.
	Polygenic behavioral abnormalities	
	Anasarca	Walrus or rubber puppies.
	Hermaphroditism	

BREED	CONDITION/INHERITANCE	DESCRIPTION/SIGNS
Cocker Spaniel (continued)	Hemophilia B, Factor IX deficiency (SLR)	Prolonged bleeding, abnormal prothrombin consumption and thromboplastin generation and reduced Factor IX. Heterozygotes with hemophilia B bleed more than heterozygotes with hemophilia A.
	Ectropion	Outward rolling lids
	Hypertrophy of the nictitans gland	
	Progressive retinal atrophy	Dilated pupils react sluggishly; night blindness progressing to blindness; atrophy of retinal vessels and increased reflectivity of tapetum lucidum
	Trichiasis	Abnormal direction of normal lashes
	Nasolacrimal puncta atresia	
	Reverse rear legs	
	Entropion	Inward rolling lids
	Patellar luxation (proposed are recessive polygenic and "multifocal inheritance")	Medial or lateral. Most common are medial, accompanied by tibial rotation on the long axis, bending of the distal end of the femoral shaft and shallow femoral trochlea; lameness at 4-6 months of age.
	Allergies	
	Seborrhea	
	Epidermal cysts	
	Lip fold pyoderma	
	Tonsil enlargement	
	Epilepsy	
	Cryptorchidism	
	Elbow dysplasia	

BREED	CONDITION/INHERITANCE	DESCRIPTION/SIGNS
Cocker Spaniel (continued)	Esophageal achalasia Retinal Dysplasia Idiopathic facial paralysis Cerebellar degeneration Renal amyloidosis Urinary calculi Chronic liver disease Primary hypothyroidism Deafness Skin neoplasia	
Collie (Scotch Colley Dog; 2 varieties— Rough and Smooth.)	Epilepsy (RP) Deafness Umbilical hernia Nasal solar dermatitis Patent ductus arteriosus Hemophilia A, Factor VIII, or AHF deficiency (SLR) Micropthalmia (result of merle to merle matings, seen in homozygous merles) Optic nerve hypoplasia	EEG may detect at an early age Protrusion of abdominal contents through umbilicus Hereditary susceptibility and lack of skin pigment predisposed to the disease Persistence and non-closure of ductus arteriosus between aorta and pulmonary artery with left to right shunt Prolonged bleeding, hemor- rhagic episodes, prolonged PTT, reduced AHF and Factor VIII Small eyes

BREED	CONDITION/INHERITANCE	DESCRIPTION/SIGNS
Collie (continued)	Recessive ectasia (Collie eye anomaly)	Excessive tortuosity of retinal dysplasia, excavation of the optic disc, retinal detachment, intraocular hemorrhage, and veriform streaks of the fundus in young dogs
	Autosomal recessive cyclic neutropenia (grey Collie syndrome)	
	Heterochromia iridis, "Walleye" (ID)	Whitish-blue iris
	Inguinal hernia	Defective formation of linea alba associated with protrusion of abdominal contents through inguinal canal
	Dwarfism	Small eyes, tiny and high-set ears, very heavy coat
	Distichiasis	An abnormal row of eyelashes
	Corneal dystrophy	
	Choroidal hypoplasia	
	Progressive retinal atrophy	Dilated pupils react sluggishly to stimuli; night blindness progressing to blindness; atrophy of retinal vessels and increased reflectivity of tapetum lucidum
	Coloboma	
	Demodecosis	
	Hidradivitis	
	Bladder cancer	
	Patent ductus arteriosus	
	Achondroplasia	

BREED	CONDITION/INHERITANCE	DESCRIPTION/SIGNS
Curly Coated Retriever	Cushings syndrome	
	Pseudocushings syndrome	
	Hypothyroid	
	Calcium metabolic disorders	
	Juvenile osteoporosis	
	Bilateral alopecia (non-thyroid)	
Dachshund (Badger Dog; Teckel; 3 kinds — Long haired, Smooth, Wirehaired)	Cleft of lip and palate (P)	Median fissures due to nonclosure of bones. Environmental and genetic factors may be involved.
	Over and undershot jaw in the Longhaired variety (R)	Abnormal relative growth of mandible and/or maxilla.
	Intervertebral disc disease	Predisposition due to breed conformation and other factors
	Osteopetrosis	Clinically similar to "swimmer" pups; radiographically uniformly dense bones and abnormal bone resorption
	Cystinuria (SLR)	Excess cystine in urine, predisposing to calculi
	Diabetes mellitus	Hereditary predisposition
	Deafness	
	Micropthalmia	Small eyes
	Ectasia syndrome	Excessive tortuosity of retinal vessels, chorioretinal dysplasia, excavation of the optic disc, retinal detachment, intraocular hemorrhage and veriform streaks of the fundus in young dogs
	Ureodermatologic syndrome	
	Renal hypoplasia	Polydipsia, polyuria

BREED	CONDITION/INHERITANCE	DESCRIPTION/SIGNS
Dachshund (continued)	Heterochromia iridis, "Walleye"	Whitish-blue iris (ID)
	Achondroplasia of the limbs (AD)	
	Keratoconjunctivitis sicca	Dry eye
	Dermoid cysts	
	Atypical pannus	
	Ectasia of sclera	Excessive tortuosity of retinal vessels, chorioretinal dysplasia, excavation of the optic disc, retinal detachment, intraocular hemorrhage and veriform streaks streaks of the fundus in young dogs
	Ununited anconeal process	
	Panniculitis	Inflammatory condition of the subcutaneous fat
	Sensory neuropathy (longhairs)	
	Uroliths	Calcium oxalate and struvate
	Idiopathic epilepsy (genetic basis)	
	Pattern baldness (inherited alopecia)	Males have bilateral alopecia of the ear pinnae: females have alopecia of the ventral body.
	Entropian	
	Hyperadrenocorticism	
	P.R.A.	
	Hypothyroidism	
	Pemphigus follaceous	

BREED	CONDITIONS/INHERITANCE	DESCRIPTION/SIGNS
Dalmatian (Coach Dog; Carriage Dog)	Uric acid stones (AR)	
	Excess uric acid excretion (R)	Predisposition to renal calculi.
	Deafness (Cochlear degeneration)	
	Globoid cell leukodystrophy	Progressive signs beginning at 3-6 months of age are pelvic stiffness or cerebellar disturbance. CSF total protein is elevated; enzyme defieciency with collections of globoid cells in the CNS.
	Muscular dystrophy (x-linked recessive)	
	Atopic dermatitis	Possibly hereditary immunologic disorder
	Glaucoma	
	Malocclusion	
	Trichiasis	Lashes which turn in or grow inward; causes epiphora
	Blue eyes	
	Bacteriuria	
	Tubular transport dysfunction	Hereditary nephropathy
Dandie Dinmont Terrier (Charlie's Hope Terrier; Mustard and Pepper Terrier)	Intervertebral disc syndrome	
	Missing teeth	
	Patellar luxation (proposed are recessive, polygenic and "multifocal inheritance")	Medial or lateral. Most common are medial, accompanied by tibial rotation on the long axis, bending of the distal end of the femoral shaft and shallow femoral trochlea; lameness at 4-6 months of age.

BREED	CONDITIONS/INHERITANCE	DESCRIPTION/SIGNS
Dandie Dinmont Terrier (continued)	Hip dysplasia	Deformed coxofemoral joints with clinical signs from none to hip lameness. Radiographically there may be shallow acetabulum, flattened femoral head, subluxation and secondary degenerative joint disease.
	Cushings syndrome	
	Shoulder subluxation and luxation	
	Elbow subluxation	
	Canine lymphoma	
Doberman Pinscher	Renal cortical hypoplasia	Polydipsia, polyuria
	Spondylolisthesis (Wobblers Syndrome)	Anterior ventral canal is narrower than the posterior canal in the "dorsoventral" direction between C_3 and C_7
	Polyostotic fibrous dysplasia	Osteophytes and cyst formation in distal metaphyses of ulna and radius.
	Von Willebrand's disease, pseudohemophilia, vascular hemophilia (ID)	Prolonged bleeding time, low Factor VIII, reduced platelet adhesiveness and abnormal prothrombin consumption time. May exhibit recurrent melena, prolonged estrual bleeding, excessive bleeding after trauma, subcutaneous hematomas.
	Missing teeth	A common problem; four or more missing teeth disqualifies dog from show ring.
	Craniomandibular osteopathy	
	Bundle of His degeneration	
	Flank sucking	
	Narcolepsy	
	Immune complex disorders	

BREED	CONDITIONS/INHERITANCE	DESCRIPTION/SIGNS
Doberman Pinscher (continued)	Glomerulopathy	
	Follicular dysplasia	Early signs are patches of erythema and alopecia on face and forelegs.
	Demodectic mange	
	Osteosarcoma	
	Dilated cardiomyopathy	Signs: lethargy, anorexia, weakness, dyspnea, vomiting.
	Elbow dysplasia	
	Artherosclerosis	
	Deafness	
	Hemophilia A	
	Persistent hyperplastic vitreons	
	Liver copper storage disease	
	Alopecia	
	Chronic active hepatitis	
English Cocker Spaniel	Generalized progressive retinal atrophy	Attenuation of retinal vessels, increased reflectivity of tapetum lucidum affecting young dogs; characterized by night blindness and progressing to blindness
	Glaucoma	
	Cryptorchidism	
	Pseudohermaphroditism	
	"Swimmers"	Characterized by inability to stand at 4-6 weeks of age
	Cataracts	
	"Short toe" anomaly	
	Deafness	

BREED	CONDITIONS/INHERITANCE	DESCRIPTION/SIGNS
English Cocker Spaniel (continued)	Hemophilia A (SLR) Juvenile amaurotic idiocy	
English Foxhound	Osteochondrosis of the spine Deafness (Cochlear degeneration)	"Anterio-posterior" herniation of intervertebral end plate into the vertebral body; stiff gait prevents proper galloping. Occurs from 7-10 months of age.
English Setter	Recessive juvenile amarauotic idiocy Hemophilia A, Factor VIII or AHF deficiency (SLR) Craniomandibular osteo-arthropathy (R) Progressive retinal atrophy Hip dysplasia (polygenic) Eclampsia Uterine inertia Deafness Hypoglycemia	Dullness and reduced vision at around 12-15 months of age developing into muscle spasms at 18 months, becoming seizures Prolonged bleeding, hemor-rhagic episodes, prolonged PTT, reduced AHF and Factor VIII Dilated pupils react sluggishly to stimuli; night blindness pro-gressing to blindness; atrophy of retinal vessels and increased reflectively of tapetum lucidum Deformed coxofemoral joint(s) with clinical signs of none to severe hip lameness. Radio-graphically, there may be shallow acetabulum, flattened femoral head, subluxation, and/or secondary degeneration joint disease. Concentration of glucose in the blood below the normal limit

BREED	CONDITIONS/INHERITANCE	DESCRIPTION/SIGNS
English Setter (continued)	Prolonged anesthesia Anaphylactic reaction to routine immunization Pyoderma Carcinoma and lymphosarcoma of oral and nasal cavity	
English Springer Spaniel (Norfolk Spaniel)	Central progressive retinal atrophy (suggested to be dominant with incomplete penetrance)	Mottling and increased reflectivity of area centralis resulting in loss of central vision, affecting dogs 3-5 years of age. Difficulty in seeing stationary objects and sight is best in dim light.
	Cutaneous asthenia, Ehlers-Danlos Syndrome (D)	Connective tissue abnormality; fragile, lax skin and hyperextensibility of joints
	Congenital seborrhea	
	Ectropion	Outward rolling lids
	Entropion	Inward rolling lids
	Factor XI (PTA) deficiency (ID)	
	Glaucoma	
	Distichiasis	An abnormal row of eyelashes
	Otitis externa	
	Primary retinal dystrophy	
	Hip dysplasia	Deformed coxofemoral joints with clinical signs from none to severe hip lameness. Radiographically, there may be shallow acetabulum, flattened femoral head, subluxation and secondary degenerative joint disease.
	Phosphofructokinase (PFK)	Enzyme deficiency; diseased red blood cells and muscle cells; intermittent dark urine after strenuous exercise
	Myasthenia gravis	

BREED	CONDITIONS/INHERITANCE	DESCRIPTION/SIGNS
English Toy Spaniel (Comforter; Spaniel Gentle; Two varieties—King Charles & Ruby Blenheim & Prince Charles)	Hanging tongue	
	Patellar luxation (proposed are recessive polygenic and multifocal inheritance)	Medial/lateral. Most common are medial, accompanied by tibial rotation on the long axis, bending of the distal end of the femoral shaft and shallow femoral trochlea. Lameness at 4-6 months of age.
	Cleft palate	Median fissures due to nonclosure of bones. Environmental and/or genetic factors may be involved.
	Umbilical hernia	Protrusion of abdominal contents through umbilicus
	Diabetes mellitus	Inability to oxidize carbohydrates due to faulty pancreatic activity; results in hyperglycemia with symptoms of thirst, hunger, emaciation and weakness
	Episodic collapse	
	Epilepsy	
	Congenital Femoral Shift	
Field Spaniel	Hypothyroidism	
	Anesthetic sensitivity	
	Pyometra	
	Hip dysplasia	
Finnish Spitz	Pemphigus foliaceous	
	Cleft palate	
	Ectasia	
	Luxated patella	
	Adult onset epilepsy	

BREED	CONDITIONS/INHERITANCE	DESCRIPTION/SIGNS
Flat Coated Retriever	Histiosarcoma Luxating patella Hip dysplasia Glaucoma Epilepsy Diabetes insipdus Megaesophagus	
Fox Terrier (Two varieties—Smooth-haired and Wire-haired)	Deafness Idiopathic epilepsey Ataxia (Due to bilateral demyeina-tion of the spinal cord) (R) Lens luxation Colonic disease Goiter (D) Recessive oligodontia Dislocation of the shoulder Pulmonic stenosis Atopic dermatitis Legg-Perthes disease Distichiasis Cataract	 Onset at 2-4 mos of age. Initially progresses rapidly, then slowly with animal being unable to walk. Produces secondary glau-coma Absence of teeth Narrow pulmonary artery at its origin Possibly hereditary immuno-logic disorder Avascular necrosis of femoral head An abnormal row of eyelashes

BREED	CONDITIONS/INHERITANCE	DESCRIPTION/SIGNS
Fox Terrier (continued)	Persistant aortic arch	Development from right aortic arch instead of left; crosses the esophagus, forming a ring with the pulmonary artery and the ligamentum arteriosum, producing esophageal stenosis
	Esophageal achalasia	
	Ectopic ureter (familial relationship)	
	Smooth—Myasthenia gravis	
	Glaucoma	
French Bulldog (Bouledogue Francais)	Hemivertebra	Asymmetric abnormal development of vertebrae which may result in neonatal death or cord compression in older puppies. Affected vertebrae become wedge-shaped due to underdevelopment of one half, resulting in scoliosis or kinked tails and crowding of ribs if present in the thoracic area.
	Brachury	Short tail
	Short skull	
	Hemophilia A, Factor VIII, or AHF deficiency (SLR)	Prolonged bleeding, hemorrhagic episodes, prolonged PTT, reduced AHF and Factor VIII
	Hemophilia B, Factor IX deficiency (SLR)	Prolonged bleeding, abnormal prothrombin consumption and thromboplastin generation and reduced Factor IX. Heterozygotes with hemophilia B bleed more than heterozygotes with hemophilia A.
	Cleft palate and lip	Median fissures due to non-closure of bones. Genetic factors may be involved.
	Elongated soft palate	

608

Breed	Conditions/Inheritance	Description/Signs
German Shepherd Dog (Alsatian; Schaferhund)	Cleft of lip and palate	Medial fissures due to nonclosure of bones. Environmental and/or genetic factors may be involved.
	Pituitary dwarfism	
	Enostenosis (Eosinophilic panostitis)	Limb pain and intermittent lameness between the ages of 6 and 12 months. Signs are persistent for two months. Subsequent recovery.
	Epilepsy (RP)	EEG may detect at an early age.
	Hemophilia A, Factor VIII, or AHF deficiency (SLR)	Prolonged bleeding, hemorrhagic episodes, prolonged PTT, reduced AHF and Factor VIII
	Renal cortical hypoplasia	Polydipsia, polyuria
	Cystinuria (SLR)	Excess cystine in the urine, predisposing to calculi
	Fibrous subaortic stenosis	Narrow aorta below its valve
	Von Willebrand's disease; pseudohemophilia; vascular hemophilia (ID)	Prolonged bleeding time, low Factor VIII, reduced platelet adhesiveness and abnormal prothrombin consumption time; may exhibit recurrent melena, prolonged estrual bleeding, excessive bleeding after trauma, subcutaneous hematomas
	Persistent right aortic arch (P)	Aortic development from right fourth aortic arch instead of left and crosses the esophagus, forming a ring around it with the pulmonary artery and the ligamentum arteriosum, producing esophageal stenosis.
	Ectasia syndrome	Excessive tortuosity of retinal vessels, chorio-retinal dysplasia, excavation of the optic disc, retinal detachment, intraocular hemorrhage and veriform streaks of the fundus in young dogs
	Bilateral cataract (D)	Opaque lenses

BREED	CONDITIONS/INHERITANCE	DESCRIPTION/SIGNS
German Shepherd (continued)	Eversion of nictitating membrane	
	Hip dysplasia (P)	Deformed coxofemoral joint(s) with clinical signs ranging from none to severe hip lameness. Radiographically, there may be shallow acetabulum, flattened femoral head, subluxation and/ or secondary degenerative joint disease.
	Conjunctival dermoid cyst	
	Behavioral abnormalities (suggested polygenic)	
	Ulcerative colitis	
	Pannus	
	Elbow dysplasia	
	Gastroenteritis	
	Malabsorption syndrome	
	Progressive posterior paralysis	Occurs in middle age to older dogs, with some predilection for males; gradual onset; asymmetric in rear limbs
	Osteosarcoma	
	Osteochondritis dissecans	
	Silica uroliths	
	Hypothyroidism (familial)	
	Deafness	
	Atopic dermatitis	
	Esophageal achalasia	
	Pancreatic insufficiency (R)	
	Nodular dermatofibrosis with renal cystadenocarcinoma	
	Uterine leiomyomas	
	Phimosis	
	Axonopathy	
	Calcinosis ciramscripta tongue	

610

Breed	Conditions/Inheritance	Description/Signs
German Shorthaired Pointer	Lymphedema	Nonpainful pitting edema, most commonly seen in the hindlegs and in severe cases, the entire body. Severe cases fatal. Moderately affected animals gradually lose edema by 3 months of age. Popliteal lymph nodes are absent or hypoplastic.
	Subaortic stenosis	Narrow aorta below its valve.
	Eversion of nictitating membrane (R)	
	Amaurotic idiocy (R)	CNS storage disease characterized at 6 months of age by nervousness and decreased training ability; at 9-12 months, progressive ataxia and impaired vision
	Pannus	
	Thrombocytopathy, platelet function defect (autsomal or incomplete dominant)	Moderate to severe bleeding diathesis, Glanzmann's disease
	Von Willebrand's disease; pseudohemophilia; vascular hemophilia (incomplete autosomal dominant)	Prolonged bleeding time, low Factor VIII, reduced platelet adhesiveness and abnormal prothrombin consumption time; may exhibit melena, prolonged estrual bleeding, excessive bleeding after trauma, subcutaneous hematomas
	Malocclusion	
	Entropion	Inward rolling lids
	Fibrosarcoma	
	Melanoma	
	Pseudohermaphroditism	
German Wirehaired Pointer	Subcutaneous cysts.	
	Malocclusion	

611

BREED	CONDITIONS/INHERITANCE	DESCRIPTION/SIGNS
Giant Schnauzer	High incidence of hip dysplasia Osteochondritis dissecans Seborrhea Von Willebrand's disease Malabsorption of cobalamin (AR) Hypothyroidism (UTI, HGE)	
Golden Retriever	Bilateral cataract (dominant)	Opaque lenses
	Cataract with microphthalmia	Opaque lenses with small eyes, associated with retinal folds
	Central progressive retinal atrophy (suggested dominant with incomplete penetrance)	Mottling and increased reflectivity of area centralis resulting in loss of central vision. Difficulty in seeing stationary objects and sight is best in dim light. Affecting dogs 3-5 years of age.
	Hemophilia A, Factor VIII or AHF deficiency (SLR)	Prolonged bleeding, hemorrhagic episodes, prolonged PTT, reduced AHD and Factor VIII
	Von Willebrand's disease; pseudohemophilia; vascular hemophilia (incomplete autosomal dominant)	Prolonged bleeding time, low Factor VIII, reduced platelet adhesiveness and abnormal prothrombin consumption time; may exhibit recurrent melena, prolonged estrual bleeding, excessive bleeding after trauma, subcutaneous hematomas
	Distichiasis	An abnormal row of eyelashes.
	Acute moist dermatitis	
	Inhalant allergies	
	Subvalvular aortic stenosis (heritable defect)	
	Hypothyroidism	

BREED	CONDITIONS/INHERITANCE	DESCRIPTION/SIGNS
Golden Retriever (continued)	Acral lick dermatitis Osteosarcoma Elbow dysplasia Muscular dystrophy (inherited) Hip dysplasia Entropion Cerebellar hypopasia Elbow osteochondrosis Diaphragmatic hernia (R)	
Gordon Setter (Black and Tan Setter)	Generalized progressive retinal atrophy (R) Tail deformities Hip dysplasia Cerebellar cortical abiotrophy Hypothyroidism	Attenuation of retinal vessels, increased reflectivity of tapetum lucidum affecting young dogs, characterized initially by night blindness progressing to blindness Deformed coxofemoral joints with clinical signs from none to severe hip lameness. Radiographically, there may be shallow acetabulum, flattened femoral head, subluxation, and secondary degenerative joint disease.

BREED	CONDITIONS/INHERITANCE	DESCRIPTION/SIGNS
Great Dane (Boarhound; Danish Dog; German Boarhound; Tiger Dog; Ulmer Mastiff)	Microphthalmia (result of merle to merle matings seen in homozygous merles)	Small eyes
	Eversion of nictitating membrane	
	Deafness (seen in homozygous merles in conjunction with ocular defects)	
	Cystinuria (SLR)	Excess cystine in the urine, predisposing to calculi
	Mitral valve defects	
	Spondylolisthesis (Wobbler syndrome)	Anterior ventral canal is narrower than the posterior canal in the "dorsoventral" direction between C_3 and C_7.
	Stockard's paralysis (P)	Preganglionic sympathetic degeneration; onset at about 3 months of age
	Heterochromia iridis "Walleye"	Blue and white iris
	Cervical calcinosis circumscripta	
	Progressive ataxia	
	Osteochondritis dissecans	Saucer shaped necrosis or flap in the posterior central portion or humeral head causing very distinct favoring of affected limb
	Necrotizing myelopathy	Acute atraumatic, flaccid paralysis of the front limbs
	Bloat	
	Metabolic bone disease	
	Osteosarcoma	
	Cerebellar hypoplasia	
	Elbow dysplasia	
	Spondylolisthesis	

BREED	CONDITIONS/INHERITANCE	DESCRIPTION/SIGNS
Great Pyrenees (Pyrenean Mountain Dog; Chien de Montagne des Pyrenees; Pyrenean Hound) For showing, back dewclaws are required.	Factor XI (PTA) deficiency (incomplete autosomal dominant)	
	Entropion	Inward rolling lids
	Hip dysplasia	Deformed coxofemoral joints with clinical signs from none to severe hip lameness. Radiographically, there may be shallow acetabulum, flattened femoral head, subluxation, and/or secondary degenerative joint disease.
	Slipped patella	
	Achondroplasia	
	Blue eyes	
	"Swimmer" puppies	Characterized by inability to stand at 4-6 weeks of age; flattened chest.
	Malocclusion	
	Missing dewclaws	
	Anophthalmia	Missing eyeballs
	Deafness	
	Brittle bone syndrome	
	Missing thoracic wall	
	Cataracts	
	Persistent hyaloid artery	
	Monorchidism	
	Cryptorchicyhism	
	Cleft palate	
	Defective heart	

BREED	CONDITIONS/INHERITANCE	DESCRIPTION/SIGNS
Greyhound One of the sight hounds. (Gre-Hound; Grig-hound; Her-hound; Laporarius Long Dog)	Hemophilia A, Factor VII or AHF deficiency (SLR)	Prolonged bleeding. Hemorrhagic episodes, prolonged PTT, reduced AHF and Factor VIII
	Predisposition to dystocia	Anatomical peculiarities, fetal death, or overnervousness of the dam
	Short spine (R)	
	Esophageal achalasia	
	Anesthesia risk	
	Lens luxation	
	Azoturia-like disease	Excessive nitrogen compounds in the urine
	Von Willebrand's disease	
	Bloat	
Harrier (Hare Hound)	Malocclusion	
Ibizan Hound One of the sight hounds.	Anesthesia risk	
	Unilateral cryptorchidism	
	Allergic reaction to several chemicals.	
	Bloat	
	Seizures (hereditary)	
	Deafness	

616

BREED	CONDITIONS/INHERITANCE	DESCRIPTION/SIGNS
Irish Setter (Modder Rhu; Red Setter; Red Spaniel)	Generalized myopathy (possibly X-linked recessive)	Stiff gait, swallowing difficulty, enlarged tongue and atrophic muscles first seen at 8 weeks of age. Serum creatinine phosphokinase and aldolase levels are high.
	Hemophilia A, Factor VIII deficiency (SLR)	Prolonged bleeding, hemorrhagic episodes prolonged PTT and reduced Factor VIII
	Persistent right aortic arch	Aortic development from right fourth aortic arch instead of left and crosses the esophagus, forming a ring around the arch with the pulmonary artery and the ligamentum arteriosum, producing esophageal stenosis.
	Quadriplegia with amblyopia (lethal) (R)	Progressive. Initially as swimmers at 3 days of age, later inability to stand and dim vision; may be accompanied by tremor and nystagmus
	Generalized progressive retinal atrophy (R)	Attenuation of retinal vessels, increased reflectivity of tapetum lucidum affecting young dogs characterized initially by night blindness and progressing to blindness
	Carpal luxation (X-linked recessive)	
	Entropion	Inward rolling lids
	Uterine inertia	
	Deformed tail	
	Cataract, juvenile cataract	
	Osteochondritis dissecans	Inflammation, both bone and cartilage; results in splitting of cartilage into the joint, especially the knee and shoulder.
	Metabolic bone disease	

BREED	CONDITIONS/INHERITANCE	DESCRIPTION/SIGNS
Irish Setter (continued)	**Idiopathic epilepsy** **Granulocytopathy**	Increased susceptibility to infection; fever gingivitis; destruction of bone in mandibles, radius and ulna
	Primary megaesophagus	
	Osteosarcoma	
	Inhalant allergies	
	Hypothyroidism	
	Hip dysplasia	
	Uredecrinatological syndrome	
Irish Terrier	**Cystinuria (SLR)**	Excess cystine in the urine, predisposing to calculi
	Tubular transport dysfunction (hereditary nephropathy)	
	Muscular dystrophy (linked x-chromosome)	
	Hereditary myopathy	
Irish Water Spaniel	**Malocclusion**	
	Hip dysplasia	Deformed coxofemoral joints with clinical signs from none to severe hip lameness. Radiographically, there may be shallow acetabulum, flattened femoral head, subluxation, and/or secondary degenerative joint disease.
	Hypotrichosis	

BREED	CONDITIONS/INHERITANCE	DESCRIPTION/SIGNS
Irish Wolfhound One of the sighthounds. (Irish Elk-hound; Irish Greyhound)	Hygroma of elbow Tail injury Rhinitis syndrome Progressive retinal atrophy Cataracts Hip and elbow dysplasia Metabolic bone disease Heart disease Osteosarcoma	Inflammation of mucous membrane of the nose
Italian Greyhound	Persistent right aortic arch. Epilepsy Increased anesthetic risk Monorchidism	Aortic development from right fourth aortic arch instead of left. Crosses the esophagus, forming a ring around it with the pulmonary artery and the ligamentum arteriosum, producing esophageal stenosis. A single testis in the scrotum
Jack Russel Terrier	Hereditary ataxia Deafness Legg perthes Luxating patella	
Japanese Chin	Monorchidism Achondropasia	A single testis in the scrotum

Breed	Conditions/Inheritance	Description/Signs
Keeshond	Epilepsy (RP)	Usually seen at 3 years of age. EEG may detect at an earlier age.
	Mitral valve defects	
	Tetralogy of Fallot (P)	Tetralogy of Fallot includes ventricular septal defect, pulmonary stenosis, dextroposition of the aorta and right ventricular hypertrophy.
	Renal cortical hypoplasia	Signs include elevated BUN, polydipsia, polyuria, anemia and weakness.
	Aberrant cilia	
	Predisposition of melanoma	
	Sebaceous cyst	
	Hypothyroidism	Deficient thyroid activity
	Conus septal defects	
Kerry Blue Terrier (Irish Blue Terrier)	Hair follicle tumors	
	Spiculosis	
	Cerebellar cortical and extrapyramidal nuclear abiotrophy.	Onset 9-16 weeks. Signs include pelvic limb stiffness and mild head tremor progressing to paralysis.
	Narrow palpebral fissure	
	Entropion	Inward rolling lids
	Keratoconjunctivitis sicca	
	Distichiasis	
	Ununited anconeal process	

BREED	CONDITIONS/INHERITANCE	DESCRIPTION/SIGNS
Komondorok (Hungarian Sheepdog)	Hip dysplasia	Deformed coxofemoral joints with clinical signs from none to severe hip lameness. Radiographically, there may be shallow acetabluam, flattened femoral head, subluxation and secondary degenerative joint disease.
	Skin problems	
	Entropion	Inward rolling lids
	Cysts	
Kuvasz	Hip dysplasia	Deformed coxofemoral joints with clinical signs from none to severe lameness. Radiographically, there may be shallow acetabulum flattened femoral head, subluxation and secondary degeneration joint disease.
	Deafness	
Labrador Retriever	Bilateral cataract	Opaque lenses
	Retinal dysplasia (R)	Jumbled, abnormally formed layers on the retina with detachment resulting in blindness
	Central progressive retinal atrophy (suggested dominant with incomplete penetrance)	Mottling and increased reflectivity of area centralis resulting in loss of central vision; difficulty in seeing stationary objects and sight is best in dim light, affecting dogs 3-5 years of age
	Hemophilia A, Factor VIII or AHF deficiency (SLR)	Prolonged bleeding, hemorrhagic episodes, prolonged PTT, reduced AHF and Factor VIII

BREED	CONDITIONS/INHERITANCE	DESCRIPTION/SIGNS
Labrador Retriever (continued)	Cystinuria (SLR)	Excess cystine in the urine, predisposing to calculi
	Carpal subluxation (XR)	Bilateral. Gene is allelic to the gene for Hemophilia A.
	Craniomandibular osteopathy	Irregular osseous proliferation of mandible and tympanic bulla; discomfort from eating and intermittent fever up to 104°F beginning at 4-7 months of age
	Dwarfism associated with retinal dysplasia	
	Deficiency of type II muscle fibers	Signs include a marked creatinuria and deficiency of muscle mass.
	Entropion	Inward rolling lids
	Hip Dysplasia	Deformed coxofemoral joints; clinical signs from none to hip lameness. Radiographically there may be shallow acetabulum, flattened femoral head subluxation, and secondary degenerative joint disease.
	Shoulder lameness	
	Shoulder dysplasia	
	Hypoglycemia	Concentration of glucose in the blood below the normal limit
	Hypothyroidism	Deficient thyroid activity
	Hypertrophic osteodystrophy	
	Missing teeth	
	Diabetes	Inability to oxidize carbohydrates due to faulty pancreatic activity; results in hypoglycemia with symptoms of thirst, hunger, emaciation, and weakness
	Melanoma	
	Prolapsed rectum	

BREED	CONDITIONS/INHERITANCE	DESCRIPTION/SIGNS
Labrador Retriever (continued)	Prolapsed uterus	
	Congenital phimosis and cutaneous mast cell tumors	
	Coloboma	
	Distichiasis	Abnormal row of eyelashes; results in irritation and epiphora
	Canine congenital hypotrichosis	
	Megaesophagus	
	Food allergy	
	Leukotrichia	
	Vitamin A resp. dermatitis	
	Dacrocystitis	
	Persistent hyaloid artery	
	Persistent pupillary membrane	
	Copper toxicosis	
	Factor IX deficiency (congenital)	Subcutaneous hematomas; profuse hemorrhage from surgical wound.
	Elbow osteochondrosis	
	Muscular dystrophy	Generalized muscle atrophy; depressed spinal reflexes; "bunny-hopping" gait.
	Receptor dystrophy	
	Associated ocular and skeletal dysplasia	
	Postnatal cerebellar	
	Cortical degeneration	
	Ununited ancoreal process	
	Epilepsy	

BREED	CONDITIONS/INHERITANCE	DESCRIPTION/SIGNS
Labrador Retriever (continued)	Liver disease and liver cirrhosis (hereditary factors) Hereditary myopathy Atherosclerosis	 Lethargy; anorexia; weakness; dyspnoea; collapse and vomiting
Lakeland Terrier (Coloured Working Terrier; Fell Terrier; Patterdale Terrier)	Lens luxation Distichiasis Ununited anconeal process Undershot jaw Cryptorchidism	 Abnormal row of eyelashes; results in irritation and epiphora Abnormal relative growth of the mandible
Lhasa Apso	Renal cortical hypoplasia (proven in this breed to be inherited) Inguinal hernia. Found in this breed to be high risk (factors not determined) Umbilical hernia Lissencephaly (Congenital absence of cerebrocortical convolutions) Distichiasis Aberrant cilia Progressive retinal atrophy	Bilateral renal cortical hypoplasia leading to uremia and secondary hyperparathyroidism; signs begin at around 1 year of age Defective formation of linea alba associated with protrusion of abdominal contents through inguinal canal Signs within first year of life; behavioral, visual and convulsive disorders Abnormal row of eyelashes; results in irritation and epiphora

BREED	CONDITIONS/INHERITANCE	DESCRIPTION/SIGNS
Lhasa Apso (continued)	Entropion (medial)	Inward rolling lids
	Patellar luxation (proposed are recessive polygenic and "multifocal inheritance")	Medial or lateral; most common are medial, accompanied by tibial rotation on the long axis, bending of the distal end of the femoral shaft, and shallow femoral trochlea; lameness at 4-6 months of age
	Lack of ADH	
	Uroliths	
	Hip dysplasia	
	Inhalant allergies	
	Congenital hypotrichosis	
	Corneal ulcers	
Maltese	Aberrant cilia	
	Hydrocephalus	
	Hypoglycemia	Concentration of glucose in the blood below normal limit
	Patellar luxation (proposed are recessive polygenic and "multifocal inheritance")	Medial or lateral; most common are medial, accompanied by tibial rotation on the long axis, bending, of the femoral shaft and shallow femoral trochlea; lameness at 4-6 months of age
	Monorchidism	A single testis in the scrotum
	Cryptorchidism	
	Deafness	
	Blindness (congenital)	
	Poor pigmentation	
	Malocclusion of misalignment	
	Hypertrophic pyloric gastropathy	

625

BREED	CONDITIONS/INHERITANCE	DESCRIPTION/SIGNS
Manchester Terrier (Black and Tan Terrier) Two varieties—Standard over 12 lbs. and not exceeding 22 lbs. and Toy.	Secondary glaucoma; luxating lens. Hypertrophic pyloric gastropathy Legg-Perthes disease Cutaneous asthenia Grand mal epilepsy	Avascular necrosis of femoral head
Mastiff (Alan; Alaunt; Bandogge; Mollossus; Tie Dog)	Vaginal hyperplasia Persistent pupillary membranes Ectropion Bloat Elbow dysplasia	Outward rolling lids
Miniature Bull Terrier	None recognized	
Miniature Pinscher (Smooth-haired Toy Pinscher)	Dislocation of the shoulder Inguinal hernia Legg-Perthes disease Progressive retinal atrophy Skin disease - lack of pigment	Defective formation of linea alba associated with protrusion of abdominal contents through the inguinal canal Avascular necrosis of femoral head Dilated pupils react sluggishly to stimuli; night blindness progressing to blindness; atrophy of retinal vessels and increased reflectivity to tapetum lucidum

BREED	CONDITIONS/INHERITANCE	DESCRIPTION/SIGNS
Miniature Schnauzer (Swergaschnauzer)	Bilateral cataract	
	Pulmonic stenosis	Narrow pulmonary artery at its origin
	Von Willebrand's disease; pseudohemophilia; vascular hemophilia (incomplete autosomal dominant)	Prolonged bleeding time, low Factor VIII, reduced platelet adhesiveness and abnormal prothrombin consumption time; may exhibit recurrent melena, prolonged estrual bleeding, excessive bleeding after trauma, subcutaneous hematomas.
	Prone to cystitis and bladder stones	
	Nephritis	
	Schnauzer comedo syndrome	Comedo—from acranial to tail head.
	Cryptorchidism	
	Sinoatrial syncope	
	Juvenile cataract	
	Legg-Perthes disease	Avascular necrosis of femoral head
	Pseudohermaphroditism	Presence of both testicles and vulva
	Esophageal achalasia	
	Juvenile renal disease (genetic basis)	
	Progressive retinal atrophy	
	Spinaliomas	
	Food allergy	
	Inhalant allergy	
	Sertoli cell tumor	
	Megaesophagus	
	Muscular dystrophy	
	Hyperlipidemia	
	Microphthalmus	
	Atherosclerosis	

BREED	CONDITIONS/INHERITANCE	DESCRIPTION/SIGNS
Newfoundland (Landseer Newfoundland is black and white and can be shown)	Subvalvular aortic stenosis (P)	Narrow aorta below its valve
	Kinked tails	
	Entropion	Inward rolling lids
	Patent ductus arteriosus	Persistence and nonclosure of ductus arteriosus between aorta and pulmonary artery with right to left shunt
	Ventricular septal defect	
	Cardiomyopathy	Spasm of the muscle around the heart cavity
	Dermoid cyst of the cornea	
	Avulsion fractures	
	Elbow dysplasia	
	Ectopic ureter	
	Ununited anconeal process	Eversion of nictitating membrane
	Bloat	
	Hot spots	
	Hip dysplasia	
	Pemphigus foliacus	
Norwegian Elkhound (Elkhound; Gray Greyhound; Grahund Grey; Elk Dog)	Generalized progressive retinal atrophy (R)	Attenuation of retinal vessels, increased reflectivity of tapetum lucidum affecting young dogs; characterized initially by night blindness leading to blindness
	Cataracts	

BREED	CONDITIONS/INHERITANCE	DESCRIPTION/SIGNS
Norwegian Elkhound (continued)	Renal cortical hypoplasia (proven in this breed to be inherited)	Bilateral renal cortical hypoplasia leading to uremia and secondary hyperparathyroidism. Signs begin at around 1 year of age.
	Subcutaneous cysts	
	Seborrhea	
	Glaucoma	
	Keratoacanthoma	
Norwich Terrier	Summer eczema	
Old English Sheepdog (English Bob-tailed Sheepdog)	Bilateral cataract (R)	
	Retinal detachment	
	Hip dysplasia	Deformed coxofemoral joints with clinical signs from none to severe lameness. Radiographically, there may be shallow acetabulum, flattened femoral head, subluxation, and/or secondary degenerative joint disease.
	Juvenile cataracts	
	Elongated tongue	
	Wobbler's syndrome (C.U.I.)	Spondylolisthesis; anterior ventral canal is narrower than the posterior canal in the dorsal-ventral direction between C_3 and C_7.
	Bloat	
	Metachondrial myopathy	Exercise intolerance
	I.M.H.A.	
	Demodicosis	

BREED	CONDITIONS/INHERITANCE	DESCRIPTION/SIGNS
Otter Hound	Platelet disorder, "Thrombocyto-pathy with giant platelets" (dominant or dominant with incomplete expression)	Mild to moderately severe bleeding; prolonged bleeding time, abnormal platelet aggregation and adhesiveness and poor clot retraction
	Hip dysplasia (severe)	Deformed coxofemoral joints with clinical signs from none to severe hip lameness. Radiographically, there may be shallow acetabulum, flattened femoral head, subluxation, and/or secondary degenerative joint disease.
	Sebaceous cysts	
	Elbow dysplasia	
Papillon (Butterfly Spaniel; Chien Ecuriel; Squirrel Dog)	Anasarca	Walrus or rubber puppies
	Patellar luxation (proposed are recessive polygenic and "multifocal inheritance")	Medial or lateral; most common common are medial, accompanied by tibial rotation on the long axis, bending of the distal end and shallow femoral trochlea; lameness at 4-6 months of age
	Entropion	Inward rolling lids
	Deafness	
Pekingese (Dragon Dog; Lion Dog; Pekin Palace Dog; Pa-Erk; Pen-Lo PaErk)	Umbilical hernia	
	Inguinal hernia (considered high risk in this breed, factors not determined)	Defective formation of linea alba associated with protrusion of abdominal contents through inguinal canal
	Hypoplasia of dens (Odontoid Process)	Either hypoplasia of dens or its nonunion with C_2 produces atlantoaxial subluxation; onset at any age producing signs ranging from neck pain to quadriplegia

BREED	CONDITIONS/INHERITANCE	DESCRIPTION/SIGNS
Pekingese (continued)	Intervertebral disc disease	Predisposition possibly due to breed conformation and other factors
	Trichiasis	Ingrown eyelashes which irritate corneal conjunctiva
	Distichiasis	Two rows of eyelashes; results in irritation and epiphora.
	Short skull	
	More prone to urolith formation	
	"Swimmers"	Characterized by inability to stand at 4-6 weeks and flattened chest
	Atypical pannus	
	Lacrimal duct atresia	Congenital absence of openings to lacrimal canal
	Microphthalmia	Abnormal smallness of eyes
	Juvenile cataract	
	Progressive retinal atrophy	Dilated pupils react sluggishly to stimuli; night blindness progressing to blindness; atrophy of retinal vessels and increased reflectivity of tapetum lucidum
	Elongated soft palate	
	Dystocia	
	Persistent penile frenulum	
	Cryptorchidism	

BREED	CONDITIONS/INHERITANCE	DESCRIPTION/SIGNS
Pembroke Welsh Corgi (Pembroke; Pembrokeshire; Ci Swadl; Welsh Heeler)	Generalized progressive retinal atrophy	Attenuation of retinal vessels, increased reflectivity of tapetum lucidum affecting young dogs; characterized initially by night blindness leading to blindness
	Cystinuria (SLR)	Excess cystine in urine predisposing to calculi.
	Predisposition to dystocia	Anatomical peculiarities, fetal death, over-nervousness of the dam
	Cervical disc disease	
	Epilepsy	
	Secondary glaucoma, lens luxation	
	Cutaneous asthenia, Ehlers-Danos syndrome (AD)	Connective tissue abnormality; fragile, lax skin and hyperextensibility of joints
	Dermoid cyst	
	Hip dysplasia	
	"Swimmers"	
	Moist dermatitis	
	Von Willebrand's	
Petit Basset Griffon Vendeen	Epilepsy	
	Hip dysplasia	
	Retinal folds	
Pharoah hound	Lymphocytic - plasmolytic gastritis	
	Gastrointestinal disorders	

BREED	CONDITIONS/INHERITANCE	DESCRIPTION/SIGNS
Pointer	Bilateral cataract (R)	
	Neurotropic osteopathy (R)	Signs at 3-9 months of age characterized by toe gnawing, self-mutilation, and low sensitivity in distal limbs; vascular degeneration; demyelination in spinal cord
	Umbilical hernia	
	Bithoracic ectromelia (possibly recessive)	Presence of a scapula only, with distal structures absent
	Progressive retinal atrophy	Pupils react sluggishly; night blindness progressing to blindness; atrophy of retinal vessels and increased reflectivity of tapetum lucidum
	Entropion	Inward rolling lids
	Calcinosis circumscripta	
	Eosinophilic Panostitis	Ear inflammation
	Sensory neuropathy	
	Deafness	
	Neuromuscular atrophy (R)	
	Hip dysplasia	
	Demodex	
	Callouses	
	Inherited dwarfism	
	Epilepsy	
	Colonic disease	

BREED	CONDITIONS/INHERITANCE	DESCRIPTION/SIGNS
Pomeranian	Patent ductus arteriosus	Persistence and nonclosure of ductus arteriosus between aorta and pulmonary artery with left to right shunt
	Hypoplasia of dens (Odontoid process)	Either hypoplasia of dens or its non-union with C_2 produces atlantoaxial subluxation; onset at any age producing signs from neck pain to quadriplegia
	Patella luxation (proposed are recessive polygenic and multifocal inheritance)	May be medial or lateral. Most cases are medial and accompanied by tibial rotation on its long axis, bending of the distal end of the femoral shaft and shallow femoral trochlea; lameness at 4-6 months of age
	Dislocation of the shoulder	
	Tracheal collapse	Decreased rigidity, elongated elastic membrane and increased circumference of the trachea; occurs most commonly in obese dogs with dome-shaped heads, well-developed necks and narrow thoracic inlets at an average age of 7 years; may be surgically corrected
	Epiphora	
	Nasolacrimal puncta atresia	
	Progressive retinal atrophy	Pupils react sluggishly; night blindness progressing to blindness; atrophy of retinal vessels and increased reflectivity of tapetum lucidum
	Open fontenal	
	Cryptorchidism	
	Glycogen storage disease	
	Elephant skin	
	Dwarfism and dystocia	

BREED	CONDITIONS/INHERITANCE	DESCRIPTION/SIGNS
Poodle (Pudel; Miniature not to exceed 15 inches; Toy not to exceed 10 inches)	Distichiasis	Two rows of eyelashes; results in irritation and epiphora
	Atopic dermatitis (possible immunologic disorder)	
	Achondroplasia (possibly recessive)	Impaired ossification of long bone cartilage producing abnormal short limbs
	Epiphyseal dysplasia	Hindleg joints of puppies sag and puppies move with swaying gait of hindquarters; radiographically, "stippling" from defective ossification of epiphyseal site with several fine foci of bone
	Osteogenesis imperfecta	
	Patent ductus arteriosus (P)	"Polygenic threshold trait"; persistence and nonclosure of ductus arteriosus between aorta and pulmonary artery with left to right shunt
	Progressive retinal atrophy	Pupils react sluggishly; night blindness progressing to blindness; atrophy of retinal vessels and increased reflectivity of tapetum lucidum
	Cerebrospinal demyelination	
	Epilepsy (AR)	EEG may detect an early age
	Ectodermal defects (Symmetrical areas of alopecia—Miniature Poodle)	Affects 2/3 of body including head, ventral trunk, dorsal pelvic region and proximal legs
	Behavioral abnormalities	
	Lacrimal duct atresia	
	Epiphora	Excessive tearing
	Microphthalmia	
	Juvenile cataracts	

BREED	CONDITIONS/INHERITANCE	DESCRIPTION/SIGNS
Poodle (continued)	Atypical pannus	
	Hemophilia A, Factor VIII or AHF deficiency (SLR)	**Prolonged bleeding, hemor-** **rhagic episodes, prolonged PTT,** **reduced AHF and Factor VIII.**
	Von Willebrand's disease	**Prolonged bleeding time, low** **Factor VII, reduced platelet** **adhesiveness and abnormal** **prothrombin consumption time;** **may exhibit recurrent melena,** **prolonged estrual bleeding,** **excessive bleeding after trauma,** **subcutaneous hematomas**
	Retinal atrophy	
	Retinal detachment	
	Hemeralopia	**Day blindness, inability to see** **effectively in bright or direct light**
	Ectopic ureters	
	Congenital deafness	
	Patellar luxation (proposed are recessive polygenic and "multi- focal inheritance")	**Medial or lateral; most common** **are medial, and tibial rotation** **on the long axis, bending of the** **distal end of the femoral shaft** **and shallow femoral trochlea;** **lameness at 4-6 months of age**
	Entropion	**Inward rolling lids**
	Intervertebral disc degeneration	
	Robertsonian translocation	
	Optic nerve hypoplasia	
	Lens-induced uveitis	
	Progressive rod-cone degeneration	
	Legg-Perthes	
	Renal dysplasia (genetic basis)	
	Narcolepsy	
	Cystinuria (SLR)	

BREED	CONDITIONS/INHERITANCE	DESCRIPTION/SIGNS
Poodle (continued)	Heart valve incompetence	
	Pyruvate Kinese deficiency	
	1 hypothyroid	
	Adult onset GH deficiency	
	Ear infections	
	Trichiasis	
	Glaucoma	
	Nonspherocytic haemolytic anemia	
	Amaurotic idiocy	
	Hairlessness	
	Persistent penile frenulum	
	Hypospadia	
	Pseudohermaphroditism	
	Cryptorchidism	
	Missing teeth	
	Cushing's disease	
	Neoplasia	
Poodle (Pudel; Standard, over 14 inches)	Distichiasis	Two rows of eyelashes; results in irritation and epiphora
	Atopic dermatitis (possible immunologic disorder)	
	Osteogenesis imperfecta	Deficient or delayed bone development; results in frequent fractures, appears at 6-8 weeks of age
	Progressive retinal atrophy	Pupils react sluggishly; night blindness progressing to blindness; atrophy of retinal vessels and increased reflectivity of tapetum lucidum

BREED	CONDITIONS/INHERITANCE	DESCRIPTION/SIGNS
Poodle (continued)	Epilepsy (suggested autosomal recessive)	EEG may detect at an early age.
	Behavioral abnormalities (suggested polygenic)	
	Lacrimal duct atresia	
	Epiphora	Excessive tearing.
	Microphthalmia	
	Juvenile cataract	
	Atypical pannus	
	Hemophilia A, Factor VIII or AHF deficiency (SLR)	Prolonged bleeding hemor-rhagic episodes, prolonged PTT, reduced AHF and Factor VIII.
	Von Willebrand's disease; pseudohemophilia; vascular hemophilia (incomplete autosomal dominant)	Prolonged bleeding time; low Factor VII, reduced platelet adhesiveness and abnormal prothrombin consumption time; may exhibit recurrent melena, prolonged estrual bleeding, excessive bleeding after trauma, subcutaneous hematomas
	Iris atrophy	
	Retinal detachment	
	Bloat	
	Sebaceous adenitis	
	Malignant neoplasm	
	Renal dysplasia (hereditary)	
	Hip dysplasia	
	Entropion	
	P.D.A.	
	Alopecia (dilute colors)	
	Hypothyroid	
	Adult onset G.H. deficiency	

BREED	CONDITIONS/INHERITANCE	DESCRIPTION/SIGNS
Portugese Water Dog	Gangliodosis or G.M.I.	
	Puppy eye syndrome	
	Addison's disease	
	P.R.A.	
	Hip dysplasia	
	Cardiomyopathy	
	Follicular dysplasia	
Pug (Chinese Pug; Carlin; Lo-Sze; Mops)	Trichiasis	Ingrown eyelashes which irritate corneal conjunctiva
	Male pseudohermaphroditism	Presence of abdominal testicles, a vulva & an os penis
	Pigmentary keratitis	
	Cleft palate and lips	Median fissures due to nonclosure of bones. Environmental and/or genetic factors may be involved.
	Elongated soft palate	
	Entropion	Inward rolling lids
	Intertrigo	Due to wrinkled head; can become infectious
	Delayed heat prostration	Recurring
	Atypical pannus formation	
	Distichiasis	Two rows of eyelashes; results in irritation and epiphora
	Legg-Perthes disease	Avascular necrosis of femoral head
	Pinched nostril	
	Med-luxating patella	
	Trichiasis	

BREED	CONDITIONS/INHERITANCE	DESCRIPTION/SIGNS
Pug (continued)	Urolithiasis Demodectic mange Obesity Encephalitis	
Puli	Temperament problems Hip dysplasia (hereditary) Deafness	Deformed coxofemoral joints with clinical signs from none to severe hip lameness. Radiographically, there may be shallow acetabulum, flattened femoral head, subluxation, and/or secondary degenerative joint disease.
Rhodesian Ridgeback (Rhodesian Lion Dog)	Dermoid sinus (dominant with "inconsistent penetrance," or recessive) Cervical vertebral deformity Hip dysplasia Lumbosacral transitional vertebral Hypothyroidism Aggression Congenital deafness	Tubular cyst in mid-dorsal line either anterior or posterior to the ridge; due to incomplete separation of skin and spinal cord during development from ectoderm Deformed coxofemoral joints with clinical signs from none to hip lameness. Radiographically, there may be shallow acetabulum, flattened femoral head, subluxation, and/or secondary degenerative joint disease.

BREED	CONDITIONS/INHERITANCE	DESCRIPTION/SIGNS
Rottweiler (Rotweil Dog; Rottweiler Metzgerhund)	Diabetes mellitus	As in humans
	Entropion	Inward rolling lids
	Ectropion	Outward rolling lids
	Hip dysplasia	Deformed coxofemoral joints with clinical signs from none to severe hip lameness. Radiographically, there may be shallow acetabulum, flattened femoral head, subluxation and/or secondary degenerative joint disease.
	Elbow dysplasia	
	Osteochondrosis	Hind leg lameness
	Muscular dystrophy	
	Kidney failure (familial)	
	Vitiligo	Asymptomatic depigmenting disease of the skin, mucosa and haircoat.
	Arthrosis of the elbow joint	
	Sesamoid disease	
	Neuroaxonal dystrophy (NAD)	
	Leukoencephalomalacia (LEM)	
	Congenital deafness	
St. Bernard (Alpine Mastiff; Two varieties—Rough and Smooth)	Stockard's paralysis (P)	
	Hemophilia A, Factor VIII or AHF deficiency (SLR)	Prolonged bleeding; hemorrhagic episodes, prolonged PTT, reduced AHF and Factor VIII
	Hemophilia B, Factor IX deficiency (SLR)	Prolonged bleeding, abnormal prothrombin consumption and thromboplastin generation and reduced Factor IX. Heterozygotes with hemophilia BA bleed more than heterozygotes with hemophilia A.

BREED	CONDITIONS/INHERITANCE	DESCRIPTION/SIGNS
St. Bernard (continued)	Eversion of nictitating membrane	
	Dermoid cysts of cornea	Thick-walled cyst containing sebaceous glands, hair follicles and sweat glands
	Aphakia with multiple colobomas	Absence of lens associated with microphthalmia, acornea, retinal detachment and anterior synechia
	Osteosarcoma	
	Hepato arteriovenous fistul.	
	Epilepsy	
	Factor I deficiency, fibrinogen deficiency, afibrinogenemia, hypo-fibrin -ogenemia.	Severe or lethal hemorrhage
	Distichiasis	Two rows of eyelashes; resulting in irritation and epiphora
	Entropion	Inward rolling lid
	Ectropion	Outward rolling lid
	Vaginal hyperplasia	
	Lip fold pyoderma	Localized; infectious
	Hip dysplasia	Deformed coxofemoral joints with clinical signs from none to severe hip lameness. Radio-graphically, there may be shallow acetabulum, flattened femoral head, subluxation and secondary degenerative joint disease.
	Metabolic bone disease	
	Genu valgum	Knees bowed medially due to rapid growth; prevalent in giant breeds
	Spleen torsion	

BREED	CONDITIONS/INHERITANCE	DESCRIPTION/SIGNS
St. Bernard **(continued)**	**Elbow dysplasia** **Deafness** **Epithelial lined cysts of anterior pituitary** **Acromegaly** **O.C.D.** **Diabetes mellitus** **Retained cartilage of distal ulna** **Lymphoma** **Gastric torsion** **Cardiomyopathy** **Hygroma** **Hypertropic osteopathy** **Idiopathic DJD** **Hot spots** **Acral lick granuloma** **Uveodermatologic syndrome**	
Saluki **One of the sight hounds (Gazelle Hound; Persian Greyhound)**	**Retinal detachment** **Progressive retinal atrophy** **Sensitive to barbiturates** **Black hair follicle dysplasia**	

BREED	CONDITIONS/INHERITANCE	DESCRIPTION/SIGNS
Samoyed **(Samojedskaja)**	**Hemophilia A, Factor VIII or AHF deficiency (SLR)**	**Prolonged bleeding, hemorrhagic episodes, prolonged PTT, reduced AHF and Factor VIII**
	Diabetes mellitus (hereditary predisposition, as in humans)	
	Pulmonic stenosis	**Narrow pulmonary artery at its origin**
	Atrial septal defects	**Hole in atrial septum**
	Progressive retinal atrophy	
	Hip dysplasia	**Deformed coxofemoral joints with clinical signs from none to severe hip lameness. Radiographically, there may be shallow shallow acetabulum, flattened femoral head, subluxation and secondary degenerative joint disease.**
	Sebaceous cysts	
	Dwarfism (autosomal recessive)	**Radiographic evidence of retarded growth apparent by 12 weeks of age.**
	Muscular dystrophy (linked to x-chromosome)	
	Hereditary nephritis (x-linked)	
	Dysplasia of pectinate ligaments	
	Uveodermatological syndrome	
	GH responsive dermatitis	
Schipperke **(Belgian Barge Dog)**	**Narrow palpebral fissure**	
	Entropion	**Inward rolling lids**
	Legg-Perthes disease	**Avascular necrosis of femoral head**
	Pemphigus foliaceous	
	Hypothyroidism	
	Dermatitis	
	Hay fever asthma	

BREED	CONDITIONS/INHERITANCE	DESCRIPTION/SIGNS
Scottish Deerhound	Gastric Torsion Torsion of the lung Torsion of the spleen O.C.D.	Bloat
Scottish Terrier	Von Willebrand's disease; pseudo-hemophilia; vascular hemophilia (D)	Prolonged bleeding time, low Factor VII, reduced platelet adhesiveness and abnormal prothrombin consumption time; may exhibit recurrent melena, prolonged estrual bleeding, excessive bleeding after trauma, subcutaneous hematomas
	Craniomandibular osteopathy	
	Achondroplasia	Imperfect ossification within the cartilage of long bones, producing dwarfism.
	Melanoma	
	Deafness	
	Scottie cramp (R)	Hyperkinetic disorder characterized by seemingly painless rigidity of limbs, back and tail muscle. Both sexes are affected. The head may be drawn between the front legs. Dog recovers in 15-30 seconds. Oral Diazapam® in doses of 0.5mg/kg given three times daily is highly effective in controlling episodes.
	Cystinuria (SLR)	Excess cystine in urine predisposing to calculi
	Primary uterine inertia	
	Ear hematoma	
	Histiocytomas	
	Thyroid problem	

BREED	CONDITIONS/INHERITANCE	DESCRIPTION/SIGNS
Scottish Terrier (continued)	Splayleg	Motor disorder
	Alexander's disease	Progressive tetraparesis
	Atopic dermatitis	
	Bladder Cancer	
	Urinary calculi	
	Luxation of lens	
	Elbow dysplasia	
	I.V.D.D.	
	Canne lymphoma	
	Pyogranulomatous and vasculitic disorder of nasal planum	
	Pyometra	
Sealyham Terrier	Retinal dysplasia (R)	Jumbled, abnormally formed layers of the retina with detachment, causing blindness
	Lens luxation	Results in secondary glaucoma
	Deafness	
	Atopic dermatitis	
Shar Pei	Undershot jaw	Abnormal relative growth of the mandible
	Stenotic nares	
	Otitis externa	Result of ears close to head, irritation
	Entropion	Inward rolling lids
	Photophobia and blepharospasm	Usually only in puppies

BREED	CONDITIONS/INHERITANCE	DESCRIPTION/SIGNS
Shar Pei (continued)	**Bowed forelegs**	
	Medial and lateral patellar luxation (proposed are recessive polygenic and "multifocal inheritance")	Medial or lateral; most common are medial, accompanied by tibial rotation on the long axis, bending of the distal end of the femoral shaft and shallow femoral trochlea; lameness at 4-6 months of age
	Hip dysplasia	Deformed coxofemoral joints with clinical signs from none to severe hip lameness. Radio-graphically, there may be shallow acetabulum, flattened femoral head, subluxation, and/or secondary degenerative joint disease.
	Interdigital erythema and pruritus	Thickening, infections and hair loss due to skin folds
	Elbow dysplasia	
	Inhalant allergies	
	Hiatal hernias	
	Idiopathic mucinosis	Pitting edema, alopecia, hyperpigmentation, severe wrinkling of head and extremities
Shetland Sheepdog (Sheltie; Peerie Dog; Toonie Dog)	**Hemophilia A, Factor VIII or AHF deficiency (SLR)**	Prolonged bleeding, hemor-rhagic episodes, prolonged PTT, reduced AHF and Factor VIII
	Ectasia syndrome (R)	Excessive tortuosity of retinal vessels, chorio-retinal dysplasia, excavation of the optic disc, retinal detachment, intraocular hemorrhage and veriform streaks of the fundus in young dogs
	Von Willebrand's disease	
	Ulcer conditions of apocrine glands	
	Familial dermatitis	

647

BREED	CONDITIONS/INHERITANCE	DESCRIPTION/SIGNS
Shetland Sheepdog (continued)	Hip dysplasia (P)	Deformed coxofemoral joint(s) with clinical signs ranging from none to severe hip lameness. Radiographically, there may be shallow acetabulum, flattened femoral head, subluxation and secondary degenerative joint disease.
	Nasal solar dermatitis	Hereditary susceptibility and lack of skin pigment predispos-ed to the disease
	Patent ductus arteriosus	Persistence and nonclosure of ductus arteriosus between aorta and pulmonary artery with left to right shunt
	Heterochromia iridis "Walleye" (D)	Blue and white iris
	Achondroplasia (probably recessive)	Dwarfism
	Cataract (AR)	
	Central progressive retinal atrophy (suggested incomplete dominant)	Mottling and increased reflectivity of area centralis resulting in lack of central vision affecting dogs 3-5 years of age; difficulty in seeing stationary objects and sight is best in dim light
	Choroidal hypoplasia	
	Coloboma	
	Epidermolysis bullosa	Onset at 2-4 mos. of age. Signs include alopecia, erythema, scaling erosions, crusting and sometimes an intact vesicle
	Hypothyroidism	
	Pemphigus foliaceous	
	Deafness	
	Bladder cancer	
	Muscular dystophy	

Breed	Conditions/Inheritance	Description/Signs
Shetland Sheepdog (continued)	Bilateral renal agenesis	
	Yeast dermatitis	
	Discord lupus	
	Uveodermatolgic syndrome	
Shiba Inu	Reflex regurgitation	
	Luxated patellas	
	Uveodermatological syndrome	
Shih Tzu	Renal cortical hypoplasia (suspected to be hereditary)	Bilateral renal cortical hypoplasia leading to uremia and secondary hyperparathyroidism; signs begin at about 1 year of age.
	Clefts of lip and palate	Median fissures due to nonclosure of bones. Environmental and/or genetic factors may be involved.
	Von Willebrand's disease; pseudohemophilia; vascular hemophilia (incomplete autosomal dominant)	Prolonged bleeding time, low Factor VII, reduced platelet adhesiveness and abnormal prothrombin consumption time; may exhibit recurrent melena, prolonged estrual bleeding, excessive bleeding after trauma, subcutaneous hematomas
	Renal dysplasia	
	Hypertrophic pyloric gastrophy	
	Entropion	
	Trichiasis	
	Dermoids	
	Third eyelid gland prolapse	
	Chronic keratitis	

Breed	Conditions/Inheritance	Description/Signs
Shih Tzu (continued)	Corneal ulcers Progressive retinal atrophy Vitriol syneresis Retinal detachment Hypospadia Achondroplasia Inhalant allergies	
Siberian Husky (Eskimo Dog; Sled Dog)	Von Willebrand's disease, pseudo-hemophilia; vascular hemophilia (incomplete autosomal dominant) Progressive retinal atrophy Corneal dystrophy Glaucoma Distichiasis Lipidosis Uveitis Zinc deficiency Congenital laryngeal paralysis Ectopic ureter Heterochromia iridis Hip dysplasia	Prolonged bleeding time, low Factor VII, reduced platelet adhesiveness and abnormal prothrombin consumption time; may exhibit recurrent melena, prolonged estrual bleeding, excessive bleeding after trauma, subcutaneous hematomas Dilated pupils react sluggishly; night blindness progressing to blindness; atrophy of retinal vessels and increased reflectivity of tapetum lucidum

BREED	CONDITIONS/INHERITANCE	DESCRIPTION/SIGNS
Siberian Husky **(continued)**	Hemophilia A Vent. septal defect Cataracts Discoid lupus Epilepsy	
Silky Terrier **(Sydney Silky)**	Tracheal collapse Patellar luxation (proposed are recessive polygenic and "multifocal inheritance") Hydrocephalus Legg-Perthes disease Cryptorchidism Diabetes mellitus Storage disease Color dilutant alopecia Yeast dermatitis Odontoid process dysplasia Occipital dysplasia Congenital cardiovascular abnomalities	Medial or lateral; most common are medial, accompanied by tibial rotation on the long axis, bending at the distal end of the femoral shaft and shallow femoral trochlea; lameness at 4-6 months of age Avascular necrosis of the femoral head
Skye Terrier **(Two varieties—prick ear and drop ear)**	Hypoplasia of the larynx (R) Ulcerative colitis Congenital kink tail (hooked on end)	Small larynx

BREED	CONDITIONS/INHERITANCE	DESCRIPTION/SIGNS
Skye Terrier (continued)	Enlarged foramen magnum Megaesophagus Allergies Autoimmune thyroid disease Skye hepatitis PC Juvenile limp	Premature closure of the distal radius
Soft-Coated Wheaten Terrier (Irish Wheaten Terrier)	Progressive retinal atrophy Dermatitis Cataracts Renal dysplasia Heart disease Hereditary neuropathy	Sensitive to grass and fleas
Spinoni Italiani	Thyroid imbalance Hip dysplasia Vaginal prolapse	
Staffordshire Bull Terrier	Bilateral cataract (R) Clefts of lip and palate Persistent hyperplastic Primary vitreous	Opaque lenses Median fissures due to nonclosure of bones. Environmental and/or genetic factors may be involved.

BREED	CONDITIONS/INHERITANCE	DESCRIPTION/SIGNS
Standard Schnauzer	Hemophilia A, Factor VIII or AHF deficiency (SLR)	Prolonged bleeding, hemorrhagic episodes, prolonged PTT, reduced AHF and Factor VIII
	Atresia of nasolacrimal puncta	
	Cataract	
	Narrow palpebral fissure	
	Pulmonic stenosis (polygenic)	
	Conjunctivitis	
	Perianal adenomas	Occurs in older dogs
	Hypothyroidism	
	Hip dysplasia	
	Follicular dermatitis	
	Benign fatty tumors	
Sussex Spaniel	Heart murmurs, enlarged hearts	
	I.V.D.D.	
Tibetan Spaniel	P.R.A.	
	Oxalate nephropathy	
Tibetan Terrier (Chrysanthemum Dog; Darjeeling Terrier)	Anesthesia sensitivity	Tibetans may require less than normal amounts
	Hypothryroidism	
	P.R.A.	
	Neuronal ceroid lipofuscinosis	
Toy Manchester (Black and Tan Terrier) Two varieties—Toy (not to exceed 12 pounds) and Standard	None recognized	

BREED	CONDITIONS/INHERITANCE	DESCRIPTION/SIGNS
Vizsla	Hemophilia A, Factor VIII or AHF deficiency (SLR)	Prolonged bleeding; hemorrhagic episodes; prolonged PTT; reduced AHF and Factor VIII
	Craniomandibular osteopathy	
	Facial nerve paralysis	
	Sebaceous adenitis	
	Hip dysplasia	
Weimaraner (Weimer Pointing Dog)	Hemophilia A, Factor VIII or AHF deficiency (SLR)	Prolonged bleeding; hemorrhagic episodes; prolonged PTT; reduced AHF and Factor VIII
	Spinal dysraphism	Begins at 4-6 weeks of age. Not progressive. Clinical signs: crouching stance; abduction of one leg, hopping gait, abnormal proprioception in hindlegs.
	Eversion of nictitating membrane	
	Umbilical hernia	Protrusion of abdominal contents through umbilicus
	Syringomyelia	
	Hip dysplasia	Deformed coxofemoral joints with clinical signs from none to hip lameness. Radiographically, there may be shallow acetabulum, flattened femoral head, subluxation, and secondary degenerative joint disease.
	Bloat	
	Undershot jaw	Abnormal growth of mandible.
	Myasthenia gravis	
	Fibrosarcoma	
	Melanoma	
	Double eyelashes	

BREED	CONDITIONS/INHERITANCE	DESCRIPTION/SIGNS
Weimaraner (continued)	Entropion Cryptorchidism Dermoid cyst of cornea Ununited anconeal process Dwarfism Cutaneous mast cell tumor XX sex reversal	
Welsh Springer Spaniel (Red and White Spaniel; Started; Tarfgi)	Hip dysplasia (infrequent) Hereditary cataract Primary glaucoma Hypothyroidism Spermatogenic arrest with azoopermia	Deformed coxofemoral joints with clinical signs from none to hip lameness. Radiographically there may be shallow acetabu- lum, flattened femoral head, sub- luxation, and/or secondary degenerative joint disease.
Welsh Terrier	Luxated lens	
West Highland White Terrier (Poltalloch Terrier; Roseneath Terrier)	Craniomandibular osteopathy (suggested to be hereditary) Globoid cell leukodystrophy. Krabbe's disease (R)	Irregular osseous proliferation of mandible and tympanic bulla. Discomfort from eating and intermittent fever up to 104°F. Begins at 4-7 months, progress- ing to 11-13 months, then may stop. Progressive signs beginning at 3-6 months are pelvic stiffness or cerebellar disturbance. CSF total protein elevated. Enzyme deficiency with collections of globoid cells in the CNS.

BREED	CONDITIONS/INHERITANCE	DESCRIPTION/SIGNS
West Highland White Terrier (continued)	Atopic dermatitis	
	Inguinal hernia, considered high risk in this breed (factors not determined)	Defective formation of linea alba associated with protrusion of abdominal contents through inguinal canal
	Legg-Perthes disease	Avascular aseptic necrosis of femoral head
	Myotonia	
	Copper toxicosis	
	Epidermal dysplasia	
	Cardiomyopathy	
	Cleft palates	
	Luxating patellas	
	Hip dysplasia	
	Cataracts	
	Seborrhea	
	Chronic liver disease	
	Cirrhosis of the liver	
	Ectopic ureter	
	Deafness	
	Fatty liver syndrome	
	Pyruvate kinase deficiency	
	K.C.S.	
Whippet (One of the sight hounds, Lightening Rag Hound; Snap Dog)	Partial alopecia	Affects 2/3 of body including head, trunk (ventral), dorsal pelvic region and proximal legs
	Cryptorchidism	
	Demodectic mange	Communicable; due to donodex in hair follicles

BREED	CONDITIONS/INHERITANCE	DESCRIPTION/SIGNS
Wirehaired Pointing Griffon	Hip dysplasia	Deformed coxofemoral joints with clinical signs from none to hip lameness. Radiographically, there may be shallow acetabulum, flattened femoral head, subluxation and secondary degenerative joint disease.
Yorkshire Terrier	Patella luxation (proposed are recessive polygenic and "multifocal inheritance")	Medial or lateral; most cases are medial and accompanied by tibial rotation on its long axis, bending of the distal end of the femoral shaft, and shallow femoral trochlea; lameness at 4-6 months of age
	Hypoplasia of dens (odontoid process)	Either hypoplasia of dens or its nonunion with C_2 produces atlantoaxial subluxation; onset at any age producing signs ranging from neck pain to quadriplegia
	Keratitis sicca, dry eye	
	Distichiasis	Two rows of eyelashes; results in irritation and epiphora
	Legg-Perthes disease	Avascular necrosis of femoral head
	Hydrocephalus	
	Melanoderma	
	Urolithiasis	
	Portocaval shunt	
	Fatty liver syndrome	
	Retinal Dysplasia	

PART III

APPENDICES AND GLOSSARY

APPENDIX 1

Breeds In Which Uroliths Are Commonly Seen[1]

CALCIUM OXYLATE	CYSTINE	URIC ACID	SILICA	STRUVITE
Miniature Schnauzer	Boxer	Dalmatian	German Shepherd	Dachshund
Miniature Poodle	German Shepherd	Yorkshire Terrier	Miniature Schnauzer	
Yorkshire Terrier	Dachshund	Miniature Schnauzer	Pekingese	
Lhasa Apso	Great Dane	Bulldog	Miniature Poodle	
Shih Tzu	Irish Setter	Beagle	Scottish Terrier	
Dalmatian	Labrador Retriever	Corgi		
Chihuahua	Miniature Poodle			
Pekingese	Scottish Terrier			
Dachshund	Corgi			
Pug				
Pomeranian				
Bichon Frise				
Boston Terrier				
Cockers				
Collie				
Beagle				
Fox Terrier				
Shetland Sheepdog				

References
1. Graves, T.K. "Bladder Stones in Dogs," *American Kennel Club Gazette*, September, 1992.

APPENDIX 2

Clinical Signs Of Canine Hypothyroidism[1]

Alterations in Cellular Metabolism And Dermatologic Diseases

- lethargy
- dry, scaly skin
- mental dullness
- coarse, dull coat
- exercise intolerance
- bilaterally symmetrical hair loss
- weight gain
- "rat tail"
- cold intolerance
- "puppy coat"
- mood swings, hyperexcitability
- hyperpigmentation
- neurologic signs
- seborrhea
- pyoderma
- myxedema

Reproductive Disorders And Cardiac Abnormalities

- infertility of either sex
- bradycardia or slow heart rate
- lack of libido
- cardiac arrythmias
- testicular atrophy
- cardiomyopathy
- hypospermia

Ocular Diseases

- aspermia
- corneal lipid deposits
- prolonged interestus interval

- corneal ulceration
- failure to have heat cycles
- uveitis
- weak, dying or stillborn pups
- kerato-conjunctivitis sicca or "dry eye"—enlarged mammary glands or
- lactation in non-pregnant bitches

Gastrointestinal Disorders And Neuromuscular Problems
- constipation
- weakness
- diarrhea
- stiffness
- vomiting
- laryngeal paralysis

Hematologic Disorders
- knuckling or dragging feet
- bone marrow failure
- muscle wasting
- bleeding

References

1. Dodds, J.W. "1990 Update on Autoimmune Diseases," *American Kennel Club Gazette*; July, 1990.

662

APPENDIX 3

Research Report on Primary Glaucoma

Effects of Risk Factors and Prophylactic Treatment on Primary Glaucoma in the Dog

Seventy dogs from 26 breeds were admitted with primary glaucoma between January 1979 and December 1983. Compared with mixed-breed dogs, eight breeds were at higher risk of developing glaucoma: Basset Hound, Beagle, Boston Terrier, Cocker Spaniel, Dalmatian, Miniature Poodle, Norwegian Elkhound and Siberian Husky. Dogs between the ages of 5 and 10 years were at increased risk. There was no predisposition for either eye to be affected first. Females were at twice the risk of males. Fourteen dogs had bilateral glaucoma. Among 46 dogs for which the number of months that the second eye remained normal was available, 24 were treated prophylactically (timolol, dichlorphenamide and for echothiopate) and 22 were not treated or had treatment stopped. Prophylactic treatment significantly extended the interval between diagnosis in the first eye and development of glaucoma in the second eye for predisposed breeds. Prophylactic treatment did not make a difference when all breeds were considered, nor did gender affect this interval.[1]

References
1. Slater, M.R. and Erb, H.N. *JAVMA* (188) 1986: 9, 1028-1030; 7 ref.

APPENDIX 4

Comparative Pathology of Canine Hereditary Nephropathies
An Interpretive Review

Hereditary nephropathies in dogs represent multiple, complex clinicopathological entities which cause renal failure in juvenile, adolescent and young adult dogs. To date, nephropathies believed to have a genetic basis have been described in 11 breeds. These disorders represent a variety of developmental, degenerative and metabolic defects. Many canine hereditary nephropathies are analogous to childhood nephropathies in man. The diseases reviewed are: agenesis (Beagle); hypoplasia (Cocker Spaniel); dysplasia (Lhasa Apso, Shih Tzu, Soft-Coated Wheaten Terrier, Poodle); primary cystic disease (Cairn Terrier); glomerulopathy (Samoyed, Doberman Pinscher); Tubulo-interstitial nephropathy (Norwegian Elkhound); tubular transport dysfunction (Basenji, Irish Terrier, Dalmatian).[1]

References

1. Picut, C.A. and Lewis, R.M. "Comparative Pathology of Canine Hereditary Nephropathies: An Interpretive Review." *Vet. Res. Comm.* 1987: II:6,561-581; 91 ref.

APPENDIX 5

Diet and Hip Dysplasia
Effects On Hip Dysplasia Incidence

Restricting the food consumption of growing Labrador Retrievers to 24% less food than their ad libitum pair-fed littermates resulted in a marked reduction in the expression of hip dysplasia. Twenty-four littermate pairs were evaluated from the time they were 8 weeks old until they were 2 years old. Hip joints of the dogs when they were 2 years old were evaluated on radiographs by use of the standard (limbs extended) position and scoring according to the Orthopaedic Foundation for Animals method and the Swedish scoring method. The incidence of hip dysplasia was 25% in the limit-fed group whereas the incidence was 71% in the ad libitum-fed group. It is concluded that these data supported the clinical recommendations to avoid overfeeding growing dogs, particularly those breeds prone to hip dysplasia, and substantiated earlier observations that limiting food intake was beneficial in preventing the expression of hip dysplasia.[1]

References
1.   "Effects of Limited Food Consumption on the Incidence of Hip Dysplasia in Growing Dogs" *JAVMA* 1992, 201:6. 857-863; 28 ref. Kealy, R.D., Olsson, S.E., Monti, K.L., Lawler, D.F., Biery, D.N., Helms, R.W., Lust, G., and Smith, G.K.

Appendix 6

Use of DNA Bar Codes to Resolve a Canine Paternity Dispute

The DNA fingerprinting method was used to resolve a canine paternity dispute. During the same estrus, a Shih Tzu bitch was inseminated by two dogs, a Shih Tzu and a Coton de Tuear. Because both breeds are alike phenotypically, it was difficult to decide whether the pups were purebred or of mixed breeding. The DNA bar codes indicated unambiguously that the two sires had fathered one pup each, thus documenting superfecundation.[1]

References

1. Georges, M., Hilbert, P., Lequarre, A.S., Leclerc, V., Hansett, R., and Vassart, G. *JAVMA* 1988, 193:9, 1095-1098; 8 ref.

APPENDIX 7

Genetic Polymorphism and Close Linkage of Two Plasma Protein Loci in Dogs

Phenotypes of an unidentified plasma protein (PA4) were determined using 2-dimensional horizontal electrophoresis in 967 dogs of 43 breeds. Two codominant, autosomal alleles (F and S) of PA4 were detected. While most breeds from middle and northeastern Asia (Akita Inu, Alaskan Malamute, Chow, Samoyed, Siberian Husky and Tibetan Terrier) had both alleles (gene frequency of S= 0.1-0.6), many of the European breeds had only the allele. Linkage studies showed that the PA4 locus was closely linked to the plasma pretransferrin 1 locus (PRT1); no recombinant was observed in 45 informative offspring studied. In nearly all breeds, the S allele of PA4 was almost always in coupling phase with the allele of PRT1.

APPENDIX 8

Gender Frequency of Canine Hip Dysplasia

The effect of gender on the frequency of dysplasia was studied in records of 4489 dysplastic dogs of a population of 22,472. The dogs were of 30 breeds and there were at least 200 dogs from each breed examined. Prevalence of dysplasia was highest in New-foundlands (29.4%) followed by Golden Retrievers (25.9%), Bernese Mountain dogs (25.3%) and Rottweilers (24.6%), and lowest in Siberian Huskies (1.3%). Prevalence of dysplasia was similar in males and females, indicating no sex predilection for hip dysplasia. Transitional vertebrae were seen in 24 (2.9%) of 818 dogs with unilateral dysplasia. Unilateral hip dysplasia occurred in 818 (18.2%) of the 4489 dogs. The frequency of unilateral dysplasia was not related to the frequency of bilateral dysplasia. There was no sex predilection for unilateral hip dysplasia.[1]

References
1. Keller, G.G. and Corley, E.A. *Veterinary Medicine.* 1989: 84:12, 1162, 1164-1166; 13 ref.

APPENDIX 9

Chest Depth/Width Ratio to Bloat

In a previous study 5802 dogs were examined for the pattern of occurrence of bloat. Pure-breed dogs were 3 times as likely to develop bloat as mixed-breed dogs, and in general, the larger the breed, the greater the risk. However, even among breeds of similar body size there were marked differences in risk. For example, the Setter breeds were at relatively high risk, while the Retriever breeds were much less likely to bloat. Also, the Basset Hound had the 6th highest risk of bloat among all pure breeds despite the fact that it usually weighs less than 50 pounds.

This pattern of breed risk led Purdue researchers to suspect that conformation of the chest (and probably abdomen) is an important factor in predisposition to bloat. Researchers hypothesized that breeds typically having a greater chest depth/width ratio would be more likely to bloat because the deeper chest and abdomen would allow the stomach and its ligaments to stretch in the ventral direction, especially when weighted down by water and ingesta. Chronic stretching would then increase the probability of twisting (volvulus, torsion), especially when the stomach is full and a rotational force is exerted, as when the dog rolls over or exercises. This hypothesis is being tested at Purdue with a second 2-year study funded by the Morris Animal Foundation, and by donations. Since the risk of bloat for many pure breeds has been determined, we now need to characterize chest size for the same breeds and compare the two measures.

Preliminary findings are very interesting. When the risk of bloat for each of seven pure breeds is plotted on the horizontal axis and the chest depth/width ratio on the vertical axis, the two measures appear to be highly correlated. There is an almost linear increase in bloat risk by breed with an increase in the chest depth/width ratio for those 7 breeds. In this example, 63% of the variation in bloat risk can be explained by a change in the chest depth/ width ratio alone! These are only preliminary results which need to be confirmed in a much larger number of dogs and dog breeds. We are measuring chest size and abdominal size in dogs that had bloat and comparing these with the same measures in dogs of the *same breed and age* that did *not* have bloat.[1]

References

1. Bloat Notes "News from the Canine Gastric Dilatation-Volvulus Research Program." School of Vet. Med., Purdue University, W. Lafayette, IN. Issue 93-2; Dec. 1993.

RADIOGRAPHS OF HIP DYSPLASIA

Courtesy of Slocum Clinic, Eugene, OR

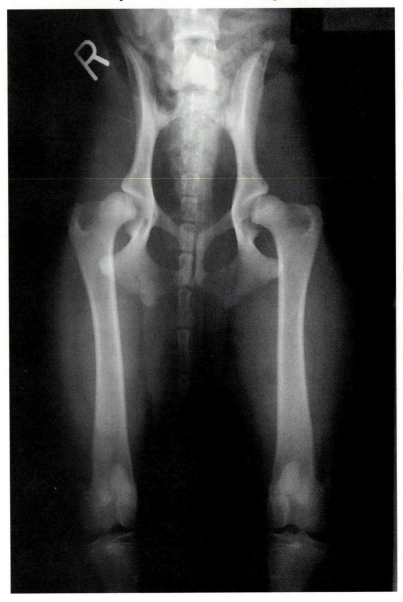

Dysplastic Hips

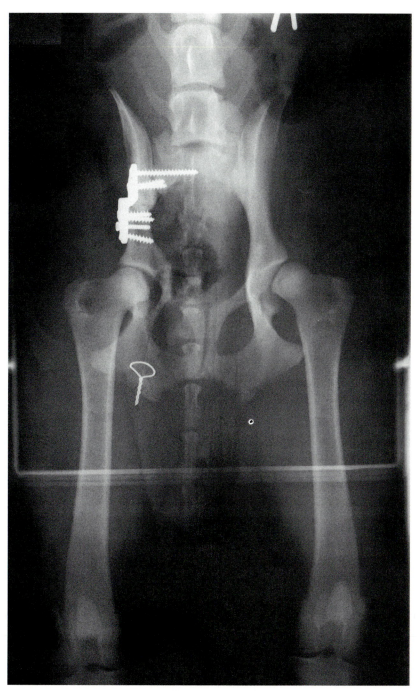

Triple Pelvic Osteotomy

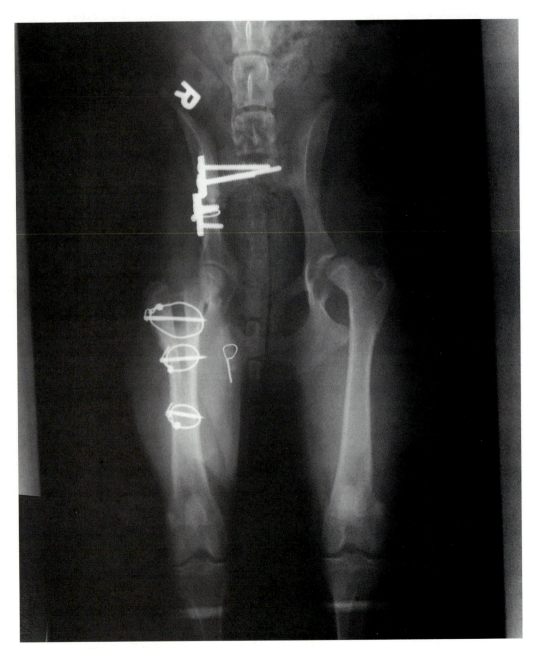

Pelvic Osteotomy And Femoral Neck Lengthening

672

APPENDIX 11

PHOTOGRAPHS OF CONGENITAL DEFECTS

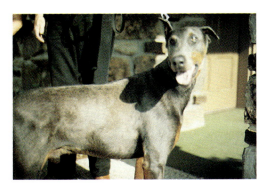

Alopecia: Associated with the gene for dilution

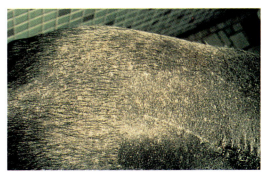

Close-up View of Alopecia

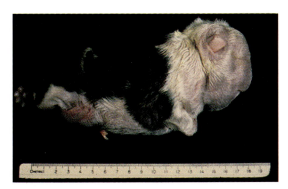

Ana Sarca: Boston Terrier

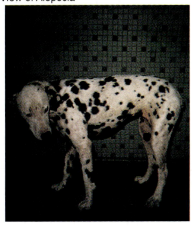

Atopy: Dalmation

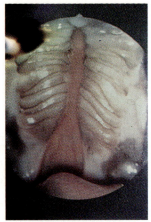

Cleft Palate: Boston Terrier

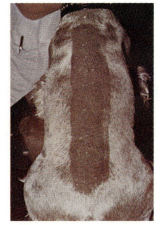

Schnauzer Commedo Syndrome

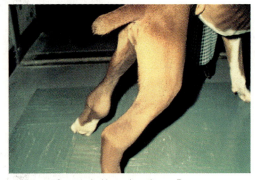

Congenital Lymphoedema: Boxer

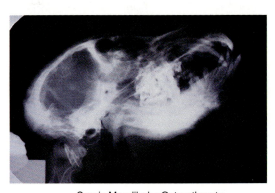

Cranio Mandibular Ostoarthropty

674

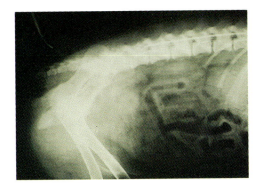
Dermoid Sinus:Communicating With Vertebral Canal

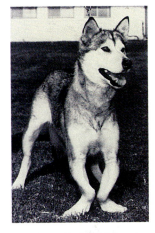
Dwarfism:Alaskan Malamute

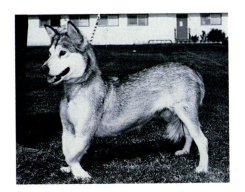
Dwarfism:Alaskan Malamute

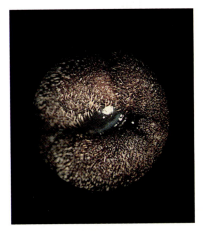
Entropion

675

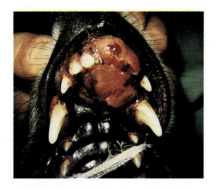

Epalis: Boxer

Hairlip: Boston Terrier

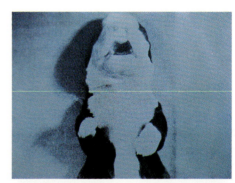

Hemivertebra: Boston Terrier

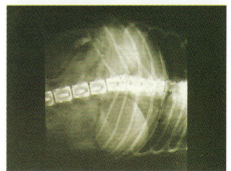

Hemophilia: Beagle

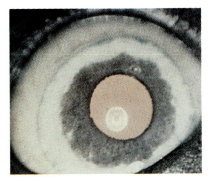

Heterochromia Iritis

Hypospadia: Boston Terrier

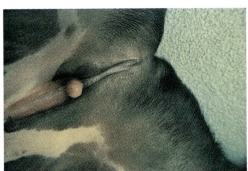

Prolapse Urethera: Bulldog
Courtesy of Dr. J. Bojrab

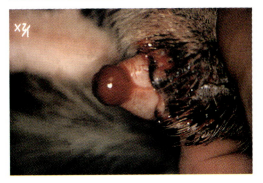

Boxer ulcer cornea

GLOSSARY

ACHONDROPLASIA: A form of dwarfism resulting from the improper ossification of long bones.

ALOPECIA: Baldness or abnormal scarcity of hair.

ANASARCA: Large edematous bodies or limbs at birth; also called walrus or rubber puppies.

ANURY: Absence of tail.

APRON: Hair longer hair on the chest than on the rest of the body.

ATAXIA: Muscle failure or irregular coordination.

ATRESIA: A body opening which is either missing or abnormally closed.

ATROPHY: Diminution of size of an organ or tissue, or decline in the normal function of a body part.

BARREL: Rib cage and body of a dog or "spring of rib..

BAT EAR: An erect, wide-based ear, rounded at the tip (e.g., French Bulldog).

BELTON: Color designation referring to spotting.

BIRD OF PREY EYE: Yellow eye.

BLANKET: The coat color on the back and upper part of the sides between the neck and the tail.

BLAZE: White markings on the face, extending between eyes and/or over muzzle.

BLOOM: When coat is in top condition.

BRACHURY: Short tail.

BREECHES: Hair on the thigh (also, culotte).

BURR: The cartilaginous projection on the inside of the ear.

BUTTERFLY NOSE: Not solid; spotted; parti-color.

BUTTON EAR: Ear folded forward close to the skull and pointing toward the eye.

CABRIOLE: Crooked front legs.

CATARACT: Opacity of the crystalline lens or the lens capsule.

COMPANION DOG (CD): Added to a dog's name as a result of three qualifying scores in AKC Novice Obedience classes.

COMPANION DOG EXCELLENT (CDX): Added to dog's name after three qualifying scores in AKC Open classes in obedience.

CHECK: More than 1/3 white coat color in a Boxer.

CHINA EYE: A bluish white iris. A fault in most breeds other than the Dalmatian, Harlequin Great Dane and Blue Merle Collie.

CHISELING: The well-defined contours in which the bony formation of the face is without fullness.

COBBY: Compact.

COW HOCKED: Top of hocks closer to each other than to the lower part of the leg.

CRANIOMANDIBULAR OSTEOPATHY: Irregular ossification of the mandible and tympanic bulla.

CRANIOSCHISIS: Soft spot in the cranium.

CROUP: The line from the pelvis to the tail set.

CRYPTORCHIDISM: The condition of the testes not descending into the scrotum.

CYSTINURIA: Excess cystine in the urine, predisposing to calculi.

DAPPLED: Refers to coat colors; brindling, tiger striping, irregularly spotted.

DEAD GRASS: Refers to coat color; varying in shade from tan to dull straw.

DEWLAP: Loose skin under the throat.

DIMPLE: Depression on either side of the breastbone, as in the Dachshund.

DISTICHIASIS: An abnormal row of eyelashes.

DOME: Rounded upper portion of the skull.

DOMINO: Reverse color marking (Afghan).

DOWN-FACED: Having the tip of the muzzle lower than the stop; downward tilting muzzle.

DROPPER: A setter-pointer cross breed.

678

DRY: Without loose skin.

DUDLEY: Yellowish or flesh-colored nose.

DYSTOCIA: Difficult labor and/or delivery of puppies.

ECTASIA (COLLIE EYE): Tortuosity of retinal vessels, with detachment and hemorrhage, excavation of the optic disc.

EPILEPSY: A condition of recurring loss of control of muscles, impairment of consciousness, and/or perturbation of autonomic nervous system.

EPIPHORA: Overflow of tears; excessive tearing.

ESOPHAGEAL ACHALASIA: Failure to relax the muscle fibers of the lower esophagus.

FEATHERING: Longer hair on belly, backs of legs, tail and ears.

FIDDLE FRONT: Crooked or bandy forelegs; a combination of being out at elbow and in at pastern.

FLEW: The lips.

FURNISHINGS: Longer growth of hair on head and body parts of certain breeds.

GAY TAIL: Tail carried above the back line.

GAZE HOUND: A sight-hunting hound.

GLAUCOMA: Increased intraocular pressure with associated lens luxation.

HEMERALOPIA: Defective vision in bright light. Also known as day blindness.

HEMOPHILIA: Prolonged bleeding. Characterized by hemorrhage and increased blood factors.

HERMAPHRODITISM: The presence of both male and female sex organs in one animal.

HETEROCHROMIA IRIDIS: More than one color in the iris. "Walleye" when the iris is blue-white.

HOMOZYGOUS: Genetically having a matching pair of alleles relating to a characteristic.

HYDROCEPHALUS: Enlarged head due to dilation of ventricles of the brain.

HYPERTROPHY: Abnormal enlargement of an organ or section of tissue.

HYPOGLYCEMIA: Concentration of glucose in the blood below the normal limit.

HYPOPLASIA: Defective or incomplete development.

IRISH MARKING: Solid-color dog with white blaze and white feet.

ISABELLA: Light fawn color.

IN-BREEDING: Mating close relatives of the same breed.

KEEL: Depth of chest below and in front of the brisket.

KERATITIS: Inflammation of the cornea.

KISS MARKS: Tan marks on cheeks and over eyes or the oval spot in the center of the back skull.

LANDSEER: Black and white Newfoundland.

LEATHER: Ears.

LINE-BREEDING: Any mating of relatives other than those prescribed for in-breeding.

LOZENGE: An oval spot of color on top of the head.

MANTLE: The coat on shoulders, back and sides.

MASK: Muzzle color.

MERLE: Bluish grey color.

MICROPHTHALMIA: Small eyes.

MISCELLANEOUS CLASS: Breeds recognized by the AKC for which no independent class is offered. They are shown against each other.

MOLERA: Incomplete ossification of the skull.

MONONEPHROSIS: Cystic degeneration of one kidney.

MYOPATHY: Referring to the diseased condition of a muscle.

OLIGODONTIA: Fewer than the normal number of teeth.

OLIGODENDROGLIOMA: A tumor of non-neural cells located at the advent of the central nervous system.

OSTEOCHONDROSIS: Saucering of the humeral head; necrosis resulting in limping gait.

OSTEOGENESIS IMPERFECTA: An inherited condition where the bones are abnormally brittle and subject to fracture.

OUTCROSSING: Mating of unrelated animals of the same breed.

OVERREACHING: Refers to a fault in gait in which the rear feet have to step outside the front feet because of excessive drive from the rear quarters.

OVERSHOT: The upper jaw protrudes beyond the lower jaw.

OSTEOPETROSIS: Uniformly dense bones and abnormal bone resorption.

PACE: A type of gait; motion of both right legs, then both left legs, causing a rolling action.

PADDING: In running gait, the action of front legs which allows a long stride by the rear legs.

PANNUS: Membrane-like vascularization of the cornea.

PARTI-COLOR: Refers to coat color; patches of two or more colors.

PENCILING: The marks or stripes dividing the tan on the toes of a black and tan hound.

PIED: Having large patches of two or more colors.

PLUME: Bushy tail carried on back.

POINTS: Markings (as with the tan on a black and tan hound)

POMPON: A rounded tuft of hair left on top of tail when tail is clipped.

PULMONIC STENOSIS: Narrow pulmonary artery at its origin.

QUADRIPLEGIA: Paralysis of all four limbs; may be progressive in as in swimmer pups.

RACY: Elongated in body and legs; light boned.

ROACH BACK: When the back curves toward the loin (convex).

ROAN: Refers to coat color; when white hairs are mixed with the predominant coat color.

ROMAN NOSE: Nose with bridge assuming a convex curve.

ROSE EAR: Ear shaped with a drop which folds over and then back.

RUDDER: Refers to the tail.

SABLE: Outer coat shaded with black over a lighter undercoat.

SADDLE: A color marking over the back.

SCISSORS BITE: Closure where the inner surface of the upper teeth is in contact with the outer surface of the lower teeth.

SELF COLOR: All one coat and pigment color.

SINGLE TRACKING: A gait in which the front tracts fall in a single line.

SLEW FEET: Feet turned out.

SMUT: In Australian Terriers, black hairs among others in the coat.

SNIPEY: A pointed muzzle.

SPLAY FOOT: Toes spread too far apart.

STILTED: Choppy, up and down gait.

STOP: The depression between the skull and the foreface.

TRACKING DOG (TD): Added to a registered dog's name when he has passed the tracking test.

THUMB MARKS: Round black spots on the tan pastern of the Manchester Terrier.

TICKED: Small color spots.

TRACE: Black hair extended from occiput to tail.

TRICHIASIS: Ingrown eyelashes which irritate the cornea. May cause epiphora.

TULIP EAR: Ear carried erect with slight forward curvature.

U.D. (UTILITY DOG): Added to a registered dog's name when he has scored a passing score three times in AKC Utility Obedience classes.

UNDERSHOT: Lower jaw protrudes beyond upper jaw.

VENT: Rectal opening

WALLEYE: Eye having blue-white iris (heterochromia iris).

WEEDY: Poorly or badly developed.

WHEATEN: Pale yellow color.

WRY MOUTH: Upper and lower teeth close off center.

680

CONTRIBUTORS TO FIRST EDITION

Consulting Editors:

Jacob E. Mosier, DVM, MS and Ralph Buckner, DVM

Affenpinscher	Ron Laughlin, DVM
	Sharon Irons Strempski
Afghan	Dr. Gerda M. Kennedy
Airedale Terrier	Barbara Strebeigh
	John B. Peterman, DVM
Akita	Mary J. Echols
Alaskan Malamute	Mary Lou Vesty
American Foxhound	Braxton B. Sawyer, THD
American Staffordshire Terrier	Thomas A. Russell, DVM
	Mitzi Ritter
American Water Spaniel	Curtis J. Fried, DVM
Australian Cattle Dog	Blain Lamont, BVMS, MRCVS
	Jim Watson
	Leila Watson
	Laura Fulton
Australian Kelpie	John Culvenor, DVM
Australian Shepherd	Robert E. Kline, DVM
Australian Terrier	John Culvenor, DVM
	Mrs. Milton Fox
Basenji	Barbara L. Henderson, DVM
	Damara Bolte
Basset Hound	Margaret W. Walton
	Calvin Moon, VMD
Beagle	John T. Refieuna
Bearded Collie	Barbara Rieseberg
Bedlington Terrier	Mrs. Marian L. Cabage
	David Haynes, DVM

Belgian Sheepdog/Belgian Malinois	Marge Turnquist
Belgian Tervuren	Mrs. Robert Krohn
Bernese Mountain Dog	R.R. Billiar
	D.G. & Grethen Johnson
Bichon Frise	John Kuenzi, DVM
	Azalia Doggett
Black and Tan Coonhound	Nina P. Ross, Ph.D
	R.C. & J.W. Koerber
Bloodhound	Robert E. Patterson, DVM
	Mrs G.E. Sinkinson, Jr.
Border Collie	Steve Weir, DVM
Border Terrier	Margaret B. Pough, MA
Borzoi	Asa Mays, Jr., DVM
	Karen K. Mays
Boston Terrier	Virginia Easton Flynn, VMD
Bouvier des Flandres	Richard Weitzman, DVM
	Marion C. Hubbard
Boxer	Loren E. Gambrel, DVM
	Lorraine C. Meyer
Briard	F. Robert Sava, DVM
	Cecily R. Collins
Brittany	Wayne Fessenden
Brussels Griffon	William F. Hanlon, DVM
	Dawn Vick Hansen
Bulldog	Richard G. Pearce, DVM
Bullmastiff	Mary Ann Deines
Bull Terrier	Forrest Rose
Cairn Terrier	Mrs Phil Shoop
Cardigan Welsh Corgi	John Culvenor, DVM
Cavalier King Charles Spaniel	Edward M. Sullivan, DVM
	Miss Elizabeth I. Spalding

Chesapeake Bay Retriever	Lorraine Berg
Chihuahua	Max E. Hurd
	Martha Hooks
	A.B. Pitman, DVM
Chow Chow	JoAnne S. O'Brien, DVM
	Georgia King Hanson
Clumber Spaniel	Fred Wingert, DVM
	Pat Behrns
Cocker Spaniel	Cheryl McNeil, DVM
Collie (Rough)	Virginia Holtz
Collies (Smooth)	Sandra K. Tuttle
Curly Coated Retriever	N. Dale Detweiler
Dachshund	Peggy Westphal
Dalmatian	James C. Blakemore, DVM
	Robert H. Schaible, Ph.D
Dandie Dinmont Terrier	Robert G. Neuhardt, MD
Doberman Pinscher	Joanna Walker
English Cocker Spaniel	Paul Layer, DVM
	Joyce Scott-Paine
English Setter	Joan R. Stainer
English Springer Spaniel	Bill and Sue Evans
English Toy Spaniel	Louis V.L. Bowers, DVM
	M. Joyce Birchall
Field Spaniel	Richard H. Squier
	Carl A. Stiefel, Jr.
Flat Coated Retriever	Sally J. Terroux
Fox Terrier	Charlotte A. Jones, MD
French Bulldog	Earl H. Harrison, DVM
	Dick and Angel Terrett
German Shepherd	Robert G. Little, Jr.,DVM
	Margaret M. Megahan
German Shorthaired Pointer	Don Sandberg

German Wirehaired Pointer	Ross D. Clark, DVM
Giant Schnauzer	William Krause, DVM
	Joan P. Anselm
	Catherine Brown
Golden Retriever	Mrs. William Herbert
Gordon Setter	Dorothy Page Whitney
	Kay Monoghan
Great Dane	Bob and Hazel Gregory
	E.P. Maynagh, DVM
Great Pyrenees	Mr & Mrs C. Seaver Smith, Jr.
	Ralph Povar, DVM
Greyhound	Richard M. Roberts, DVM
	Glen Harbert, DVM
	Elsie S. Neustadt, MD
Harrier	Wayne E. Nelson
Ibizan Hound	Nan Kilgore
Irish Setter	Lucy Jane Meyers
Irish Water Spaniel	Marion Hopkins
Irish Wolfhound	Brig. Gen. Alfred W. DeQuoy
Italian Greyhound	M.B. Schwartz, DVM
	Audrey F. Sutton
Japanese Spaniel	Ross D. Clark, DVM
Keeshond	W.J Rosskopf, Jr.,DVM
	Nan Greenwood
Kerry Blue Terrier	Beatrice Schlesinger
	Melvin Schlesinger
Komondor	J.C. Blumenthal, DVM
	Joy C. Levy
Kuvasz	Mary Jane Sepmeier, DVM
Labrador Retriever	Roy J. Brinkman, DVM
	Maureen Gamble
	Nolan Gross, DVM
Lakeland Terrier	Donald Webb, DVM
	Patricia Rock, MS

Lhasa Apso	D.G. Carlson, DVM
	Dr. Robert J. Berndt
Maltese	D.G. Carlson, DVM
	Dr. Robert J. Berndt
Manchester Terrier	C. E. Sawyer, MD
Mastiff	Marie A. Moore
Miniature Bull Terrier	Ross D. Clark, DVM
Miniature Pinscher	Buris R. Boshell, MD
Miniature Schnauzer	Harry L. Quick, DVM
Newfoundland	T.D. Vincent, DVM
	Barbara Rouleau
Norwegian Elkhound	William L. Austin, DVM
	Nina P. Ross, Ph.D
Norwich and Norfolk Terrier	C.R. Hower, VMD
	Constance S. Larrabee
Old English Sheepdog	L.D. Naranche, DVM
	Oren D. Bush, DDS
Otter Hound	Hugh R. Mouat, DVM
	Margaret B. Pough, MA
Papillon	Richard W. Esquivel, DVM
	Catherine Davis Gauss
Pekigese	Nigel Aubrey-Jones
Pembroke Welsh Corgi	Neil H. McLain
	Mary Gay Sargent
Pointer	Robert F. Parker, DVM
	Mrs. Harry Hirschberger
Pomeranian	Don Hohmann, DVM
	Norma Creider
Poodle--Standard	Francis P. Fretwell
Poodle--Toy and Miniature	Ross Clark, DVM
Pug	Donald Pfeifer, MD
Puli	L.A. MacLeod, DVM
	Mrs. Sylvia Owen

Rhodesian Ridgeback	Loraine H. Hulbert
	R.M. Bloom, DVM
	E. Clough, VMD
	D.E. Martinelli, DVM
Rottweilers	Curtis Giller, DVM
	Marthajo Rademacher
Saint Bernard	Barbara Straw, DVM
Saluki	Asa Mays, DVM
	Winafred B. Lucas, Ph.D
Samoyed	Mary Lou Grattius
	Patricia J. Hritzo
Schipperke	V. Frances Griggs
Scottish Deerhound	Gayle Bontecu
Scottish Terrier	Barbara Kingsbury
Sealyham Terrier	D.C. Smith, DVM
Shar Pei	John S. McKibben, DVM, Ph.D
	Walter Dugan Skinner
Shetland Sheepdog	Lincoln Kutsher, VMD
	Constance B. Hubbard
Shih Tzu	Ross D. Clark, DVM
Siberian Husky	Kathleen Kanzier
Silky Terrier	John Culvenor, DVM
Skye Terrier	Olga Smid
Soft-coated Wheaten Terrier	Jacqueline Gottlieb
Staffordshire Bull Terrier	Ross D. Clark, DVM
Standard Schnauzer	William D. Jones, DVM
	Mary Cole Schofield
Sussex Spaniel	T.A. Luley, DVM
	George and Marcia Deugan
Tibetan Terrier	Irving G. Cashell, VMD
	Mrs. Henry Murphy
Vizsla	Shirley Brown

Weimaraner	Donna Wainwright
Welsh Springer Spaniel	Will K. Weichell, DVM
	Bruce and Sylvia Foreacre
Welsh Terrier	Donald M. Walsh, DVM
	Mrs Susan P. Fitzwilliam
West Highland White Terrier	John T. Marvin
Whippet	Mrs W.P. Wear
Wirehaired Pointing Griffon	John S. McKibben, DVM
	Teresa L. and Michael W. Lewis
Yorkshire Terrier	Ross D. Clark, DVM